# PSYCHIATRIC NURSING

A Psychotherapeutic
Management Approach

# PSYCHIATRIC NURSING

## A Psychotherapeutic Management Approach

### Norman L. Keltner, EdD, RN

Associate Professor
University of Alabama
School of Nursing
Birmingham, Alabama

### Lee Hilyard Schwecke, RN, MSN

Associate Professor and Doctoral Candidate
Indiana University
School of Nursing
Indianapolis, Indiana

### Carol E. Bostrom, RN, MSN

Lecturer
Indiana University
School of Nursing
Indianapolis, Indiana

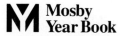 Mosby
Year Book

St. Louis   Baltimore   Boston   Chicago   London   Philadelphia   Sydney   Toronto

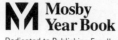
**Mosby**
**Year Book**
Dedicated to Publishing Excellence

*Editor:* Linda L. Duncan
*Developmental Editor:* Mary Espenschied
*Project Supervisor:* Barbara Merritt
*Editing and Production:* CRACOM Corporation
*Design:* Elizabeth K. Fett

Printed in the United States of America

Mosby–Year Book, Inc.
11830 Westline Industrial Drive, St. Louis, Missouri, 63146



**Library of Congress Cataloging-in-Publication Data**

Keltner, Norman L.
    Psychiatric nursing:a psychotherapeutic management approach/
  Normal L. Keltner, Lee Hilyard Schwecke, Carol E. Bostrom.
      p.      cm.
    Includes bibliographical references and index.
    ISBN 0-8016-3309-5
    1.   Psychiatric nursing.   2.   Psychotherapy.   3.   Nurse and patient.
  I.   Schwecke, Lee Hilyard.   II.   Bostrom, Carol E.   III.   Title.
    [DNLM: 1.   Models, Psychological.   2.   Nurse—Patient Relations.
  3.   Psychiatric Nursing.   4.   Psychotherapy—nurses' instruction.      WY
  160 K29p]
  RC440.K36          1991
  610.73'68—dc20
  DNLM/DLC
  for Library of Congress                                              90-13574
                                                                            CIP

GW/GW/RRD   9   8   7   6   5   4   3   2

# Contributors

**Veda Marie Boyer, RN, MS**
Director of Nursing Services
Indiana State Department of Mental Health
Indianapolis, Indiana

**Patricia Clunn, EdD, ARNP, CS**
Professor
School of Nursing
University of Miami
Miami, Florida

**Mary Jo Kasselman, RN, PhD**
Professor
Department of Nursing
California State University
Bakersfield, California

**Bette R. Keltner, RN, PhD**
Professor
School of Nursing
University of Alabama
Birmingham, Alabama

**Janet C. Kirsch, EdD, RN**
School of Nursing
Indiana University
Indianapolis, Indiana

**Peggy Tracy Leapley, RN, PhD**
Associate Professor
Department of Nursing
California State University
Bakersfield, California

**Sue Main, RN, CS, DNS**
Clincial Nurse Specialist
Community Hospital North
Psychiatric Pavilion
Indianapolis, Indiana

**Cleo Metcalf, CNAA, MSN, RN**
Associate Chief
Nursing Service—Education
Martinez Veterans Affairs Medical Center
Martinez, California

**Dorothy Dick Meyer, BSN, JD**
Staff Attorney
Greater Bakersfield Legal Assistance Inc.
Bakersfield, California

**Mira Kirk Nelson, EdD, RN, C**
Assistant Professor
Harris College of Nursing
Texas Christian Unviersity
Fort Worth, Texas

**Patricia Nord, RN, C**
Administrative Manager
Psychiatric Department
Kern Medical Center
Bakersfield, California

**MaryLou Scavnicky-Mylant, RN, CPNP, PhD**
Associate Professor
School of Nursing
University of Wyoming
Laramie, Wyoming

**Gale R. Woolley, ARNP, EdD**
Associate Professor, Sr.
Department of Nursing Education
Miami-Dade Community College
Miami, Florida

# Preface

Psychiatric nursing practice and education have gone through many changes in the past decade, and with these changes comes the need to make understandable and meaningful information accessible to nurses and students. The philosophy of this text stems from our experience as practicing nurses and educators and our belief that we truly understand what nurses and students need and want to further their nursing education. Unlike textbooks that attempt to cover every aspect of psychiatric nursing and that superficially cover many important topics, this book focuses on practical, essential information that nurses need to effectively care for patients and successfully interact with other members of the health care team.

*Psychiatric Nursing: A Psychotherapeutic Management Approach* takes a practical, clinical approach to nursing, integrating clinical realities with the theory taught in schools of nursing and emphasizing those duties for which nurses primarily are responsible. We also have striven to differentiate therapy from therapeutic interventions. Students after 6 to 8 weeks of training can function therapeutically, but they are not therapists. To become a therapist takes years of extensive training. The focus in this text is on the therapeutic skills that fall within nursing's domain.

The model of psychotherapeutic management presented in this book is unique in its simplicity and its application to practice. Its three components, which follow, are based on an understanding of psychopathology:

- The therapeutic nurse-patient relationship
- Psychopharmacology
- Milieu management

These three concepts are explored as they relate to the clinical psychiatric setting (Units Two to Four). In addition, within Unit Five these components are applied consistently to major disorders, thus providing a framework for nursing care and decision making.

## ORGANIZATION

The text is organized in seven units. Unit One, Introduction to Psychiatric Nursing, explores the evolution of psychiatric nursing, addressing important historical, theoretical, and legal issues. The psychotherapeutic management model, which serves as the framework for the rest of the book, is presented in Chapter 3. Unit Two focuses on the first component of the psychotherapeutic management model: the therapeutic nurse-patient relationship. The unit opens with a general discussion of communication and the development of the one-on-one therapeutic relationship, followed by principles of therapeutic communication applied to aggressive patients and groups of patients. Unit Three presents an in-depth discussion of psychopharmacology, addressing the six major classes of drugs used in psychiatric treatment. Unit Four contains three chapters devoted to milieu management, including a chapter on roles of the psychotherapeutic manager. Unit Five provides consistently organized discussions of the major classifications of disorders presented in the American Psychiatric Association's *Diagnostic and Statistical Manual of Mental Disorders* (third edition, revised). Unit Six discusses two other therapies used in the clinical setting: behavior therapy and somatic therapy. The book concludes with a unit on special populations in psychiatric nursing, including victims of violent behavior, children and adolescents, the elderly, and patients with AIDS.

## FEATURES

With students in mind, we have provided a number of tools to facilitate understanding and promote clinical competence:

- *Learning objectives* point students to important concepts within each chapter.
- *Sample care plans,* organized around the five-step nursing process and the psychotherapeutic managment model, guide students in developing individualized care plans for the patients.
- *DSM-III-R, NANDA, and PND-I diagnostic classification systems* have been presented to reflect up-to-date clinical terminology.
- *Study questions* help students review important concepts presented throughout the text.
- Numerous *summary boxes* and tables highlight key information in an easily accessible format.
- A *glossary* at the end of the book presents common psychiatric terms and definitions.
- The *latest references* have been provided to reflect current research in psychiatry and psychiatric nursing.

We have made every attempt to avoid the use of sexist pronouns, where possible, using plural nouns and pronouns. Sometimes, however, to avoid awkwardness of style, we have referred to the nurse as "she" and the patient as "he."

Norman L. Keltner
Lee Hilyard Schwecke
Carol E. Bostrom

# Acknowledgments

The writing of *Psychiatric Nursing: A Psychotherapeutic Management Approach* represents several years of work and reflects the influence of many nurses on my career. For their help I am especially indebted to Jo Bacci and Jeanne Lough, my first instructors in the psychiatric technician program at Stockton State Hospital; Dan Ramsey, Willie Smith, and Mitchell Patterson, good friends and fellow students in the nursing program at Delta College in Stockton; Vi Torres, instructor and later department head at Delta College, who encouraged me when I needed it; John Bergey, a psychiatric nursing instructor at Fresno State University; Cleo Metcalf, a colleague and friend at the Veterans Hospital in Fresno; Jacqueline Johnson, who introduced me to academia; Maura Carroll, a true mentor during my years at California State University, Stanislaus, in Turlock, California; Susan Leddy, who gave me my first teaching position at the University of Wyoming; and Opal Hipps, a mentor, friend, and thoughtful listener at Baylor University. Two nonnurse academicians, Marshal Shlafer, Professor of Pharmacology at the University of Michigan, and Anthony Hines, Dean of Engineering at the University of Missouri, were an inspiration to me because I saw in them the academic work ethic lived out. I am also grateful to the administration and to Steve Arvizu, Dean of Graduate Studies and Research at California State University — Bakersfield, who were supportive of my work in several tangible ways.

I also want to express my appreciation to my family. My wife, Bette, has been a critical sounding board and an understanding source of encouragement during the preparation of this book. My children, Sara, Amanda, and Alex, have been patient and helpful to Dad all the way. Finally I dedicate my effort to the memory of two who would have considered it the most significant book in the history of nursing: My mom, Gladys, and my dad, Lawrence, who were always proud of me.

**N.L.K.**

We would like to express tremendous appreciation to Carol Hash for the extensive typing and proofreading she did, often under unfair time pressures. We thank Sandra Wood, RN, MSN, for all her content evaluation and editing assistance. A special thank you is extended to David Wagner, MD, for his helpful content suggestions.

This book would not have been possible without the hundreds of students, patients, university colleagues, and hospital personnel who have helped us over time to expand our knowledge and develop more effective interventions and strategies.

**L.H.S. and C.E.B.**

A loving thank you to my children, Janson and Renee Schwecke, for their patience and for taking on more responsibilities in the past two years. A special thank you to my parents, Mildred and Lawrence Hilyard, who always believed in me and supported my efforts. I only wish my mother could have lived to see this book in print.

**L.H.S.**

I wish to thank my husband, Paul, for his support and patience and my children, Melanie, Elizabeth, and Jonathan, for their understanding and helpfulness. To each of them I give my love and appreciation.

**C.E.B.**

We would like collectively to acknowledge our indebtedness to the many reviewers from nursing programs around the country for their insight and direction during the writing process. Linda Duncan, Senior Editor at Mosby–Year Book, has been a constant source of inspiration to us. Linda liked our ideas from the very beginning and was helpful every time we spoke to her. Another person who has made this book a reality is Mary Espenschied. Mary worked very hard in developing this book. She edited our writing, provided suggestions, and reinforced our thinking on various ideas.

**N.L.K**
**L.H.S**
**C.E.B**

# Contents

**22**  Organic Mental Syndromes and Disorders, 389
**Mira Kirk Nelson**

## UNIT SIX  Special Therapies in Psychiatric Nursing

### 26  Behavior Therapy, 515
**Sue Main**

### 27  Somatic Therapies, 528
**Norman L. Keltner and Cleo Metcalf**

## UNIT SEVEN  Special Populations in Psychiatric Nursing

### 28  Victims of Violent Behavior, 543

## APPENDIXES

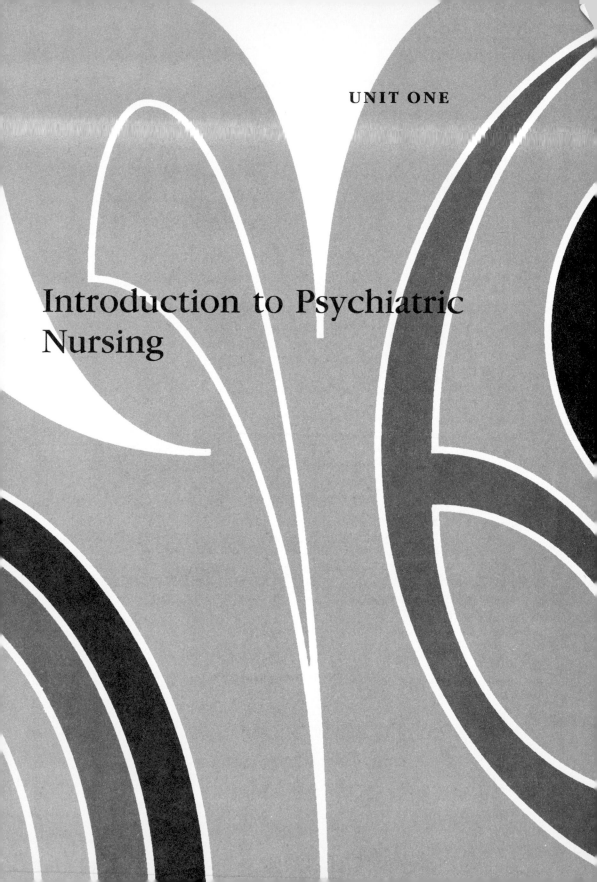

UNIT ONE

# Introduction to Psychiatric Nursing

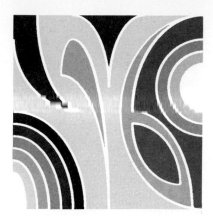

## CHAPTER 1

# Historical Issues in Psychiatric Care

LEARNING OBJECTIVES

After reading this chapter you should be able to

- Explain the history of psychiatry as a foundation for current psychiatric nursing practice
- Identify the significant changes occurring during the period of enlightenment
- Describe the contributions of the early scientists to the current understanding of mental illness
- Describe the impact psychotropic drugs have had on psychiatric care
- Describe the immediate and long-term effects of the community mental health movement
- Describe the steps in psychiatric nursing over the past 50 years that have led to today's psychiatric nursing environment

According to several psychiatric epidemiologists (Regier et al., 1988), 15.8% of Americans 18 years of age and older are affected by a mental disorder. Accordingly, psychiatric nurses provide one of the most important services in health care today. Table 1-1 gives a breakdown by percentages of the psychiatric diagnoses prevalent at any one time in our society.

## BENCHMARKS IN PSYCHIATRIC HISTORY

The modern era of psychiatric care can be traced from events occurring in England and France near the end of the eighteenth century, a time referred to as the Enlightenment. Before this time the mentally ill were often regarded as wild animals. Rosenblatt (1984) writes of the ABCs of community response during this time: assistance, banishment, confinement. Assistance was the least restrictive approach. Assistance, such as food and money, often enabled the family to maintain its integrity as a unit. Banishment occurred in some communities, particularly when the deranged were strangers. Banishment led to wandering bands of "lunatics . . . living no one cared how, and dying no one cared where" (Rosenblatt, 1984). The infamous *Ship of Fools,* boatloads of the mentally disordered cast out to sea to find their "right minds," occurred during this period. In America during colonial times wandering bands without shelter, food, or care drifted from village to village, occasionally finding acceptance but more often encountering rejection and hostility.

Confinement was the most restrictive method of dealing with the mentally ill. Men and women were often chained and indiscriminately mixed, the old with the young, men with women, the insane with criminals or paupers. They were thought to be immune to normal biologic stressors, such as cold, heat, and hunger (Foucault, 1967), and suffered accordingly. Patients were placed on display for the amusement of the public and their "helpers." For example, until 1770 a small fee was charged visitors at St. Mary of Bethlehem Hospital (Bedlam) in England, and at Bicêtré in France the attendants served as ringmasters with actual whips to "encourage" their

**TABLE 1-1**   Prevalence of mental disorders in the United States

| Diagnosis | Percentage of population over 17 years of age |
|---|---|
| Anxiety disorders | 7.3 |
| Mood disorders | 5.1 |
| Alcoholism | 2.8 |
| Drug abuse | 1.3 |
| Obsessive-compulsive disorder | 1.3 |
| Schizophrenia | 0.7 |
| Antisocial disorder | 0.5 |
| Manic-depressive disorder | 0.4 |
| Somatization | 0.1 |

From Regier DA et al: One-month prevalence of mental disorders in the United States, Arch Gen Psychiatry 45:977, 1988. © 1988 by the American Medical Association.

"patients" to perform (Rosenblatt, 1984). These warehouses for the tormented discouraged outside intrusion and attracted "employees" who were at the bottom levels of both social and moral society, but as the late 1700s approached, a day of enlightenment dawned, the establishment of the asylum.

Four different periods—the late eighteenth century, the late nineteenth century, the 1950s, and the 1960s—seem to stand out as benchmarks in the evolution of modern psychiatric care (Table 1-2). The four periods are designated as benchmarks because at these times there was a significant change in thinking concerning the mentally ill in which certain individuals or specific events played a dominant role. After each period consequent events occurred that were important in their own right; yet their inspirational source can be traced to the aforementioned benchmarks.

**TABLE 1-2**    Benchmark periods in psychiatric history

| Period | People or event | Significant change in thinking | Result(s) |
|---|---|---|---|
| *Enlightenment:* Late eighteenth, early nineteenth centuries | Pinel (1745-1826) unchaining the men at Bicêtre (1793) Tuke (1732-1822) establishing the York Retreat | The insane were included in the family of man—no longer to be chained and beaten as animals. The dignity of man was upheld. | The asylum movement. |
| *Scientific study* of the mind and mental illness: Late nineteenth century | Freud (1856-1939) psychoanalysis, the unconscious, the importance of early life experiences | Man could be studied, and that study held promise for treating and curing mental health problems. | The study of the mind and treatment approaches to psychiatric conditions flourished. |
| *Psychotropic drugs:* 1950s | Chlorpromazine (Thorazine) (1952) Imipramine (Tofranil) (1959) | Some mental illnesses are caused by biochemical imbalances. If we can find the biochemical problem through research, we can find a pharmacologic cure. People would no longer need to be confined. | A factor in the development of CMHC. The term *least restrictive alternative* evolved from this important discovery. |
| *Community mental health:* early 1960s | Community Mental Health Centers Act (1963) | Individuals do not need to be hospitalized away from home and community. People, all people, have the right to be treated in their own community. | Pro's and con's on the results: Intervention in familiar surroundings has helped many people. Homelessness is linked to deinstitutionalization. |

## Period of enlightenment

The modern era of psychiatric care began with two men, Philippe Pinel in France and William Tuke in England. In 1793 Pinel became superintendent of the French institution Bicêtré (for men) and later the Salpêtrière (for women). He was dismayed by the conditions he found. Soon after assuming leadership, he unchained the shackled, clothed the naked, fed the hungry, and did away with whips and other instruments of cruel treatment. At that same time in England, Tuke was planning a private facility using moral treatment for the mentally ill because he deplored the conditions he witnessed in public facilities. In 1796 the York Retreat opened for patients. These two men accounted for this first benchmark of modern psychiatric care. One (Pinel) was motivated by scientific considerations. The other (Tuke) was motivated by his Quaker religious orientation.

**Asylum.** The concept of asylum developed from the humane efforts of Pinel and Tuke. The term *asylum* can mean protection, social support, or sanctuary from the stresses of life. A touring Russian gymnast pleading for asylum is a good example of this definition of asylum. Asylum can also be defined as a place, a physical location, or a state of mind. It was the first definition that motivated Pinel, Tuke, and other like-minded individuals. They understood that the mentally ill decompensated under stress, so they sought to provide an environment relatively free from psychosocial stressors. Their language has little appeal today, for example, "madness," "lunacy," "insanity," "idiocy," "feeblemindedness," yet these terms were not used in a pejorative sense. They were accepted terms of the day. These early reformers were driven by a desire to improve the lot of abandoned, mentally disordered persons. They were driven by a desire to provide asylum or sanctuary.

Dorothea Dix (1802-1887) was the first major reformer in the United States. She was instrumental in developing the concept of asylum and played a direct role in opening 32 state hospitals. Her efforts are invariably described as a crusade. Several years before launching her "crusade" she visited Tuke's York Retreat. Undoubtedly her impressions of his moral treatment influenced her own concerns for the pain and suffering she had witnessed in her native land. Dix believed the greater citizenry, as represented by the government, had an obligation to their mentally ill brothers and sisters. She proposed to alleviate suffering with adequate shelter, nutritious food, and warm clothing.

The first asylum in the United States, the Eastern Lunatic Asylum in Williamsburg, Virginia, was founded in 1773. Others followed, such as the Frankford Asylum near Philadelphia (1813), the Bloomingdale Asylum in New York (1818), and the Hartford Retreat in Connecticut (1824). The Philadelphia and New York asylums were established under Quaker influence and thus can be traced to Tuke (Rosenblatt, 1984).

This period of enlightenment was short lived. Within 100 years of the establishment of the first asylum the reformers were being assailed as misusers and abusers of their charges. Maltreatment and corrupt practice were viewed as the norm by a public willing to generalize the faults of some to all. State hospitals were beset with problems. The first definition of asylum (sanctuary) had materialized as hospitals set apart from cities, usually in a rural setting. These once sought-after characteristics came to be viewed as liabilities. The patients were *isolated geographically, isolated from family,* and *isolated from follow-up care.* While the reformers were still talking asylum, the world was beginning to think treatment. The term *asylum* had taken on the unflattering second definition as a place, an undesirable place.

In 1855 the New York County Superintendents for the Poor resolved to remove insane persons from poorhouses and jails and place them in institutions where "treatment" was available. By 1890 New York State had passed the State Care Act, which formally removed the insane from the poorhouses to the state hospital (Gralnick, 1986). It was official: Institutions for the insane were no longer to be called asylums but were to be called hospitals, by inference places for treatment.

**Beginning of psychiatric nursing.** It was at this time (about 100 years ago) that the official history of psychiatric nursing began. Linda Richards, the first American psychiatric nurse, was a graduate of the New England Hospital for Women. She spent a great part of her professional career developing nursing care in psychiatric hospitals and also directed a school of psychiatric nursing at the McLean Psychiatric Asylum in Waverly, Massachusetts, in 1880. Within 10 years, because of her efforts, more than 30 asylums had developed schools for nurses.

## Period of scientific study

The move in thinking from sanctuary to treatment is linked to the second benchmark in psychiatric care, which is personified by Sigmund Freud (1859-1939). Toward the last third of the nineteenth century a number of men of science devoted themselves to understanding the mind and mental illness. The fruits of their labor held great promise, some of which is still unfulfilled. Nonetheless, the efforts forever changed the world's view of mental illness. Mental illness need not just be suffered, however humanely patients are treated, but can be alleviated. In a sense, psychiatric care was popularized.

**Early scientists.** Although Freud had the greatest impact on the world's view of mental illness, scientifically he did not work or think in a vacuum. Other men and women had tremendous impact on this new enthusiastic and optimistic approach to mental illness. Emil Kraepelin (1856-1926) made tremendous contributions to classification of mental disorders. He was a true scientist; his descriptions of schizophrenia are classics and are valuable reading today. Eugene Bleuler (1857-1939) contributed the term *schizophrenia* to our vocabulary. He also added a note of optimism to the treatment of schizophrenia. Still others, many of whom were colleagues or disciples of Freud, made significant contributions to the emerging field.

Freud's contributions still influence modern psychiatric care today. Although for a number of years it was popular to belittle his accomplishments, doing so belied any discernment of the underpinnings of much current psychotherapy. To paraphrase Sir Isaac Newton (1642-1727), if we see far today, it is because we stand on the shoulders of giants.

Freud described human behavior in psychological terms. He developed a theory of motivation; he established the usefulness of talking (catharsis); he explained the importance of dreams; and he proposed to unlock the hidden parts of the mind. He introduced new terms that are now daily fare, such as *psychoanalysis, id, ego, superego, free association.* He was able to do this because he felt free to study man as he might study any animal. Darwin's work gave him permission to view man in this context. From Freud's study evolved the work of others, including those who learned from and studied with Freud himself. Alfred Adler, Carl Jung, Ernest Jones, Otto Rank, Helene Deutsch, Karen Horney, and Freud's daughter, Anna Freud, all made significant and, in most cases, lasting contributions to the field of psychiatry.

But Freud inspired others than just those around him. Society is indebted to him for inspiration—even those who have not agreed with his thinking. He challenged us to look at man objectively. Other dynamic theories, as well as behavioral (Watson, Wolpe, Skinner), somatic (electroshock therapy 1937, psychosurgery 1935), and biologic theories, were ripples of his arguments. He fostered a milieu of thinking about the mind and about mental disorders that profoundly influenced the next generation of theorists. (Freud's and selected other theorists' models of behavior are presented in more detail in Chapter 2.)

## Period of psychotropic drugs

From this milieu of theory development and scientific thought came the third benchmark, which began with the discovery of psychotropic drugs in the 1950s. Chlorpromazine (Thorazine), an antipsychotic drug, was introduced first and imipramine (Tofranil), an antidepressant, was introduced a few years later. Their impact has been powerful. Persons who seemed beyond reach became less agitated and experienced a reduction in psychotic thinking. Depressed persons regained normal feelings. Hospital stays were shortened, and hospital environments improved, since there was less noise and less agitation. Many persons who worked in state hospitals before the advent of psychotropic drugs describe the confusion and hostility as deafening and "crazy." One person stated that he had to "fight his way onto the unit in the morning and fight his way off at night." Many believed these to be truly miracle drugs. But, as with previous promises made, these were broken also. Unit Three is devoted to an understanding of the role of psychotropic drugs in the treatment of mental disorders.

## Period of community mental health

It would be inaccurate to conceptualize one benchmark period coming to a complete halt as the next one developed. There is much overlapping of trends as advocates of one view struggle on while more dynamic forces emerge elsewhere. As the various treatment approaches were being developed in the milieu derived from Freud's theories, the state hospital system continued its plunge into psychiatric Siberia. Critics grew. The popular movie *The Snake Pit* portrayed a mindless, ineffective, and at times cruel system of care. In an even more devastating exposé, the book *The Shame of the States* by Albert Deutsch (1948) vividly painted with words and photographs the deplorable conditions in several large state hospitals around the country.

Legislators were watching, reading, and listening. Legislation was passed that would change the approach to psychiatric care. In 1946 President Truman signed the National Mental Health Act, which enabled the establishment of the National Institute of Mental Health (1949). In 1947 the Hill-Burton Act legislated funds to build general hospitals with psychiatric units. This began the effort to intervene early and shorten the length of care.

In 1961 the Joint Commission on Mental Health and Mental Illness appointed by President Kennedy published a report entitled "Action for Mental Health" (1961). The report urged increased support for the state hospital system, recognizing along with others a need for improved treatment of this population. The supporters of this document were drowned out by opponents of the state hospital system. In fact, the more outspoken critics of the existing system pronounced it the very cause of mental illness.

Instead of more monetary support for the state hospital system, a convergence of forces set the stage for this fourth benchmark. The public's declining confidence in the state hospital system, the failure of various treatment approaches to eradicate mental illness, the legislative climate that had begun in the 1940s, a new emphasis on the civil rights of the mentally ill, and the newfound faith in psychotropic drugs led to the enactment of the Community Mental Health Centers (CMHC) Act in 1963, which virtually destroyed the state hospital system. A deliberate shift from institutional to extrainstitutional care was made. In a word, the deinstitutionalization of the state hospital system population was the goal. The aforementioned problem of *geographical isolation* was countered with community treatment centers and community living arrangements (e.g., half-way houses). *Isolation from family* was dealt with by keeping the mentally disordered close to the family. *Isolation from follow-up care* was remedied by definition: various levels of care were available in the community.

Community mental health programs were proposed to meet the needs of all persons living within the boundaries of a geographic catchment area and had the following goals:

- Emergency care offered on a 24-hour basis
- Inpatient care for persons needing short-term hospitalization
- Partial hospitalization in the form of day treatment centers
- Outpatient care
- Consultation and education for the area served by the center

**Effect on nursing.** The community mental health movement broadened the scope of psychiatric nursing. No longer did the psychiatric nurse simply work in the hospital or inpatient setting. A whole new world of opportunities became available to the psychiatric nurse, from working with the chronically mentally ill to working with the "worried well" and beyond to social issues. This professional evolution of care had both positive and negative effects. On the positive side, it made nurses more understanding of all humanity and broadened professional vision. Perhaps one of the finest dimensions of psychiatric nursing resulted: our concern for the whole person. Mental health was no longer a concern reserved for a few miserable, unfortunate souls but was a legitimate concern for all of us, all the time. A negative effect was the resultant confusion about mental illness. A softening of the criteria resulted in more and more "problems" being claimed as legitimate concerns of mental health professionals. As the public and public leaders became confused about what was or was not a mental health problem, the scope of community mental health concerns grew even wider. Inevitably the status of inpatient psychiatric nursing suffered as newer, more visible roles with less disabled patients became available to nurses.

## DEINSTITUTIONALIZATION

Deinstitutionalization is the depopulating of the state mental hospitals. State hospitals reached their peak census in 1955 and then slowly began the process of trimming their census rolls. It is important to understand that the impetus for deinstitutionalization began before 1963. In fact, it began before 1955. The roots of this process began with the growing concerns about asylum and were nurtured by some of the events previously discussed. A more subtle factor was psychiatry's and psychiatric nursing's growing disillusionment with the chronically mentally ill and an embracing of the "worried well."

These factors clearly laid the groundwork for deinstitutionalization; however, it was federal actions that fully detonated the process. First, as discussed above, was the CMHC Act. The second federal action was the legislation that provided the mentally disabled person with an income while he was living in the community. This legislation was named Aid to the Disabled (ATD) and is now called Supplemental Security Income (SSI). State governments soon found ATD, even when supplemented by the state, to be less costly than state hospitalization. Perhaps the final piece in the deinstitutionalization movement was the change in commitment laws. Out of concern for the civil rights of mental patients, involuntary commitment to the state hospital became difficult. The state had to demonstrate that the "accused" was a clear danger to himself or to others. These sweeping changes were reactions to years of injustice wherein the person said to be mentally ill could be detained and involuntarily committed for long periods of time with little recourse. (The reader is referred to Rosenhan's classic study [1973] to appreciate just how difficult it was for a "sane" person to be discharged from a mental hospital.) The stage was set for rapid depopulation of the state hospitals.

### Depopulation of state hospitals

The state hospital population reached its peak in 1955, with 560,000 patients. By 1986 the state hospital population had dropped to 120,000 patients (Bachrach, 1986). This represents a drop of 80%. Even more dramatic, the 560,000 patients in 1955 represented 0.3% of the U.S. population (based on a 1955 population of 165 million), while the 120,000 state hospital patients in 1986 represented only 0.05% of the U.S. population (based on a 1986 population of 239 million).

The general rate of reduction nationally was 1% to 2% a year from 1955 to 1965 and about 5% per year between 1965 and 1975 as the federal events of 1963 began to be felt (Morrissey et al., 1986). This decline has resulted in the closing of more than 50 state hospitals since 1970 (Frank, 1989). Those patients "left behind" require a high level of care, have few social relationships, and are psychotic. For the most part, they are involuntarily detained young men who are acutely ill and dangerous (Dorwart, 1988). Although deinstitutionalization has slowed in the last few years, its effect on the public mental hospitals is still profound. *Recidivism,* a term traditionally used to describe repeat criminal offenders, is now being used to describe the "revolving door" effect of persons cycling and recycling through the community agency.

## Community effects

The effects of deinstitutionalization are also felt in community agencies. For example, emergency room use by acutely disturbed persons has increased dramatically in the absence of the "old" system. Emergency psychiatric services are sagging from the load they carry. General hospital psychiatric units are overwhelmed at times with the continuous flow of patients being admitted and discharged. (The average stay of patients in some county facilities is less than 4 days.) Their mission has expanded as they have had to offset the shrinking state hospital. Compared to the patients of the 1960s and 1970s, today's patients are more aggressive and assaultive (Cohen and Marcos, 1989). Emergency rooms have become holding areas or short-term, acute outpatient treatment settings for patients needing (but not wanting) to be admitted to a psychiatric unit. During the 1980s visits of psychiatric patients to emergency rooms climbed 400% to 500% in some cities. One large general hospital recorded a rise in emergency psychiatric visits from 100 to 2600 per year between 1972 and 1982 (Kaskey and Ianzito, 1984).

Many mental health professionals are pleased with the depopulating of state hospitals. Others, while pleased, see such problems as the increased use of community emergency services as a cause for concern. Still others, those who never supported the deinstitutionalization concept, are satisfied their minority position has been vindicated.

## HOMELESSNESS

"Probably nothing more graphically illustrates the problems of deinstitutionalization than the shameful and incredible phenomenon of the homeless mentally ill" (Lamb, 1988). Homelessness is not new. It just seems to be because of media attention. The media focus, however, is a reflection of real increases in this population. The former view (when homeless people were not making headlines) held that homeless people (mostly men) were skid row bums. The current view has been altered considerably. It is now believed the homeless are people (now men, women, and children [families]) who have been displaced by social policies over which they have no control. The estimates about the dimension of the "problem" range from 200,000 to 3 million plus on any given day. Estimates concerning the prevalence of mental illness among this population also vary. The New York State Office of Mental Health (Community Services Society, 1982) found less than one fourth of the homeless needed mental health services, while Bassuk (1983) stated 90% of those he interviewed had a diagnosable mental illness. Most experts believe 25% to 50% of adult homeless have a psychosis and that 33% to 50% are alcoholics.

Homeless people may live exclusively on the streets, the so-called street people, or they may make use of community shelters. A possible third group are those who are able to stay in cheap hotels—sometimes referred to as "psychiatric ghettos"—for a short while between nights in less accommodating surroundings.

Homelessness, besides being an end product of chronic mental illness, probably exacerbates it as well. Stated another way, many chronically ill persons drift down to the streets because of their inability to succeed in a competitive society, and once they get to the streets, the stresses of the homeless life compound their mental health problems. They are in a no-win situation. And, as with many societal problems, some groups seem to fare worse than others. As Carter (1986) points out, "The rush to depopulate state mental institutions resulted in the dumping of many socially unskilled and economically deprived black chronic patients on poverty-ridden black communities. . . . Society's preoccupation with protecting the mentally ill from the abuses of mental health professionals has contributed to the misuse of the criminal justice system to control socially unacceptable behavior." Carter believes black people, who rely heavily on public psychiatric institutions, have been inordinately affected.

Proponents of deinstitutionalization argue that these problems are not inherently a part of depopulating state hospitals but have resulted because the money has not followed the patient out of the hospital. Inpatient psychiatric treatment still accounts for 70% of mental health dollars in the United States (Goldstein and Horgan, 1988), so, they argue, community mental health has never been given the financial base to realize its promise. Critics, on the other hand, point to the homeless and the disproportionate effect felt by some minority groups as evidence of a need for change. Homelessness is more than a lack of shelter, they maintain. Homelessness is a lack of support systems, support systems that were available in the public mental hospital system.

## EVOLUTION OF PSYCHIATRIC CARE CONCERNS

Psychiatry in general lost interest in the chronically mentally ill as a result of the influx of psychoanalysts in the 1930s and 1940s (Miller, 1984). As Freud himself had discovered, his analytic approach was most helpful to persons with less severe problems and was not particularly helpful to psychotic patients. It is human nature to seek out what one does well and to avoid what one does not do so well. Thus, as more and more psychiatrists and psychiatric nurses were influenced by Freudian thinking, there was a natural pulling away from the chronically mentally ill and a refocusing on those more amenable to this treatment approach. Public mental hospitals lost prestige, as did the physicians and nurses working in them. Within the psychiatric nursing fraternity, staff psychiatric nurses were not as highly valued as those psychiatric nurses working in the therapist role. As participants in a self-fulfilling prophecy, the devalued inpatient psychiatric nurses in public hospitals in many cases became as they were viewed.

The mainstream of psychiatry and psychiatric nursing turned from the chronically disturbed patient to individuals with lowered self-esteem, those who were striving to reach their potential, those who had not developed the ability to trust, the existentially unhappy (Detre, 1987). In a phrase, psychiatry turned toward the "worried well." Psychiatry changed its focus from one extreme of the psychiatric care continuum (the chronically mentally ill) to the other (the worried well) over a few decades.

Social issues started to emerge as legitimate professional concerns. Psychiatry and psychiatric nursing became interested in such issues as poverty, racism, alternate life-styles, and sexism at the professional level. It is the perception of some clinicians that this process of enlightenment and social relevance further distanced the main-stream of psychiatric care from those most in need of that care. This may be particularly true of the nurse psychotherapist. Pelletier (1984), in his interesting article "Nurse Psychotherapists: Who Do They Treat," found that most of their patients were women and that therapy focused on women's experience in today's world, that is, lack of awareness of body or feelings, physical or sexual abuse, a spouse's infidelity, conflict with a mother or other family members over issues of dependence or independence, alcoholism, marital separation or divorce, and alienation from a parent or child. Pelletier refers to those treated as "well clients" dealing with situational reactions. Medication was not mentioned, and he suggests that nurse psychotherapists might not find it "feasible" to shoulder the responsibility associated with psychotic patients. In practice, this means that some of the best-trained psychiatric nurses are not available for the psychiatric patients most in need of their help.

## NURSING EDUCATION

The first psychiatric nursing textbook was written by Harriet Bailey in 1920. The title of the book, *Nursing Mental Diseases,* reflected the appropriate terminology of the day.

An important distinction about psychiatric nursing is that it was not brought into the greater nursing fold until the 1940s. Because psychiatric nurses were trained in state hospitals, they could work only in state hospitals. In 1937 the National League for Nursing (then called the National League for Nursing Education) recommended psychiatric nursing be made a part of the curriculum of general nursing programs. As the views of the major theorists, such as Sullivan (see Chapter 2) with his "interpersonal psychiatry" and Maxwell Jones (see Chapter 15) with his "therapeutic milieu," became prominent, the role of psychiatric nurses grew.

As psychiatric nursing developed, others recognized its contribution to psychiatric care. Psychiatric nursing was one of four professional groups (along with psychiatry, psychology, and social work) given money for training in the 1946 National Mental Health Act. These monies enabled more nurses to be trained in basic psychiatric nursing (undergraduate) and spurred specialization at the advanced level (graduate).

The views of two important figures in psychiatric nursing in the '50s shaped and gave direction to psychiatric nursing practice and contributed to a professional climate. Hildegarde Peplau (1952, 1959, 1962) developed a model for psychiatric nursing practice. Her book *Interpersonal Relations in Nursing* and article "Interpersonal Techniques: The Crux of Psychiatric Nursing" influence practice to this day. Her approach, heavily influenced by Harry Stack Sullivan, emphasized the interpersonal dimension of practice. She also wrote a history of psychiatric nursing that carefully traced the unfolding of the profession. Peplau may be the single most important historical figure in psychiatric nursing. A more complete review of her thinking is found in Chapter 6.

Another influential figure was June Mellow (1953, 1967, 1986). Mellow viewed nursing therapy as taking place in an "experiential-action medium" in which the nurse and the patient share the factors in the environment. Her approach focuses on psychosocial needs and patient strengths. As Peplau and Mellow (and others) began to articulate what psychiatric nurses do, the profession experienced another surge forward in its quest for professional accountability.

### Nursing research

One effect of the Community Mental Health Centers Act in 1963 was a broadening of the scope of psychiatric nursing practice and a consequent increased responsibility for improving practice. Psychiatric nursing looked to research as an answer to improving practice. Previously most "psychiatric nursing" research was conducted by nonnurses. By the early 1970s this had changed so that most psychiatric nursing research was conducted by nurses (Pearlmutter, 1985).

By 1974 a psychiatric nursing conference, after reviewing professional developments between 1946 and 1974, suggested that future nursing research focus on one-on-one relationships, group work, milieu therapy, and family therapy (Pearlmutter, 1985), Research is now an integral part of psychiatric nursing practice. This reasearch is communicated in journals dedicated exclusively to psychiatric nursing: *Perspectives in Psychiatric Care* (1963), *Journal of Psychosocial Nursing and Mental Health Services* (1963), *Issues in Mental Health Nursing* (1979), and *Archives of Psychiatric Nursing* (1987).

### STANDARDS OF PRACTICE

In 1973, standards of care were developed by the American Nurses' Association's Division of Psychiatric and Mental Health Practice. That document was revised in 1982. The revised "Standards for Psychiatric and Mental Health Nursing Practice" reflect the current state of knowledge and the wider range of professional practice. These standards of care apply to all settings where nurses practice psychiatric nursing. Two standards are specifically applicable to advanced practitioners, for example, clinical specialists. In addition to this standardization of care, an effort to classify the areas of concern for psychiatric nursing has been developed. A panel of psychiatric nursing leaders continues to work on nursing diagnoses.

### CERTIFICATION OF COMPETENCY

One of the latest developments in the evolution of psychiatric nursing has been the decision of the American Nurses' Association (ANA) to provide certification for those nurses who meet established criteria. This step represents a major milestone. In effect, the ANA endorses the certified nurse as competent at certain levels. Certification is available at both the generalist and clinical specialist levels. As of 1987 the ANA reported 8214 generalists and 2756 clinical specialists (ANA, 1988). Psychiatric nurses have evolved from caretakers to clinical specialists, from custodians to psychotherapists, from asylum-educated to doctorally prepared practitioners. The professional vision and contributions to care have changed dramatically in these 100 years.

Extremes in professional thinking are beginning to be resolved. Although some nurses still focus their interventions on the "worried well," most focust their attention on the multitudes of persons in the middle of the continuum—the millions who suffer from phobias, obsessions, anxiety, substance abuse, sexual dysfunction, and so on. The chronically mentally ill remain underserved in many areas, but that is changing also.

## KEY CONCEPTS

1. Understanding the principles of psychiatric nursing is important since over 15% of the population is affected by mental health problems.
2. Modern psychiatry can be traced through four benchmark eras: the period of enlightenment, the period of scientific study, the period of psychotropic drugs, and the period of community mental health.
3. Historically, the mentally ill were banished and confined, but the *period of enlightenment* ushered in an era in which the mentally ill were treated humanely.
4. The asylum movement (providing asylum from the hostile world) grew out of the humane emphasis of the period of enlightenment and resulted in development of the state hospital system.
5. During the *period of scientific study* such men as Freud, Kraepelin, and Bleuler studied man objectively; this resulted in both psychodynamic and biological understandings of mental disorders.
6. During the *period of psychotropic drugs* antipsychotic drugs (chlorpromazine [Thorazine] in the early 1950s), antidepressant drugs (imipramine [Tofranil] in the late 1950s), and other drugs were developed and greatly contributed to the treatment of specific mental disorders.
7. As a result of several converging factors (e.g., the potential of psychotropic drugs, a hostile public opinion about state hospitals), the *period of community mental health* began.
8. Deinstitutionalization, changing the locus of treatment from the state hospital to the community, is a product of the community mental health movement.
9. A high percentage of the nation's homeless have a diagnosable mental disorder, and critics of deinstitutionalization place some of the blame for homelessness on the community mental health movement.

### REFERENCES

American Nurses' Association: Certification catalog, Kansas City, 1988, The Association.

American Nurses' Association: Standards of psychiatric and mental health nursing practice, Kansas City, 1982, The Association.

Bachrach LL: The future of the state mental hospital, Hosp Community Psychiatry 37:467, 1986.

Bassuk EL: The homeless problem, Sci Am 241:40, 1984.

Carter JH: Deinstitutionalization of black patients: an apocalypse now, Hosp Community Psychiatry 40:677, 1989.

Cohen NL and Marcos LR: The bad-mad dilemma of public psychiatry, Hosp Community Psychiatry 40:677, 1989.

Community Service Society: Who are the homeless? A study of randomly selected men who use the New York City shelters, Albany, NY, 1982, The Society.

Detre T: The future of psychiatry, Am J Psychiatry 144:621, 1987.

Deutsch A: The shame of the states, New York, 1948, Harcourt Brace.

Dorwart RA: A ten-year followup study of the effects of deinstitutionalization, Hosp Community Psychiatry, 39:287, 1988.

Foucault M: Madness and civilization (translated from the French), New York, 1967, New American Library.

Frank RG: The medically indigent mentally ill: approaches to financing, Hosp Community Psychiatry 40:9-12, 1989.

Goldstein JN and Horgan CM: Inpatient and outpatient psychiatric services: substitutes or complements, Hosp Community Psychiatry 37:433, 1986.

Gralnick A: The asylum snare, Hosp Community Psychiatry 37:433, 1986.

Joint Commission on Mental Illness and Health: Action for mental health: final report, New York, 1961, Basic Books.

Kaskey GB and Ianzito BM: Development of an emergency psychiatric treatment unit, Hosp Community Psychiatry 35:1220, 1984.

Lamb HR: Deinstitutionalization at the crossroads, Hosp Community Psychiatry 39:941, 1988.

Mellow J: An exploratory study of nursing therapy with two persons with psychoses (master of science thesis), Boston, 1953, Boston University School of Nursing.

Mellow J: Evolution of nursing therapy through research, Psychiatr Opinion 4:15, 1967.

Mellow J: A personal perspective of nursing therapy, Hosp Community Psychiatry 37:182, 1986.

Miller RD: Public mental hospital work: pros and cons for psychiatrists, Hosp Community Psychiatry 35:928, 1984.

Morrissey JP, Witkin MJ, and Bethel HE: Trends by state in the capacity and volume of inpatient services, state and county mental hospitals, United States, 1976-1980, Series CN10, Pub ADM 86-146, Rockville, MD, 1986, National Institute of Mental Health.

Pearlmutter DR: Recent trends and issues in psychiatric—mental health nursing, Hosp Community Psychiatry 36:56, 1985.

Pelletier LR: Nurse-psychotherapists: Whom do they treat? Hosp Community Psychiatry 35:1149, 1984.

Peplau H: Interpersonal relations in nursing, New York, 1952, G.P. Putnam's Sons.

Peplau H: Principles of psychiatric nursing. In Arieti S, editor: American handbook of psychiatry, vol. 2. New York, 1959, Basic Books Inc, Publishers.

Peplau H: Interpersonal technique: the crux of psychiatric nursing, Am J Nurs 62:50, 1962.

Regier DA, Boyd JH, Burke JD, et al: One-month prevalence of mental disorders in the United States, Arch Gen Psychiatry 45:977, 1988.

Rosenblatt A.: Concepts of the asylum in the care of the mentally ill, Hosp Community Psychiatry 35:244, 1984.

Rosenhan DL: On being sane in insane places, Science 179:250, 1973.

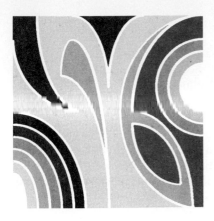

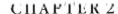

## CHAPTER 2

# Theoretical Models for Working with Psychiatric Patients

LEARNING OBJECTIVES

After reading this chapter you should be able to

- Compare and contrast major theoretical models that contribute to the understanding of psychiatric patients and their behaviors.
- Identify key concepts of the major theoretical models.
- Describe the relevance of each theoretical model to psychiatric nursing practice.
- Describe the five axes of the Psychiatric Classification System.

The following theoretical models of human behavior have been selected for discussion in this chapter because they provide basic concepts for working with psychiatric patients: psychoanalytical, developmental, interpersonal, rational-emotive, reality, and stress models. These models are summarized in Table 2-1. The American Psychiatric Association's *Diagnostic and Statistical Manual of Mental Disorders, Third Edition Revised (DSM-III-R)* is discussed briefly . The authors of the DSM-III-R have attempted to provide a document free of theoretical bias. While it is important for nurses to understand the theoretical models presented in the chapter, it is also important to recognize that the DSM-III-R, the official diagnostic manual in American psychiatry, does not endorse any of the models.

## PSYCHOANALYTICAL MODEL

The psychoanalytical model is a theory of personality that originated with Sigmund Freud. It emphasizes man's unconscious processes or psychodynamic factors as the basis for motivation and behavior. Freud believed that the personality is formed in early childhood and that knowledge of how an individual's drives, instincts, psychic energy or libido, and psychosexual attitude are formed during the first 6 years of life is crucial to an understanding of his personality.

### Key concepts

**Personality processes.**  The personality consists of three processes: the id, the ego, and the superego. These three segments function as a whole to bring about behavior. When they function in harmony with each other, the individual experiences stability. When disharmony occurs, the individual is in conflict. The individual is all id at birth, wanting to experience only pleasure. This instinctual drive is known as the pleasure principle. Seeking pleasure involves primary process thinking, which enables the individual to strive for pleasure through the use of fantasy and images. The id is compulsive and without morals. The ego controls id impulses and mediates between the id and reality. The ego focuses on the reality principle and strives to meet the demands of the id while maintaining the well-being of the individual by distinguishing fantasy from environmental reality. The second process, the ego, comprises rational, logical thinking and intelligence. The ego is that part of the personality that experiences anxiety and uses defense mechanisms for protection. Heredity and environmental factors, along with maturation, influence the formation of the ego.

The superego is concerned with right and wrong and is the conscience. It provides the ego with an inner control to help cope with the id. The superego is formed from the internalization of what parents teach their children about right and wrong through rewards and punishments. The person's self-esteem is affected by whether he perceives himself as doing what is good or right. Guilt and inferiority are experienced if he cannot live up to parental standards. Inner conflict results when the id, the ego, and the superego are striving for different goals.

**Consciousness.**  Freuds' concepts of the levels of consciousness are central in an understanding of problems of personality and behavior. *Consciousness* or material

**TABLE 2-1**　Therapeutic models

| Model | Assumptions | Goals/approaches | Dialogue |
|---|---|---|---|
| Psychoanalytical (Freud) | Individuals are motivated by unconscious desires and conflicts. Personality is developed by early childhood. | *Insight* into unconscious conflicts and processes Personality reconstruction | Patient: All women hate me. Immediate response: Tell me about one woman you are having trouble with. |
| | Illness results from childhood conflicts and ego defenses inadequate to cope with anxiety. Change is a process of *insight.* | Use of free association, dream analysis, and analyses of transference and resistance | *Insight*-oriented response: Tell me about your relationship with your mother. |
| Developmental (Erikson) | Biological, psychological, social, and environmental factors influence personality development throughout the life cycle. | Mastery of developmental tasks through achievement of insight; continued development through death | Patient: I can't do anything right. Help me. |
| | *Growth* involves resolution of critical tasks at each of the eight developmental stages. | Analysis of developmental issues, fears, and barriers to *growth* to achieve insight | Immediate response: I hear your doubt in yourself. But I did see you make a positive decision this morning. |
| | Lack of resolution of tasks results in incomplete development and difficulties in relationships. Change involves reexperiencing and resolving developmental crises. Change is a process of *growth* | Facilitation of mastery of developmental tasks with support and problem-solving | *Growth*-oriented response: I can help you look at ways to develop your self-confidence. |

*Continued.*

**TABLE 2-1**  Therapeutic models—cont'd

| Model | Assumptions | Goals/approaches | Dialogue |
|---|---|---|---|
| Interpersonal (Sullivan, Peplau) | Interpersonal relationships and anxiety facilitate development of the self system. | Development of satisfactory relationships and maturity | Patient: I can't sit still. I'm too nervous. |
| | Development occurs in stages with changing types of relationships. | Relative freedom from the interference of anxiety | Immediate response: Let's take a walk for a few minutes. |
| | Faulty patterns of relating interfere with security and maturity. | Learning effective interpersonal skills | *Reeducation* response: Let's talk about what kind of things make you nervous and what you can do about them. |
| | Security operations protect against anxiety and interfere with learning. | Examination of current interpersonal difficulties | |
| | Change is a process of *reeducation*. | Use of therapist-patient relationships as a vehicle for analyzing interpersonal processes and testing new skills | |
| | | Consensual validation, validation, reality testing, and reflecting positive appraisals | |
| Rational-emotive (Ellis) | An individual has value simply because he exists. | Substitution of *rational* beliefs for irrational ones | Patient: My wife makes me so angry. |
| | Individuals have potential for *rational* and irrational thinking. | Elimination of self-defeating behaviors | Immediate response: What did your wife do that you chose to get angry about? |
| | Irrational beliefs produce irrational emotions and behaviors. | Increased responsibility for feelings, behaviors, and change | *Rational-emotive* response: What is self-defeating about the statement you just made? |
| | Change involves changing beliefs in order to change feelings and behaviors. | Challenging of irrational beliefs | |
| | Change is a process of *rational* thinking. | Cognitive homework | |
| | | Role playing and testing out new behaviors | |

| Reality (Glasser) | An individual's most basic psychological needs are to be loved (to be involved) and to feel worthwhile (to have respect from self and others). | Facing reality and developing standards for behaving responsibly | Patient: The stupid doctor revoked my weekend pass. |
| | Meeting these needs must be done responsibly and within the context of reality. | Greater maturity, conscientiousness, and responsibility | Immediate response: What did you do that showed you were not ready for a pass? |
| | Responsibility is fulfilling one's own needs without interfering with others fulfilling their needs. | Being accountable for one's behaviors | Relearning response: What behaviors do you think will be necessary before you will be given a pass? |
| | Illness results from irresponsible behavior. | Being open, warm, honest, authentic, and accepting of the patient as a person | |
| | Change is a process of *relearning*. | Becoming deeply involved with the patient | |
| | | Focusing on current behaviors and consequences | |
| | | Confronting irresponsible behaviors | |
| | | Assisting with relearning of responsible behaviors | |
| Stress (Selye, Lazarus) | A stress is any positive or negative occurrence or emotion requiring a response. | Developing effective coping mechanisms | Patient: I'm so tense I can't sleep. |
| | Stress produces physiological and psychological responses. | Reduction of bodily tensions | Immediate response: Have a relaxation exercise I can show you |
| | Inadequate handling of stress can lead to physical and/or mental illness. | Increasing resources and social supports | *Problem-solving* approach: You've said you're worried about seeing your family tomorrow. Let's talk it out what you might say to them. |
| | Change is a process of *problem solving* | Stress management | |
| | | Biofeedback | |
| | | Relaxation training | |

within our awareness is only one small part of the mind. The *unconscious* is a larger area and consists of memories, conflicts, experiences, and material that have been repressed. It cannot be recalled at will. *Preconscious* material refers to memories that can be recalled to consciousness. Freud believed that by uncovering unconscious material the individual would gain an understanding of his behavior, which would enable him to make choices about his behavior and thus improve his mental health. To bring the unconscious into awareness, psychoanalytical therapy uses dreams, hypnosis, free association, and projective techniques that will bring to awareness repressed thoughts and feelings. Insight into the meaning of symptoms and behaviors facilitates change.

**Defense mechanisms.**   The ego usually copes with anxiety by rational means. When anxiety is painful, the individual copes by using defense mechanisms. Used moderately, defense mechanisms are *normal* methods that people use to protect the ego and to diminish anxiety. When these mechanisms are used excessively, however, the individual is unable to face reality and does not solve his problems. Defense mechanisms are primarily unconscious behaviors; however, some are within voluntary control. Some common defense mechanisms are described in Table 2-2.

Painful feelings connected with childhood conflicts are usually repressed. Later in life, as similar conflicts are once again experienced, repression fails, and these feelings emerge, causing anxiety and discomfort. Freud defined three kinds of anxiety: reality, moral, and neurotic. Reality anxiety stems from an external real threat. Neurotic anxiety deals with the fear that instincts will cause one to do something for which he will be punished. Moral anxiety deals with guilt that is experienced if one does something contrary to his conscience. These types of anxiety form the basis of many mental illnesses.

**Goals of psychoanalysis.**   The goals of Freudian psychoanalytical therapy are to make the unconscious conscious so that the individual can work through the past and understand his behavior. By overcoming resistance and repression, childhood experiences can be analyzed. Uncovering causes of current behaviors will lead to insight. Only then will the individual be able to decrease his self-defeating behaviors and change his character.

### Therapist's role

The therapist uses free association and dream analysis to uncover unconscious material. The analyst uses free association with patients so that repressed material can be identified and interpreted to patients. Doing so leads to increased insight into underlying dynamics of behaviors. Interpretation or translation of repressed material uncovers additional unconscious data. Dream analysis helps the patient uncover the meaning of his dream, which also increases awareness about present behavior. Patients' inconsistencies and resistance to therapy are confronted. Transference (see Chapter 6) occurring in the relationship is used to encourage projection and working through of feelings that would otherwise remain unconscious.

### Relevance to nursing practice

In brief therapeutic encounters the nurse is able to recognize and understand maladaptive defense mechanisms used by the patient. In an ongoing nurse-patient re-

**TABLE 2-2** Defense mechanisms

| Defense mechanism | Definition | Normal use | Patient example |
|---|---|---|---|
| Repression | Unconscious and involuntary forgetting of painful ideas, events, and conflicts | A car accident victim is unable to remember details of the impact. | Mrs. Young, a victim of incest does not know why she has always hated her uncle. |
| Denial | Unconscious refusal to admit an unacceptable idea or behavior | A nursing student refuses to admit that she is flunking out of school despite F's in two courses. | Mr. Davis, who is alcohol dependent, states that he can control his drinking. |
| Suppression | Voluntary exclusion from awareness, anxiety-producing feelings, ideas, and situations | A student states, "I cannot think about my wedding tonight. I have to study." | Michelle states to the nurse that she is not ready to talk about her recent divorce. |
| Rationalization | Attempts to make or prove that one's feelings or behaviors are justifiable | A student states, "I got a C on the test because the teacher asked poor questions." | Mr. Jones, a paranoid schizophrenic, states that he cannot go to work because he is afraid of his coworkers instead of admitting that he is mentally ill. |
| Intellectualization | Using only logical explanations without feelings or an affective component | A wife states to her husband that a dented car fender is much better than a completely wrecked car and garage door. | Mrs. Mann talks about her son's death and bout with cancer as being mercifully short without showing any signs of sadness. |
| Identification | A conscious or unconscious attempt to model oneself after a respected person | When a little girl dresses up like her mother to play house, she tries to talk and act like her mother. | Sheila states to the nurse, "When I get out of the hospital, I want to be a nurse just like you." |
| Introjection | Unconsciously incorporating wishes, values, attitudes of others as if they were your own | While her mother is gone, a young girl disciplines her brother just like her mother would. | Without realizing it, a patient talks and acts like his therapist, analyzing other patients. |
| Compensation | Covering up for a weakness by overemphasizing or making up a desirable trait | An academically weak high school student becomes a star in the school play. | A schizophrenic patient who is unable to talk to other patients becomes known for his expressive poetry. |
| Reaction formation | A conscious behavior that is the exact opposite of an unconscious feeling | An older brother who dislikes his younger brother sends him gifts for every holiday. | Miss Marla, who unconsciously hates her mother, continuously tells her how wonderful her mother is. |

Continued.

**TABLE 2-2   Defense mechanisms—cont'd**

| Defense mechanism | Definition | Normal use | Patient example |
|---|---|---|---|
| Sublimation | Channeling instinctual drives into acceptable activities | An adolescent arrested once for stealing later opens a business installing security systems in banks. | A former perpetrator of incest who fears relapse initiates a local chapter of Parents United. |
| Displacement | Discharging pentup feelings to a less threatening object | A husband comes home from work and yells at his wife after a bad day at work. | Mrs. Faust screams at another patient after being told by her psychiatrist that she cannot have a weekend pass. |
| Projection | Blaming someone else for one's difficulties or placing one's unethical desires on someone else | A teenager comes home late from a date and states that her friend did not bring her home on time. | Katrina states that she used marijuana while on pass because her boyfriend made her smoke it. |
| Conversion | The unconscious expression of intrapsychic conflict symbolically through physical symptoms | A student awakens with a migraine the morning of a final examination and feels too ill to take it. She does not realize that 1 hour of cramming left her unprepared. | Mr. Jenson suddenly develops impotence after his wife discovers he is having an affair with his secretary. |
| Undoing | Doing something to counteract or make up for a transgression or wrong doing | After spanking her son, a mother bakes his favorite cookies. | After eating another patient's cookies, Mrs. Donnelly apologizes to the patients, cleans the refrigerator, and labels everyone's snack with their names. |
| Dissociation | The unconscious separation of painful feelings and emotions from an unacceptable idea, situation, or object. | A young wife talks about her husband's extensive gambling debts as if they were nothing to be concerned about. | A patient tells the nurse that when she was sexually molested as a child, she felt as if she were outside of her body watching what was happening without feeling anything. |
| Regression | Return to an earlier and more comfortable developmental level | A 6-year-old wets the bed at night since the birth of his baby sister. | Mr. Hivey isolates himself in his room and lies in a fetal position since his admission. |

lationship, the nurse points out maladaptive mechanisms and works with the patient to decrease these behaviors and increase adaptive ones. In a long-term relationship the patient can be assisted with learning to think, feel, and behave according to his own individual values, beliefs, and needs and not according to someone else's. The patient also needs assistance with accepting his desires and drives as normal human phenomena over which he need not feel guilt or shame.

## DEVELOPMENTAL MODEL

Erik Erikson built upon Freud's psychoanalytic model by including psychosocial and environmental influences along with the psychosexual. His developmental model spans the total life cycle from birth to death, instead of ending with adolescence. He believed that each of his eight stages of development allowed opportunities for growth up to the acceptance of one's own death.

### Key concepts

Each stage was described by Erikson as an emotional crisis involving positive and negative experiences. Growth or mastery of critical tasks was the result of having more positive than negative experiences. Nonmastery of tasks inhibited movement to the next stage. Erikson believed that man's drive to live and grow was opposed by a drive to return to comfortable earlier states, even the one before birth; therefore, he saw regression as a possibility.

Implied, but not clearly described in his model, is the concept of partial mastery of critical tasks in development. The degree of mastery of each stage is related to the degree of maturity attained by the adult. Defects in development carried from one stage to the next progressively interfere with functioning until the individual is no longer capable of growing without emotionally returning to the earlier stages to resolve the crisis. For example, a person may develop enough trust in others to engage in superficial relationships but not be able to develop intimacy with a spouse. Another person may have enough initiative to accept a job but lacks the industry to stay with it. An environmental or social tragedy can shake the early foundations of development, such as when divorce from a spouse threatens the individual's sense of trust in others and results in doubts in oneself.

Mastery of the critical tasks of each stage occurs more easily when it is chronologically appropriate. Overcoming delayed or incomplete development is difficult but possible.

### Relevance to nursing practice

Most psychiatric patients evidence developmental delays or only partial mastery of developmental stages preceding the stage expected for their chronological age. To help a patient master tasks necessary for overcoming development problems, the nurse conducts an assessment of the patient's level of functioning. This involves interpretations of verbal and nonverbal behaviors to identify the degree of mastery of each stage up to the patient's chronological age. The behavioral manifestations of problems are clues to issues to be addressed in working with the patient. Although

Erikson focused on the polarities of each developmental stage (e.g., trust-mistrust), as if the "positive" pole were the desirable task to be accomplished, it is now recognized that the extremes of either pole produce problems in functioning. For example, being overly trusting can result in an individual's being repeatedly taken advantage of by others (Table 2-3). Nursing interventions with specific developmental issues are discussed in Chapter 6 on the nurse-patient relationship and in the chapters on specific disorders.

**TABLE 2-3**   Adult manifestations of Erikson's eight stages of development

| Life stage | Adult behaviors reflecting mastery | Adult behaviors reflecting developmental problems |
|---|---|---|
| Trust vs mistrust (0 to 18 months) | Realistic trust of self and others<br>Confidence in others<br>Optimism and hope<br>Sharing openly with others<br>Relating to others effectively | Suspiciousness of others<br>Testing of others<br>Fear of criticism and affection<br>Dissatisfaction and hostility<br>Sense of others being evil<br>Fear of sharing and asking for help<br>Projection of blame and undesirable feelings<br>Withdrawal from others<br>*or*<br>Overly trusting of others<br>Being gullible<br>Being naive<br>Sharing too quickly and easily |
| Autonomy vs shame and doubt (18 months to 3 years) | Self-control and will power<br>Realistic self-concept and self-esteem<br>Pride and sense of goodwill<br>Cooperativeness<br>Generosity tempered with withholding<br>Delayed gratification when necessary | Self-doubt and self-consciousness<br>Dependence on others for approval and sense of worth<br>Feeling of being exposed<br>Fear of being attacked<br>Sense of being out of control of self and one's life<br>Obsessive-compulsive behaviors<br>Jealousy<br>*or*<br>Excessive independence or defiance<br>Denial of problems<br>Unwillingness to ask for help<br>Impulsiveness and inability to wait<br>Reckless disregard for the safety of self and others |

Table compiled by Lee Schwecke and Sandra Wood, Indiana University School of Nursing, 1988.

**TABLE 2-3**   Adult manifestations of Erikson's eight stages of development    cont'd

| Life stage | Adult behaviors reflecting mastery | Adult behaviors reflecting developmental problems |
|---|---|---|
| Initiative vs guilt (3 to 5 years) | An adequate conscience<br>Initiative balanced with restraint<br>Appropriate social behaviors<br>Curiosity and exploration<br>Healthy competitiveness<br>Sense of direction<br>Original and purposeful activities | Passivity and apathy<br>Excessive compliance<br>Self-restriction and self-denial<br>Unreasonable or excessive guilt or embarrassment for actions, ideas, and mistakes<br>Assuming a role as victim<br>Self-punishment<br>Reluctance to show emotions<br>Underachievement of potential<br>Absence of sense of direction<br>*or*<br>Good plans or ideas but lack of follow-through<br>Little sense of guilt despite actions<br>Expansive expression of emotions (such as jealous rage)<br>Labile emotions<br>Showing off<br>Excessive competitiveness |
| Industry vs inferiority (6 to 12 years) | Sense of competence<br>Completion of projects<br>Pleasure in diligence and effectiveness<br>Ability to cooperate and compromise<br>Identification with admired others<br>Joy of involvement in the world and with others<br>Balance of work and play | Feeling unworthy and inadequate<br>Poor work history (quitting jobs, lack of promotions, absenteeism, decline in productivity)<br>Work viewed as only an obligation<br>Inadequate problem-solving skills<br>Manipulation of others to provide for self<br>Violation of other's rights<br>Inability to cooperate or compromise or to assist others<br>Lack of friends of the same sex<br>*or*<br>Overly high achieving<br>Reluctance to attempt new things for fear of failing<br>Feeling unable to gain love or affection unless totally successful<br>Perfectionistic<br>Being a workaholic and taking little time for recreation<br>Excessive organization of one's life |

*Continued.*

**TABLE 2-3**   Adult manifestations of Erikson's eight stages of development—cont'd

| Life stage | Adult behaviors reflecting mastery | Adult behaviors reflecting developmental problems |
|---|---|---|
| Identity vs role diffusion (12 to 18 to 20 years) | Confident sense of self<br>Emotional stability<br>Commitment to career planning and realistic long-term goals<br>Sense of having a place in society<br>Establishing relationships with the opposite sex<br>Fidelity to friends<br>Development of personal values<br>Testing out adult roles | Lack of or giving up of long-term goals, beliefs, and values<br>Lack of defined roles or loss of productive roles<br>Lack of confidence<br>Feelings of confusion, indecision, and alienation<br>Vacillation between dependence and rebellion<br>Superficial, short-term relationship with the opposite sex<br>*or*<br>Dramatic overconfidence<br>Acting out behaviors, including alcohol and drug use<br>Showy display of sex role behaviors |
| Intimacy vs isolation (18 to 25 to 30 years) | Ability to give and receive love<br>Development of commitments and mutuality with others of both sexes<br>Collaboration in work and affiliations<br>Sacrifices for others<br>Responsible sexual behavior | Persistent aloneness/isolation<br>Emotional distance in all relationships<br>Prejudices against others<br>Lack of established vocation—many career changes<br>Seeking of intimacy through sexual encounters (equating sex with intimacy)<br>*or*<br>Imposing too much togetherness in opposite sex relationships<br>Possessiveness and jealousy<br>Dependency on parents, spouse or both<br>Abusiveness toward loved ones<br>Inability to try new things socially or vocationally (staying in routine or mundane job and activities) |

## INTERPERSONAL MODEL

Harry Stack Sullivan (1953) developed a comprehensive examination of interpersonal relationships called the Interpersonal Theory of Psychiatry. He considered the healthy person as a social being with the ability to live effectively in relationships with others. Mental illness was viewed as any degree of lack of awareness of processes in one's interpersonal relationships. Relationships were viewed as the source of anxiety and maladaptive behaviors as well as personality formation.

**TABLE 2-3**    Adult manifestations of Erikson's eight stages of development—cont'd

| Life stage | Adult behaviors reflecting mastery | Adult behaviors reflecting developmental problems |
|---|---|---|
| Generativity vs stagnation or self-absorption (30 to 65 years) | Productive, constructive, creative activity<br>Personal and professional growth<br>Parental and societal responsibilities<br>Caring guidance of others | Self-centeredness and self-indulgence<br>Exaggerated concern for appearance and possessions<br>Lack of interest in the welfare of others<br>Lack of involvement in community or professional activities or organizations<br>Loss of interest in marriage, extramarital affairs, or both<br>*or*<br>Too many professional or community activities to the detriment of family<br>Too little time for self |
| Integrity vs despair (65 years to death) | Feelings of self-acceptance<br>Sense of dignity, worth, and importance<br>Adaptation to life according to limitations<br>Valuing one's life<br>Sharing of wisdom<br>Exploration of philosophy of life and death | Sense of helplessness, hopelessness, worthlessness or uselessness, meaninglessness<br>Regression<br>Loneliness<br>Withdrawal and focusing on past mistakes, failures, and dissatisfactions<br>Contempt for self and others<br>Sense of being too old to start over<br>Suicidal ideas or apathy<br>Fear of focusing on death<br>Inability to occupy self with satisfying activities (hobbies, volunteer work, social events)<br>*or*<br>Inability to reduce activities appropriately<br>Overtaxing strength and abilities<br>Feeling indispensable<br>Denial of death as inevitable |

## Key concepts

Sullivan conceived of the personality as an energy system having a main goal of reducing tension. He identified three types of tension: the *tension of needs* (stemming from the physiochemical requirements of life), the *tension of anxiety* (stemming from interpersonal situations), and the *tension of need for sleep.* Theoretically, a person could vary from a state of complete lack of tension (euphoria) to a state of terror as a result of extreme tension, but Sullivan doubted that the pure extremes existed very long after birth. The relaxation of the tension of needs is experienced as *satisfaction,* and the relaxation of the tension of anxiety is experienced as *interpersonal security* (Sullivan, 1953).

**Self-system.** Sullivan labeled the personality a "self-system" that develops relatively enduring patterns (dynamisms) for avoiding or minimizing anxiety during interpersonal encounters and the meeting of biologic needs. He believed that anxiety could be communicated empathetically from one person to another. Anxiety activates behaviors that reduce it and helps the individual differentiate among experiences (a process of learning). Severe anxiety (or panic) does not convey information and produces confusion, even to the point of amnesia (Sullivan, 1953). Less severe anxiety informs the individual of the different situations that cause and relieve tension. As the self-system is developing in infancy, it is initially organized into the "good me" when needs are satisfied, the "bad me" when needs are unmet and anxiety persists, and "not me" when anxiety is severe and information is not completely integrated into the personality on a conscious level. These three personifications of self develop in response to the caregiver's behavior and level of anxiety. If the caregiver is calm, tender, and satisfies the infant's needs, he or she is perceived as a "good" person, and the infant experiences "good me." If the caregiver is anxious and does not satisfy the infant's needs, he or she is perceived as a "bad" person, and the infant experiences "bad me." If the caregiver is anxious and uncaring, the anxiety communicated to the infant may be severe enough for the infant to have a "not me" experience. As the infant moves to early childhood and develops language, the separate personifications of the caregiver and the self as good and bad begin to fuse into a sense of a whole individual with different behaviors in different situations. However, feedback from others (reflected appraisals) continues to shape the child's view of himself (self-concept) in positive and negative ways.

**Modes of experiencing.** Sullivan identified ways individuals learn about others, relationship, and the world: the prototaxic, parataxic, and syntaxic modes of experiencing (Sullivan, 1953). The *prototaxic mode* is the infant's first type of experiencing and involves feelings, bodily sensations, and images, all of which last only a short while. These are "now" experiences, which are not connected to each other or to past experiences. In the *parataxic mode* of experiencing, events that occur nearly simultaneously are perceived with a cause-and-effect relationship. For example, a child who sneezed just before his mother dropped a dish would believe his sneeze caused the dish to drop. With age and the development of language, the child moves into the *syntaxic mode* of experiencing in which experiences are logically connected and differentiated into past, present, and predictions of the future. Meaningful relationships are possible as this mode develops.

In mental illness the syntaxic mode of experiencing may be lost as the patient regresses to the parataxic mode. The patient commonly distorts the actual characteristics of a current person and sees instead characteristics of persons from his past. This is called parataxic distortion. A remembered experience may become related causally to a current event as well. In severe psychosis the patient may regress to the prototaxic mode of experiencing with a fragmented perception of reality and flight of ideas. Discussion of cause and effect or problem solving is impossible.

Since the infant is unable to avoid the "bad" caregiver or the anxiety-producing situations, mechanisms called security operations develop for protection against the anxiety. In *somnolent detachment*, one goes to sleep to avoid the anxiety. *Apathy is an emotional detachment or numbing, even though the experiences are remem-*bered. *Selective inattention* is a process of tuning out or not noticing details associated with anxiety-producing situations. *Dissociation* prevents situations from being integrated into conscious awareness. Another operation to reduce anxiety is to convert it to anger. The powerlessness experienced with anxiety is exchanged from a temporary feeling of power associated with anger directed outwardly. While these security operations protect against anxiety, they also interfere with the learning that normally occurs in interpersonal interactions (the socialization processes). *Focal awareness* or the ability to grasp the details and meanings of situations and the behaviors of others is necessary for adequate learning. Also necessary for learning is *consensual validation,* a process of verifying the accuracy of perceptions and meanings of events with others involved in those situations.

**Personality development.** Sullivan's model included a sequence of personality development focusing on tools or behaviors needed to accomplish developmental tasks. In infancy (birth to 1½ years), for example, crying is a tool used to establish contact with others so that one can learn to count on others. In childhood (1½ to 6 years), language assists with learning to delay the gratification of needs. In the juvenile period, competition, compromise, and cooperation are tools for developing relationships with peers. In preadolescence (9 to 12 years), collaboration and the capacity for love assist in the development of a chum relationship with a person of the same sex. These same tools, plus sexual desire, facilitate learning to establish relationships with members of the opposite sex in early adolescence (ages 12 to 14). The independence developed in early adolescence moves toward interdependence in late adolescence (ages 14 to 21), and the individual learns to form a lasting sexual relationship (Sullivan, 1953). Sullivan's development model did not describe changes beyond late adolescence.

## Therapist's role

For Sullivan, the focus of therapy was on the patient's current interpersonal relationships and experiences with the goal of developing maturity and satisfactory relationships relatively free from anxiety. The therapist-patient relationship is a vehicle for analyzing the patient's interpersonal processes and testing out new skills in relating. The therapist takes an active role as a "participant observer" in experiencing the patient's interpersonal problems. Although the focus of therapy is on the patient's here-and-now problems, distortions created by past experiences, especially "not me" experiences, are often revealed. The therapist helps correct these distortions with clear communications, consensual validation, and presentation of reality. In challenge to a patient's negative self-image, the therapist presents appraisals of the patient as a worthwhile, respectable person with rights, dignity, and valuable abilities. The focus of sessions is often on loneliness, fear of rejection, clarifying emotions and their causes, use of anxiety for learning about self and others, management of interpersonal frustrations, and development of self-respect.

### Relevance to nursing practice

Hildegard Peplau played a significant role in applying Sullivan's concepts to nursing practice. Peplau saw a major goal of nursing as helping patients reduce their anxiety and convert it to constructive action. She elaborated on and applied to nursing Sullivan's concept of degrees of anxiety ("pure" euphoria, mild anxiety, moderate anxiety, severe anxiety, panic, terror states, and "pure" anxiety) (Peplau, 1963). She described the effect of mild anxiety through panic levels on perception and learning. (See Chapter 18, "Anxiety-Related Disorders," for descriptions.) She saw the nurse as helping a patient decrease his insecurity and improve his functioning through an interpersonal relationship that was like a microcosm of the way the patient functioned in other relationships. Some applications of Sullivan's work as proposed by Peplau are presented in Chapter 6.

## RATIONAL-EMOTIVE THERAPY MODEL

Albert Ellis's rational-emotive therapy (RET) model focuses on thinking and behaving rather than on the expression of feelings. It uses a cognitive approach based on an individual's ability to think, judge, decide, analyze, and do. Unlike Freud, who saw symptoms of disturbance as having been produced by past childhood experiences, Ellis views the individual's present meanings, attitudes, and philosophies as needing modification or change. "Whatever his parents' behavior may have been, he no longer has to take them seriously, to agree with their criticisms of him, and to keep castigating himself" (Ellis, 1973). An individual should value himself simply because he exists and should not judge himself by how he performs or is rated by himself and others.

### Key concepts

Ellis believes that individuals think both rationally and irrationally and that the *irrational beliefs* or thoughts are what get people into trouble because they maintain self-defeating behaviors. He also believes individuals are capable of understanding their limitations and can change their values and beliefs while challenging their self-defeating behaviors. Emotional disturbances are produced by the repetition of irrational thoughts that keep dysfunctional behaviors operant. Blaming ourselves and others and thinking and feeling that something is "bad" maintain emotional disturbance. RET teaches individuals to stop blaming themselves and to accept themselves as they are with flaws and imperfections. Anxiety can be avoided by learning to change inappropriate emotions and self-defeating behaviors. RET attacks an individual's problem from a cognitive, emotive, and behavioral standpoint by using the A-B-C theory of personality. A is the *activating event*; B is the *belief about A;* and C is the *emotional reaction.* A (event) does not cause C (emotions); rather B (our irrational beliefs about A), causes C. Intervention then is aimed at B, our irrational beliefs, and is called D or disputing and changing irrational beliefs (Ellis, 1973).

According to Ellis (1973), the following are some irrational beliefs that all individuals subscribe to:

- The need to feel loved and approved by everyone
- The need to be totally competent in order to be considered worthwhile
- The sense that we have little ability to change or control our feelings
- The influence of our past should definitely determine our feelings now
- Viewing things as catastrophic when we are rejected or treated unfairly
- Thinking people who are obnoxious should be blamed as being rotten or bad
- It is easier to be passive in life than to face up to difficulties and responsibilities
- Life is awful if we do not solve problems with the right or precise solution

## Therapists' role

Because patients have many irrational "shoulds," "oughts," and "musts," the therapist challenges these beliefs actively and directly. He educates patients about changing irrational beliefs to rational ones by demonstrating how illogical their thinking is. He uses humor to confront the patient's irrational thinking and explains how to replace it with rational thinking to reduce dysfunctional feelings and behaviors. The process of therapy focuses on and emphasizes the present. Patients learn to take responsibility for their ideas and behaviors and work to eliminate disturbing behaviors.

The therapist accepts the patient as he is and does not allow the patient to rate or condemn himself. Homework assignments are given to focus on positive statements and behaviors. Books on RET are assigned as part of the educational process. New positive self-statements are encouraged to enable the patient to begin to think, feel, and behave differently. Role playing and modeling are also employed.

## Relevance to nursing practice

Nurses help patients to change irrational beliefs and reduce stress and anxiety. Patients have many self-deprecating or negative feelings about themselves that the nurse can dispute by pointing out specific positive qualities. Awareness of these qualities or aspects can facilitate a patient's belief that he is worthwhile and has valuable characteristics. Self-blame and guilt can be reduced and patients can feel better about themselves. Patients who project blame can be shown that they alone are responsible for their behaviors. For example, the alcoholic is very skillful at blaming others for his problems when, in fact, he alone is responsible for continuing to drink and for the problems encountered as a result of his drinking.

Other patients who continually function according to "shoulds," "musts," and "oughts," can be taught to be more self-centered in doing what they as individuals want and believe in. They need not condemn themselves for being their own persons. Their anxiety and hostile feelings toward themselves and others can be eliminated if they can achieve a feeling of comfort about themselves.

## REALITY THERAPY MODEL

William Glasser developed reality therapy because he believed all patients and delinquents shared the common characteristic of denying "the reality of the world around them" instead of fulfilling their needs responsibly within the context of reality.

He defined responsibility as "the ability to fulfill one's needs, and to do so in a way that does not deprive others of the ability to fulfill their needs" (Glasser, 1965, p. xv). Glasser recognized that he could not change a patient's history or past relationship problems but that he could help him change his current behaviors so his future could improve. He found that improved responsibility led to improved mental health.

## Key concepts

According to Glasser, all individuals continually strive to meet their needs. The two major psychological needs are to love and be loved (to have relatedness) and to feel worthwhile (to have respect from self and others). Implied in these needs are the need for identity and involvement. A child develops a positive identity by being involved with others who teach rights, wrongs, and responsibility while conveying to the child that he is worthwhile. The child then learns to be comfortable with and enjoy being around others.

Unfortunately, individuals do not always strive to meet their needs responsibly. There may be an "incapacity or failure at the interpersonal level of functioning" (Glasser, 1965). Glasser believed that illness resulted from behaving irresponsibly rather than the reverse; anger, fear, depression, and anxiety are also the result of irresponsible behavior in relationships. Common forms of irresponsible behavior are violations of one's morals, values, or standards; misinforming others about one's self or needs (being dishonest); shunning others because of fear of rejection; lying to oneself by rationalizing and excusing one's own behavior; not accepting the consequences of one's behavior; blaming others for problems; and, eventually, losing contact with reality (by denying it). Suicide and denial are major ways of avoiding reality and responsibility. Short-term pleasures such as those derived from alcohol and drugs also interfere with long-term satisfaction and happiness.

## Therapist's role

The goal of reality therapy is to help patients face reality and then to develop responsible behavior patterns so that their needs for love and worth can be met. Directing patients "toward greater maturity, conscientiousness, and responsibility" improves the patients' potential for long-term happiness and pleasure (Glasser, 1965). Glasser emphasized the need for the therapist to be authentic, open, honest, responsible, and deeply involved with patients. Initially the patient needs warmth and uncritical acceptance as a worthwhile person who is cared about even though his irresponsible behaviors and excuses for those behaviors are not accepted. The unrealistic and irresponsible behaviors are actively confronted, even disciplined, while the patient as a person and his positive behaviors are supported. The patient repeatedly evaluates whether what he is doing is getting him what he wants and whether others are hurt in the process. The patient is asked to choose more effective behaviors and to design specific, realistic plans for trying them out. Plans that are not successful are revised until accountability and responsibility are achieved.

## Relevance to nursing practice

Psychiatric nurses are regularly involved in helping patients identify reality and what interferes with the effective meeting of their needs. Reality testing is a common nursing intervention. Nurses are routinely responsible for explaining the rules of the unit and for outlining the expected or appropriate and inappropriate behaviors. The milieu of the unit is normally designed to foster improvements in independence and responsibility, which are rewarded with increases in privileges and freedom. Setting limits on unacceptable (irresponsible) behaviors benefits the patient in the long run.

Even without labeling behaviors as irresponsible, nurses are accustomed to helping patients examine the consequences of specific behaviors, especially in current relationships. Supportive confrontation encourages patients to make their own decisions about changes, choose their own solutions, and test out new behaviors. This type of relearning process is described in Chapter 6 on the nurse-patient relationhsip.

## STRESS MODELS

Stress theories provide nurses with a framework for understanding how stress affects individuals and their responses. The ability to deal or cope with stress adaptively leads to problem solving or conflict resolution, whereas the inability to cope effectively or adaptively may result in physiologic or mental disorders and even death.

### Key concepts

**Selye's stress-adaptation theory.** Selye defined stress as the wear and tear on the body. He developed a framework, *stress-adaptation theory,* to explain what occurs physiologically to a person who is responding to stress. Selye viewed a stressor as any positive or negative occurrence or emotion requiring a response. Inevitably, man's interaction with the environment produces stress. The type of response elicited depends on the individual's perception of the stressor. However, Selye discovered that by objectively measuring structural and chemical changes in the body, many persons demonstrated the same symptoms regardless of stressor. These changes became known as the general adaptation syndrome (GAS), and they occurred in three stages: alarm, resistance, and exhaustion. Selye did not elaborate on the psychosocial changes, but his three stages can be correlated with the levels of anxiety. The three stages of GAS are summarized in Table 2-4.

In this text the psychosocial changes will be emphasized since sleep and weight disturbances are primarily the only physical changes that nurses can assess and evaluate.

*Alarm reaction.* The impingement of any kind of stressor on the individual activates the "fight or flight" mechanism. The individual experiences an increase in alertness to focus on the immediate task or threat and mobilizes his resources and defenses to concentrate his energies on the particular stressor. The levels of anxiety experienced are mild (1+) to moderate (2+). Learning and problem solving can occur. If the stressor continues or is not adaptively or effectively resolved, the individual experiences the next stage.

**TABLE 2-4**  The stress adaptation syndrome

| Stage | Physical change | Psychosocial changes |
|---|---|---|
| **STAGE I:** Alarm reaction<br>Mobilization of the body's defensive forces and activation of the "fight-or-flight" mechanism | Release of norepinephrine and epinephrine causing vaso-constriction, increased blood pressure, and increased rate and force of cardiac contraction<br>Increased hormone levels<br>Enlargement of adrenal cortex<br>Marked loss of body weight<br>Shrinkage of the thymus, spleen, and lymph nodes<br>Irritation of the gastric mucosa | Increased level of alertness<br>Increased level of anxiety<br>Task-oriented, defense-oriented, inefficient, or maladaptive behavior may occur |
| **STAGE II:** Stage of resistance<br>Optimal adaptation to stress within the person's capabilities | Hormone levels readjust<br>Reduction in activity and size of adrenal cortex<br>Lymph nodes return to normal size<br>Weight returns to normal | Increased and intensified use of coping mechanisms<br>Tendency to rely on defense-oriented behavior |
| **STAGE III:** Stage of exhaustion<br>Loss of ability to resist stress because of depletion of body resources | Decreased immune response with suppression of T cells and atrophy of thymus<br>Depletion of adrenal glands and hormone production<br>Weight loss<br>Englargement of lymph nodes and dysfunction of lymphatic system<br>If exposure to the stressor continues, cardiac failure, renal failure, or death may occur | Defense-oriented behaviors become exaggerated<br>Disorganization of thinking<br>Disorganization of personality<br>Sensory stimuli may be misperceived with appearance of illusion<br>Reality contact may be reduced with appearance of delusions or hallucinations<br>If exposure to the stressor continues, stupor or violence may occur |

From Kneisl CR and Ames SW. Adult health nursing: a biopsychosocial approach, Menlo Park, Calif., 1986, Addison-Wesley.

*Stage of resistance.*   In this stage the individual strives to adapt to stress. For adaptation to occur, use of coping and defense mechanisms is increased. Problem solving and learning are difficult but can be accomplished with assistance. Psychosomatic symptoms begin to develop. The levels of anxiety experienced are moderate (2+) to severe (3+). If the individual is overwhelmed by the stressor, he experiences the next stage.

*Stage of exhaustion.* Stress that lasts too long, overwhelming stress, or the total inability to cope results in exhaustion. Anxiety is experienced at the severe (3 + ) to panic (4 + ) level. The individual's defenses are exaggerated and dysfunctional. His personality becomes disorganized, his thinking illogical, and his decision making ineffective. Delusions and hallucinations can occur with sensory misperception and a greatly reduced orientation to reality. The individual may become violent or suicidal or may even be completely immobilized. With immobilizaton, he can experience a severe level of anxiety but not appear to be visibly anxious. Death can occur if exhaustion continues without intervention.

**Lazarus's interactional theory.** In contrast to Selye's emphasis on the physiologic effects of stress, Lazarus focuses on the psychological aspects. He viewed psychological stress as "a relationship between the person and the environment that is appraised by the person as taxing or exceeding his or her resources and endangering his or her well-being" (Lazarus and Folkman, 1984). Lazarus believes that the basis of an individual's coping is not due to anxiety per se but to the appraisal of threat. "Anxiety is the response to threat" (Lazarus, 1966). The significance of the threat or what it means to the individual is of primary importance. Stressors are perceived differently by different individuals. For one person an event may be viewed as a challenge, but for another it may be a severe threat or problem. This personal evaluation of a stressor or event is based on cognitive appraisal. "Through cognitive appraisal processes the person evaluates the significance of what is happening for his or her well-being" (Lazarus and Folkman, 1984).

There are three kinds of cognitive appraisal: primary, secondary, and reappraisal. *Primary appraisal* refers to the judgment an individual makes about an event. What does it mean to him? How does it affect him? With *secondary appraisal* the individual evaluates what he can do about it. He looks at possible strategies or solutions for his use as well as resources and supports. *Reappraisal* is simply appraisal made after new or additional information has been received.

Numerous personal and environmental factors influence appraisal. Commitments and beliefs are particularly relevant in secondary appraisal. An individual's views of what he holds to be important and meaningful along with what he is working toward or striving for influence his appraisal of a stressor. Personal feelings and emotions give clues about values and beliefs. A seemingly appropriate solution may not be useful because it conflicts with an individual's values and beliefs. For example, a passive wife may be unable to be assertive and confrontative with her husband because she was taught and believes that women should be quiet and submissive to their husbands. She also would not be able to bear her husband's wrath and anger.

Stressful events often create demands with which the individual cannot effectively cope. Sometimes personal resources or social supports are not adequate. Even if supports and resources are available, values, beliefs, and norms may prohibit their use. For example, a man may want to assertively state his views to his employer but feels that he cannot since his employer is his father-in-law and he fears his wife's reaction. At times a person may view a particular threat as negative because of past experiences or conflicts. Preferred methods of coping are sometimes used but are ineffective in resolving the problem and may actually lead to or result in more problems. Ineffective coping and the creation of additional problems will result in additional stress and lead to physical or mental illness or both.

### Relevance to nursing practice

Stress theories provide a framework for the nurse to assess the effects of stress on patients and their coping processes. To assist the patient with developing adaptive or effective coping methods, palliative, maladaptive, and dysfunctional behaviors must be identified and processed with the nurse so that the patient is aware of the consequence of his behavior. Palliative mechanisms decrease the emotions without solving the problems. Maladaptive mechanisms do not manage the emotions sufficiently and do not solve the problems. Dysfunctional mechanisms create new or additional problems. (For additional explanation, see Chapter 18.)

A patient's appraisal of his stressors or problems will include what the stressors mean to him, what resources or supports he has to help him cope, and how his beliefs and values influence his coping. In considering what the stressor means to the patient, the nurse can facilitate cognitive restructuring or problem solving by helping the patient to choose adaptive and appropriate coping behaviors. At times the nurse will need to help initiate, encourage, and motivate the patient to use adaptive behaviors. The patient and the nurse can then evaluate the effectiveness of strategies used. When the patient is exhibiting behaviors found in Selye's stage of exhaustion or is primarily using dysfunctional coping, the nurse is able to assess the patient's inability to take constructive action and the necessity for making decisions on behalf of the patient. After the patient gains some control over his behavior, he can benefit from stress management, problem solving, relaxation training, and biofeedback, depending on which method is needed.

### PSYCHIATRIC CLASSIFICATION SYSTEM MODEL

The American Psychiatric Association's *Diagnostic and Statistical Manual of Mental Disorders, Third Edition Revised* (DSM-III-R), is an official classification of mental disorders and health problems. The individual is evaluated on five axes:

- Axis I       Clinical syndromes and V codes (conditions not attributable to a mental disorder that are a focus of attention or treatment)
- Axis II      Personality and developmental disorders
- Axis III     Physical disorders and conditions
- Axis IV      Severity of psychosocial stressors
- Axis V       Global assessment of functioning

Axes I and II include all the psychiatric diagnoses. Sometimes predominant personality traits are listed on axis II when a full personality disorder is not evident. It is possible to have multiple diagnoses on axes I and II. Each diagnosis is assigned its own code number (see Appendix A). Axis III includes present physical conditions that relate to axes I and II diagnoses or have a bearing on treatment.

Axis IV assigns code numbers to reflect the severity of acute or enduring psychosocial stressors. The codes range from 1, meaning none, to 6, meaning catastrophic (see Appendix A).

Axis V, the global measurement of functioning scale, considers psychological, social, and occupational functioning. The code ranges from 90, meaning absent or minimal symptoms, to 1, indicating persistent inability to function (see Appendix A).

The physician or psychiatrist is responsible for assigning the diagnoses and prescribing appropriate medications for conditions on Axes I, II, and III. The behaviors related to those diagnoses require nursing interventions. Axis IV identifies present stressors or problems that may or may not be related to the other diagnoses but are of a concern to the patient. Axis V assesses illness-related behaviors and symptoms often needing immediate nursing intervention. The data found on all five axes contribute to the holistic assessment of patients and provide a foundation for nursing interventions.

## KEY CONCEPTS

1. Concepts from various theoretical models provide frameworks for understanding patient behaviors and problems.
2. Extensive use of defense mechanisms and maladaptive coping behaviors are assessed and understood by the nurse as inhibiting healthy or adaptive responses. The nurse then helps the patient develop adaptive coping responses or behaviors.
3. Unresolved developmental issues interfere with the patient's ability to solve problems and meet his own needs. Therefore they must be addressed in the nurse-patient relationship.
4. Peplau used Sullivan's concepts of anxiety as a critical part of her framework in the nurse-patient relationship.
5. Stress and anxiety can be reduced by changing and replacing irrational beliefs with rational ones.
6. Facing reality and responsibility for self are major goals of reality therapy.
7. Stress models explain many of the physiological and psychological manifestations.
8. Although Axes I through III are diagnosed by the physician, all axes provide information useful for nursing interventions.

## REFERENCES

Brill AA, editor: The basic writings of Sigmund Freud, New York, 1938, Random House.

Ellis A: Humanistic psychotherapy: the rational-emotive approach, New York, 1973, The Julian Press.

Erikson EH: Childhood and society, New York, 1963, W. W. Norton & Co.

Erikson EH: Identity: youth and crisis, New York, 1968, W. W. Norton & Co.

Field WE, editor: The psychotherapy of Hildegard E. Peplau, New Braunfels, Texas, 1979, PSF Productions.

Freud S and Strachey J, editors: The ego and the id, New York, 1960, W. W. Norton & Co.

Freud S: The problem of anxiety, New York, 1936, W. W. Norton & Co.

Glasser W: Reality therapy: a new approach to psychiatry, New York, 1965, Harper & Row.

Kneisl CR and Ames SW: Adult health nursing: a biopsychosocial approach, Menlo Park, Calif., 1986, Addison-Wesley.

Lazarus RS: Psychological stress and the coping process, St. Louis, 1966, McGraw-Hill Book Co.

Lazarus RS and Folkman S: Stress, appraisal, and coping, New York, 1984, Springer Publishing Co.

Lego S: The one-to-one nurse-patient relationship, Perspect Psychiatr Care 18(2):67, 1980.

Peplau HE: Interpersonal relations in nursing, New York, 1952, G.P. Putnam's Sons.

Peplau HE: Talking with patients. Am J Nurs 60:964, 1960.

Peplau HE: A working definition of anxiety. In Burd SF and Marshall MA, editors: Some clinical approaches to psychiatric nursing. Toronto, 1963, The Macmillan Co.

Selye H: The stress of life, St. Louis, 1956, McGraw-Hill Book Co.

Sullivan HS: Interpersonal theory of psychiatry, New York, 1953, W. W. Norton & Co.

Thompson L: Peplau's theory: an application to short-term therapy. J Psychosoc Nurs 24(8):26, 1986.

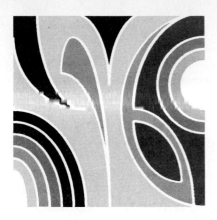

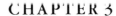

## CHAPTER 3

# Psychotherapeutic Management

LEARNING OBJECTIVES

After reading this chapter you should be able to

- Describe the components of psychotherapeutic management.
- Articulate why these components are of equal importance therapeutically.

## PSYCHOTHERAPEUTIC MANAGEMENT

In 1979 Koldjeski wrote: "Psychiatric nurses must clearly demonstrate the exact nature of their practice and must differentiate their practice from the practice of other nonmedical mental health personnel." Following Koldjeski's prescription, psychotherapeutic management was proposed as a model to clarify and distinguish the role of the psychiatric nurse (Keltner, 1985). Of the five basic categories into which psychiatric treatment can be divided—words (which encompass all forms of psychotherapy), drugs, environment, somatic therapies, and behavioral conditioning—psychotherapeutic management emphasizes three: psychotherapeutic nurse-patient relationship (words), psychopharmacology (drugs), and milieu management (environment), all of which must be supported by a sound understanding of psychopathology (Fig. 3-1). For example, a person with schizophrenia in an inpatient setting profits most when a therapeutic nurse-patient relationship, psychopharmacology, and a well-managed milieu are available. When one component is missing from the equation, the patient's treatment is compromised. Ordinarily, when psychotropic drugs are subtracted from this equation, the patient will decompensate. Likewise, if drugs and therapeutic communication are available (perhaps from only a few motivated staff members) but the overall environment is poorly managed, the patient

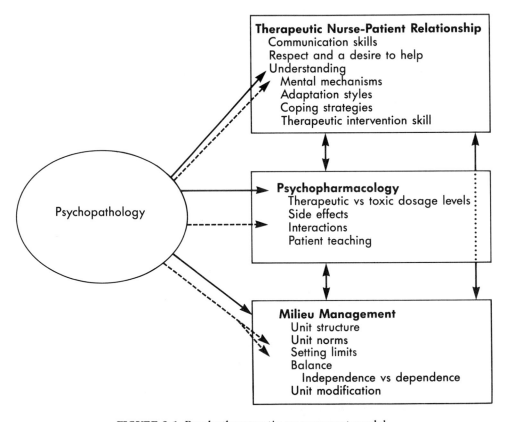

**FIGURE 3-1** Psychotherapeutic management model.

is left to fend for himself, thus draining him of internal resources needed for healing. When an inpatient receives only drug therapy but is denied therapeutic interaction opportunities in a well-managed milieu, we return to the inadequacies of custodial care. In other words, all the components of the psychotherapeutic management equation must be present if the patient is to fully realize the benefits of effective nursing intervention. Psychotherapeutic management endeavors to bring balance to practice and, with balance, role clarification, thus providing a valuable approach to both inpatient and outpatient settings. Each individual interaction finds greater meaning within the broader construct of psychotherapeutic management.

Psychotherapeutic management owes a conceptual debt to Mellow's (1967) experiential-action model and follows the recommendations of a 1974 psychiatric nursing conference (Pearlmutter, 1985).

*THE THERAPEUTIC NURSE-PATIENT RELATIONSHIP* Part of the "knowing," in the Koldjeskian sense, is the ability to differentiate therapy from being therapeutic. We propose that the art of therapy is the domain of graduate-level psychiatric nurses and that the art of being therapeutic is the domain of undergraduate-level psychiatric nurses.

Role confusion begins with unrealistic expectations for the nurse-patient relationship. If, as this model suggests, the nurse-patient relationship is but one of three important components, then it follows that it is not necessarily the most important. At times it may be the most important, but at other times it is not. When it is overemphasized, a distortion in psychiatric nursing practice can develop, for example, the psychiatric nurse who eschews psychotropic drugs. Unit II, "Therapeutic Nurse-Patient Relationship," is devoted to this first dimension of psychotherapeutic management. The different emphases placed on words and the wide range of styles within the domain of words are discussed, specifically communication (Chapter 5), the nature of the nurse-patient relationship (Chapter 6), the aggressive patient (Chapter 7), group interaction (Chapter 8), and consultation-liaison nursing (Chapter 9).

*PSYCHOPHARMACOLOGY* Unit III, "Psychopharmacology," is devoted to communicating the contribution of psychotropic drugs to psychiatric nursing, the responsibilities of the nurse, and essential information about these drugs. Psychopharmacology is an important dimension in psychotherapeutic management, as psychotropic drugs have enabled millions of persons to live more fulfilling lives, although clearly drugs are not always indicated. In the inpatient setting that provides 24-hour care the nurse is in an advantageous position to assess side effects, to evaluate desired effects, and generally to intervene before serious drug-related problems occur. In addition, the nurse dispenses medications and makes decisions regarding p.r.n. medications. Thus it is incumbent upon the nurse to be knowledgeable about psychopharmacology.

*MILIEU MANAGEMENT* Unit IV, "Milieu Management," recognizes the impact on patients of their surroundings and deals with the five environmental elements nurses must consider in creating a therapeutic milieu: structure, norms, limit setting, balance, and unit modification. "The interpersonal environment in which a patient lives may be therapeutic or nontherapeutic depending almost entirely on the interest and ability of the [nursing] staff" (Kyes and Hofling, 1974). Human beings are incapable of not interacting with their environment. Nurses are the primary molders of psychiatric patients' treatment environment. Nurses are the consistent force in the milieu. In managing the milieu, nurses serve multiple roles: they work with patients individually, lead groups, participate in community meetings, coordinate medical care (with physicians), make discharge arrangements, and work with families. In addition, nurses provide leadership in interdisciplinary team meetings and are the professionals who most often implement team decisions (Keltner, 1985). Talbot and Miller (1966) state: "An ideal psychiatric hospital is not merely a sanctuary, a cotton-padded milieu that emphasizes the fragility, the incompetence, the helplessness, the bizarreness of patients. It is a sane society when it permits the optimal use of the intact ego capacities through its social organization, its social supports, and its community values." Nursing's strength lies in its ability to shape the environment and its availability to intervene when crises occur.

## PSYCHOPATHOLOGY

Unit V, "Psychopathology," provides the foundation on which the three components of psychotherapeutic management rest. It facilitates therapeutic communication in the nurse-patient relationship and lays the groundwork for an understanding of psychopharmacology and milieu management. Schizophrenia and other psychoses, mood and anxiety-related disorders, organic mental disorders, personality disorders, drug and alcohol abuse, and eating disorders are dealt with in the various chapters.

## SPECIAL THERAPIES

Unit VI, "Special Therapies in Psychiatric Nursing," includes a chapter on behavior therapy and one on somatic therapy. Behavior therapy includes all forms of behavior conditioning, such as desensitization and reciprocal inhibition. Somatic therapies include electroconvulsive therapy and psychosurgery. Somatic and behavioral therapies are important dimensions of psychiatric care but do not have the universal clinical applications of the other categories of psychiatric treatment and thus are not emphasized in this text.

## SPECIAL POPULATIONS

Unit VII, "Special Populations in Psychiatric Nursing," contains chapters dealing with the victims of violence, mental health issues in children, and the elderly.

## KEY CONCEPTS

1. Psychotherapeutic management is a model of care that clarifies the nature of psychiatric nursing and differentiates psychiatric nursing practice from the practice of other disciplines.
2. The components of psychotherapeutic management include a therapeutic nurse-patient relationship, psychopharmacology, and milieu management supported by a basic understanding of psychopathology.

3. The *therapeutic nurse-patient relationship* emphasizes the importance of the nurse's understanding of basic principles of therapeutic communication.
4. Being therapeutic is different than providing therapy in that therapeutic inter-actions should occur during usual patient contact while therapy indicates a more formal and structured interaction.
5. *Psychopharmacologic* understanding is important to the nurse because nurses administer medication, make decisions about p.r.n. medication, and evaluate for therapeutic and adverse responses to medication.
6. Because man is incapable of not interacting with his environment, *milieu management* is an important nursing consideration. Nurses are uniquely responsible for developing the patient's environment.
7. The milieu is composed of five environmental elements: unit structure, unit norms, limit setting, balance, and unit modification.
8. An understanding of *psychopathology* facilitates the nurse-patient relationship, lays the groundwork for understanding psychopharmacology, and provides a theoretical structure for milieu management.

## REFERENCES

Keltner NL: Psychotherapeutic management: a model for nursing practice, Perspect Psychiatr Care 23:125, 1985.

Koldjeski D: Mental health and psychiatric nursing and primary health care: issues and prospects. Proceedings of the Fourth National Conference in Graduate Education in Psychiatric and Mental Health Nursing. Kansas City, Mo, 1979, American Nurses' Association.

Kyes J, Hofling C: Basic psychiatric concepts in nursing, ed 3, Philadelphia, 1974, J. B. Lippincott, p.455.

Mellow J: Evolution of nursing therapy through research. Psychiatr Opinion 4:15, 1967.

Pearlmutter DR: Recent trends and issues in psychiatric–mental health nursing. Hosp Community Psychiatry 36:56, 1985.

Talbot E, Miller SC: The struggle to create a sane society in the psychiatric hospital. Psychiatry 29:165, 1966.

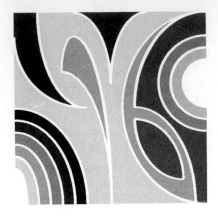

## CHAPTER 4

# Legal Issues

PATRICIA NORD AND DOROTHY DICK MEYER

LEARNING OBJECTIVES

After reading this chapter you should be able to

- Identify significant court decisions in psychiatric care.
- Distinguish the categories of commitment.
- Recognize the competing interests between individual rights and the state's interest in maintaining the health and safety of its citizens.
- Understand the legal, constitutional rights of patients.
- Describe the liability of the nurse in issues such as wrongful commitment and duty to warn.
- Define the terms that apply to the legal issues involved in health care.

The legal issues in the treatment of the mentally ill have evolved over the centuries and have paralleled the advances of legal jurisprudence in the industrialized countries. Societies through the ages and up to the present time have grappled with balancing the rights of the individual against the rights of society at large.

This chapter focuses on the laws that attempt to balance the basic rights of the individual against society's interest in being protected from persons who, because of mental disorder, present a threat of harm. The fundamental rights accorded each individual flow from various amendments to the Constitution of the United States and from the constitutions of individual states. Following are the specific rights from which the rights of mental patients are derived:

1. Freedom from unreasonable search and seizure
2. Right of privacy
3. Freedom of choice and self-determination (e.g., the right to accept or refuse medical treatment)

There are four major categories of legal issues in the treatment of the mentally ill person that are of importance to the psychiatric nurse:

1. Precedent-setting legal milestones in psychiatric care
2. Commitment issues
3. Patient rights
4. Nursing liability and related issues

Additionally, nursing implications will be presented throughout the chapter to help the student understand the significant nursing tasks associated with selected legal issues.

## PRECEDENT-SETTING LEGAL MILESTONES IN PSYCHIATRIC CARE

Before specific legal issues in psychiatric nursing are addressed, it is important to briefly review significant milestones in the evolution of legal thought. Society has not always been concerned with the individual rights of the mentally ill person. In fact, it can be argued that in no other area of nursing practice has the patient been so deprived of personal rights, freedom of choice, and dignity. The student is encouraged to review Chapter 1 to appreciate the impetus for the humane care and legal protection of mentally ill persons today. Since the evolution of psychiatric legal thought parallels the evolution of psychiatric treatment presented in Chapter 1, historical information presented there will not be repeated.

Many rulings have influenced our current legal view of mental illness. Those presented below, although they in no way form an exhaustive list of major court decisions, do reflect decisions that have shaped and formed our mental health system and are part of an ongoing process to accomplish the following legislative objectives:

- End inappropriate, indefinite, and involuntary commitment of mentally ill persons
- Provide prompt evaluation and treatment of mentally ill persons
- Guarantee and protect public safety

- Safeguard individual rights through judicial review
- Provide individualized treatment, supervision, and placement services by a conservatorship or guardianship program for gravely disabled persons
- Encourage the full use of all existing agencies, professional personnel, and public funds to accomplish these objectives and to prevent duplication of services and unnecessary expenditures

The following eight rulings have had a significant influence on our mental health treatment system:

1. The *M'Naghten rule (1843)* states that a man who does not understand the nature and implications of his criminal actions because of insanity cannot be held legally accountable for those actions. This ruling was based on the case of Daniel M'Naghten, a Scotsman who felt persecuted by the ruling political party and attempted to kill the prime minister. Although he failed to kill the prime minister, he did shoot the prime minister's secretary. He was ruled *not guilty by reason of insanity* and was committed to an asylum. This case has provided a basis for legal decisions in American courts since 1851.

2. *Rouse v Cameron 373 F2d 451 (DC Cir 1966)* was a case in which a man who pleaded not guilty by reason of insanity to the charge of illegally carrying a dangerous weapon was committed to a mental institution. After 4 years he argued that he was not receiving treatment (and therefore could not improve enough to be considered discharged). The court ruled that he had the *right to treatment*.

3. *Griswold v Connecticut (1965) 381 U.S. 479* was the case in which the United States Supreme Court first recognized that a *right of personal privacy* exists under the Constitution of the United States. This case involved the issue of whether the state of Connecticut had the right to prohibit the giving of birth control information to married couples. A majority of the Court held that the Ninth Amendment supports the creation of "peripheral rights" not expressly mentioned in the Bill of Rights including the right of privacy. Subsequent cases dealing with various aspects of treatment for mental disorders utilized this ruling.

4. *Wyatt v Stickney 344 F Supp 373 (MD Ala 1972)* was another case involving *right to treatment*. In this case the entire mental health system of Alabama was sued for an inadequate treatment program. The court ruled that the Alabama mental health system must do the following at each institution:

- Stop the use of patients for hospital labor needs
- Ensure a humane environment
- Develop and maintain minimum staffing standards
- Establish institutional human rights committees
- Provide the least restrictive environment for each patient

5. *Rogers v Okin 478 F Supp (D Mass 1979)* was a case in which patients at Boston State Hospital sought the *right to refuse treatment*. The hospital forced nonviolent patients to take medications against their will. The court

based its decision on the constitutional right to privacy. Furthermore, this decision required patients or their guardians to give informed consent be-fore drug treatment could begin. This case has significant implications for nurses who are tempted to "force" patients to take medications for "their own good."

6. *Rennie v Klein (3d Cir 1983) 720 F2d 266* was a case in which a man claimed his rights were violated by the hospital when he was forced to take psychotropic medications. He won the *right to refuse treatment*. The ruling contained several significant statements concerning patient rights. The essence of these statements is the legal obligation of mental health professionals to obtain informed consent before administering psychotropic medications.

7. *Meier v Ross General Hospital (1968) 69 Cal 2nd 420* was a case that established the *duty to warn of threatened suicide*. A physician was found liable for the death of his patient who committed suicide by jumping headfirst through an open window of his room. Prior to admission the patient had attempted suicide by slashing his wrists. The physician was deemed liable for not protecting the patient from his own actions.

8. *Tarasoff v The Regents of the University of California (1976), 17 Cal 3d 425* expanded the liability of a mental health professional even further. The court established a *duty to warn of threats of harm to others*. In this case a patient confided to the therapist that he intended to kill an unnamed, but readily identifiable girl when she returned from spending the summer in Brazil. The therapist notified campus police and requested their assistance in confining the man. The officers took the patient into custody but released him because he appeared rational. Shortly after her return from Brazil, Tatiana Tarasoff was killed by the man, Prosenjit Poddar. Her parents successfully sued the University of California claiming that the therapist had a duty to warn their daughter of Poddar's threats.

## COMMITMENT ISSUES

All states have commitment procedures for the treatment of persons suffering from a diagnosable mental disorder. There are basically three types of commitments for psychiatric care: voluntary, involuntary, and the commitment of incapacitated persons. (See Box 4-1 for the definition of key terms.)

### Voluntary commitment

By far, most persons with a mental health problem seek help voluntarily. Although specific procedures may vary from hospital to hospital, basically the person or his therapist requests admission and signs the appropriate documents. When the person is ready to leave the treatment setting, he signs himself out. Most states have a grace period that allows the professional staff the time and opportunity to assess the patient before he leaves voluntarily. Rather frequently a voluntary patient wanting to sign himself out of the hospital is placed on an involuntary commitment status because the staff's assessment indicates a need for further treatment.

**Box 4-1**
## KEY TERMS

**Assault** an offer or threat to touch another without consent.

**Battery** a touching of the person of another, of his clothes, or anything else attached to his person without consent.

**Civil law** this part of the legal system is concerned with the legal rights and duties of private persons. Civil lawsuits can recapture monetary loss from professionals who have been guilty of false imprisonment, defamation of character, assault and battery, or negligence.

**Conservator or guardian** a legally appointed person who controls the affairs of a gravely disabled person, including the right to consent or refuse psychiatric treatment.

**Gravely disabled** a person who is unable to provide food, clothing, or shelter for himself because of a mental illness.

**Informed consent** providing the patient with information about a specific treatment including its benefits, side effects, and possible risks that will enable him to make a competent and voluntary decision.

**Involuntary commitment** a commitment status in which a person who has the legal capacity to consent to mental health treatment refuses to do so and is involuntarily detained for treatment by the state. Three categories of involuntary commitment are: evaluation and emergency care, certification for observation and treatment, and extended or indeterminate care.

**Least restrictive alternative** an environment that provides the necessary treatment requirements in the least restrictive setting possible. For example, a hospital setting is more restrictive than a board and care setting. If the board and care setting provides the necessary treatment requirements for a person then that environment would represent the least restrictive alternative.

**Malpractice** negligence by a professional. Malpractice is a civil action that can be brought against a nurse if she has breached a standard of care that a reasonably prudent nurse would meet.

**Negligence** the failure to do that which a reasonably prudent and careful person would do under the circumstances, or the doing of that which a reasonable and prudent person would not do.

**Probable cause** sufficient, credible facts which would induce a reasonably intelligent and prudent person to believe that a cause of action exists.

**Voluntary commitment** a commitment status in which the patient or his conservator/guardian requests treatment and signs an application for that treatment. This person is free to sign himself out of the hospital also.

## Involuntary commitment

Involuntary treatment means that an individual who has the legal capacity to consent to mental health treatment refuses to do so. In every state, persons who are considered *dangerous to self or others* because of a mental disorder can be involuntarily treated for that mental disorder. In about half the states a third criterion, *gravely disabled*, is also cause for involuntary treatment. There are three common categories of involuntary treatment: evaluation and emergency care, certification for observation and treatment, and extended or indeterminate care. Involuntary treatment, not surprisingly, is the area of psychiatric care where most legal issues develop.

**Evaluation and emergency care.** Individuals who meet any one of the above three criteria can be involuntarily detained for evaluation and emergency treatment in most states. Typically an authorized person, such as a police officer, will sign documents placing the person under involuntary care. The length of the involuntary status varies from state to state, with 72 hours or so being close to the average.

*Nursing implications.* Since the length of this involuntary treatment period is prescribed by law, the staff must scrupulously adhere to legal time constraints. The nursing staff must be absolutely aware of when the emergency treatment period is over and prepare the patient for discharge at that time. The patient may be asked to remain in the facility voluntarily, and if he refuses, he may be asked to sign out against medical advice (AMA). The following case study provides a realistic vignette for the involuntary detention of a person.

> **Case study.** Joey Youngblood, a 45-year-old truck driver, after taking a large number of "uppers" (amphetamines) on his cross country trip became irrational at a truck stop. He began yelling and accusing the waitress of trying to poison him. He became suspicious of everyone and sat in a corner booth trembling but vigilant. He refused to leave and became threatening when approached by the truck stop management. The police arrived and after a brief struggle with Mr. Youngblood took him to the county hospital for involuntary hospitalization for 72 hours.

**Certification for observation and treatment.** Each state has laws governing involuntary treatment for mental disorders that provide for the certification for observation and treatment of mental illness. These state laws authorize a qualified expert to determine if a person has a treatable mental disorder. A mental disorder can be defined as a condition that substantially impairs the person's thoughts, perception of reality, emotional process, judgment, or behavior. In most states a qualified expert might include a physician, a psychiatrist, a master's prepared nurse or social worker, or a psychologist. A treatable mental disorder indicates that the problem is amenable to and can improve in response to treatment. For example, someone who is hearing voices telling him to kill himself would meet this criterion, whereas someone who is simply angry and threatening to kill someone would not.

During the certification process a complaint or a *probable cause* statement is written indicating that the person is a danger to self or others or is gravely disabled. The probable cause statement is required by the Fourth Amendment of the Constitution of the United States, which prohibits "search and seizure of a person without probable cause." In this context, probable cause means facts must be known that would lead an ordinary person to believe that the person detained is mentally disordered and is a danger to self or others or is gravely disabled. The probable cause hearing is not held for the purpose of determining whether the person is mentally ill but whether there is just cause to keep the person for treatment against his will.

If it is determined that probable cause exists, the person can be detained for observation and treatment. The person must be informed of his rights upon being certified for this level of involuntary care. The length of this observation and treatment period varies from state to state. In California a patient can be held involuntarily for 14 days, whereas in West Virginia a patient can be held for 6 months.

*Nursing implications.* If there is no legal basis for continued commitment, the person must be released. The hospital staff may suggest voluntary admission at that point and if it is refused may require the patient to sign out AMA. The nurse is often responsible for assuring AMA forms are signed and that a follow-up appointment for continued treatment on an outpatient basis is scheduled.

**Extended or indeterminate commitment.** The extended or indeterminate commitment is reserved for those persons who continue to need psychiatric care of a prolonged nature but who refuse to seek such help voluntarily. Typically, extended hospitalizations last from 60 to 180 days. Indeterminate hospitalization can last much longer. Most states require that a patient being recommended for an extended or indeterminate commitment be brought before a hearing officer. This system of checks and balances decreases the possibility of a person's being "railroaded" into a mental hospital and assures the person of full legal protection.

### Commitment of incapacitated persons

In most states there is a procedure for establishing a conservator or guardian for gravely disabled persons (the conservatee). The definition of gravely disabled is an inability to provide food, clothing, and shelter for oneself because of a mental illness. This does not mean that all people living on the streets are gravely disabled. However, the person with money in his pocket who cannot negotiate arrangements for food or shelter is gravely disabled.

The appointment of a conservator or guardian is a serious legal matter, and full legal protection under the law is provided for persons being evaluated for conservatee status. The proposed conservatee is entitled to representation by a private attorney or a court-appointed public defender to challenge conservatorship. If a conservator or guardian is appointed, he is given broad powers including the right to order the conservatee to receive psychiatric treatment. Although technically the patient might be receiving treatment against his will, there is a legal distinction between this commitment and an involuntary commitment. That legal distinction is based on the premise that the conservator now speaks for the patient; hence the treatment is not involuntary.

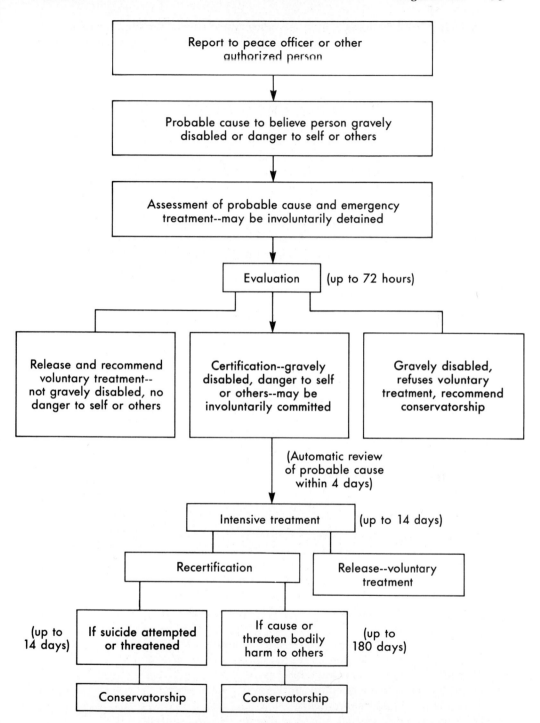

**FIGURE 4-1** Flow chart for certification procedure.

**Nursing implications.** Since the conservator speaks for the conservatee, the nurse must gain consent from the conservator for decisions other patients on the unit could consent to themselves. For instance, a newspaper reporter may want to interview patients about hospital living conditions. Although other patients could agree or refuse to participate on their own, a conservatee would need permission from the conservator. A nurse who forgets to gain conservator approval may face legal consequences.

## PATIENT RIGHTS

Box 4-2 contains a list of rights that a patient should be afforded even if he is being treated involuntarily. The specific rights vary somewhat from state to state, but all are derived from a bill of rights established in 1980 by the federal Mental Health Systems Act. This congressional action recommended to state governing bodies a set of basic patient rights that most states either fully or partially support. A list of patient rights should be prominently displayed for all to see and explained to every patient on admission.

### Suspension of patient rights

Occasionally it is necessary to suspend a right for the protection of the patient or of others.

**Nursing implications.** If a right is suspended, the nurse must clearly document that if the patient were allowed to continue to exercise the specific right, the patient could do harm to himself or to others. For example, a suicidal patient may have

**Box 4-2**
### MOST COMMONLY ADOPTED PATIENT RIGHTS

1. Right to treatment in the least restrictive alternative
2. Right to confidentiality of records
3. Right to freedom from restraints and seclusion
4. Right to give or refuse consent to treatment
5. Right to access to personal belongings
6. Right to daily exercise
7. Right to have visitors
8. Right to use of writing materials and uncensored mail
9. Right to use of telephone
10. Right to access courts and attorneys
11. Right to employment compensation
12. Right to be informed of rights
13. Right to refuse electroconvulsive therapy or psychosurgery

right of access to personal belongings suspended because it is felt that he might attempt to harm himself with those objects. The nurse must document the concern and the suspension of this right in the nurse's notes.

## Right to treatment in least restrictive alternative

Persons with mental health problems have the right to have those problems treated and to have them treated in the least restrictive alternative available. This "right" has emerged from court decisions previously mentioned. In particular, patients who are held against their will should not be detained and then not treated.

**Nursing implications.** The nurse does not usually make the decision about which treatment setting the patient will enter. However, the nurse has treatment responsibilities and could be held liable if the patient is not receiving adequate treatment. The following case study illustrates the issue of the right to treatment in the least restrictive alternative.

> **Case study.** Thelma Brown, a 76-year-old female with a history of mental illness, is admitted to the county hospital psychiatric unit. She was found wandering near her home in a confused state but is of no obvious danger to self or others. Her married son cannot accept her into his home but agrees that she may not be able to go back home to live on her own. Ms. Brown insists upon going back home, however, and her case is heard before the court. The court rules that she does not need commitment to a psychiatric unit but does need supervision in a less restrictive environment. The unit social worker finds an agreeable placement in a senior citizen's board-and-care facility for Ms. Brown.

## Right to confidentiality of records

All information and records obtained in the course of providing services to either voluntary or involuntary recipients of services are confidential. The Colorado Society of Clinical Specialists in Psychiatric Nursing (1990) has developed guidelines for psychiatric nurses to follow when they are dealing with the issue of confidentiality:

1. Keep all patient records secure.
2. Carefully consider the content of record entries.
3. Release information only with written consent.
4. Disguise clinical material when it is used for teaching.
5. Maintain the anonymity of research subjects.

**Nursing implications.** When confidential information is released, the nurse should document that release in the nursing notes. She should include the date and circumstances under which such disclosure was made, the names and relationships to the patient of the persons or agencies to whom such disclosures were made, and the specific information disclosed. Most states provide legal redress for the patient should a nurse willfully disclose confidential information. The confidentiality of the patient's records should not be confused with doctrine of privileged communication. Under this doctrine a psychiatrist is not obliged to reveal the contents of sessions with the patient. This privilege is based on the public's understanding of the need for trust between a physician and patient. Most states do not include nurses under this provision.

### Right to freedom from restraints and seclusion

The proper procedure for dealing with harmful behavior is to try calming the patient verbally at first. Chapter 8 carefully traces the steps to follow in working with an aggressive patient. When it is determined that verbal and psychopharmacological interventions are not adequate to stem the patient's aggressiveness, seclusion or seclusion with restraint may be required. Seclusion is defined as the process of isolating a person in a room with the door locked. Restraint means controlling a person's physical activity by mechanical devices such as leather restraints.

**Nursing Implications.**  The use of seclusion and restraint continues to be both a legal and an ethical problem for nurses (Craig, et al., 1989). Because it is unlawful to seclude or restrain a person without justification, the nurse must have a physician's order and carefully document the following:

1. Type of restraint
2. Reason for restraining the patient
3. Length of time to be restrained, for example, "4-Point leather restraint STAT for assaultive behavior until calm."

The patient must be checked every 10 to 15 minutes with appropriate documentation and must verify the need for continued restraint at that same time interval. The case on p. 57 study provides a typical scenario with the appropriate nursing interventions.

### Right to give or refuse consent to treatment

The final patient right to be explored is the right to give or refuse consent to treatment. Court rulings mentioned previously provide the legal precedents for the patient's right to a treatment. The *Rogers v Okin* case provided the foundation for a patient's right to refuse treatment. This right is of most concern to patients and staff when the issue of medication is involved.

Voluntary patients have long been recognized to have the right to refuse treatment. If a voluntary patient believes that the treatment he is receiving is helpful he can accept it; if he believes that it is not helpful, he can refuse it. Involuntary patients, on the other hand, have not always been understood to have the same ability to refuse treatment. In the case of medications, many involuntary patients through the years have been forced to take medications against their will. Legally it is now recognized that an involuntarily admitted patient does not lose his right to give informed consent to the administration of psychotropic drugs. The key issue is whether the patient has the capacity to give informed consent to the administration of these drugs. The court makes the determination but does not respond to issues of need or alternative treatments. Once the court decides that a person is not competent to understand the need for treatment, medications can then be imposed upon that person. How this decision is implemented varies from state to state.

In cases of a psychiatric emergency, medications can be given without consent to prevent harm to the patient or to others.

**Case study.** Abel Keiver, a 28-year-old man, was brought to the inpatient unit by the city police department after he was found wandering around the local college campus acting in a bizarre and agitated manner. He had been stopping students and asking questions such as "What is college?" "What is learning?" He was disheveled and dirty and was threatening people. Campus police detained Mr. Keiver until the city police arrived. Mr. Keiver told police that he was hearing voices telling him to cut off his arms and his legs. He could not produce a realistic plan to provide for his own food, clothing, and shelter and was brought to the emergency room for evaluation.

Since his admission to the unit (5/18/90) Mr. Keiver has been extremely preoccupied with internal stimuli and delusional ideation, including thoughts of self-mutilation and aggression toward others. He refuses to discuss plans for his discharge stating that, "I am going to die here." Mr. Keiver has required restraint and seclusion on several occasions because of his aggressive behavior. The nursing progress record (Box 4-3) and the restraint and seclusion nursing notes (Box 4-4) provide a record of his behavior and the nursing responses to that behavior.

The nursing staff, after making the decision to place Mr. Keiver in restraint and seclusion, must then make sure that they have complied with a checklist for seclusion and restraints similar to the one that follows:

| | | | | |
|---|---|---|---|---|
| 1. | Documentation of justification | Yes | No | NA |
| 2. | Physicians order | Yes | No | NA |
| 3. | Type of restraints | Yes | No | NA |
| 4. | Duration | Yes | No | NA |
| 5. | Every 15 minutes checked by staff | Yes | No | NA |
| 6. | Every 1 hour checked by RN | Yes | No | NA |
| 7. | Patient's Rights Denial Form | Yes | No | NA |
| 8. | Fluids every hour | Yes | No | NA |
| 9. | Limbs exercised every 2 hours | Yes | No | NA |
| 10. | Patient's rights advocate notified after 8 hours | Yes | No | NA |

<hr>

## Box 4-3
### NURSING PROGRESS RECORD

| Date | Time | Format |
|---|---|---|
| 5/20/90 | 0210 | Pt has continued to pace hallway, dayroom, and his room. At 0045 was asking for sleep meds. Pt stated the best way to get well was walking. |
| | 0315 | Pt refuses to go to room and try to rest. Pacing dayroom and at times kneeling as if in prayer. |
| | 0430 | Pt asleep on top of bed, naked with door open. |
| | 0830 | Pt refusing medication. Appears very agitated. |
| | 0930 | Pt very agitated, tearing up another patient's magazine and throwing into trash. Placed in seclusion. |
| | 1030 | Escalation of agitation. When staff went into room to check on Mr. Keiver he swung at staff and attempted to bite the nurse. Placed in 4-point restraint by 4 female and 2 male staff members. Pt stated that he was being "raped" and that "Christ lives in me." Haldol 5 mg IM and Cogentin 2 mg IM given. |

### Box 4-4
## RESTRAINT AND SECLUSION NURSING NOTES

| Date | Time | Checked | Water | Food | Observations |
|------|------|---------|-------|------|--------------|
| 5/20 | 0930 | | | | Pt placed in seclusion because of agitated threatening behavior. |
| | 0945 | ✔ | | | Pt pacing in room. Crying and shouting. |
| | 1000 | ✔ | | | Pt remains agitated and threatening. |
| | 1015 | ✔ | | | Pt cursing at staff. |
| | 1030 | ✔ | | | Pt placed in 4-point restraint because of combative behavior. Placed face down. |
| | 1045 | ✔ | ✔ | | Pt still agitated and threatening. Water given. |
| | 1100 | ✔ | | | Vital signs 130/90, 90, 20. Pt continues to ramble about Jesus and being raped. |
| | 1115 | ✔ | | | Pt continues to threaten staff entering room. |
| | 1130 | ✔ | | | RN checked pt. Pt angrily cursing at RN. |
| | 1145 | ✔ | ✔ | ✔ | Pt hallucinating, crying, stating that he hears his baby crying. Refused lunch tray at this time. |
| | 1200 | ✔ | | | Pt incoherent but not crying. |
| | 1215 | ✔ | | ✔ | O.J. given. 130/98, 112, 20. |
| | 1230 | ✔ | | | Pt growing calmer but states still hears baby crying. Limbs exercised. |
| | 1245 | ✔ | ✔ | | Pt states he is trying to get the bad thoughts out. |
| | 1300 | ✔ | | | Pt appears to be asleep. |
| | 1315 | ✔ | | | Pt states he likes the medication he was given. |
| | 1330 | ✔ | | | Pt appears to be asleep. |
| | 1345 | ✔ | ✔ | | Pt apologized for hitting staff member. |
| | 1400 | | | | Pt released from restraints. States he can control himself now. Appears to be much calmer. |

**Nursing implications.** Nurses administer medications to patients. Since it is not uncommon for patients to refuse medications and nurses to coax them into taking medications, nurses must be sure that they do not coax so hard that they are actually forcing medications upon a person. It is also not always clear what constitutes a psychiatric emergency. Nurses may be liable should their interpretation of a psychiatric emergency differ from that of another professional or that of a judge. The following case study illustrates the dilemma associated with a patient refusing medication.

> **Case study.** Joyce Zimmerman is a 44-year-old female with an admitting diagnosis of bipolar illness. This is her sixteenth admission to the county hospital psychiatric unit. The staff know Ms. Zimmerman well, having helped her through periods of manic behavior many times before. Historically, Ms. Zimmerman is angry, assaultive, and refuses medications. She says nasty things to staff and is particularly rude to Hispanic and black staff members. Although all staff recognize that she is mentally ill, her remarks are so biting at times that some staff have difficulty maintaining a professional posture. Although no one has ever been seriously hurt by Ms. Zimmerman, her attempts to slap and choke people has both patients and staff on edge. The physician has ordered lithium carbonate 300 mg t.i.d. and chlorpromazine 50 mg IM q4h p.r.n. for assaultive behavior. Ms. Zimmerman has refused the lithium, and the nursing staff continue to give chlorpromazine when her behavior justifies doing so. The consensus of both nursing and medical staff is that Ms. Zimmerman will not improve until she starts taking her lithium on a regular basis, yet her illness is instrumental in her refusal of that medication. The staff requested a court hearing to evaluate Ms. Zimmerman's competency and the need for the appointment of a guardian. (The student is reminded that in an emergency the nursing staff is permitted to medicate an assaultive patient without consent. However, the staff is not permitted to medicate a patient against his will at other times even when that behavior [e.g., hallucinations, extreme withdrawn behavior] indicates a need for pharmacological intervention).
>
> At the hearing the physician testified concerning his evaluation of the patient; nursing documentation was reviewed; and Ms. Zimmerman appeared with a court-appointed representative. During the proceedings Ms. Zimmerman stated that she had been sodomized by a black technician on the unit and that she knew President Bush personally. Furthermore, she made various grandiose claims that substantiated to the court the truth of the medical and nursing staff testimony. The court appointed a guardian for Ms. Zimmerman. The guardian agreed with the staff's assessment that Ms. Zimmerman should take the psychotropic medications prescribed by the physician, and should she refuse to do so, the nursing staff was to administer those drugs to her.
>
> One week after the court order, Ms. Zimmerman was joking with the staff, taking medications voluntarily, and anticipating her return to the board-and-care facility where she lived.

## NURSING LIABILITY AND RELATED ISSUES
### Malpractice

Psychiatric nurses are responsible for many significant decisions in the care of psychiatric patients. Lapses in attention to specific legal constraints on their practice can result in liability suits against them and their employer. Areas of concern that can lead to lawsuits include inappropriate dissemination of confidential information, illegal confinement, failure to obtain consent for medication and other treatments, inadequate treatment, medication errors, and the duty to warn of threatened suicide or harm to others. Malpractice is a civil action that can be brought against a nurse if she has breached a professional standard of care (Beck et al., 1988). A malpractice case rests on establishing the violation of the standard of care that the patient is entitled to once the nurse-patient relationship is initiated. The standard of care is the care a reasonably prudent nurse would give. These issues are potential sources of malpractice suits against the nurse, and legal rulings have, in many cases, established parameters of appropriate professional behavior by which the nurse will be compared.

### Duty to warn of threatened suicide or harm to others

Mental health professionals have a duty to warn of threatened suicide or harm to others based on a number of court rulings including the Tarasoff and Meier cases mentioned previously. The mental health professional is caught between her duty to protect the confidentiality of her communication with a patient and her responsibility as a professional to society.

**Nursing implications.** A nurse who is aware of a patient's intention to harm himself or others must communicate that information to other professionals and take steps to protect the potential recipient of that harm. Documentation in the patient's record is crucial to effective communication of this information. If the nurse fails to take prudent action, she can be held liable under several court decisions.

> **Case study.** Bill Chance, age 26, was brought to the hospital by city police. He was found outside the city library ranting and raving about Satan. He was admitted to the unit with a diagnosis of schizophrenia, paranoid type. He states that he has electricity in his blood and that he has super powers. Although he was not displaying weapons at the time, the police found and confiscated a gun from Mr. Chance. During a conversation with the nurse on the third day after admission, he tells the nurse that his ex-girlfriend works at the city library and that he was going there to kill her for leaving him. He will not admit to no longer having those impulses. Upon team review both the police and Mr. Chance's ex-girlfriend are warned of his threats.

### Civil remedies for wrongful involuntary commitment

Persons who are wrongfully committed to a psychiatric facility have several types of civil suits they can file against mental health professionals:

- **False imprisonment:** lack of probable cause, confining a patient so that he has no way of escape, inappropriate use of restraint and seclusion, not allowing a voluntary patient to leave when he is ready.
- **Assault and battery:** force used in unlawful detention, inappropriately forceful restraint (battery), telling a patient you are going to force him to take medication (assault).

- **Malicious prosecution:** defamation by original informant such as the police officer who initiated the evaluation and emergency treatment, the person who certifies the patient for further treatment
- **Negligence:** absence of measures to prevent harm to patient.

## Documentation

The nursing staff is responsible for completing a variety of forms that document the progress of the patient and serve as a legal record of the treatment he received. Nursing notes, restraint and seclusion forms, medication records, and physician order sheets are but a few of the forms required. Careful attention to these records promotes communication among staff, enhances treatment, diminishes treatment errors (e.g., medication errors), and reduces liability claims.

The psychiatric nurse, because she has the most patient contact and because of the unique contributions of nursing to psychiatric care, is in a position to positively influence the legal issues confronting those involved in that care today.

## KEY CONCEPTS

1. Our understanding of the rights of mentally ill persons has evolved over the centuries. Today, based upon several legal decisions, the mentally ill person's protection from unreasonable hospitalization has been established.
2. These landmark cases triggered several states to legislate the end of inappropriate, indefinite, and involuntary commitment to mental hospitals.
3. There are three categories of commitment:
   a. Voluntary, the person requests hospitalization.
   b. Involuntary, a person with the legal capacity to consent refuses to do so and is treated against his will.
   c. Commitment of an incapacitated person, the treatment of a person who does not have the legal capacity to consent to treatment.
4. Involuntary commitment can take three forms: a brief evaluation and emergency care form, an intermediate certification for observation and treatment form, and a longer extended or indeterminate form.
5. Patients under psychiatric care have many rights guaranteed by the Constitution of the United States and the constitutions of individual states. These rights flow from the following basic rights: the freedom from unreasonable search and seizure, the right of privacy, and the freedom of choice and self-determination.
6. Seclusion and restraint are special procedures for dealing with assaultive and dangerous patients in which these patients can be isolated or mechanically restrained to prevent injury to the patient, other patients, or staff.
7. Patients, even involuntarily admitted patients, must give informed consent before they are given psychotropic drugs, and they retain the right to refuse medication. Except for emergency situations, involuntarily admitted patients cannot be given medication against their will without judicial approval.
8. Psychiatric nurses are at legal risk for civil action if they are guilty of false imprisonment, assault and battery, malicious prosecution, or negligent harm.

9. Mental health professionals have a duty to warn the potential victim of a psychiatric patient should that patient, in the course of treatment, reveal an intent to harm another person.

10. All information and records obtained in the course of providing services to either voluntarily or involuntarily admitted mental patients are confidential.

## REFERENCES

Beck CK, Rawlins RP, and Williams SR: Mental health-psychiatric nursing, St. Louis, 1988, The C. V. Mosby Co.

Colorado Society of Clinical Specialists in Psychiatric Nursing: Ethical guidelines for confidentiality, J Psychosoc Nurs 28:43, 1990.

Craig C, Ray F, and Hix C: Seclusion and restraint: decreasing the discomfort, J Psychosoc Nurs 27:16, 1989.

Klerman GL: The psychiatric patient's right to effective treatment: implications of Osheroff v. Chestnut Lodge, Am J Psychiatry 147:409, 1990.

# The Therapeutic Nurse-Patient Relationship

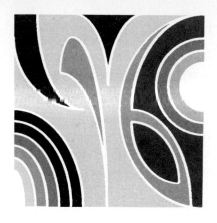

## CHAPTER 5

# Communication

BETTE R. KELTNER

LEARNING OBJECTIVES

After reading this chapter you should be able to

- Distinguish between social and therapeutic communication.
- Identify goals of therapeutic communication.
- Discuss critical therapeutic communication issues.
- Know a variety of techniques that facilitate client-centered communication.
- State common obstacles that interfere with therapeutic communication.

Communication is an interaction between two or more persons. It involves the exchange of information, which can be concrete or highly abstract, by simple or highly sophisticated means between a sender and a receiver. The product of communication is a message to be interpreted by the recipient. Communication connects and organizes human beings. The universal human need for interpersonal communication forms the foundation for civilization. In ancient times verbal communication alone provided a meaningful connection to the past. As cultures became literate, the role of the elderly as keepers of history was supplanted.

Words (verbal or written) and behaviors (nonverbal) are the primary channels for communication. The evolution of human communication has resulted in a written language and technology that can transcend obstacles of time and distance. These communication methods can dramatically alter a society. For instance, we observe, marvel at, and may feel threatened by the many changes that occur because of computerized capabilities, such as new words, individualized learning, information access, and rapid analytic abilities. Social roles, such as the role of the elderly, also are influenced by applied communication methods.

Nurses are professionals who have a contract with society to provide health care for its members in need. We rely on communication as pivotal to analysis, collaboration, and delivery of services. Health professionals share a broad undergraduate education that forms a common culture (Hirsch, 1986) essential to interdisciplinary understanding. These professionals also share a vast, complex body of scientific knowledge that is applied to resolve human needs. Nurses are responsible for the mastery of a significant share of this knowledge and are expected to communicate this information effectively with both the most (i.e., colleagues) and least educated members of society. Consequently nursing requires a sound education and a solid foundation for effective communication to work with these varied groups. For nurses who work with psychiatric patients, patients with alterations in thinking and behavior, the challenge of communication is even greater.

## CATEGORIES OF COMMUNICATION

In psychiatric nursing the important categories of communication are writing, speech, and behavior. In psychiatric nursing the goal is not only to understand the patient and assure that he can understand you but also to teach him more effective communication skills for interaction with mainstream society.

### Written communication

Since written material is a primary means of acquiring and sharing information, mastery of language skills is imperative. All professions require some form of written reports, instructions, or the sharing of findings and ideas. Vocabulary, grammar, and organization of ideas are critical skills. The degree of participation in any work setting, as well as leadership, is dependent on language skills.

### Speech and behavior

Besides sound, oral communication includes the mannerisms that modify the message. The timbre and tone of voice have meaning. The rate of speech and the emphasis affect the message. The body and the environment may also become incorporated into the message of words. For example, the nurse can express sincere concern or caring with and without words of concern. It is important for verbal and nonverbal communication to be congruent (Carran and Kraus-Mayer, 1989). The nurse's level of confidence is also communicated.

**Communicating with confidence.** Whether the nurse is responding to parents in an emergency room, to a question from a physician, or to a signal for help from a mentally distraught patient, the ability to send a message of confidence is fundamental to good nursing care. This certainly is not a "know-it-all" attitude but one that reassures the recipient that here is a professional who has a mastery of meaningful abilities. Hesitation, tentativeness or timidity, habitually trailing sentences, and rapid, high-pitched speech all suggest insecurity and cause distrust. Not all decisions must be made immediately, and most patients realize that no one person knows everything. However, to not recognize the need for confident reassurance in patients who are anxious and in pain (physical or psychic) indicates a poor understanding of the importance of communication in nursing practice. Reassurance is achieved not through platitudes (i.e., you're going to be OK, Mr. Smith) but through competence, realistic promises that can be kept, and confident communication.

## Interpretation of communication

Interpretation of a message is filtered through a person's knowledge and experience. Some aspects of communication clearly are more commonly understood than others. Words generally are more precisely understood than behaviors. Words are emphasized because they are the vehicles of expression most easily described and categorized (Havens, 1986). However, anyone who has studied a foreign language appreciates that nuances are often lost in translation because of the limitations of words. It is said that John Steinbeck's widow was traveling in Nagasaki and entered a bookstore with a sign that indicated English was spoken there. On inquiring as to whether the store carried any of Steinbeck's works, she was reassured that one book was particularly popular—"Angry Raisins." The book was *The Grapes of Wrath*.

It is important that nurses also have a broad knowledge of cultures, cues, and content to accurately interpret and respond. It is vital that one acquire the ability to look beyond the superficial without becoming trapped in the "parlor psychiatry" ploy of assigning covert meanings to everything from sneezes to scratches. The content and context of communication cannot be overlooked.

## THERAPEUTIC COMMUNICATION

It is clear that everyone is capable of communicating. Why, then, do professionals have books and classes teaching them how to communicate? Social or personal styles of communicating are not appropriate in the therapeutic situation. It is essential to differentiate between therapeutic communication and social communication. Therapeutic communication functions as a treatment for persons in need. This treatment may be *ancillary, primary,* or *singular,* but the interactions between the professional and the patient exist to help the patient. *Ancillary* uses of communication include communicating with any person who receives nursing care. A critically ill patient should experience expert communication as part of nursing care that may be chiefly technological. For a knowledge deficit or some mental illnesses, communication is a *primary* therapeutic mode to impart knowledge, to evoke understanding, or simply to interact. Some therapies rely *solely* on communication to help the patient. These are discussed in Chapter 2.

### Therapeutic versus social communication

Therapeutic communication is highly stylized (Zinberg, 1987) and occurs with a plan and a purpose. Social communication involves equal disclosure of personal information and intimacy, and both parties enjoy equal opportunities for spontaneity. Therapeutic communication focuses on the patient but is planned and directed by the professional. It is stylized in the sense of specific guidelines but typically does not use the same words and sequence for each patient. In social exchanges both participants seek to have personal needs met, whereas the needs of the patient are the focus of therapeutic communication. Therapeutic communication relies on patient disclosure of personal and sometimes painful feelings with the professional at an emotional distance near enough to be involved but objective enough to be helpful. When working with a depressed patient, a professional should come away feeling "sadness" but not "despair." In a social relationship a friend may share feelings of anger and aggression toward a mutual friend with the expectation that the feelings will be kept confidential. In therapeutic communication it must be understood that while confidentiality will be respected, a professional is obligated at times to share information within the professional community. The nurse is a patient's advocate, not a patient's friend.

### Dynamics of therapeutic communication

Therapeutic communication requires attention to multiple interacting factors. At the core of communication are the words and nonverbal behaviors relating to the patient's health needs that are exchanged between patient and nurse. Fig. 5-1, a Venn diagram, illustrates key dimensions of participants in communication that should be understood. It is important to view the patient and oneself as a whole. It is also important to focus on those aspects of the patient that need intervention. In this manner the nursing process operates to effectively provide nursing care: assessment, diagnosis, planning, intervention, and evaluation define therapeutic communication (see Box 5-1).

Therapeutic communication is referred to as synergistic. This means that ongoing exchanges between patient and nurse on a particular subject (say, dependency) are not merely additive but have increased meaning and influence as the dialogue continues. This is analogous to the chemical effect of codeine and aspirin when they are taken together: the effect is greater than if each of these drugs is taken separately (Pluckman, 1978, p. 9).

**Balance in communication.** Havens (1986) refers to the "contagion of affect" (e.g., manic patients produce excited wards; paranoid patients can cause staff to

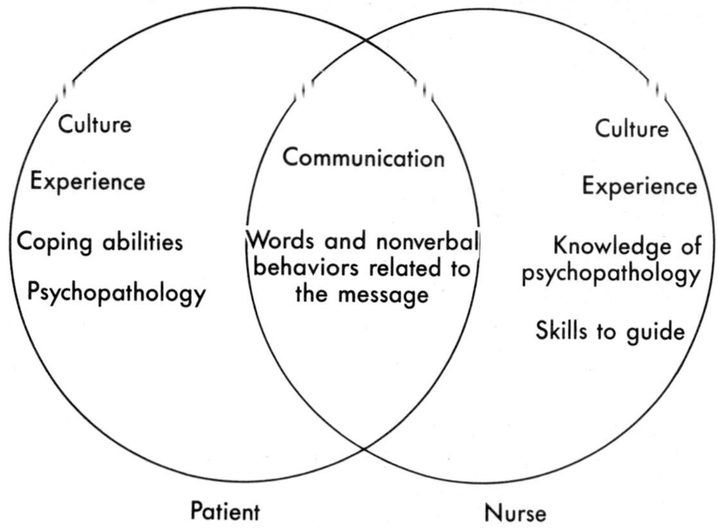

FIGURE 5-1 Essential and influencing variables of the therapeutic communication environment.

become argumentative) and considers it a "dangerous sign" if a health care worker is not affected by patients. For example, if the nurse is not "down" when caring for a suicidal patient, she may not have come close enough to aid the suffering person. The result of this "contagion" in the clinical setting is an underworld of strong emotional tones that shape and move the participants. Professionals can grasp these forces and use them to clinical advantage (Havens, 1986). For the nurse to achieve balance it is necessary to establish a working distance that is close enough to make separation meaningful but not so close as to make separation "impossible" (Havens, 1986).

The client-centered approach is the approach taught in many nursing programs because it has been demonstrated to be useful in many different clinical settings, and it helps the nurse achieve balance. This method helps the patient express feelings and ideas and develop personal problem solving skills. In the client-centered approach the professional guides a conversation to a goal using few words. This method became so popular that jokes about a therapist's "hmmmmm" and constant repeating of a patient's words underscored some frustrations that can occur if the approach is mechanical and not well balanced. Havens (1986) stated that it took years to get therapists to "shut up," and now we're trying to get them talking again. Previous prohibitions against giving advice or offering explanations have been changed by many professionals, who find that limited use of these two mechanisms does not compromise the client-centered approach. The client-centered approach can promote self-discovery and insight; it can foster a sense of success and control and can lead to new problem-solving and coping skills.

**Environmental considerations.** The environment can facilitate or impede therapeutic communication. Nurses often have much control over the environment.

Box 5-1

# THERAPEUTIC COMMUNICATION TECHNIQUES

## ASSESSMENT

### Techniques fostering descriptions

- **Silence** planned absence of verbal remarks to allow patient to think and say more

    Facing the patient; maintaining eye contact; conveying interest and concern in facial expressions.

- **Active listening** paying attention to all of patient's verbal and nonverbal communications; identifying recurrent patterns of thinking, feeling, and behaving

    Facing the patient; maintaining eye contact; conveying interest and concern in facial expressions.

- **Questioning** using open-ended questions to achieve relevance and depth in discussion

    Who? What? Where? When? What did you (they) say? Do? What happened? Tell me about it?

- **General leads** using neutral expressions to encourage continued talking

    Go on. Ummm. I'm listening. I hear what you're saying.

- **Restating** repeating exact words of patient so he is reminded of what he has said or knows that he is heard

    I heard you say you were going home soon. You say your mother wasn't happy to see you?

- **Verbalizing the implied** rephrasing of patient's words to highlight an underlying message

    *Patient:* There is nothing to do at home. *Nurse:* It sounds as if you might feel bored at home.

- **Clarification** asking the patient to restate, elaborate on, or give an example of an idea

    What do you mean by "feeling sick inside"? Give me an example of when you feel "lost."

---

## NURSING DIAGNOSIS

### Techniques fostering analysis and conclusions

- **Making observations** putting into words what is seen to encourage a discussion

    You seem restless. I noticed you had trouble making a decision about . . . .

- **Presenting reality** offering a view of what is real and what is not

    I don't hear any voices other than yours and mine. This is a decision you will have to make for yourself.

- **Verbalizing the implied** (see above)

- **Encouraging description of perceptions** asking for the patient's view of situations

    What do you think is happening to you right now? What kinds of situations are you anxious about?

NURSING DIAGNOSIS—cont'd

## Techniques fostering analysis and conclusions—cont'd

- **Placing an event in time or sequence** asking for relationships among events

  When did you do this? Then what happened? What led up to ... ?

- **Encouraging comparisons** asking for similarities and differences among feelings, behaviors, and events

  How does this compare to last time? What is different about the way you responded today?

- **Identifying themes** asking patient to identify recurrent patterns in thoughts, feelings, and behaviors

  So what do you do each time you argue with your wife? What is the major feeling you have about all women?

- **Summarizing** reviewing the main points and conclusions

  Let's see, so far you have said ....

## Techniques fostering interpretation of meaning and importance

- **Focusing** pursuing a topic until its meaning or importance is clear

  Tell me more about these feelings. What bothers you about ... ?

- **Interpreting** giving the nurse's view of the meaning or importance of something

  It sounds as if this is very important to you.

- **Encouraging evaluation** asking for the patient's view of the meaning or importance of something

  So what does this all mean to you? How important is it for you to change this behavior?

## PLANNING

## Techniques fostering problem solving and decisions

- **Suggesting collaboration** offering to help the patient solve problems

  Let's see if we can figure out an answer.

- **Encouraging goal setting** asking patient to decide on the type of change needed

  What do you think needs to change?

- **Encouraging consideration of options** asking the patient to consider pros and cons of possible options for change

  What would be the advantage of trying ... ? What might happen if you ... ?

- **Encouraging decisions** asking the patient to make a choice among options

  Which is the best alternative for you? What would work best?

- **Encouraging formulation of a plan** asking for step by step actions that will be needed.

  What exactly will it take to carry out your plan? What else do you need to do?

*Continued.*

### Box 5-1
## THERAPEUTIC COMMUNICATION TECHNIQUES—cont'd

**IMPLEMENTATION**

**Techniques fostering carrying out of plans**

• **Testing out new behaviors**
1. **Rehearsing** verbally describing what will be said and done.

Tell me exactly what you will say to your wife on Saturday.

2. **Role playing** practicing behaviors with the nurse playing a particular role.

I'll play your wife. What do you want to say to me?

• **Supportive confrontation** acknowledging the difficulty in changing but pushing for action

I know it isn't easy to do this, but I think you can do it.

• **Limit setting** discouraging nonproductive feelings and behaviors and encouraging productive ones

You're slipping into your aggressive tone again. Try it again more assertively.

• **Giving feedback** pointing out specific behaviors and giving impressions on reactions

When you said . . . , I felt . . . . I thought you conveyed anger when you said . . .

**EVALUATION**

• **Possibly repeating steps of nursing process** evaluation may involve repeating the steps of the nursing process to get a description of what happened, conclusions about successes, and ideas for changing the plans.

• **Encouraging evaluation** encouraging the patient to evaluate his actions

How well did it work when you tried . . . ?

In fact, Nightingale underscored this when she asserted that nursing's task was to put the patient in the best environment for nature to heal him. The act of sitting to listen to a distraught patient, providing privacy for a grieving family, or introducing a depressed patient to short episodes of small-group interaction are examples of interventions that use the environment to achieve a therapeutic communication goal. Likewise, the environment may foster assessment of patient needs and formulation of a diagnosis. Poor physical hygiene is an environmental cue that confirms the existence of a problem.

*Proxemics* refers to the way in which people use environmental space in interaction. Typically, boundaries for public and social communication are more distant than those for personal or therapeutic communication. Nursing practice may violate these social conventions when a nurse and a patient must communicate in close proximity to each other before a therapeutic relationship has been formed. The nurse should be aware of this and assist the patient to feel more comfortable talking to a "stranger" just centimeters away. Sometimes it is helpful to complete a physical task, such as examining a patient's ears, and then to step back and face the patient before discussing the findings rather than to attempt a conversation "head to head." Proxemics may be used in a therapeutic manner also. Family sculpture is an activity in which a person places family members in a "living" snapshot pose that may suggest how comfortable he or she is with each member (Keltner and Gillett, 1983).

**Biological considerations.** Biological integrity influences the nature of the therapeutic communication process. Some mental problems have biological causes that create situations requiring understanding and modification of communication. For example, persons with multiple sclerosis may experience mood fluctuations and extreme fatigue. Certain sensory limitations (blindness, hearing loss) may compromise communication, necessitating compensatory measures such as slow face-to-face speech for lip reading. Developmental disabilities may seriously limit the ability to comprehend and remember. Carefully constructed simple sentences with a single main idea may have to be repeated several times. Evaluation of the effectiveness of communication at frequent intervals is a good way to determine the best pace for the patient.

**Cultural considerations.** Culture directly influences behaviors and interpretations. Words and behaviors have meanings that vary among individuals and also among cultural groups. Each of us learns to express ourselves in a family unit, which reflects a larger cultural group experience. For example, visitors notice a health care team enter the rooms of two patients. After the team leaves the first room the person is hysterical and sobbing. After they leave the second room the patient is quiet and subdued. From the patients' reactions the observers could not know that each person had just been informed of the same serious diagnosis. Pain or anxiety may be communicated to the nurse differently by patients who are black, Hispanic, and Chinese. The nurse needs to be sensitive to the message and may need to elicit more information from the patient to clarify the message.

In recent years, efforts to improve cultural sensitivity and increase knowledge about diverse groups and their values have greatly benefited nursing practice. However, in the case of disadvantaged minorities, it is possible to be culturally sensitive but to lack the skills essential for dealing with the patient's health needs. Persons of disadvantaged ethnic or social groups have complex problems requiring interventions from highly skilled professionals. Many minority groups suffer from inadequate health services because the professionals who care for them are ill prepared to cope with high-risk, vulnerable patients with complex illnesses. Focusing exclusively on an understanding of culture compromises the care these patients receive (American Indian Physicians, 1988). A culturally sensitive approach would allocate expert resources and technologies to compensate for the multiple forces of deprivation that interfere with achievement of good health.

**Kinesic considerations.** Kinesics is the study of body movements. *Body language* is a popular term that reminds us that facial expressions, eye movements, gestures, and mannerisms have meaning. Facial expressions have been called the "language of emotion" (Havens, 1986). In certain cultures body language is used to indicate a person's feelings. Gaze aversion is often used to disengage or avoid communication. Crossing the arms over the chest occurs many times when a person feels defensive. However, this also occurs many times when a person is cold. It is important that the nurse be sensitive to these cues and interpret them in a global context of the therapeutic communication. If the message seems inconsistent or confusing, exploring the meaning of body language may be useful. For example, the nurse might say, "Many times when people back away from a person, they do it because they are afraid. Is there something that makes you fearful?" For many of us, body language sometimes communicates our feelings and sometimes merely reflects a habit. The nurse must become aware of her own "body habits" and consider possible meanings associated with these behaviors. Behaviors that communicate caring, confidence, and calmness should be cultivated. Sensitivity and understanding of kinesics is important in interpreting messages from a patient but should be viewed as cues rather than as diagnostic.

## THERAPEUTIC TECHNIQUES

Therapeutic techniques are a means of helping patients and not ends in themselves. Techniques are used to accomplish therapeutic goals. Careful consideration should be given to the choice of a technique. Selection of any method should be based on goals and should not be made indiscriminately. The techniques presented in Box 5-1 are arranged according to the steps of the nursing process, which they tend to facilitate. Some techniques may be versatile enough to be used in more than one step.

### Speech patterns

The simplest form of interpersonal speech, the declarative sentence, can evoke feeling:

> "It was a nice day in August."
> "No, it was raining."

The statement was made, and the patient was stimulated to add, correct, or erase.

The most powerful form of verbal communication is the statement of fact or possibility. One does not have to be correct to evoke responses, i.e., the intent may be to jog the memory, as multiple-choice questions do. A statement can put shy or suspicious persons at ease, so they do not feel pressured. The nurse should realize that even the most tactful question in the world is still inquisitive and requests an answer. Questions, which students are prone to overuse, can be balanced by a simple declarative statement.

*Reflection* is a technique in which the nurse restates or repeats the patient's statement. This method can encourage clarification or continuation of the same thoughts. If the nurse is uncertain about the message or feels a need to focus on understanding a particular thought, it may be helpful to ask the patient to clarify. The nurse can simply state "This is what I understand you to be saying    " and allow the patient to clarify in his or her own manner. Feedback and reinforcement are similar techniques. *Feedback* is any response to a sender of a message. *Reinforcement* is a message, by word or action, that gives approval and encouragement. When a patient expresses his feelings about a situation, the nurse can offer reinforcement—for example, by nodding, by acknowledging that putting feelings into words helps in coping with those feelings, or by reflecting the statement. These techniques can be overdone, and the nurse should never become so preoccupied with her own use of words that she becomes more interested in her own remarks than in the patient's.

## Rhythms

The identification of rhythms or themes is important. There is a mutual integration of the clinical situation with professional theories and techniques (Margulies and Havens, 1981). The repetition of words, phrases, and behaviors may form patterns that reveal the inner (intrapsychic) and outer (interpersonal) worlds (Zinberg, 1987). This takes time and comes only a little more quickly with experience.

Everyone is familiar with the hocus-pocus jokes about psychotherapists who can discern a person's entire childhood history from that person's description of an episode of indigestion. One should not accept superficial intellectualizations as an authentic representation of understanding. "Parlor psychiatry" makes quick and facile connections without understanding patterns, rhythms, and content of patient relationships (Zinberg, 1987). A purpose of therapeutic communication is to comfort by our presence, not to startle by our great insights. In clinical settings in which interpretation is emphasized, "a patient may wait for the next insight with fists clenched; small wonder, for it is rarely good news" (Havens, 1986). Interaction with the patient involves the subtle establishment of boundaries through rhythms. The patient's words or silence forms patterns. The identification of themes and rhythms frames a foundation for a gradual, thorough understanding of patient needs.

## Summarizing

Another skill useful in therapeutic communication is the ability to summarize. Summarizing involves the selection of important points that have been recognized, distilling them, and possibly even linking them to points that have arisen in previous communications. "Listing" ("there seem to be three major areas in which you have difficulty") helps to maintain focus. Summaries are customary at the conclusion of therapeutic communication but may also be helpful during a conversation to aid the nurse in guiding a discussion into productive arenas.

## Advice

Although early psychoanalysts frowned on the giving of advice to patients, many contemporary therapists often find the giving of advice to be valuable. The professional gives advice based not on his own values, needs, and aspirations but on informed knowledge of a situation (Winston et al., 1986). The rationale for advice should be made explicit—not "You should go to AA!" but rather "You ought to go to AA because most people in your circumstances have a better chance of staying sober with AA." When a professional is consulted by a patient who becomes disorganized in response to minimal stress and the professional tells her to first get dressed and then straighten her home, he or she is providing structure and help with routine. Many times patients want to depend on a professional. Requests for advice are usually best handled by helping the patient consider alternatives, keeping in mind that patients, like all of us, have many reasons for rejecting advice (Winston et al., 1986). A good rule is to avoid pointing out to people something that is painfully obvious; if patients were prepared to see the obvious, they would (Zinberg, 1987).

## Objectivity

For the comfort of both patient and nurse the professional should be considered invulnerable in the psychological sense; that is, the patient can say wounding, hurtful things or express undying affection or gratitude without fear of reprisal or acceptance. Few things are more destructive than the patient's perception that a professional is weak in the sense that he or she takes the patient's feelings at face value and is directly affected by them. The capacity to remain objective by no means represents infallibility. A professional who never says anything wrong is not doing enough.

Often patients (and occasionally nurses) want to believe that the unusual frankness in the therapeutic relationship is directly transferable to social situations (Zinberg, 1987). It is not. Therapeutic communication is unique in this respect.

## Confidence

Mental disorder or distress is a situation that needs a calm, confident, professional approach. Short, simple sentences with eye contact and awareness of one's own body language are useful in conveying confidence. A slow, low-pitched voice sets a tone of control. Identify yourself. Actions such as hands on hips, arms tightly folded, hesitant speech, or an uncertain attitude undermine the goal of organizing energies to focus on the patient's problems. The nurse may give information, explain, reflect, clarify, reassure, orient, and observe signs and symptoms as she establishes an atmosphere of confidence for the patient (Kendrick and Webber, 1986).

## Record keeping

Although record keeping may not be thought of as communication and often is burdensome, therapeutic communication is most effective when adequate record keeping is maintained. Besides providing other professionals with a progressive account of the patient, records assist the nurse to organize and understand dimensions of communications that may not have been evident as the transaction occurred. Computer technology has improved record keeping by permitting easy cross referencing and information retrieval. Computers have even been used as therapy for depression by focusing patients' attention on an activity and increasing their self-esteem (Kane, 1989). (See discussion of written patient assessments in Chapter 6.)

# COMMON OBSTACLES TO THERAPEUTIC COMMUNICATION

In the same manner that therapeutic communication moves the patient toward a goal, certain messages create barriers to reaching that goal. Several barriers occur frequently because of lingering nervous mannerisms or carryover of social expectations to the therapeutic situation. It is the nurse who must recognize and overcome any habitual communication obstacle that could interfere with effective therapeutic communication. Therapeutic communication involves the use of oneself. Thus many personal feelings are evoked that can be personally disturbing for the new nurse.

It is not unusual for the student or the new clinician to experience fear when she is communicating with people experiencing severe psychic or physical stress. Fear compromises therapeutic communication. The nurse may become preoccupied with or worried about such questions as "Could this be me? My brother does this sometimes; does that mean he's crazy? What if this patient gets angry with me?" Therapeutic communication relies on the resolution of most of these issues. College students and those establishing new nursing careers have possibly had little time for introspection. Even if it is "integrated" into a curriculum, self-examination becomes only another task. It is imperative, however, that the psychiatric nurse anticipate and understand her personal values and vulnerabilities. This is accomplished over time and, ideally, under the supervision of nurses who are sensitive to the evolution of self-awareness. The new nurse can profit not only from analyzing technique and content from patient interactions but also from analyzing her own feelings that accompany the interactions. (See Chapter 7, "Working with the Aggressive Patient," for further discussion on self-awareness.)

## Nurses' insecurity

Often nurses erect obstacles to communication because they feel insecure. In an attempt to achieve security, the nurse may assume a parent type of role toward the patient. Emrich (1989) reports that many staff-patient interactions are parental, illness maintaining, and disconfirming. Parental responses can be manifested by remarks that are *consistently* nurturing, critical, or condescending. A nurse generally falls into one of these three patterns and avoids the feelings of insecurity for herself. However, it is clear to experienced nurses that any of these patterns impede the patient's progress toward understanding and coping.

## Inappropriate responses

The nurse's response to a message should be based on assessment and knowledge of the situation. It is particularly common for inexperienced nurses to act on assumptions that reflect social rather than therapeutic standards. The inexperienced nurse may withdraw from the patient who is angrily cursing rather than confront him with his behavior, or she may become caught up in the fears and accusations of a paranoid patient and thereby reinforce the symptoms handicapping the patient. Nervous laughter and inappropriate smiles are not uncommon when a nurse is uncomfortable with a situation. New or unsympathetic persons will occasionally laugh when listening to distressed patients. They are being antipathetic; that is, they have uttered the sound farthest removed from the patient's expression. This can be compared to the patient who laughs at a point of distress to establish distance from himself by failing to empathize with himself (Havens, 1986). Inappropriate responses create an obstacle to therapeutic communication, which exists to help the patient improve his mental health.

Another common obstacle is *evasion* or avoidance of direct discussion of a topic that is introduced or implied. This occurs often in social communication, where some subjects are taboo and especially where pursuing a line of thought would embarrass or provoke unpleasant feelings. It is often necessary to pursue such subjects to ascertain the history or the present emotional forces of the patient. Standard social responses to cliches can interfere with therapeutic communication. It is common for a patient to say to a nurse, "I have to tell you something very important if you promise not to tell anyone." This may be a promise that cannot be kept. Nurses should not get involved with bargaining (Kendrick and Webber, 1986). Even "therapeutic" skills can be abused. The nurse may become preoccupied with what she wants to say next instead of listening to the patient. Silence is an important therapeutic skill, but one that can be overdone, particularly if the nurse "puts" the patient in charge of pacing to avoid the responsibility herself.

Inappropriate apologies, such as "I'm sorry to call you, doctor, but your patient is having a crisis," do not accurately represent the message a nurse may want to get across. Tentativeness is a similar problem. "I sort of need to take your blood pressure" or "I think your doctor wants you to take this medication" does not clearly communicate that these activities are crucial to the patient's well-being. Habitual trailing sentences are often a problem. Sometimes this may be done therapeutically for effect to evoke response from a patient, but it is often a mannerism that implies insecurity. Poor grammar, such as the use of double negatives, can confuse communication between the patient and the nurse.

## THERAPEUTIC COMMUNICATION ISSUES

Several therapeutic models emphasize or endorse particular therapeutic communication skills. Each formulates techniques that use these skills in various degrees or sequences. The models may reflect different philosophies about treatment or may be used effectively for certain patient problems more than for others. Certain issues are fundamental to therapeutic communication: setting limits, listening, power, goal-directed communication, and dealing with conflict.

### Setting limits

Therapeutic communication is structured by setting limits. Rules and boundaries form this structure. Honesty, appropriate means of expression, and confidentiality are examples of this structure. Above all, therapeutic communication strives to *avoid pretense.* Honesty is a fundamental ground rule. The professional should not agree, as people so regularly do in ordinary social situations, in order to avoid conflict. It can be important to ask questions or seek definitions. In social communication, being agreeable is important to intimacy and getting along. Being agreeable is not necessarily therapeutic. A patient should be able to express frustration and anger, but within the boundaries established by the professional. Striking out or threatening is outside the limits of therapeutic communication. The professional therapeutic relationship is not lost, limited, or terminated by disagreement. The patient may reveal serious problems, knowing that the professional will remain constant in caring for him even when not agreeing with him

## Listening

One of the most important therapeutic communication skills is listening. To the beginning professional this hardly seems like a skill. However, listening with only deliberate thoughtful interjections is very different from listening in social communication. Here most of the "action" seems to be coming from the patient. Listening involves careful attention to words and behaviors, with responses that encourage the patient to continue in avenues that will be productive in terms of insight, information, or problem solving. It is actually one of the most difficult skills to master because therapeutic listening is not passive, serving merely as a sounding board, but is active in that the nurse is engaged to the point that she can guide a conversation in a certain direction with but few words. Listening is hard work. Concentration is certainly a skill that is refined with experience. A professional becomes more and more sensitive and quick to recognize important cues.

When one is highly attuned to the patient through therapeutic listening, the use of adjectival exclamations as punctuation marks ("awful!" "wonderful!") may be useful. Impersonal comments, such as "how wonderful!" or "terrible," can be used to convey acceptance. These statements imply support rather than ascribe an expressed state to the patient. Empathy may lead a nurse further to state, "I feel terrified when I realize what you were experiencing" instead of stating, "You feel terrified." When we empathize we reduce the patient's burden of feeling (Havens, 1986). The language of empathy moves a nurse into the patient's space. This is noninvasive if empathy is accurate, if it is the patient's feeling that is experienced and not the nurse's feeling. Empathy aims at merger or identity with feelings rather than working at a distance. Identity of feelings allows the nurse to understand the patient without taking on the same feelings. It is appropriate at times, however, to draw back a bit and not attend too intently. If the nurse senses she is losing her objectivity, she has crossed over from empathy to sympathy and needs to draw back.

## Power

Mental illness is a particularly powerful emotional force. Power can only be opposed powerfully. Therefore a professional must have power and use it (Havens, 1986). The patient's progress is impeded if the nurse seems unwilling to use her resources to help him. Disclaimers such as "we all have equal power on this unit" are confusing. Slogans like this have a nice appeal, but nurses do make decisions for patients at times. Neither the patient nor the professional should overwhelm the other.

## Goal-directed communication

Guidance toward a goal is a hallmark of therapeutic communication that requires a mastery of abilities and considerable experience. A nurse draws on much knowledge to know what information to elicit for a competent assessment and diagnosis. It takes much practice to comfortably use words that evoke responses from patients.

One technique is to use open-ended questions rather than to phrase queries in such a way that they can be answered "yes" or "no." Goal-directed communication sets the stage for rapid development of the therapeutic process (Carmona, 1988). A general goal always is to facilitate help-seeking behaviors and to mitigate obstacles to normal growth (Ursano and Halen, 1986). At times guidance means that the nurse places herself in the background to facilitate the patient's growth (Sandman, Norberg, and Adolfsson, 1988).

## Conflict

It is not unusual for any nurse, but especially one who works with mentally ill or troubled persons, to find herself in a conflict situation. Patient agitation levels decrease if the patient senses that the nurse is calm and confident (Kendrick and Webber, 1986). It is important to discuss with the patient the cause of the agitation, and this is most easily accomplished with quiet, firm direction. Conflict between staff members may occur more often in environments with strong emotional undertones, and the same methods should be applied in these situations to resolve problems.

## KEY CONCEPTS

1. Therapeutic techniques are skills to help people, not goals in themselves.
2. Therapeutic communication occurs with a plan and a purpose, whereas social communication involves equal levels of intimacy and opportunity for spontaneity.
3. Therapeutic communication differs from social communication because it focuses on the patient rather than on the "give-and-take" experience.
4. Goals of psychiatric nursing are to understand the patient, to assure that he can understand the nurse, and to teach more effective communication skills.
5. These goals are accomplished as the nurse permits the patient to express widely divergent emotions while demonstrating a stable affect and sense of direction.
6. It is important to balance several issues in therapeutic communication so as to achieve an appropriate working distance without creating an artificial atmosphere.
7. Therapeutic techniques avoid pretense by clearly establishing rules of honesty, boundaries for acceptable behavior, and a sense of purpose.
8. Listening is a therapeutic communication technique that requires careful concentration and limited thoughtful comments in order to guide the conversation toward a goal.
9. The client-centered approach attempts to elicit self-discovery, insight, and problem solving from the patient.
10. Professionals are responsible for the flow of therapeutic communication and must recognize communication barriers in order to use appropriate therapeutic techniques.
11. Some common obstacles that interfere with therapeutic communication are nervous mannerisms, evasion, and assumption of a parental role with the patient.

## REFERENCES

Carmona P: Changing traditions in psychotherapy, Clin Nurse Specialist 2(2):105, 1990.

Emrich K: Helping or hurting? Interacting in
the psychiatric milieu. J Psychosoc Nurs
27(12):26, 1989.

Farran CJ and Keane-Hagerty E: Communicating
effectively with dementia patients. J Psychosoc
Nurs 27(5):13, 1989.

Havens L: Making contact: uses of language in
psychotherapy. Cambridge, Mass., 1986, Harvard University Press.

Kane G: Computers and psychiatric clients.
J Psychosoc Nurs 27(3):12, 1989.

Keltner B and Gillett P: Family sculpture, J Nurs
Educ 23(8):361, 1983.

Kendrick DW and Webber G: When in seclusion,
Am J Nurs 86(10):1117, 1986.

Margulies A and Havens L: The initial encounter:
what to do first. Am J Psychiatry 138(4):421,
1981.

Moore L, Van Arsdale P, Gitterberg J, and Aldrich
R: The biocultural basis of health, Prospect
Heights, Ill., 1987, Waveland Press.

Pluckman M: Human communication: the ma-
trix of nursing, New York, 1978, McGraw-Hill
Book Co.

Sandman PO, Norberg A, and Adolfsson R: Verbal
communication and behavior during meals in
patients. J Adv Nurs 13:571, 1988.

Ursano R and Hales R: A review of brief
individual psychotherapies. Am J Psychiatry
143(12):1507, 1986.

Weiner M: Practical psychotherapy. New York,
1986, Brunner/Mazel.

Zinberg N: Elements of the private therapeutic
interview. Am J Psychiatry 144(12):1527,
1987.

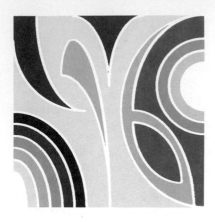

# The Nature of the Nurse-Patient Relationship

LEARNING OBJECTIVES
After reading this chapter you should be able to

- Outline Peplau's stages of the nurse-patient relationship.
- Describe what it means to be therapeutic.
- Describe the stages of a therapeutic nurse-patient relationship.
- Identify major tasks of each stage of the nurse-patient relationship.
- Recognize strategies of crisis intervention.
- Describe the relevance of common issues in the nurse-patient relationship.
- Recognize verbal strategies in interacting with patients.
- Relate nursing process to psychiatric nursing practice.
- Identify components of written patient assessments.

Hildegard Peplau defined nursing as "a significant, therapeutic, interpersonal process. . . . Nursing is an educative instrument, a maturing force, that aims to promote forward movement of personality in the direction of creative, constructive, productive, personal, and community living" (1952, p. 16).

## PEPLAU'S STAGES OF THE NURSE-PATIENT RELATIONSHIP

Peplau believed the nurse and the patient began as strangers and moved in stages to become collaborators in problem solving. Although stages in a nurse-patient relationship have been given various names by various authors, Peplau's concept and descriptions remain valid. In the *stage of orientation,* the patient feels a need and seeks help. The nurse helps the patient understand his problems and accept the help available. The nurse actively works to develop trust and the relationship itself. In the *identification stage,* there is clarification of perceptions and expectations about the relationship. There is further definition of problems and identification of tentative solutions. The nurse is alert to signs of dependence, independence, and interdependence. In the *exploration stage,* the patient becomes more motivated to use assistance from available resources in resolving problems. The patient may engage in testing of the nurse and may fluctuate between dependence and independence. Peplau believed the *resolution stage* needed close attention to avoid destroying the benefits gained from the relationship. Focus is on the growth that occurred and on helping the patient develop self-responsibility for setting new goals. The entire relationship is seen as growth promoting and as a learning experience for nurse and patient (Peplau, 1952).

Peplau (1952) proposed various roles as applications of Sullivan's work (see Chapter 2): as a *resource* person, the nurse provides information; as a *counselor,* she helps patients explore feelings and problems; as a *surrogate,* she helps them examine old feelings about past relationships; and as a *technical expert,* she coordinates professional services available to the patients. Peplau also described how nurses could be participant observers and show acceptance, listening skills, clarification, interpretation, and consensual validation in relating to patients.

## BEING THERAPEUTIC

Many factors influence the relationship between a nurse and a patient, and various therapeutic activities can be used within the relationship to facilitate successful patient adaptation. Behavioral theory perspectives provide a background for discussion of patient needs, types of nurse-patient contacts, and duration of the relationship. No single theoretical model is effective with every patient, in every situation, or with every kind of problem. Each model has value for selected patients and problems. Even patients with the same psychiatric diagnosis will have somewhat different manifestations of symptoms, given their unique history, current life situation, and emerging needs. Each patient is a unique, worthwhile, holistic being struggling with internal needs and external realities. By relating individually to each patient, the nurse employs selected strategies to help the patient cope with needs and struggles.

The nurse's relationship with a patient comprises a series of goal-directed interactions in which the nurse uses verbal and nonverbal communications to convey a willingness to listen, a genuine respect for the patient, a desire to help, and an understanding of the patient as a person, his problems, and his needs (Strupp, 1973). Nursing process is the tool with which the nurse assesses patients' problems, selects interventions, and evaluates the effectiveness of care. In psychiatric nursing, nursing process is grounded in knowledge of the nature of therapeutic relationships, concepts and processes of psychopathology, milieu management, and psychopharmacology (Keltner, 1985). A nurse's basic education provides the knowledge and skills for being therapeutic in encounters with patients; special training as a psychotherapist is not required.

Psychotherapists receive specialized training, generally focused on a particular therapy model that attempts to explain the causes of mental illness and offers specialized techniques for achieving patient outcomes. Psychotherapists are more interested in formalized, ongoing sessions than they are in brief therapeutic encounters. Sessions have a specified time, place, and length and a designated fee. Psychotherapists are selective in their choice of patients and are restrictive in that they have rules for conducting sessions.

In contrast, nurses engaging in therapeutic activities, especially in an inpatient setting, recognize that each encounter with a patient is part of an overall therapeutic picture: a therapeutic milieu (Keltner, 1985). Patients discuss real problems and practical solutions and practice skills needed in real-life situations in preparation for their return to the community. Brief encounters offer an opportunity to process feelings and thoughts as they occur to the patient. Validation and feedback are available quickly. Many patients are unable to tolerate intense, ongoing therapy but can benefit from consistent therapeutic encounters with one or more nurses, even if the hospitalization lasts only a few days.

## THERAPEUTIC RELATIONSHIPS

Although not so formalized as therapy, brief therapeutic relationships are planned, patient centered, and goal directed. The nurse purposefully and carefully guides the conversations toward the patient's exploration of problems, issues, and needs and then selects therapeutic strategies to facilitate awareness, decisions, changes, or comfort. Along with showing concern, compassion, and interest, the nurse maintains an objectivity that the patient may lack. The nurse may share some personal data, such as age, marital status, or title, but rarely discloses personal problems. Occasionally a brief self-disclosure may help a patient clarify specific issues or feel more "normal." ("When I feel depressed, it's usually because I'm angry and not expressing it for some reason. Do you think you might be angry about something?" Or "Sometimes, I'm afraid to tell my husband something because I don't know how he will react. Is there anything that is hard for you to talk to your wife about?") Therapeutic self-disclosure facilitates patient comfort and openness but never burdens the patient with the nurse's problem.

Informal or recreational encounters with patients (card game, craft class, ward party) may be spontaneous but therapeutic. The nurse observes inappropriate social behaviors or lack of skills; then helps patients use their "free time" to develop social and verbal skills, to reality test, and to get feedback and support for new behaviors (Morris and Myton, 1986). Activities help patients reduce anxiety and body tension, develop a sense of competence, and engage in risk taking (Morris and Myton, 1986).

Encounters are opportunities to demonstrate ways of handling situations: "Well, we didn't win this hand, but I'm enjoying the game anyway." "I've made that mistake before too. I can show you how to correct it." "Everyone has a right to his or her opinion. I'll listen to yours and then you can hear mine."

The nurse-patient relationship is not a social relationship (see Chapter 5). A social relationship involves companionship, mutual support, intimacy, and equal disclosure of personal information. Although a nurse may relate informally with a patient, the maintenance of objectivity and goal directedness is crucial. Patients, especially those with a history of unsatisfying relationships with others, may misinterpret the nurse's interest and concern. Patients often ask (or wish to ask) the nurse to be a friend or to go out on a date. When this occurs, the nurse reminds the patient of her role and takes the opportunity to discuss the patient's need for friendship, love, and support.

## DEVELOPMENT OF A THERAPEUTIC RELATIONSHIP

Therapeutic relationships vary in depth, length, and focus. A brief therapeutic encounter may last only a few minutes, focusing on a patient's *immediate* need, *current feeling,* or an *observed behavior.* In contrast, in a long-term hospitalization or program the relationship may last 6 months or more, with weekly meetings focusing on underlying causes of behaviors, developmental issues, or long-term problems.

In an acute-care setting the patient relates to many nurses and staff members each day. In this situation, progress in a nurse-patient relationship is the responsibility of each nurse. One nurse admits the patient to the unit and begins the relationship. Another nurse may discharge the patient and complete the termination. In between, shift reports, care plans, and progress notes help each nurse work with the patient toward the same goals. This therapeutic relationship is generally described in terms of three stages of development: orientation, working, and termination.

### Orientation stage

The orientation stage involves learning about the patient and his initial concerns and needs. It also involves the patient's learning the role of the nurse. The patient is informed of the general purpose of talking with the nurses. The initial purpose may be stated as broadly as "identifying a problem you want to work on," "helping you figure out what has been happening to you lately," or "getting to know what has been bothering you." Once the patient's problems become more evident, the nurse collaborates with the patient to define a more specific area to pursue, such as learning to be assertive or processing feelings about a divorce. Then each nurse working with the patient focuses on some aspect of this goal.

It is important that each nurse let the patient know that she cannot solve problems or make decisions for him. The nurse can, however, ask questions to help the patient look at realistic options so he can make his own decisions.

In a longer-term relationship with one nurse, arrangements are made for when and where to meet, for how long, and how often. This might be for 45 minutes twice a week in an office off the unit. In brief encounters on a unit the nurse still needs to be aware of the need for privacy and should suggest moving to an un-crowded area to talk. It helps the patient to know how much time the nurse can spend with him (usually 30 minutes or less) and that the relationship will end at the time of the patient's discharge.

Regardless of the formality or length of the relationship, the nurse (each nurse) actively encourages the patient to feel comfortable in the relationship. Trustwor-thiness is shown by the nurse's being honest about intentions, being consistent, and keeping promises. Warmth, interest, and concern are conveyed with words and congruent body language. Clear, specific communications decrease confusion and suspiciousness. Confidentiality is explained in terms of patient information being shared *only* with the immediate unit staff who are involved in the patient's care.

Many patients are afraid or unable to approach the nurses, so reaching out and initiating conversations is important. Quiet, withdrawn patients often are overlooked because they cannot ask for assistance. A nurse's offer to listen and help conveys to the patient that he is a worthwhile person who is respected.

Initially the nurse is nonconfrontational, in that she does not openly challenge what the patient is saying. That would interfere with trust and with data collection. (Supportive confrontation is discussed in the working stage.)

**Beginning assessment.** The initial sessions with the nurse (or nurses), in-cluding the intake interview, provide an opportunity for a beginning assessment of the patient's needs, coping strategies, defenses (mental mechanisms), and adaptation styles (Keltner, 1985). The patient's recurring thoughts, feelings, and behaviors are clues to problem areas. It is important to assess the degree of awareness of problems and the ability or motivation to change. Although assessment is ongoing and pro-gressive over time, tentative goals are based on the most immediate needs or prob-lems. (For many facilities, the initial care plan must be written within 24 hours of admission.)

Between interviews, there are many opportunities to observe the patient and his behaviors in activities, during meals, with other patients during free time, and at medication times. The family may contribute information as well. Assessment tools may be used. (See Appendix C for examples of formal assessment tools.)

**Management of emotions.** When patients are admitted, they typically are experiencing painful emotions, such as fear, grief, anger, ambivalence, confusion, shame, embarrassment, or guilt. They are often afraid of losing control of themselves or of being viewed as weak for expressing feelings. Nurses sometimes are unsure how to handle patients' feelings. A way to keep feelings from escalating is to talk about them directly. Since the patient is likely to try to conceal or minimize feelings, the nurse must be alert to indirect references, nonverbal cues, and voice tones. The nurse can then identify the feeling and ask for validation: "I'm getting the impression you are angry. What are you feeling right now?"

In dealing with feelings, especially anger, it is helpful to remember that the feeling is created not by the nurse but by some situation or significant person in the patient's life. A patient may displace anger onto the nurse at first. However, if confronted with the anger, the patient is more likely to recognize the real source and decrease this projection. Patients need to understand that feelings are natural but that the way they are expressed can cause a problem. Belittling or minimizing a patient's emotions is inappropriate, as is false reassurance, such as "Everything will be alright." In fact, the patient may feel worse for a while as he begins to face his emotions; thus such reassurance is dishonest as well as inappropriate.

Conveying empathy is a way of helping patients deal with emotional pain. Empathy is an objective understanding of how the patient feels or sees his situation. Empathy comes from actively listening to the patient's perspective about his experiences. Empathy conveys a hope for improvement: "I hear how painful this is for you and would like to try to help you deal with the situation in a productive way." With sympathy, the nurse feels the same feelings as the patient, and the objectivity is lost. Sympathy often leads to comforting or reassuring the patient or to pity for the patient. Either way, the outcome for the patient is a sense of "poor me, I have a right to stay this way." This is not to say that sympathy is always inappropriate; people who do share a mutual loss will experience mutual sympathy.

Once a patient is able to talk directly about emotions, the focus can be on coping more effectively with them. In the orientation stage it is not possible to resolve the problem creating the feelings, but it is possible to temporarily reduce the feelings to a tolerable level by using palliative coping mechanisms. Explaining the experiences and feelings to an empathetic listener helps, but if ventilation intensifies the feelings, distracting the patient from that topic may be necessary for a while. Adequate rest and nutrition reduce the impact of tension on the body. Physical exercise and relaxation techniques also alleviate some of the tension a patient may be feeling. Although palliative mechanisms are less desirable than adaptive ones in the long run, the goal at this stage is to prevent loss of control or total retreat from pain.

**Providing support.** As with empathy, support begins in the orientation stage and continues throughout the relationship with a patient. Support confirms the patient's worth and rights as a human being. This includes avoiding value judgments of the person (as bad, stupid, crazy, lazy), even if the patient has made poor choices. It acknowledges that no one is perfect and that making mistakes is human. Learning from mistakes is beneficial. Support focuses realistically and concretely on the patient's abilities and strengths: not "You're a good person," but "I like the way you helped that other patient find his room." Patients need recognition of their healthy actions and feelings. A patient's dependence is tolerated until he is capable of being more independent, but any independent actions are pointed out. Support includes realistic hope and promises, such as "I don't have an answer right now, but I will work with you to find one."

**Providing structure.** A major strategy in the orientation stage is providing structure for the patient. If the patient is losing control of his thoughts, feelings, or behavior, the nurse has the responsibility of taking temporary control. This may mean offering a p.r.n. medication, directing the patient to a quieter, less stimulating place, or staying with the patient at a comfortable distance. If these measures are not effective, seclusion or restraints may be indicated. In contrast, providing structure also includes decreasing the withdrawal and isolation of a quiet, nonparticipating patient. Spending time with this patient, even in silence at times, is important. The nurse can also suggest activities, such as watching television or taking a walk together.

A major facet of providing structure is *limit setting*. (See also Unit IV, "Milieu Management.") It is in the patient's best interest to decrease or stop dysfunctional behaviors. The nurse accepts the patient as a person while discouraging self-defeating behaviors. The patient's rights and self-esteem need protection, but so do those of others around the patient. Limit setting involves pointing out the behavior and its negative effect and suggesting an alternative behavior. For example, if the patient is self-deprecating, the nurse points out the patient's negative comments and how they affect his feelings about himself and suggests that the patient point out something positive about himself.

The behaviors that typically need immediate intervention are verbal and physical aggression, self-destructive behaviors, fire setting, noncompliance with rules and medications, alcohol or drug use, manipulation of others, inappropriate touching of others, indecent exposure, attempts to leave the hospital without permission, and failure to eat or sleep. Continuous rumination over painful feelings or disturbed thought processes is nonproductive and self-perpetuating. The nurse listens to the content and the process of negative feelings or delusions long enough to understand the messages or themes conveyed, but then she begins to distract the patient to more productive topics. Limit setting is a kind but firm strategy: "I know you are angry right now, but I'm having trouble understanding the situation because of all the swearing; please try to stop." Or, "I realize these thoughts are really important to you, but there are other areas I need to know about so I can help you."

The transition from the orientation stage to the working stage is not smooth or firmly defined. The patient's anxiety may increase when he is working on issues, and he may return to more superficial matters for awhile.

## Working stage

When the strategies of the orientation stage are successful and the patient is ready, the work toward behavior change can begin. However, change may not be the goal for some patients, especially the chronically ill. Instead, stabilization on medications, reduction of symptoms, and development of supportive relationships in and outside of the hospital are valid goals. Especially for patients with chronic schizophrenia, the ability to relate to someone is an important goal (Goering, 1988). For other patients there is enough awareness, motivation, and trust in the nurses to begin to explore problems, identify possible solutions, and test out new behaviors.

The process of changing behavior is difficult. Peplau (1963) identified the process of learning as necessary for change (see Table 6-1). The first step of *observation* is a prerequisite, since without awareness of a problem there is no motivation to change. The way the nurse knows how well a patient understands his problems is to ask the patient for in-depth, detailed descriptions of situations, thoughts, feelings, and behaviors. The *analysis* step is then necessary to encourage accuracy in the patient's conclusions about the problems. It is one thing for a patient to describe

**TABLE 6-1**   Questions to facilitate patient learning

| Steps of learning* | Process | Types of questions |
|---|---|---|
| **ASSESSMENT** | | |
| Observation | Awareness | • Who? What? Where? When?<br>• What did you (they) say (or do)? |
| Description | Sequence and completeness | • What happened when . . . ?<br>• Then what happened?<br>• Tell me about . . . . |
| **NURSING DIAGNOSIS** | | |
| Analysis | Accuracy in conclusions | • What did you think about . . . ?<br>• What is the connection between . . . ?<br>• What happens each time . . . ? (How?) (Why?) |
| Interpretation | Meaning and importance | • What bothers you about . . . ?<br>• What kind of problem is it to . . . ?<br>• How serious do you think . . . is for you?<br>• How relevant is . . . ? |
| **PLANNING** | Problem solving and choosing actions | • What needs to change? In what ways?<br>• What would work better?<br>• What are the advantages and disadvantages of . . . ?<br>• What might happen if you . . . ?<br>• What will help you try . . . ?<br>• What concerns you about trying . . . ? |
| **IMPLEMENTATION (testing out)** | Trying new thinking, feeling, behavior | Practice in role play<br>Practice in real situation |
| **EVALUATION** | Repeat the assessment and nursing diagnosis steps | See questions above |

*The Steps of Learning were originally identified by H.E. Peplau in *Some Clinical Approaches to Psychiatric Nursing,* edited by Burd, S.E., and Marshall, M.A. Toronto; 1963. The Macmillan Co.

the type and sequence of arguments he has with his wife; it is another process to conclude that he is afraid of losing control over his wife. Even when a patient is able to identify the problem accurately, he may not automatically decide his behavior is worth changing. The *interpretation* step leads to a decision that change is necessary and appropriate.

Problem solving is the crux of the *planning* step. Patients are guided in decisions about change, in developing and considering alternative solutions, and in formulating a method for carrying out the plan. The *testing-out* step involves actually trying the new behavior or solution in a safe environment with the nurse and then in a real situation. The nurse can ask the patient to rehearse what he will say and do in an upcoming situation: "Tell me what you will say to your daughter this weekend." Practice allows the patient to get feedback and modify his plan. Role playing is another way of practicing behaviors. The nurse plays the role of the person with whom the patient is having difficulty. The nurse assesses the patient's communications and behaviors and helps him handle the situation effectively.

Feedback is part of the step of *evaluating* the success of new behaviors or solutions to problems. The objective is to determine whether modification or a different approach is needed. The nurse gives feedback in a constructive manner and helps the patient learn to ask for and use feedback appropriately. Effective behaviors are more likely to continue if their benefits are discussed and reinforcement is given. Destructive behaviors are more likely to be identified if the patient is taught to evaluate the effect of his actions on himself and others.

**Data collection.**  Nurses facilitate awareness, analysis, and interpretation by in-depth but selective exploration of issues and by identifying priority issues. Patients may be overwhelmed by focusing on too many problems at once. The nurse helps the patient make sense out of his confusion by directing the data collection and focusing on manageable and changeable issues. It is frustrating both to the patient and to the nurse to spend time and energy exploring an unchangeable problem, such as rehashing what the patient *could have* done to prevent the divorce instead of focusing on what he *can do* now to make new friends.

**Reality testing and cognitive restructuring.**  Reality testing is an important strategy in the analysis, interpretation, and planning phases. It helps the patient see reality more clearly and objectively where there may have been past distortions or inaccuracies. Reality testing is not a matter of arguing a point of view but of presenting one so the patient can consider another option. It is constructive, not destructive, feedback: "I know the voices seem real to you, but I don't hear any." "You make it sound as if all men are alike, and I don't see it that way."

The goal of reality testing is cognitive restructuring: helping the patient see other viewpoints that will help him adjust his view to be more realistic. The patient might need to redefine how he interpreted a situation or change his perception of another person's behavior (Takla, 1985). He might need to give up an "irrational belief" in favor of a more rational one, such as changing from "I have to be perfect" to "It's OK to make mistakes; I can learn from them." It could also mean giving up an unrealistic goal for a more appropriate one. At times the redefinition involves discovering that anger is really fear.

**Supportive confrontation.**  Supportive confrontation is similar to reality testing but has a broader focus than specific perceptions, interpretations, or feelings. It is aimed at contradictions, discrepancies, responsibility, accountability, independence, and behavioral change. It combines support with a push for constructive, productive action. The support acknowledges fears, pain, ambivalence, and how hard it is to change, while the confrontation includes hope and confidence that an action is possible.

- Giving up alcohol is a scary idea, but by participating in this program, you can get the information and support needed to do it.
- I hear your ambivalence, but taking the risk has much to offer.
- We all like to be taken care of once in a while, but making our own decisions helps our self-esteem.

Supportive confrontation challenges the patient to meet his own needs appropriately and to be accountable for his own feelings, behaviors, and decisions. Confrontation without support is generally perceived as an attack and is nonproductive. It is avoided because it is often what the patient has experienced from others at home, school, or work.

   **Promoting change.**  In addition to problem solving and supportive confrontation, there are other strategies to facilitate change. One is to change the balance of the risk/benefit ratio. Any change has a risk of failure, loss of a comfortable habit, potential rejection, or even creation of new problems. The potential benefits are growth, self-satisfaction, improved relationships, and a healthier self-esteem. Change is more likely if the risks are low and the potential for benefits is high. The nurse can help decrease the risks by discussing ways to overcome them. Short-term and long-term benefits also need to be discussed. Well-thought-out and rational decisions are more likely to result in change. Patient-initiated change with concrete plans and actions tends to be more successful than change imposed by others. Practicing or rehearsing with the nurse builds confidence for trying a new behavior with others. Support and acceptance of the change by the patient's friends and family will help. Support groups can be particularly useful. Timing of change is also an issue; the patient is more likely to change when he is ready and motivated. Pushing for change too quickly is frustrating for all concerned.

   **Teaching new skills.**  Wanting to change is not sufficient; one must know how to change. A patient cannot change from being passive to being assertive if he does not know what assertion is or sounds like. Skills that a nurse takes for granted may not have been learned by a patient. Common skills patients need to learn are relaxation; stress, conflict, and anger-management techniques; assertiveness; decision-making processes; and communication, social, and community living skills. At times the skill training must begin at a basic, concrete level. One patient's first exercise was to approach another patient and *read* from his 3 × 5 inch card: "Hi, my name is Bill, and I'm from Greenfield. What's your name?" Skills are taught in small steps with frequent intermittent opportunities for practice and feedback. Homework assignments can be used; for example, the nurse might suggest that between sessions the patient practice a particular skill and report the results at the next session.

### Termination stage

In inpatient settings and even in longer-term relationships the "work" and changes are rarely completed because patients are discharged or move and nurses change units or jobs. However, there are strategies that facilitate a healthy ending of the relationship for both the patient and the nurse. If all the nurses involved with the patient are not available to discuss termination, the one assigned to discharge the patient can implement the strategies.

**Evaluation (or summary) of progress.** The nurse guides the discussion to help the patient identify *for himself* the specific changes in thoughts, feelings, and behaviors that have occurred. Even small steps toward long-term goals are discussed. It is important to reinforce the changes and strengths of the patient. Areas or issues still needing work are outlined, but with the caution that the patient should not try to change everything at once. The patient is encouraged to set priorities for these issues and reasonable time frames for action.

**Synthesizing what has occurred.** Synthesizing focuses on the more indirect outcomes of the relationship, such as more open communications or more appropriate expression of feelings. As a result of the relationship, patients often feel more comfortable in initiating interactions, making requests, and expressing opinions, even if these were not discussed during the nurse-patient encounters. Increased participation and socialization need to be recognized as well. As the nurse points out the accrued benefits of the relationship, the patient is encouraged to form other relationships with future counselors and new friends.

**Referrals.** For problems that need continuing attention after discharge, referrals are made to appropriate resources, such as doctor's offices, clinics, self-help groups, or community agencies. The resources provide support and foster continued change.

**Discussion of termination.** Regardless of the length, frequency of contact, or intensity of the nurse-patient relationship, it is important to discuss the participants' reactions to it. Feelings may be positive, ambivalent, or negative, and they may vary in degree. The more superficial the relationship, the more likely the reactions will be mild. However, the relationship may mean more to the patient than it does to the nurse. Therefore this loss may be significant to the patient. Patients may experience anger or fear at not having the support and acceptance provided by the nurse. Some patients may even avoid any discussion of termination. Even so, the nurse should make an attempt to "make it official" by saying "goodbye" and stating her feelings about the relationship. She serves as a role model for the patient who is at the time unable to discuss termination. The feelings of the nurse are important and open to discussion (but not to the point of burdening the patient with the nurse's issues). The nurse may feel as if she is abandoning the patient, especially if trust building was difficult for the patient.

## CRISIS INTERVENTION

Crisis intervention does not fall into any one stage of the nurse-patient relationship, because it is appropriate at any time a crisis occurs, even in the inpatient setting. Any "stressful event or hazardous situation" has the potential for precipitating a crisis (Lindemann, 1956). A crisis differs from stress in that it results in a period of severe disorganization due to the failure of the individual's usual coping mechanisms or the lack of his usual resources. Feeling totally out of control of one's life is extremely disturbing and motivates the patient to escape the pain (Caplan, 1961).

## Individual reactions

The patient's anxiety generally rises to a severe or panic level during a crisis. There is a sense of overwhelming helplessness and hopelessness when nothing seems to be working. The patient may feel immobilized and either gives up or keeps trying the same, ineffective coping methods. A person in a crisis state needs and is generally receptive to help. During the period of disorganization there is a natural tendency to depend on others for guidance and assistance. (Trust is less of an issue at this time.) With the right kind of help at the right time, the patient can generally overcome the problem, regain equilibrium, and return to "normal" within 4 to 6 weeks. It is common for the patient to learn new coping skills, develop new or improved relationships with others, and begin functioning better than before the crisis occurred. This is the reason crisis is said to have growth-promoting potential (Aguilera and Messick, 1982).

The disorganization period of a crisis is so distressing that it cannot be tolerated emotionally or physically for more than 4 to 6 weeks. If the right kind of help is not available and the crisis is not successfully resolved in that time period, the person is likely to (1) become exhausted and physically ill, (2) adopt dysfunctional coping patterns that manage the intense feelings without solving the problems (become emotionally ill), or (3) attempt suicide to escape the pain. Dysfunctional patterns of coping tend to persist unless the person seeks intensive counseling for a prolonged time. It takes less time and is more effective to intervene *during* the crisis to *prevent* the development of dysfunctional coping patterns.

## Strategies of crisis intervention

Strategies of crisis intervention aim at dealing with the immediate cause and at bolstering emotional security rather than at underlying issues and long-term resolution (Aguilera and Messick, 1982). Emotion management and support are valuable parts of crisis intervention, preventing further decompensation or a suicide attempt. Pointing out irrational thought processes and supportive confrontation aid in moving the patient to immediate decisions and actions to relieve the immediate problem and the accompanying sense of helplessness. The patient may need kind, firm directions and assistance in finding external resources when he is feeling overwhelmed and immobilized. Alternate ways of coping are sought (Aguilera and Messick, 1982).

Working with a person in crisis is demanding and intense for a short period of time, usually a few days to a few weeks. Therefore it is essential to involve others who can be with and help the person. These others are taught to help and to find resources if they lack knowledge. As the crisis subsides, support persons and community resources continue to be important for assistance, especially since the risk of suicide can persist for 2 to 3 months after the crisis has abated. This period is valuable for counseling aimed at learning adaptive coping strategies.

## ISSUES IN THE NURSE-PATIENT RELATIONSHIP
### Violent behavior

In working with inpatients, nurses sometimes encounter concerns that result from and influence relationships with the patient. Fear of violent behavior and of being injured is of concern with the few patients who do not respond to the verbal diffusing of anger or who feel extremely threatened by staff (usually because of internal thought disturbances). There are precautions to take for protection:

- Stay out of striking distance (which also reduces the threat to the patient).
- Do not touch a patient without his approval.
- Do not go into a room alone with a patient until he is in control of his behavior and you know him fairly well.
- Sit by the door with the door opened until the patient is in control of his behavior.
- Change the topic temporarily if the patient's behavior is escalating.
- Leave the patient temporarily if he is agitated and asking to be left alone.
- Call for staff assistance if the patient is losing control.

(Chapter 7 discusses working with aggressive patients.)

### Invasion of privacy

Another concern at times is invasion of privacy. Psychiatric nurses investigate intensely personal areas of patients' lives, such as values, beliefs, feelings, intimate relationships, and sexuality. The focus may also be on legally sensitive areas, such as incest, spouse abuse, and drug use. Although these are areas patients need to work on, they are not easy to discuss. The nurse enhances the patient's ability to be open and honest by explaining about a sensitive area, by asking questions in a kind, matter-of-fact manner, and by reiterating a desire to help the patient.

### Saying the wrong thing

Sometimes a nurse is afraid of harming a patient by "saying the wrong thing." Patients do not "fall apart" or explode because of a single mistake by the nurse if the nurse's overall attitude is positive and helpful. However, patients are sensitive to malicious intent and rejection. The nurse's mistake can actually become a therapeutic encounter as the nurse becomes a role model in how to admit and apologize for a mistake. Patients often have trouble doing this with persons they care about. It is appropriate for the nurse to be honest about what she does not know (Morris and Myton, 1986) and to offer to seek out the information for or with the patient. It sometimes can be beneficial for a patient to teach a nurse something (for example, about the nuances of his illness or about a recreational game). The nurse then becomes a role model as a learner (Morris and Myton, 1986).

### Conflicting values

Occasionally conflicts arise between a nurse's and a patient's beliefs or values. Both can state their views in a discussion, but arguing is inappropriate. A better approach is to help the patient examine the effects or outcomes of his beliefs on his overall life, relationships, and happiness. The patient may believe he has the right to drink as much and as often as he wants because it is legal. He may need to look at the effects on his marriage, job, health, and economic status. It is not necessary to agree with or like every patient's beliefs, values, or behaviors to be an effective nurse. It is important for the nurse to be aware of her own stance on issues and to understand the patient's point of view *as he sees it.* There is no need for a patient to change a belief or a behavior if it is not causing problems for himself or others around him. Beliefs and behaviors that have positive effects need reinforcement.

## Collaboration

The axiom in nursing of involving the patient in his own care has relevance in psychiatric nursing as well. Patients have a right to make decisions about their care (Loomis, 1985). When a patient recognizes his problems and needs, desires to change, and asks for assistance, the nurse is able to collaborate with the patient on goals and plans for the changes. Collaboration generally produces more effective and longer-lasting change than does coercion or simple compliance (Shillinger, 1983). Unfortunately, there are instances when collaboration is not possible, such as when the patient denies having any problems and refuses help. When the patient has an obvious disturbance in thought processes (as with severe hallucinations or delusions), he may be incapable of collaborating in his care until these subside. At times the only goal a patient will agree to work on is "to get out of the hospital." This mutually agreed-on goal provides an opening for discussion of behavior changes necessary before discharge can occur.

## INTERACTIONS WITH SELECTED BEHAVIORS

Certain problem behaviors, such as anger and withdrawal, have already been discussed under the stages of the nurse-patient relationship. The purpose of this section is to discuss interventions with selected behaviors appropriate for brief encounters with patients. Longer-term interventions are discussed in the chapters dealing with the psychiatric disorders.

## Hallucinations

The initial approach with a patient who appears to be listening to or talking with "voices" is to comment on his behavior: "You look as if you are listening to something. What do you hear?" If the patient acknowledges hearing something the nurse cannot hear, the nurse can say, "I don't hear anything. Tell me what you hear." The early assessment of hallucinations is of the content of messages that reveal dynamics of the patient, such as themes of powerlessness, guilt, loneliness, or suicide. Once the content is known, there is no need to focus on the hallucinations; doing so could reinforce them: "I know the voices are important to you, but let's talk about your loneliness right now."

## Delusions

The initial approach with respect to delusions is clarification of meanings, such as, "Who do you think is trying to hurt you?" or "Tell me about this power you think you have." As with hallucinations, delusions are not discussed once the meanings are clarified. The underlying themes reflected in the delusions are more appropriately addressed in interventions, such as helping the patient who says she is a queen feel important in realistic ways.

### Incoherent speech patterns

Disturbed thought processes are evident in speech, and the approach is to try to clarify the meanings of the communications. However, the severely ill patient is unable to be more clear, and repeated questions will only increase his anxiety. Medications generally clear the thought disturbances within a week. Until then the nurse spends a short time with the patient regularly without pressuring or frustrating him.

### Manipulation

Common manipulations are for attention, sympathy ("poor me"), control, and dependence (for others to take responsibility). Often manipulation is not recognized until it has already "worked." Then the nurse may experience anger or embarrassment. The initial approach is to point out what is happening (or has happened): "I'm getting the feeling you would like me to tell you what to do. What scares you about this decision?" or "You are experiencing a lot of pain and would like me to relieve it for you. Let's talk about what *you* can do to relieve it." Limit setting is useful with manipulative patients. A power struggle with the patient is useless. Helping a patient relate effectively with others is more fruitful.

### Crying

Unless crying is a manipulative gesture or prolonged and unproductive, it should be allowed, even encouraged verbally and nonverbally. By saying, "It's OK to cry" or quietly offering a tissue, the nurse gives the patient permission to cry and relieves tension (McGreevy and Van Heukelem, 1977). Privacy should be provided. The nurse should be as quiet and unobtrusive as possible until the crying has ceased (McGreevy and Van Heukelem, 1977). Then the patient is offered an opportunity to talk about what precipitated the tears.

### Sexual innuendos or inappropriate touch

Patients generally stop these behaviors when asked and when they are reminded that they are inappropriate. The nurse then discusses the underlying need. If they do continue, the limit setting can be stronger: "I want to talk to you but not if you continue to touch me. If you don't stop, I will have to leave and come back later." It may also help to pair a sexually acting-out patient who has poor impulse control with a staff member of the same sex until he is further along in treatment.

### Uncooperativeness

According to Busch (1987), there may be at least three styles of the "noninvolved client":

1. **Resistant:** the patient who is afraid to face emotions, clings to his defenses, and is afraid to change.
2. **Reluctant:** the patient who was coerced or forced to get treatment and claims he does not need it (denial).
3. **Uncommitted:** the patient whose goals for treatment are incompatible with the treatment modality or the therapist's beliefs.

The approaches in brief encounters with each style are as difficult as the long-term approach. Listening, reflecting, and clarifying what is heard without pushing are appropriate for identifying the underlying causes of the misbehaviors (Smith, 1987). Then, as possible, the causes, fears, and outcomes of their behaviors are discussed. Trust is often an issue for these patients, so measures to increase trust plus much patience from the nurse will be needed.

## Depressed affect

When the patient is expressing sadness and a negative attitude about everything, the nurse sometimes experiences sadness and sympathy for the patient. Patience, frequent contact, and empathy are more appropriate. The patient's feelings are acknowledged, but rumination is discouraged. Personal hygiene and gradual involvement in activities are encouraged. Major decisions are postponed until emotions subside and thinking is more logical.

## Suspiciousness

When a patient is suspicious, he may be afraid of everyone, everything, and every interaction around him. It is therefore important to communicate clearly and congruently. Misinterpretations by the patient are clarified, but arguments over differences in opinion are avoided. Rationales or explanations for rules, activities, occurrences, noises, and requests are offered regularly. The patient's participation is encouraged but not forced in order to avoid increasing his fears.

## Hyperactivity

Excessive physical and emotional activity in a patient is upsetting to the staff, to other patients, and often to the patient himself. Even unintentionally the patient may harm himself or others (see previous discussion of violence). The patient needs to be in a quiet area with minimal auditory and visual stimulation. Physical activity, such as walking or using a stationary bicycle, may help drain excess energy. The nurse must remain calm, speak slowly and softly, and respect the patient's personal space. Directions are given in a kind, simple, but firm manner.

## Transference

Transference involves the unconscious emotional reaction a patient has in a current situation that is really based on old childhood relationships and experiences. An example would be the patient perceiving the nurse as feeling and acting as his mother did, regardless of how the nurse is really acting (Schroder, 1985). Transference may explain feelings patients exhibit that do not fit in the current context of a situation or that are out of proportion to the situation. The main issue of transference is the wish to be taken care of and to have needs met (Schroder, 1985). Transference may be severe in the form of delusions or may be more generalized, as in stereotyping of all males as aggressive and all females as submissive. Transference can be positive if the patient views the nurse as helpful and caring. Negative transference is more difficult to deal with because of the unpleasant emotions, such as anger and fear, that interfere with treatment (Schroder, 1985).

Nurses may experience transference reactions with patients, coworkers, and doctors. Guilt or anger about not helping a particular patient or anger toward a demanding patient may be an unconscious transference response (Schroder, 1985). Countertransference (reactions based on the nurse's past experiences) may occur in response to a patient's transference after a relationship is established. These feelings will interfere with the nurse's ability to be therapeutic. A positive reaction might lead to the nurse's being sympathetic and unable to confront the patient appropriately. A negative reaction could lead to avoidance or rejection of the patient. In either case, the nurse's behavior is not therapeutic.

The first intervention in brief encounters is to recognize the transference or countertransference. This is difficult because of the unconscious processes involved. Coworkers are more likely to recognize the phenomenon initially and give feedback to the nurse about it. Once the reaction is recognized, the nurse can seek assistance in examining the countertransference issues. The nurse needs to examine her feelings, reactions, and behaviors before she will be able to interact more appropriately with the patient. The transference reactions of the patient also must be examined gently but directly. The nurse must be open and clear about her genuine reactions when the patient is misperceiving her behavior. The nurse also states what she can and cannot do for the patient who is seeking to have his needs met by her. Limit setting is useful when the patient acts inappropriately toward the nurse. Redirection of needs to more appropriate persons can also be a helpful intervention. For example, "I can't be your girlfriend, but let's talk about who you can seek out as a girlfriend after discharge."

## NURSING PROCESS

In psychiatric nursing, use of the nursing process has the same goal as in other areas of nursing: "patient-centered, goal-directed action" (Van Servellen, 1982). Care is adapted to the patient's unique needs. Individualized care is first based on a detailed assessment of the patient.

*ASSESSMENT* On admission the assessment begins with an intake interview that includes an assessment of mental status (see Box 6-1). Some patients are too ill to participate in or complete this interview. In such cases as much as possible is gleaned from the behaviors exhibited. One can describe behaviors without knowing or identifying their causes (for example, anxiety level, degree of withdrawal, thought disturbances as reflected in speech, voice tone, and general appearance). Causes and dynamics can be elicited later in order to form a better basis for a treatment plan (Parsons, 1986). Even when the initial assessment is relatively complete, each encounter with the patient involves a continuing assessment, which may or may not be congruent with the initial assessment. No one acts or feels the same way 24 hours a day, 7 days a week. The ongoing assessment begins with an investigation of what the patient is saying or doing at the moment: "You have been sitting alone for awhile. What have you been thinking about? You mentioned being worried; what about?"

When the nurse decides to investigate a patient's behavior, it is valuable to explore the following:

- The context or situation that precipitated the behavior
- What the patient was thinking at the time
- What the patient was feeling then and now
- Whether the behavior makes sense in that context
- Whether the behavior was adaptive or dysfunctional
- How this episode fits with the total picture of the patient
- Whether a change is needed

*NURSING DIAGNOSIS* Nursing diagnoses, or a problem list, are based on conclusions about the dynamics of the patient's verbalizations and behaviors. Regardless of the format or style of nursing diagnosis expected in a particular setting, the diagnoses or list of problems should be specific and point to a desired patient outcome. "Ineffective coping with stress" gives little idea of what behavior needs to change. "Avoidance of decisions about housing because of divorce" gives a clearer indication of the issue on which the patient needs to work. Another nursing diagnosis model would state the same problem as "ambivalence due to divorce as evidenced by avoidance of decisions about housing." The more specific the diagnosis or problem statement, the more specific the goals will be.

*PLANNING* A goal specifies an adaptive behavior to be substitued for a dysfunctional one. It is unrealistic to expect a patient to change his negative self-esteem to a positive one during a short inpatient stay. A more realistic behavioral goal would be to ask the patient to write a list of his strengths, abilities, or positive qualities. This goal is achievable and measureable. Goals may be either short term or long term. Short-term goals are those achievable in perhaps 1 to 3 weeks, during an inpatient stay. Long-term goals relate to issues that require follow-up counseling after discharge. For example, a patient's short-term goal may be to identify her fears about relationships with men. The longer-term goal is to decide on ways of responding to potential dating situations that would decrease her fears and enable her to handle a dating situation.

*IMPLEMENTATION OR INTERVENTION* In the psychiatric setting nursing interventions involve few "hands-on" activities other than giving medications. Instead, the verbal strategies discussed in this chapter and in Chapter 5 are used to guide patients in solving problems for themselves. Psychiatric nurses primarily are facilitators and educators.

*EVALUATION* The more realistic and measurable the goals, the greater the likelihood the patient and the nurse will have a sense of progress. A major problem with evaluating care in psychiatric nursing is expecting too much change too soon. Especially in acute-care settings, it is difficult to see patients go home before "all their problems are solved." Even when short-term goals are met, the patient has other unsolved problems. If the short-term goals were related to learning better skills, such as communication, problem solving, and social skills, the patient will be able to continue his progress after discharge. The nurse also evaluates the quality of her interventions and her professional behaviors.

## WRITTEN PATIENT ASSESSMENTS
### Intake interview

Each psychiatric hospital, unit, clinic, and program has its own version of an intake or nursing assessment form, which usually includes a mental status assessment. Box 6-1 briefly outlines the typical components of an initial patient assessment.

Systems and medical problems are reviewed to identify the need for medical orders or special nursing care or diets; allergies are listed. Current medications with dosages, frequency, and time of last dose are important. Potential for withdrawal from medications or other drugs is a risk to be noted.

Since most facilities have an intake form or checklist, the results of the interview do not have to be written in a narrative form. There may be an expectation of summarizing the critical content in an admission note in the progress notes.

### Nursing care plans

The initial care plan may be updated at any time but begins with one or two behavior-oriented problems to be addressed immediately, such as suicide, aggression, self-mutilation, escape, withdrawal or isolation, delusions, hallucinations, impulsive or compulsive acts, suspiciousness, uncooperativeness, or altered thought processes. Updated care plans are often developed by the treatment team, which may include the psychiatrist, nurses, social worker, psychologist, activity therapists, and nutritionist.

### Progress notes

The form of charting in progress notes (Box 6-2) varies in each setting, but the components are basically the same.

Charting is an important way to communicate with team members so that care is consistent and goal directed. Charting is also a way of evaluating the effectiveness of treatment plans (Parsons, 1986).

### Process recording

Peplau used process recordings in her writings to show applications of concepts and examples of interventions. She emphasized the use of communication skills as the means to help patients learn and solve problems. Process recordings are a tool for learning about effective work with patients. They provide a means of assessing and analyzing communication skills, identifying patient themes, and evaluating the effectiveness of interventions. Audio- or videotape recordings are more accurate but are not usually possible in most settings or with many patients. Written process recordings may begin with notes taken during the interview or may be done totally by recall afterward.

Box 6-1
## INITIAL PATIENT ASSESSMENT

**Demographic data:** Full name, sex, age, date of birth, address, marital status, family members' names and ages, and sometimes religious preference.

**Admission data:** Date and time of admission and whether the patient is admitted voluntarily or under a type of commitment procedure.

**Reason for current admission:** The current problems as perceived by the patient include stressors, difficulty with coping, and any "emergency behaviors," such as suicidal ideas or attempts, aggression toward others, destructive behaviors, or escape risk.

**Previous psychiatric history:** Dates, reasons for admissions, and types of treatment and their effectiveness.

**Drug and alcohol use/abuse:** Amount, frequency, and duration of use, past and present, of legal and illegal substances.

**Disturbances in patterns of daily living:** Sleep, intake and elimination, sexual activity, work, leisure, self-care, hygiene.

**Support systems:** Amount of contact with others, types of relationships, availability of support.

**General appearance:** Type and appearance of clothing, cleanliness, physical condition, posture.

**Behaviors during the interview:**
- Anger—how it is expressed: covertly, overtly, verbally, physically.
- Degree of cooperation in interview.
- Social skills: positive ones as well as unpleasant habits, shyness, withdrawal, intrusiveness.
- Amount and type of motor activity: psychomotor retardation, agitation, restlessness, tics, tremors, hypervigilance, or lack of motor activity.
- Speech patterns: amount, rate, volume, pressure, mutism, slurring, stuttering.
- Degree of concentration and attention span.

**Orientation:** To time, place, person and level of consciousness.

**Memory:** Recent and remote, amnesia, blackouts, confabulation.

**Thought processes reflected in speech:** Blocking, circumstantiality, loose associations, flight of ideas, perseveration, tangential ideas, ambivalence, neologisms.

**Thought content:** Helplessness, hopelessness, worthlessness, guilt, suicidal ideas and plans, homicidal thoughts and plans, suspiciousness, feelings of persecution, phobias, obsessions, compulsions, preoccupations, antisocial attitudes, blaming of others, poverty of content.

**Hallucinations:** Visual, auditory, other.

**Delusions:** Of reference, influence, persecution, grandeur, religious, somatic.

**Intellectual functioning:** Use of language and knowledge, abstract vs concrete thinking (proverbs), calculations (serial sevens).

**Affect/mood:** Anxiety level, elevated mood, depressed mood, labile mood, blunted or flat affect, inappropriate affect.

**Insight:** Degree of awareness of problems and causes.

**Judgment:** Soundness of problem solving and decisions.

**Motivation:** Degree of motivation for treatment.

# Nursing Care Plan

WEEKLY UPDATE: ___7-7-90___

NAME: ___Anita Jarvis___                    ADMISSION DATE: ___6-21-90___

DSM-III-R DIAGNOSIS: ___296.22 Major depression, melancholic type___

**ASSESSMENT:**
***Areas of strength:*** Has family who cares. Had good work record; asking for help; thinking abstractly.
***Problems:*** Unable to get out of bed and care for self; suicide thoughts but no plan; decreased socialization and support; impending divorce.

**DIAGNOSES:** Suicidal thoughts related to separation from husband. Fear of living alone related to pending divorce. Sense of helplessness and hopelessness related to lowered self-esteem.

|  | Date met |
|---|---|
| **PLANNING:** | |
| ***Short-term goals:*** | |
| Patient will verbalize that she is no longer suicidal. | 6-30-90 |
| Patient will verbally express guilt and anger at husband and situation. | 6-25-90 |
| Patient will phone friend and children for assistance. | 6-23-90 |
| ***Long-term goals:*** | |
| Patient will decide where to live after discharge. | 7-6-90 |
| Patient will describe resources and ability to support self. | In progress |

**IMPLEMENTATION/INTERVENTION:**
***Nurse-patient relationship:*** Initiate suicide precautions as a nursing measure; monitor energy level and suicidal ideas; offer support as feelings are expressed; reinforce strengths.
***Psychopharmacology:*** Amitriptyline 25 mg p.o. t.i.d.
***Milieu management:*** Encourage patient to stay out of room; encourage attendance at self-esteem, assertiveness, problem-solving, and recreational groups.

**EVALUATION:** Patient will stay with daughter after discharge; patient called employer and requested extended sick leave; patient will see outpatient counselor in mid-July

**Box 6-2**
## PROGRESS NOTES

- **Subjective content:** what the patient says about his thoughts, feelings, behaviors, and problems.
- **Objective data:** what the nurse observes or measures, such as appearance, nonverbal behaviors, and vital signs.
- **Analysis or conclusions:** what the nurse's impressions are of what the patient is experiencing or demonstrating in behavioral or descriptive terms (not medical diagnosis). Defenses, mood, and issues are identified. Depressed mood and paranoid ideas can be discussed but not "depression" and "paranoia" as illnesses. Saying the patient conveys a depressed mood is different than saying he has a major depression disorder. Conclusions may also be described or noted about the changes (regression or progress) in the patient and responses to medications.
- **Plan:** what the nurses or other team members can do to intervene with the problems described in the progress note.

A process recording is a record of an encounter with a patient that is as nearly verbatim as possible. It generally includes the nonverbal behaviors of the nurse and the patient as well as verbal interaction. Analysis of the interaction patterns and content may be included next to each written statement or may be summarized at the end of the process recording. The process recording may be analyzed by the nurse herself or shared with someone who can give constructive feedback on problem areas and strategies for improvement. The recording *is a learning tool,* not an end in itself, which can be used periodically for professional learning or growth. A sample process recording (Box 6-3) is presented along with a sample intake interview (Box 6-4), nursing care plan, and progress note (Box 6-5) related to the same "patient."

## Box 6-3
## SAMPLE PROCESS RECORDING

| Nurse | | Patient | |
| --- | --- | --- | --- |
| Verbal | Nonverbal | Verbal | Nonverbal |
| Mrs. Jarvis, my name is Janet. I'm a staff nurse on this unit. | Standing facing and looking at patient, arms at side with papers in hand. | (silence) | Sitting at table. Looking at floor. Hands folded in lap. |
| Mrs. Jarvis, please come with me to the office. I'd like to learn more about you and tell you about the unit. | (same as above) Takes one step backward and turns slightly. | (silence) | Slowly stands up. Picks up purse. Stands, still looking at floor. |

(Nurse leads the way to office, walking slowly but slightly ahead of the patient. The patient follows without looking up at the nurse. In the office the nurse sits in chair at desk and opens a folder of papers. The patient sits in chair at side of desk, holding her purse with both hands on her lap.)

| Nurse Verbal | Nurse Nonverbal | Patient Verbal | Patient Nonverbal |
| --- | --- | --- | --- |
| Would you prefer to be called Mrs. Jarvis or Anita? | Has pen in hand ready to write. Other hand flat on desk. Looking at patient. | (pause) Anita | (same as above, looking at floor) |
| Anita, we will be better able to help you if we know more about you. What has happened recently in your life? | (same as above) | (pause) I couldn't get out of bed. (pause) I was so tired. | Turns head slightly, still looking at floor. No smile or frown. |
| How long were you feeling so tired? | Writing and looking at paper. | I don't know. (pause) A week, I guess. | (same as above) |

## Box 6-3
## SAMPLE PROCESS RECORDING—cont'd

| Nurse | | Patient | |
|---|---|---|---|
| Verbal | Nonverbal | Verbal | Nonverbal |
| What happened a week ago? | Looking at patient. Moves tissue box toward patient. | (pause) My husband (pause) left. | Tears in eyes. Tries to open purse. |
| I can see this is difficult for you to talk about (pause). What did he say when he left? | Looking at patient. Both arms on desk. | That he was fed up. (pause) That he wanted a divorce. | Nods head. Raises eyes slightly but still not looking at nurse. Starts to cry. Gets tissue. Occasional sobs. Holding tissue. |
| What did you say to him? | Turns slightly toward patient. One arm on desk. Other arm on arm of chair. | I don't know. I don't remember. (pause) Maybe I asked him to stay. | |
| Then what happened? | (same as above) | It's all a blur. I think I cried all day. | (same as above) |
| Who did you talk to? | (same as above) | No one. (pause) I'm alone. My kids are married and gone. I just stayed in bed. | Same but sobbing less often. |
| When you were feeling so tired, did you have any thoughts of killing yourself? | (same as above) | (pause) I was so scared of being alone. I thought I'd rather be dead than alone. | Looks at nurse for first time. Both hands in lap. |
| How did you think about killing yourself? | (same as above) | I couldn't think of anything. I didn't know what to do. | Looks at floor again. Fumbling in purse. |

*Continued.*

**Box 6-3**

## SAMPLE PROCESS RECORDING—cont'd

| Nurse | | Patient | |
|---|---|---|---|
| **Verbal** | **Nonverbal** | **Verbal** | **Nonverbal** |
| Are you still thinking about suicide? | Hands patient another tissue. | Not really. (pause) But I still wish I was dead. I don't know what to do. | Blows nose and then puts hands in lap. Looks at nurse. |
| While you are here, we are going to help you consider some options about what you can do, so you will not feel so alone and scared. (pause) | Leans forward. Looking at patient. Both hands on lap. | (silence) | Looks at floor again. Crying has stopped. Looks at nurse. |
| It will help us if I ask you some questions. | Turns back to papers, ready to write. | OK. | |

## Box 6-4
### INITIAL NURSING ASSESSMENT (Intake Form)

**Name:** Anita Jarvis      **Sex:** Female      **Age:** 46
**Date of birth:** 6/27/44      **Marital Status:** Separated; married 26 years

| **Family members: Name** | **Relationship** | **Age** |
| --- | --- | --- |
| David Jarvis | Son | 24 |
| Beth Samuels | Daughter | 23 |
| Brian Jarvis | Husband | 48 |

**Date and time of admission:** 6/30/90      3:15 PM

**Type of admission:** Voluntary; brought by son

**Reason for current admission:** Husband left approximately 1 week ago. Patient has felt fatigued and spends most of the day in bed. Son found his mother yesterday and called the crisis clinic. Patient was seen today, and admission was recommended. Patient admits to suicidal thoughts but has no plan. She presently wishes she were dead. Patient is afraid to live alone.

**Previous psychiatric history:** None.

**Drug and alcohol use/abuse:** Patient denies use of drugs (illegal and over the counter) and medicine except for aspirin. States she usually has one to two drinks per week; occasionally three to four drinks when at a social gathering.

**Disturbances in patterns of daily living:**

    **Sleep:** In bed 14 to 16 hours per day but sleeps only 3 to 4 hours a night.

    **Intake and elimination:** Has not cooked a meal in 1 week but has eaten every day—mostly sandwiches and snack food. Had small bowel movement yesterday. No problem with voiding.

    **Sexual:** Decreased frequency and pleasure progressively over last year because of marital problems.

    **Leisure:** No activities, except TV, in last 1 to 2 months. Used to enjoy bowling, cards, and travel.

    **Self-care:** Patient states she is normally a good housekeeper and takes good care of herself. In last 2 to 3 weeks she has not cleaned house or done laundry. Last shower was a week ago.

    **Work:** Patient called in sick 8 days ago. Previously had a good work record as a computer programmer.

    **Support systems:** Progressive decline in socializing during last 6 months. No phone calls or visits with children in last 2 weeks until yesterday when son arrived. Limited support except for children. Patient states she used to have one close friend (seen a month ago) but she is afraid she has alienated her. Is not close to her parents and younger brother, all of whom live out of state.

*Continued.*

**Box 6-4**

## INITIAL NURSING ASSESSMENT (Intake Form)—cont'd

**General appearance:** Dressed appropriately for season; clothes are clean but unpressed. Hair is uncombed. Slouched shoulders. Pale. Blank expression.

**Behaviors during interview:**

  **Anger:** Covert anger evident but not expressed.

  **Cooperation:** Slow to respond but cooperative.

  **Social skills:** Withdrawn, no unpleasant habits, reduced socialization prior to admission.

  **Motor activity:** Movement is slowed, crying at times; no tics or tremors noted.

  **Speech patterns:** Amount is reduced with slowed rate and soft tone.

  **Concentration/attention span:** Exhibits decreased concentration; easily distracted by stimuli; slight shortening of attention span.

**Orientation:** Aware of person, place, and time.

**Memory:**

  **Remote:** Complete with good detail.

  **Recent:** Difficulty organizing sequence but mostly complete except for last week.

**Thought processes:** No disturbances noted except ambivalence toward divorce.

**Thought content:** Is expressing helplessness, hopelessness, guilt, suicidal thoughts without a plan, and covert anger. Also fears being alone.

**Hallucinations:** None reported.

**Delusions:** None reported or evident.

**Intellectual functioning:** College education evident in vocabulary. Calculations and proverbs were not done. Abstract thinking is evident in discussion of "love" and "fidelity."

**Affect:** Blunted with depressed mood. Anxiety level is moderate.

**Insight:** Aware of problems in facing divorce but not yet able to describe factors leading to separation.

**Judgment:** No impairment until past week when she became unable to make decisions, take action, or seek support.

**Motivation for treatment:** Wants help with depression, tiredness, and handling divorce. Is unable to state what type of help she needs.

**Box 6-5**
## SAMPLE PROGRESS NOTE

| Date & Time | Narrative |
| --- | --- |

**Date & Time**
6/21/90  3:15 PM

**Narrative**

46-year-old white female voluntarily admitted to 3N, accompanied by son. Initial nursing assessment is completed.

**S:**  Patient states she has been tired and staying in bed most of the day since husband left a week ago. States she is unsure of what led to the separation and cannot face living alone. Has thoughts of suicide but no plan. "I still wish I was dead." Describes decrease in socialization and support. Saw one friend a month ago. Did not contact children about separation and is not close to her own family. Verbalizes that she doesn't know what to do about the impending divorce and her future.

**O:**  Exhibits blunted affect, limited eye contact, slowed motor activity and speech (occasionally cries). A "no suicide contract" was signed and placed in chart.

**A:**  Expressing helplessness and hopelessness. Guilt is evident, but patient cannot describe feelings. Anger is barely evident at this point. Suicidal but lacks energy to plan. Support is available but not perceived as such.

**P:**  1. Approach and sit with patient frequently.
2. Encourage expression of feelings as tolerated in small doses.
3. Monitor energy level and suicidal ideation.
4. Encourage attendance at group meetings.

## KEY CONCEPTS

1. The nurse uses verbal and nonverbal communications to convey a willingness to listen, genuine respect, a desire to help, and an understanding of the patient as a person with unique problems and needs.
2. The nurse-patient relationship is a series of goal-directed interactions focused on the patient's thoughts, feelings, behaviors, and potential solutions to problems.
3. Nursing process is the tool with which the nurse assesses each patient's problems, selects and carries out specific interventions, and evaluates the effectiveness of care.
4. The patient's relationship with staff nurses progresses in definable stages: orientation, working, and termination.
5. Each stage of the nurse-patient relationship involves specific tasks needed to facilitate its progress.
6. Crisis intervention strategies concentrate on the immediate precipitant, physical safety, and emotional security.
7. Issues and patient behaviors interfering with progress of the nurse-patient relationship need to be addressed by the nurse.
8. In psychiatric nursing practice, the roles of facilitator and educator are primary functions of the nurse.
9. The written patient assessments, care plans, and progress notes provide an important means of ensuring consistency and continuity of care.
10. Process recordings are a learning tool to facilitate professional growth.

## REFERENCES

Aguilera DC and Messick JM: Crisis intervention: theory and methodology, ed 4, St. Louis, 1982, The C.V. Mosby Co.

Busch PV: Therapy with the noninvolved client. J Psychosoc Nurs 25(11):21, 1987.

Caplan G: An approach to community mental health. New York, 1961, Grune & Stratton.

Cohen S: Mental status assessment. Am J Nurs 81(8):1493, 1981.

Duncan BL and Solovey AD: Strategic-brief therapy: an insight-oriented approach. J Marital Family Ther 15(1):1, 1989.

Forchuk C and Brown B: Establishing a nurse-client relationship. J Psychosoc Nurs 27(2):30, 1989.

Gallop R and Wynn F: Difficult young adult chronic patients: reevaluating short-term clinical management. J Psychosoc Nurs 24(3):29, 1986.

Goering PN and Stylianos SK: Exploring the helping relationship between the schizophrenic client and rehabilitation therapist. Am J Orthopsychiatry 58(2):271-280, 1988.

Hay MA and Nelson LM: Client classification: a needs approach. J Psychosoc Nurs 26(12):23, 1988.

Jenny J: Classifying nursing diagnoses: a self-care approach. Nurs Health Care 10(2):83, 1989.

Kahn EM: Psychotherapy with chronic schizophrenics: alliance, transference, and countertransference, J Psychosoc Nurs 22(7):20, 1984.

Kaplan HI, Freedman AM, and Sadock BJ: Comprehensive textbook of psychiatry, ed 3, Baltimore, 1980, Williams & Wilkins Co.

Karshmer JF: Rules of thumb: hints for the psychiatric nursing student. J Psychiatr Nurs Ment Health Serv 20(3):25, 1982.

Keltner NL: Psychotherapeutic management: a model for nursing practice. Perspect Psychiatr Care 23(4):125, 1985.

Lindemann E: The meaning of crisis in the individual and family. Teachers College Record 57:310, 1956.

Loomis ME: Levels of contracting. J Psychosoc Nurs 23(3):9, 1985.

McGreevy A and Van Heukelom J: Caring, the neglected dimension. Nurs Digest, 5.61, 1977.

Morris MM and Myton CL: Ego function: enhancement through social interaction, J Psychosoc Nurs 24(12):17, 1986.

Parsons PJ: Building better treatment plans. J Psychosoc Nurs 24(4):9, 1986.

Peplau HE: Interpersonal relations in nursing. New York, 1952, G.P. Putnam's Sons.

Peplau HE: A working definition of anxiety. In Burd SE and Marshall MA, editors: Some clinical approaches to psychiatric nursing. Toronto, 1963, The Macmillan Co.

Peplau HE: Psychotherapeutic strategies. Perspect Psychiatr Care 6(6):264, 1968.

Schroder PJ: Recognizing transference and countertransference. J Psychosoc Nurs 23(2):21, 1985.

Scott AL: Human interaction and personal boundaries. J Psychosoc Nurs 26(8):23, 1988.

Shillinger FL: Locus of control: implications for clinical nursing practice. Image 15(2):58, 1983.

Small SM: Outline for psychiatric examination. East Hanover, NJ, 1980, Sanday.

Strupp HH: On the basic ingredients of psychotherapy. J Consult Clinical Psychol 41:1, 1973.

Sullivan-Taylor L: Policemen and nursing students: crisis intervention team. J Psychosoc Nurs 23(9):26, 1985.

Takla MA: Paradoxical intervention in psychiatric nursing practice. Perspect Psychiatr Care 23(4):141, 1985.

Topf M: Verbal interpersonal responsiveness. J Psychosoc Nurs 26(7):8, 1988.

Topf M and Dambacher B: Teaching interpersonal skills: a model for facilitating optimal interpersonal relations. J Psychiatr Nurs Mental Health Serv 19(12):29, 1981.

Van Servellen G: The concept of individualized care in nursing practice. Nurs Health Care 3(9):482, 1982.

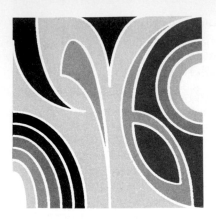

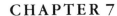

# Working with the Aggressive Patient

PATRICIA CLUNN, LEE HILYARD SCHWECKE, AND
CAROL E. BOSTROM

LEARNING OBJECTIVES
After reading this chapter you should be able to

- Describe the differences between anger, aggression, passive aggression, and assertiveness.
- Define assault and battery, legal and social.
- Describe the animal, individual, social-psychological, and sociocultural models of aggression.
- Describe the five stages of the assault cycle.
- Explain the verbal nursing interventions with anger and nonviolent aggression.
- Match the external control interventions with the escalation and crisis phases of the assault cycle.
- Describe the nursing care of patients in seclusion and restraints.
- Explain the functions needed to support a staff victim of patient assault.

Anger is a normal human emotion that is crucial for individual growth and a factor present in all relationships. When handled appropriately and expressed assertively, it is a positive creative force leading to problem solving and productive change. When channeled inappropriately and expressed as verbal or physical aggression, it is a destructive and potentially life-threatening force. Physical aggression is also called assault, battery, or violence. Anger may also be expressed indirectly as passive aggression (e.g., sarcasm) or internalized, and it may lead to unpleasant emotional and physical problems.

The focus of this chapter is on the individual patient's expressions of anger with nursing staff and with other patients in inpatient psychiatric settings. However, it is important for nurses to recognize that anger and aggression occur in any setting, including emergency rooms, medical and surgical units, nursing homes, community health settings, and clinics. Aggressive patient behaviors occurring in nonpsychiatric settings are usually unanticipated and very disturbing. Nonpsychiatric staff may be unfamiliar with predicting and preventing aggression and may be unprepared for managing it. Psychiatric nursing staff are normally trained in assessing and defusing anger and in safe management of aggressive behaviors.

## EXTENT OF THE PROBLEM

There is an alarming increase in the incidence of family, child, spouse, and elderly abuse in American society (Gelles, 1987). The overcrowding of U.S. jails has, to an extent, contributed to the increase in aggressive incidents in hospital settings. Alcohol and drug abusers are often taken to a hospital instead of to jail. The increase in the use of crack cocaine has also contributed to the increase in violence (Cohen, 1989).

McNeil et al. (1989) examined the correlation of threats of aggression before admission with assault-related events after admission. Of the 253 patients, 60 had made threats to attack someone during the 2 weeks before admission. Of these, 50 patients (83.3%) were involved in an assault-related incident at least once during the first 72 hours of admission. Of the remaining patients (193) who had made no threats of attack before admission, 71 (36.8%) were involved in an assault-related event. It is crucial to note that of the 253 patients studied, 94% had been committed on a 72-hour emergency-detention court order.

In studying the behaviors of black and white patients in 12 public urban psychiatric settings, Lindsey et al. (1989) found miniscule differences in dangerous behaviors between voluntarily and involuntarily admitted black patients. However, involuntarily admitted white patients showed higher levels of dangerous behavior than did voluntarily admitted white patients. Janofsky et al. (1988) found voluntarily admitted patients to be more verbally threatening (36.1%) than physically assaultive (14.8%).

## RELATED CONCEPTS
### Anger

Anger is a normal response to something a person perceives as a frustration of desires or a threat to one's needs. It is a derivation of anxiety and includes feelings of powerlessness and helplessness that may be rational or irrational. Anger may be justified or unjustified, conscious or unconscious, intentional or unintentional.

While everyone experiences feelings of anger on occasion, open displays of anger are discouraged and are considered socially inappropriate in our society. American children are usually punished for expressions of anger and are taught to deny or repress these, as well as other, strong emotions. This can be observed in the difficulties encountered in dealing with frustrations and temper tantrums that American children exhibit when compared, for example, with Oriental or Vietnamese children. When adults in this culture inappropriately express their anger toward the person they perceive as causing their anger, the recipient responds with fear and frustration and avoids that person if possible. The recipient may also feel helpless, guilty, defensive, or angry. At times the recipient may fight back, retaliate, seek revenge, or hold a grudge.

Anger, in its early stages, is healthy when it is verbally expressed appropriately to the person perceived as causing the anger. Usually these angry verbalizations represent the person's intense effort to keep and protect a relationship by communicating difficulties and painful misunderstandings. (See Box 7-1 for other common precipitants of anger.)

The more important a person or situation is to an individual, the more intense the anger. Individuals seldom become angry over situations or others who are not important to them.

Angry behaviors span a continuum from mild irritation and arguing, to verbally or physically abusing self or others, to uncontrollable violence. Many individuals throw things in anger, displacing their anger on to objects (see Box 7-2). The repression or suppression of anger adds to the potential for verbal or physical aggression.

### Definitions of assault and battery

**Legal assault and battery.** The legal definition states that assault is any threatening behavior that conveys a "clear and immediate danger of physical injury to person." Carrying out the threat of injury is defined as battery. Battery includes hitting, kicking, hair pulling, chair throwing, biting, and scratching but does not include verbal abuse (Smith, 1981) or physical aggression toward objects. Nurses have the right, professionally and legally, to use physical force to prevent patients from injuring themselves and others. Nursing interventions are based on the least-restrictive-alternative principle that is emphasized in the American Nurses Association Standards for Psychiatric and Mental Health Nursing. This principle states the nurse will "set limits in a humane and least restrictive manner" to assure the safety and security of patients and others. The legal definition also provides a "rationale for avoiding the use of physical force to achieve compliance in situations where there is not a clear and immediate danger of physical injury" (Smith, 1981, p. 34).

**Social assault and battery.** The social definition modifies the legal one. Social norms allow certain illegal assaults without legal consequences within relatively vague constraints. What is tolerated depends on who is assaulted by whom, when,

**Box 7-1**
## COMMON PRECIPITANTS OF ANGER

Threat to:
   Self-esteem
   Health or safety
   Sense of control
   Sense of security
Loss of:
   Relationships
   Possessions
Conflict with significant person
Unmet goals
Frustration of needs or wants
Criticism by others
Interference by others
Not getting one's way
Being attacked or confined
Inability to effectively communicate
   feelings and needs
Confusion
Misperceptions of others' intentions
Suspiciousness of others
Overwhelming stress
Economic decline or unemployment
Victimization

History of being abused
Membership in violent subculture
Poor impulse control
Loss of inhibitions (with alcohol or
   drugs)
Prolonged insomnia
Withdrawal from alcohol or drugs
Endocrine or metabolic disorders
Toxic reactions
Temporal lobe epilepsy
Toxic reactions
Organic brain dysfunctions
Brain tumors
Disorientation
Manic excitement
Panic attack
Perception distortions or illusions
Paranoid ideation
Delusions
Hallucinations

and where and on the degree of injury resulting from the battery. For example, battery that causes no visible injury and that does not require hospitalization may be socially permitted, as when children of the same size fight during a sports event. Men may be allowed to assault each other in an inner city bar but not in an expensive restaurant. Parents are allowed to physically discipline children, but children are not allowed to hit back (Smith, 1981).

On a psychiatric unit, assault is never tolerated, but norms usually allow controlled physical aggression, such as using a punching bag or foam bats. If a patient does hit a staff member, the staff member is not allowed to strike back. The patient can be restricted with seclusion or restraint without legal consequences. A patient may be allowed (but carefully monitored) to hit his pillow but should be stopped if he begins to damage furniture.

## Box 7-2
## EXPRESSIONS OF ANGER

| Objective | | Turned Inward | |
|---|---|---|---|
| **Turned outward** | **Passive aggression** | **Subjective** | **Objective** |
| Verbalization of | Impatience | Feeling upset | Crying |
| anger | Pouting | Tenseness | Self-mutilation |
| Irritation | Sulking | Feeling let down | Suicide |
| Pacing with agi- | Frustration | Unhappy | |
| tation | Pessimism | Feeling hurt | |
| Swearing | Annoyance | Disappointment | |
| Hostility | Resentment | Guilt | |
| Contempt | Jealousy | Inferiority feelings | |
| Rigid posture | Bitterness | Sense of failure | |
| Clenched fists | Complaining | Humiliation | |
| Tense facial ex- | Deceptive | Somatic symptoms | |
| pression | sweetness | Feeling of harrass- | |
| Cynicism | Unreasonable- | ment | |
| Insulting remarks | ness | Envy | |
| Intimidation | Intolerance | Feeling violated | |
| Bragging about | Resistance | Feeling alienated | |
| prior violence | Stubbornness | Feeling demoralized | |
| Provocation | Intentional for- | Feeling depressed | |
| Sadistic | getting | Resignation | |
| Maliciousness | Noncompliance | Feeling powerless | |
| Verbal abuse | Procrastination | Helplessness | |
| Temper tantrums | Antagonism | Hopelessness | |
| Violation of others' | Belittling | Desperation | |
| rights | Sarcasm | Apathy | |
| Screaming | Fault finding | | |
| Deviance | Manipulation | | |
| Rage | Power struggles | | |
| Argumentativeness | Unfair teasing | | |
| Overt defiance | Sabotage of | | |
| Threats: words or | others | | |
| weapons | Domination | | |
| Damage to property | | | |
| Assault | | | |
| Rape | | | |
| Homicide | | | |

## Verbal aggression

In addition to physical aggression and battery, anger may be shown outwardly in verbal aggression (see Box 7-5). Most of the research indicates, in line with the earlier literature, that verbally aggressive acts tend to have a repetitive pattern and are among the major warning signs of assault and battery. Verbal expressions of aggression also tend to provoke unproductive counterreactions. Escalation of aggressive content seldom results in a constructive solution to a problem.

Persons who are verbally aggressive tend to deny their other feelings, such as fear or guilt, and to express anger instead. They destroy relationships with angry outbursts in their need to control others and situations. They do not respect others, and if they achieve their goals, it is by intimidation. They waste energy in many arguments and defensive behaviors. Their distress is demonstrated by power struggles and frequent unpleasant arguments. For verbally aggressive persons (as well as for those who assault others), the long-term results are loss of self-respect, relationships, and jobs.

Social norms may influence the degree and amount of verbal aggression tolerated. At a sporting event, fans are allowed to scream, swear, and be verbally abusive, especially toward referees and umpires. The same behaviors toward an employer are not tolerated. A brother may verbally pick on his sister, but he puts a stop to the same behavior of a neighbor toward his sister.

On a psychiatric unit the quiet mumbling or swearing by a patient with schizophrenia or a patient with organic brain syndrome may be ignored. The louder swearing of a patient who is in contact with reality is not tolerated, especially if directed toward a patient who is unable to respond assertively. If two relatively competent patients are arguing, staff members may not intervene, except with brief suggestions, to allow the patients the positive experience of conflict resolution. If one of those patients is less competent, staff members might stop the argument as soon as it begins.

## Passive aggression and passivity

Passive-aggressive persons express their anger indirectly and undermine others in a variety of subtle, evasive ways. Passive persons turn their anger inward, are unaware of their underlying anger, and see themselves as good, kind, congenial, and helpful. Passivity and passive aggression, like most problems with aggression, are attributed to early childhood socialization experiences. Experts theorize that the parents of these persons are usually aggressive toward their children and yet at the same time block the children's need to express anger directly. Given the small child's intense dependency needs, the child learns to conceal or express his anger in indirect ways, as by being stubborn, forgetful, procrastinating, negative, pessimistic, noncompliant, sarcastic, antagonistic, and complaining, and by sabotaging and blocking other's goals.

Persons whose behaviors are passive deny their anger and displace it with feelings of fear. They damage, destroy, or avoid relationships and opposing circumstances as a defense. They cannot say "no" and feel that others take advantage of them. They waste energy by setting up and repeating nonassertive situations that were not adequately resolved in their past. They seldom achieve their goals and show signs of their distress with low self-esteem, helplessness, hopelessness, depression, substance abuse, physical illnesses, and suicide attempts.

They frustrate others and, vicariously, stimulate the anger and aggression they deny in themselves. The dynamics of both passive and aggressive persons stimulate or "trigger" the acting out of patients who have problems controlling their aggressive impulses; thus these patients are often the unwitting provocative victims on inpatient units. The inciting of anger in other patients is not tolerated, and staff intervention is appropriate.

### Asssertiveness

One of the widely accepted methods for learning how to replace aggressive, passive-aggressive, and nonassertive behaviors with healthy assertiveness is assertiveness training. Assertiveness training is aimed at teaching the individual the behavioral repertoire needed to interact successfully with others while maintaining one's and another's rights. It employs a variety of behavior-modification techniques, such as relaxation training and role playing.

Assertive persons are aware of their feelings of fear and anger, respect themselves and others, and build productive relationships. They use their energy constructively to achieve goals.

### DEVELOPMENTAL VIEW OF AGGRESSION

Frequently hostile persons are described as being in "a rage," a term most professionals use to describe irrational (infantile) responses, which are the most primitive form of aggressive expressions. Rage reactions are present in the infant's loud, uncontrollable crying and screaming, profuse perspiration, difficulty in breathing (sometimes turning "blue"), and flailing of arms and legs.

Children move from infantile rage to "temper tantrums." With the progression of impulse control and maturing of the coordination, children are able to direct their anger at an object. Children learn to focus unpleasant feelings on persons or situations perceived to be responsible for the discomfort of "hurt" feelings. By the early school-age years, children assault and hit one another quite frequently (Smith, 1981).

Normally, preadolescents learn to restrict childish tendencies for hitting each other and translate aggressive impulses to competitive sports, character assassinations, slander, sarcasm, practical jokes, and destructive gossip. By adolescence, fighting is controlled and purposeful. Group cooperation is emphasized in competitive activities, accounting for the tendency for teenage groups to deteriorate pathologically to "gangs" or cults (Smith, 1981).

Under usual circumstances in American culture, as age increases, the ability to control impulses also increases. Between the ages of 22 and 45 years, almost all expressions of aggression and fighting occur within the family, taking the form of spouse, elder, and child abuse. After the age of 45 years, people seem to stop fighting until around the age of 70, when aging may result in diminished impulse control (Smith, 1981) and cognitive impairment (Meddaugh, 1990), and expressions of aggression again emerge as a problem.

## Gender and aggression

Males, traditionally, are more aggressive than females, and differences are attributed to biology, hormones, culture, learning, and, most important, societal perpetuation of male role dominance. Men patients striking out at women nurses are often responding in their usual, habitual way toward women's actions. Historically, until recently, women were viewed as the property of men in their families (fathers, husbands). Statistics hold that between 25% and 30% of all male-female relationships include male violence and abuse toward women. In the United States, women are at higher risk of being violently assaulted by men with whom they have significant relationships than by strangers, and the most dangerous place for females is in their homes (see Chapter 28).

## ETIOLOGY OF AGGRESSION
### Animal models

Darwin was one of the first to study animal aggression, the results of which were published in his *Survival of the Species.* Darwin posited that animal aggression had a positive function in strengthening animal and human species through natural selection and the "survival of the fittest" (Lanza, 1983).

Freud's death-instinct theory drew on Darwin's theory, saying instincts were present in animals and man, and also emphasized the positive aspects of human aggression for mastery and survival. Freud's death-instinct theory held that all human beings wish to return to a state of nothingness, the state from which they emerged. The more powerful the death instinct, the greater the need to direct aggression outward toward others (Freud, 1962). When individuals cannot discharge aggression outwardly to others, aggression is turned inward and becomes self-destructive or is manifested as guilt, anger at self, or depression.

Lorenz's (1981) extensive research on animal territoriality and body buffer space has been applied to human behavior, showing that human beings have defined space "zones." As with animals, these zones increase when persons feel threatened, and research findings indicate that individuals who are potentially violent require five times the body buffer zones of persons who are nonviolent. The clinical implications of this are for nurses to "stand away" from patients who are struggling to maintain control and to give them the opportunity to regain self-control.

## Individual, social-psychological, and sociocultural models

Individual theories explain violence as some quality of the person and use biologically based explanations of aggression.

> Violent behavior is a neurological dysfunction or abnormality and . . . may be due to congenital conditions, permanent injury or transient neurological states. Specific physical conditions considered to cause violence include (1) organic brain disease, such as tumors of the frontal or temporal lobe or temporal lobe epilepsy; (2) cerebral vascular accidents; (3) head injuries; and (4) reactions to drugs and alcohol (Braun, 1981, pp. 26-27).

> Changes in serotonin levels are related to changes in affective behavior in general and aggressive behaviors in particular (Lanza, 1983, p. 12).

Social-psychological theories focus on the interaction of individuals with their social environment and locate the source of violence in interpersonal frustrations or self-concepts that reflect the appraisals of others. Sociocultural theories focus on social structures, norms, values, institutional organizations, and systems operations to explain individual violence. Box 7-3 summarizes the theories of aggression.

## Stress models

Stress provides the best framework for nurses' understanding and intervening in intense emotional reactions, such as aggression, anxiety, panic, fear, and phobic attacks. Stress-driven aggression involves a chain of responses due to neurophysiological actions and reactions known as the general adaptation syndrome (GAS), which is explained in Chapter 2. Research with experienced nurse clinicians who frequently and successfully assess patients' potential for violence found that these assessments usually relied on the stage of the stress response the patient was experiencing and on the extent of the patients' autonomic "fight" options in the fight-or-flight response (Clunn, 1983).

**Assault cycle.** Smith's stress model (1981) includes the assault cycle with five stages of a predictable pattern or chain of aggressive responses to emotional or physical stress. In instances in which patients are repeatedly assaultive, it can be observed that their behavior patterns are ritualistic, stereotypical, and automatic. As the acuity of the aggressive response increases, there is a comparable decrease in the patients' problem-solving abilities, creativity and spontaneity, and behavioral options. The five-phase assault cycle adapted from Smith (1981) includes the following:

1. *Triggering phase:* the stress-producing event occurs, resulting in a number of stress responses. These include muscular tension, changes in voice quality, signs of readiness to retaliate, tapping, pacing, repeat verbalizations, noncompliance, restlessness, irritability, suspiciousness, perspiration, tremors, glaring, a change in breathing.
2. *Escalation phase:* responses represent escalating behaviors that indicate movement toward loss of control. These include a pale or flushed face, screaming, swearing, high agitation, hypersensitivity, threats, demands, clenched fists, tautness, loss of reasoning ability, provocative behaviors.
3. *Crisis phase:* a period of emotional and physical crisis in which a full-blown battery occurs. It includes fighting, hitting, kicking, scratching, throwing things.
4. *Recovery phase:* a period of cooling down in which the person slows down and returns to normal responses. Behaviors may include accusations, recriminations, lowering of the voice, and change in conversation content.
5. *Postcrisis depression phase:* this phase includes crying, apologies, reconciliatory interactions. Repression of assaultive feelings may convert to hostility that later appears as negative actions such as passive aggression.

## Box 7-3
# OVERVIEW OF THEORETICAL DETERMINANTS OF AGGRESSION

### Individual or biological theories

**Psychopathology:** Attributes deviations to individual biological and physiological differences, such as genes, chromosomes, instincts, traits, and/or organic structures. Basis for pharmacological interventions (Tardiff, 1982). Delusions, hallucinations, illusions, and misperceptions are indicators for concern.

**Alcohol or drugs:** There is little scientific evidence supporting the belief that alcohol and drugs *cause* aggression and violence. As "disinhibitors," patients on drugs or alcohol show weakened judgment, perceptions, and impulse control. Most experts consider aggression and violence not a function of drugs but a convenient excuse to express unacceptable feelings and behaviors (Gottheil, 1983).

### Social psychological theories

**Frustration-aggression:** Postulates aggressive behaviors occur when a goal is blocked or inhibited (Dollard et al., 1939; Berkowitz, 1962). While cultural forces may inhibit or accentuate how aggression is "acted out," the tendency to respond aggressively is inherent in all human organisms. The self-concept is involved and threatened, resulting in angry feelings.

**Social learning:** Assumes aggression is the product of successful learning situations. The person has learned the responses of aggression and violence and what stimuli are to be followed by violence. Violence can be learned through imitation (Bandura, 1973); learning norms that approve of aggression and violence (Campbell, 1984); and viewing violence with an appropriate role model (Barnett, 1977). These social learning theories are drawn on to explain why aggression and violence tend to become personal as well as family patterns expressed across generations.

**Clockwork orange:** Named for Burgess's (1962) book, holds that various aggressive or violent acts are due to boredom, thrill seeking (Cohen, 1955), or stress seeking (Kagan et al., 1982); used to explain delinquency. Tension is seen as an essential element in relationships, and if a certain amount of tension and stress are not present, people act out to "stir things up" (Zuckerman, 1978).

Adapted from Gelles RJ and Straus MA: Determinants of violence in the family: toward a theoretical integration. In Wesley R, Burr R, Hill R, Ivan Nye IF, and Reiss, IL: Contemporary theories about the family. New York, 1979, The Free Press, pp. 568–569.

*Continued.*

Box 7-3
# OVERVIEW OF THEORETICAL DETERMINANTS OF AGGRESSION—cont'd

## Sociocultural theories

**Functional:** Theory holds that while aggression and violence can cause injury and sometimes death, they fulfill certain social functions (Lorenz, 1981). Functions identified by Coser (1956) include (1) as an area of achievement and (2) as a catalyst for action. Aggression and violence are thus important to the maintenance and adaptability of the group to changing circumstances and important to its survival (Simmel, 1955).

**Culture of violence:** Social values and norms provide meaning and give direction to violent acts, thus facilitating or bringing about aggression and violence in situations specific to the norms and values of the specific culture or subculture (Landau, 1984). Explains why some sectors of a society, or different societies, are more violent than others, for example, different groups have different cultural rules that legitimize or require violence (Kagan et al., 1982).

**Conflict:** Theory is based on the assumption that conflict is an inevitable part of all human associations and views individual actors, groups, or organizations as seeking to further their own interest rather than participating in a consensus-equilibrium-seeking system. Theory explains why there is conflict and violence in the most integrated and solidaristic human groups. Violence is likely to occur when other modes of pursuing individual or group interests break down because of faulty conflict management at the confrontation stage.

**Resource:** Based on the assumption that all social systems "rest to some degree on force or its threat" (Goode, 1971). Asserts violence and threats of violence are fundamental to the organization of all social systems. The greater the resources a person can command, the more force he can muster: however, the more resources a person can command, the less he will actually deploy the force in overt ways (Holm, 1983).

**General systems:** Cybernetic feedback loop, which assumes systems attempt to keep key variables stable (Straus, 1973), explains ways in which aggression and violence are stabilized and managed. Systems are viewed as goal seeking, purposive, adaptive. Violence is a system product or output (Steinmetz, 1977).

## ASSESSING AND INTERVENING WITH KEY VARIABLES OF AGGRESSION
### The nurse

Nurses working with psychiatric patients who may "act out" need to be aware of their own aggressive impulses, how they deal with their anger, and how they channel it into constructive, productive actions. Nurses also need to know the kinds of patient situations and behaviors that trigger anger in them. It is important they know how they respond to verbal threats and to patients showing anxiety, fear, panic, and assaultive crises. It is unwise for nurses who fear they may lose control of their own anger and impulses to intervene with patients who are experiencing problems with aggression. Nurses cannot defuse the patient's anger or aggression when they are in a similar state, and they may intensify the patients' emotions by the unwitting interpersonal transmission of their emotions to the patient.

Potential patient assaults often evoke the nurses' fear of being hurt or of inflicting pain on others. While a patient is being restrained, body and hand contact with the patient, whether of the same or the opposite sex, may have subtle, threatening sexual overtones (Lions, 1983) or may bring back hazy memories of childhood battles. When patients become aggressive, nurses may experience frustration, a feeling of professional inadequacy, or a sense of failure.

Some nurses believe their participation in physical control of the patients will damage their chances of developing or continuing a therapeutic relationship with the acting-out patient; in most cases, however, just the opposite is true. Potential patient assaults provide the nurse with opportunities to demonstrate and convey to the patient that she can help him regain control and deal more constructively with the stresses in the environment that caused his initial problem and hospitalization. If the patient's behavior is viewed as a form of communication, then acting out should alert the staff to the fact that the patient's inner controls are failing and that he needs assistance to regain impulse control.

### The environment

There are variables in the milieu of a facility that may contribute to the development and escalation of aggression. An environment with excessive stimuli may increase the anxiety and agitation levels of some patients and interfere with restful sleep. Overcrowding and lack of sufficient space may decrease a sense of privacy and personal space. Ideally, units should have both quiet rooms and activity rooms to meet different patients' needs at different times. Colors, lighting, and decor of certain rooms can be used purposely to enhance relaxation and composure.

Resources for energy-draining activities, such as exercise equipment and sports areas, may be useful in preventing escalation of aggression. Boredom may also be relieved by structured and unstructured diversionary activities, such as movies, games, cards, crafts, and therapeutic and recreational reading materials. Staffing needs to be sufficient for monitoring patients and supervising activities. Tolerance of a degree of pacing and smoking may reduce tension, but an excess of these activities may disturb other patients.

The philosophies and policies of a facility affect both the milieu and patient behaviors. Excessive or unfair restriction of rights and privileges may lead to tension and rebellion. Reasonable yet flexible rules reduce the risk of power and control issues between staff and patients. Policies and rules can contribute to the structure, predictability, and consistency of the milieu. Staff's degree of use of chemical controls, seclusion, and restraints may lead to a sense of safety and security *or* convey an atmosphere of punishment.

## The patient

There are specific times that patients are more likely to become aggressive or assaultive: change of shifts, mealtimes, visiting hours, in elevators and during transportation to the outside areas, and periods of change and admission. Hospitalization is a stress-producing situation (Lazarus, 1984) that may escalate the patient's anger, anxiety, and the admitting symptoms. For example, paranoid patients may see the nursing staff as part of a plot to restrict them; compulsive patients may become more stereotyped and rigid, overreacting when they cannot repeat compulsive behavior in the hospital.

Many aspects of the admission process itself are threatening to the patient and can undermine the little impulse control the patient has left. Admission interviews, unavoidably, focus on emotionally charged issues, personal searches, the removal or restriction of personal items, physical examinations, and meeting unfamiliar professionals. The patient enters a new environment with many other patients and rules. Nurses need to be sensitive to the stress of the admission process and to integrate the patient slowly into the unit. When patients have a history of assault or are currently agitated, it is important to delay all but essential procedures and decrease the stimuli and stress as much as possible.

Patients may be disruptive to each other, especially those who are hyperactive, intrusive, openly sexual, manipulative, or threatening or who exhibit bizarre behaviors. Staff members are responsible not only for helping these patients control their behaviors but also for helping the other patients learn assertive responses for handling such situations.

Change is especially unnerving for patients who have great dependency needs and shaky impulse control. Change of staff, shifts, and ward routines; admissions and discharges of other patients; other patients acting out; and transfer to other areas are all potential trigger factors. Even positive changes in the patient's status may be experienced by the patient as a loss of support, care, and protection, as when patients are transferred to less restrictive units or discharged back to the community. All physical moves, status changes, and changes in treatment, such as medications, should be carefully explained in advance. Rapid changes cause the most anxiety, and the nurse needs to convey support and confidence that the patient has the coping skills to deal with the event.

Aggressive acting-out behavior is one way patients have of telling the staff that change is highly threatening. Fear of change may be the reason patients do not ask for more freedom, such as passes. Requests for more freedom may be the way the patient is testing the staff. To understand the meaning of the admission or change experience for the patient, it is important that the nurse have certain information about the patient to assist the patient in adjusting to his changed role. The information needed can be obtained from the patient verbally and by observation of him as he interacts with staff and other patients on the unit and with his social support system and significant relationships during visiting times. Documentation should include the patient's habitual coping patterns and personal eccentricities. Specific examples of communications alerting staff to potential triggers of aggression include "thinks all female nurses are going to be mean to him, like his mother;" "abuses men as his father abused him;" "gets upset whenever the female doctor is here;" "gets terrified whenever men are around." Other information includes the times and places a patient seems to be especially vulnerable, such as when mother visits, in large groups, when alone with a staff member of the opposite sex, or when in the bathroom.

The patient's admitting diagnosis and coexisting medical conditions may provide clues to potential aggression. Patients with a diagnosis of schizophrenia, mania, substance abuse, or an organic brain disorder have a higher incidence of aggression after admission (McNeil et al., 1989; Janofsky et al., 1988). Patients with antisocial, passive-aggressive, and borderline traits may also have aggressive tendencies. Medical problems especially associated with aggressive outbursts are brain injury to the temporal lobe, epilepsy (in the postictal state), and tumors. Patients who suffer from intellectual or neurological impairments that limit their ability to communicate with or understand others in the environment are at high risk of assault.

Factors in a patient's background that are particularly relevant in an assessment of aggression potential are a history of family (or cultural) violence, abuse, or gross disorganization. Other indicators are the patient's history of truancy, fire setting, impulsivity, previous assaults, and destruction of property. A particularly relevant indicator is a specific threat of violence made 2 weeks before admission.

Some facilities use a five-point scale to assess a patient's potential for violence at admission. The scale provides a rating and related interventions (Box 7-4).

## NURSING INTERVENTIONS IN ANGER AND NONVIOLENT AGGRESSION

Three factors to consider in intervening with anger and nonviolent or verbal aggression are the *source* and the *target* of the patient's anger and the *likelihood of escalation.* A patient may be angry about a situation or a person outside the hospital but is directing his anger inward as depression or suicidal ideation. Although angry at someone or at a situation outside, another patient might be showing it as passive aggression and aiming it at no one in particular. A third patient might express the anger openly and loudly in a particular situation. In these instances the anger is likely to be defused by talking about it directly each time it is apparent.

On the other hand, a patient may be angry at someone or about a current situation on the unit, angry about an outside situation but displacing it onto staff, threatening suicide with an available object, or responding to internal stimuli, such as hallucinations, delusions, or physiological disruptions. In these situations there is a greater possibility that the patient will lose control of his anger.

The nursing interventions in both escalating and nonescalating anger begin with

### Box 7-4
## FIVE-POINT SCALE FOR ASSESSING POTENTIAL FOR VIOLENCE

| | | |
|---|---|---|
| 0 | Nonviolent | Presenting no danger of violence to others |
| 1 | Low potential for violence | Presenting slight violence potential and slight danger to others; needs verbal defusing of feelings and stress management |
| 2 | Moderate potential for violence | Potentially violent with the likelihood of injuring others if state is aggravated; requires a controlled environment and supervision and medication |
| 3 | High potential for violence | Presenting a danger to others, with a high likelihood of violence; requires restriction, supervision, and immediate intervention, including medications and a quiet room, to avoid injury to others |
| 4 | Violent | Encountered in a violent assault episode, presenting danger to other persons; needs immediate protective measures of seclusion, restraint, and medication |

Adapted from Clunn PA: Nurses' assessment of a person's potential for violence, doctoral dissertation, New York, 1975, Columbia University Teachers' College.

an assessment *at a safe distance.* Chapter 6 on the nurse-patient relationship describes normal precautions to take with any patient in a potentially unpredictable situation, such as staying between the patient and an exit and using body language that is the least threatening to the patient. Warmth and empathy are essential, but there may also be a need for firm limit setting to help the patient contain his behavior to a safe level: "I want to let you talk, but put the ashtray down first." "We need to go to the other room to talk." Or "Stay here. I don't want you to leave the unit."

If the patient is less verbal, less direct, or overly controlling his anger, the nurse needs to take an active, supportive, and directive role in facilitating ventilation and then problem solving. Initially the nurse may have to point out specific behaviors and ask the patient to explain the situation. (For example, "I hear a lot of sarcastic remarks; what happened during your phone call?" or "You look so down right now; what are you thinking about?") Getting a full description of the situations, thoughts, and feelings will require more questioning and patience. The general progression is still to ask for a description of the situations, thoughts, and feelings before moving to problem solving. For the patient who is turning anger inward, it is also appropriate to ask if he is thinking about suicide.

It is helpful to ask the patient to assess his own potential for acting on his anger. "How likely are you to try to hurt your wife when you are angry?" "How serious are you about killing yourself?" If, during the assessment and ventilation process, the anger does not gradually diffuse or the patient begins to become irrational and out of control, interventions based on the assault cycle become necessary.

## NURSING INTERVENTIONS BASED ON THE ASSAULT CYCLE

The goal of all interventions based on the assault cycle are to strengthen the patients' impulse control. Nurses need to demonstrate that attempts to use least restrictive measures (talking and medications) were employed before the more restrictive interventions of seclusion and restraints. Patient responses at each stress level and to each progressively restrictive intervention should be included in documentation. In almost all cases, verbal strategies should be used before physical interventions. Although interventions with patients who are potentially assaultive are usually unpleasant for nurses, studies show that many patients appreciate and want the staff to provide the external controls they lack and need, such as seclusion. Calm, positive approaches convey to patients that they are expected to cope, and this attitude supports healthy functioning.

### Triggering phase

The patient's responses are nonviolent and present no danger to others in the "trigger phase." The behavior reflects his usual physiological and psychological coping and defense mechanisms. It is important to know how the nurse and the environment are perceived by the patient and the likelihood of the patient's acting on these perceptions. If the patient's stressor is another person in the immediate environment, the two can be separated and talked with individually by two nurses.

To facilitate ventilation, emphasis is on support, with the use of an empathetic, nondirective, concerned technique. The nurse speaks in calm, clear, simple statements avoiding any challenge of the patient. Aggressive, confrontive, threatening approaches at this time usually result in escalation of the patient's aggression and weakening of his struggle for self-control. While ventilation is encouraged, the patient is reminded to stay in control of himself. The patient's loss of control is socially embarrassing for him and counterproductive, leaving him with feelings of vulnerability and loss of autonomy. To protect the dignity of the patient and the rights and safety of others, the patient can be asked to move to a quieter area, or other patients may be asked to leave.

When the ventilation subsides, problem solving can begin to identify alternative solutions. If, however, the ventilation has not been particularly productive, it is important to offer the patient alternatives that allow him to express threatening emotions safely and yet help him regain control and a sense of self-esteem. He can punch pillows, tear up telephone books, pound clay, or walk up and down the hall with the nurse and also have some calming medications.

## Escalation phase

If the tension-reduction strategies fail and the patient becomes irrational and begins to swear, scream, and threaten, the nurse needs to take control of the situation. At a safe distance the nurse calls the patient by name and states in a calm, firm manner that she can see the behaviors indicating loss of control. She does not threaten punishment but offers help by taking charge on behalf of the patient, who is unable to do so at present. The nurse avoids sudden movements and loud tones to avoid an appearance of an attack.

If the patient has orders for p.r.n. antianxiety or antipsychotic medications, an oral dose can be offered early in the escalation phase. If the oral dose is refused or if the excalation is rapid, an intramuscular medication may be necessary. Among the oral antianxiety medications, lorazepam (Ativan) and alprazolam (Xanax) are the drugs of choice because they take effect rapidly and have fewer side effects. They may occasionally lower the patient's inhibitions and aggravate his behaviors (Turpin, 1983). Lorazepam may also be given intramuscularly. Among the antipsychotic medications, the high-potency ones, haloperidol (Haldol), fluphenazine (Prolixin), and thiothixene (Navane), have less sedating qualities but help decrease the agitation (Turpin, 1983).

The patient is kindly but firmly told that he must go to a quiet room with the nurse. Given the principle of least restrictive alternative, time out in a quiet room is offered first (Glynn et al., 1989). If this measure is ineffective, then more restrictive measures may be instituted when the patient actually begins to lose control. Other staff members may be called to be on "standby" but should try to remain out of the patient's view initially. Clinical research has shown that the mere presence of another person, especially a silent observer, is interpreted by the patient as representing someone who supports his position. Thus it is important that other staff members in the patient's view, but at a greater distance from the patient, also speak and support the verbal input of the nurse who is intervening. When patients are potentially violent, their physical proximity to others is perceived as being much closer than it actually is.

The nurse in direct contact with the patient decides whether the patient is able to respond to directions in a reasonable time. If the patient is not responding to directions to control himself or to move to a quiet, safe place, the nurse than asks for staff assistance for a stronger "show of determination" to take control. This involves having four to six staff members within sight of the patient but still at a greater distance from the patient than the primary nurse, so they do *not* appear ready to attack the patient. Often when the patient becomes aware of the other staff members and is informed that the staff *will* take control if he does not comply with directions, the patient is able to gain reasonable composure and cooperate with the nurse's request. Then he is often willing to take the medications and go to the quieter room. If not, the patient has usually come close to entering the crisis phase.

## Crisis phase

This phase is reached when the patient is approaching an attack on the environment, other patients, himself, or the staff. Verbal limits are ineffective, and external control by the staff is essential. In such emergency or crisis situations, immediate seclusion, restraint, or the administration of "stat" medications becomes necessary. These actions should be supported by standing emergency protocols approved by the physicians and hospital and should be carefully and thoroughly documented in the patient's record. Most facilities have an alarm or buzzer system to alert staff to the need for assistance.

**Seclusion.** Seclusion is the process of placing the patient alone in a specially designed lockable room from which he can be observed through a window (Kirkpatrick, 1989). Nurses usually make the decision to initiate and terminate the seclusion of patients according to the established protocols and are almost always involved in the care of the patient during seclusion. The principle of seclusion is containment: restricting the person so he does not hurt self or others, providing isolation and decreasing stimulation (Kalogiera et al., 1989). Agitation and disruptive behaviors are the major reasons for seclusion; thus seclusion may be viewed as a preventive strategy to avoid aggressive assaults and not just as a response measure. Violent behaviors are the second most commonly given reason for seclusion. Research indicates that about two thirds of the patients' behaviors during seclusion are nondisturbed, cooperative, or sleeping (Kirkpatrick, 1989). Thus seclusion provides an intensive care environment in which a patient's behavior and treatment can be more carefully monitored. Most patients report that the seclusion experience makes their behavior better; "time out," closer supervision, quiet interactions, and medication are therapeutically positive.

The degree of seclusion varies according to the current status of the patient. When the patient is voluntarily able to choose "time out," especially if he is already on regular medicine, he may be able to go to his own room and stay voluntarily without a locked door. This degree of seclusion may be relatively brief (Glynn et al., 1989). If he is less cooperative, two staff members might escort him, without bodily contact, to a seclusion room that contains only a bed (bolted to the floor) and a mattress. This kind of room decreases stimuli, protects the patient from injury, prevents destruction of property, and provides privacy for the patient. The security window allows observation of the patient, and the door, lockable from the outside, keeps the patient from leaving the room. Dangerous articles—belts, sharp objects such as pens and keys, shoes, and eyeglasses—are taken from the patient.

**Crisis response team.** Psychiatric emergencies must be dealt with in coordinated and organized ways, and it is important that the staff or crisis response team have the opportunity to role-play their approach in advance of a crisis. A crisis response team is usually composed of members of the psychiatric staff on inpatient units and is summoned to the unit by a code (similar to the codes used in a medical emergency). The team is called when the unit staff has exhausted other intervention strategies or when there is an unexpected assaultive incident. The team places the patient in seclusion (and restraints, if needed) after the patient has been confined and controlled. All staff members need to master self-protection techniques against such behaviors as kicking, hitting, and biting. Facilities that do not use codes or external teams usually provide aggression-management programs for students and staff, and most employees are required to periodically update these skills, just as with other emergency skills, such as cardiopulmonary resuscitation.

The staff must take immediate action when assaults occur. Six to eight staff members are needed to *safely* control a patient and assure there will be no injury to staff, patient, or other patients on the unit. It is important not to underestimate the number of staff needed because of the size, age, or sex of the patient. In recent research, many staff members said they were "surprised" at the strength and power of many patients who unexpectedly assaulted them (Clunn, 1988). Some agencies now include patients' previous athletic interests and accomplishments, such as weight lifting and black belts, on the admission form.

Although details of the procedures are not described here, a general outline of events is presented. To prepare for external control of a patient, staff members remove glasses, rings, earrings, pens, watches, keys, and anything that could cause injury to the patient or to themselves. Furniture and objects that can be used as weapons are removed from the area. One staff member becomes the team leader to organize and direct the planned, coordinated approach while one continues talking with the patient. At least one of the staff members gets the other patients to a safe place and stays with them.

**Restraint.** The team approaches the patient calmly in a show of force. The patient is told that the team is there to help and that they will not hurt the patient and will not let him hurt anyone. Initially, two team members approach the patient from the front and take control of his arms so they can guide him to the seclusion room. If the patient struggles, the other staff members quickly take control of the patient's legs and head so the patient can be carried to the room. Physical contact is protective and defensive, not aggressive and attacking. One staff person opens doors, moves obstacles, and brings the restraint cuffs. A nurse prepares the intramuscular medication. Once in the seclusion room, the patient is usually placed on the bed on his stomach or back. Four or more of the staff members hold the patient's extremities and head securely without hyperextending any joints. Wrist and ankle restraints, often made of leather lined with sheepskin, are applied to all four extremities and buckled to the frame of the bed. The arms are tied in a position at the patient's side, not above his head. The restraints are tight enough to inhibit slipping out of them but not tight enough to interfere with circulation. A waist restraint and a restraint between the ankles are applied only if the patient is at risk of injury because of fighting the restraints. Before staff members leave the patient, he is observed for his ability to move safely in the restraints. Medications may be administered at this time.

**Care of patients in seclusion or restaints.** When a patient is placed in seclusion or restraints, intensive nursing care is instituted. The patient is to be free of all belongings, all things that could harm him, and all objects that he could use to harm others. The patient is monitored closely every 15 minutes, with at least two staff members entering the room, announcing who they are and the purpose of the visit. The patient's mental status, response to and side effects of medications, hydration, nutrition, elimination, range of motion, vital signs, and hygiene are monitored. Immediate attention to any injuries resulting from the incident or from the restraints is critical and requires documentation. Every 1 to 2 hours the restraints are removed, one at a time for 10 minutes each. A minimum of two staff members are present during the release and range of motion. A change of position and skin care are also important. Stimuli are reduced by restricting visitors, phone calls, and diversional materials, such as radios and magazines.

## Recovery and depression phases

The patient is assured that he is not being punished while in seclusion. Patients need to be assisted in relaxing, sleeping, and benefiting from these phases of cooling down and reconciliation. The patient's time in restraints or seclusion should be a supportive, restorative time. Once the patient is calm and in control, he is encouraged to discuss what happened in the episode of losing control and alternatives for handling a similar situation in the future.

The patient is ready to be released from restraints when he shows signs of self-control, decreased anxiety and agitation, stabilization of mood, increased attention span, reality orientation and judgment, regulation of sleep, and normalization of sleep patterns. He may be kept in the seclusion room a brief time to assess his reaction to release from the restraints. Patients need assistance to reenter the ward, and nurses need to make efforts to help other patients accept them back.

After the patient is restrained and secluded, the staff should meet, ensure that there were no staff injuries, evaluate how they handled the situation, and give each other mutual support and feedback. Feelings and attitudes are discussed, along with suggestions for improved use of procedures. These debriefing meetings provide the unit staff ongoing in-service opportunities to monitor their reactions as well as augment their own skills. Careful documentation of the patient's behaviors before, during, and after the incident and a rationale for physical control interventions, seclusion, and restraint are essential legal protections for the nurse. These may be recorded as "incident reports" and should be written after all concerned have calmed down. Staff perceptions are compared for accuracy. Documentation is descriptive, sequential, organized, and specific in terms of what was seen, heard, felt, and said by whom, who was notified, and actions taken and to be taken. The request for and granting of a physician's order for seclusion and restraint are also recorded.

Other patients' reactions to a restraint and seclusion situation need to be openly discussed and explored. Patient government and inpatient groups provide excellent opportunities for the patients to share their concerns, reactions, and fears of losing control. It is important to tell the other patients that staff is providing control and care until the patient can control his behavior.

## STAFF AS VICTIMS OF ASSAULT

Most incidents of patient outbursts of anger do not result in restraint procedures, but when they do, the process is always a difficult one for the staff as well as for the patient. Staff and the patient are understandably drained physically and emotionally. The process of debriefing and recovery is complicated if a staff person has been injured.

Emotionally, being injured by a patient is similar to being a victim of any crime (see Chapter 28). Such an occurrence can destroy the staff member's sense of trust in others and sense of control of her life. The staff member often expresses feelings of being vulnerable, responsible for the incident, less competent, and unworthy (Dawson et al., 1988). The assault may be minimized, and feelings may even be denied if emotional support and debriefing are not provided at a later time (after the medical examination and treatment are completed). If the injured staff member is away from work for a period of time, the rest of the unit staff may not realize that their emotions have subsided much more than those of their injured colleague. To ensure that the staff victim achieves emotional resolution of the incident, some facilities have developed a formalized process of follow-up. Trained staff members, who understand the dynamics of assault, the common responses of victims, and supportive interventions, keep in touch with the injured person. The needs of the victim determine the frequency and number of meetings that occur. The goal of this process is to facilitate emotional resolution, help the person remain productive, and decrease the chance of resignation (Dawson et al., 1988).

## KEY CONCEPTS

1. Anger is a normal human emotion that may be expressed assertively, passively, passively-aggressively, and aggressively.
2. Verbal and physical aggression, especially assault and battery, require safe, immediate interventions based on the principle of least restrictive alternative.
3. Social norms may modify the legal definition of assault and battery and tolerate certain behaviors in certain situations.
4. The animal, individual, and social-psychological models of aggression offer explanations of the development of aggression.
5. Factors within the nurse, the environment, and the patient affect the development and expression of anger.
6. The assault cycle describes the predictable phases of aggression: the triggering, escalation, crisis, recovery, and depression phases.
7. Nursing interventions with anger and nonviolent aggression concentrate on ventilation to defuse the anger and then on problem solving to identify ways of handling the causes of the anger appropriately.
8. Tension reduction, medications, physical control, seclusion, or restraints become necessary in the escalation and crisis phases of the assault cycle.
9. Patients in seclusion and restraints require intensive physical and emotional nursing care.
10. Staff members who are injured by a patient may require assistance in recovering.

### REFERENCES

American Nurses' Association: Code of ethics for professional nurses, Kansas City, Mo., 1980, The Assocition.

American Nurses' Association: Standards of psychiatric and mental health nursing, Kansas City, Mo., 1982, The Assocation.

Bandura A: Aggression: a social learning analysis, Englewood Cliff, N.J., 1973, Prentice Hall.

Bellak, L: The concept of acting out: theoretical considerations. In Abt LE and Weissman SL, editors: Acting out, ed 2, Northvale, N.J., 1987, Jason Aronson, Inc.

Berkowitz L: Aggression: a social psychological analysis, New York, 1962, McGraw-Hill.

Binder RL and McNiel DE: Victims and families of violent psychiatric patients, Bull Am Acad Psychiatry Law 14:131, 1986.

Braun L: Theoretical frameworks for understanding violent behavior. In Babich K, editor: Assessing patient violence in the health setting, Boulder, Colo., 1981, Western Interstate Commission for Higher Education.

Burgess A: A clockwork orange, New York, 1962, Ballantine Books.

Campbell J: Theories of violence, In Campbell J and Humphreys J, editors: Nursing care of victims of family violence, New York, 1984, Reston.

Chesser AS: The assaultive patient. Part I., Nursing intervention, Adv Psychiatr Ment Health Nurs 1:1, 1982.

Clunn PA: Nurse's assessments of a person's potential for violence: use of grounded theory in developing a nursing diagnosis. In Kim M, McFarland G, and McLane A, editors: Classification of nursing diagnosis; proceedings of the fifth national conference, St. Louis, 1984, The CV Mosby Co.

Clunn PA: Nurses assessments of violence potential, In Babich K, editor: Assessing patient violence in the health care setting, Boulder, Colo., 1981, Western Interstate Commission for Higher Education.

Clunn PA: Nurses' assessment of a person's potential for violence, doctoral dissertation, New York, 1975, Columbia University Teachers' College.

Clunn, PA: Unpublished research, 1988.

Cohen AK: Delinquent boys: the culture of the gang, New York, 1955, Free Press.

Cohen NL and Marcos LR: The bad-mad dilemma for public psychiatry, Hosp Community Psychiatry 40(7):677, 1989.

Comas-Diaz L and Griffith EEH, editors: Clinical guidelines in cross-cultural mental health, New York, 1988, John Wiley.

Coser LA: The functions of social conflict, New York, 1956, Free Press.

Dawson J, et al: Response to patient assault: a peer support program for nurses, J Psychosoc Nurs 26(2):8, 1988.

Dollard JLW et al: Frustration and aggression, New Haven, Conn., 1939, Yale University Press.

Freud S: Beyond the pleasure principle, standard edition, London, 1962, Hogarth Press.

Fromm E: Anatomy of human destructiveness, New York, 1973, Basic Books.

Gelles, RJ: Family violence, ed 2, California, 1987, Sage.

Glynn, JM, et al: Compliance with less restrictive aggression control procedures, Hosp Community Psychiatry 40(1):82, 1989.

Goode, WJ: Force and violence in the family, J Marriage Family 33:624, 1971.

Gottheil E, editor: Alcohol, drug abuse and aggression, Springfield, Ill, 1983, Charles C Thomas.

Holm O: Four factors affecting perceived aggressiveness, J Psychol 114:227, 1983.

Janofsky JS, Spears S, and Neubauer DN: Psychiatrist's accuracy on predicting violent behaviors on an inpatient unit, Hosp Community Psychiatry 39(10):1090, 1988.

Jones MK: Patient violence: a report of 200 incidents, J Psychosoc Nurs 23(6):12, 1985.

Kagan S, Knight GR, and Romero SM: Culture and the development of conflict resolution style, J Cross Cultural Psychol 13:43, 1982.

Kalogjera IJ, et al: Impact of therapeutic management on use of seclusion and restraint with disruptive adolescent inpatients, Hosp Community Psychiatry 40(3):280, 1989.

Kirkpatrick H: A descriptive study of seclusion, Arch Psychiatr Nurs 3:3, 1989.

Krakowski M, Volavka J, and Brizer D: Psychopathology and violence: a review of the literature, Compr Psychiatry 27:131, 1986.

Lanza ML: Origins of aggression, Psychosoc Nurs Mental Health Serv 21(6):10, 1983.

Laudau SF: Trends in violence and aggression: a cross cultural analysis, Int J Compar Soc 25:133, 1984.

Lazarus IRS and Grolkman SR: Stress, appraisal and coping, New York, 1984, Springer.

Lindsey KP, Paul GL, and Mariatto MJ: Urban psychiatric commitments: disability and dangerous behavior of black and white recent admissions, Hosp Community Psychiatry 40(3):286, 1989.

Lions JR and Reid WH, editors: Assaults within psychiatric facilities, New York, 1983, Grune & Stratton.

Lorenz KZ: The foundations of ethology, New York, 1981, Springer-Verlag.

Manglass L: Psychiatric interventions you can use in emergency, RN, 49:38, November, 1986.

McFarland BH, et al: Chronic mental illness and the criminal justice system, Hosp Community Psychiatry 40(7):719, 1989.

McNeil DE, Binder RL, and Greenfield T: Predictors of violence in civilly committed acute psychiatric patients, Am J Psychiatry 145:965, 1988.

McNeil DE and Binder RL: Relationship between preadmission threats and later violent behavior in acute psychiatric inpatients, Hosp Community Psychiatry 40(6):605, 1989.

Meddaugh, DI: Reactance: understanding aggressive behavior in long-term care, J Psychosoc Nurs 28(4):28, 1990.

Mills MJ: Civil commitment; the relationship between perceived dangerousness and mental illness, Arch Gen Psychiatry 45:770, 1988.

Munns DC: A validation of the defining characteristics of the nursing diagnosis "potential for violence," Nurs Clin North Am 4:711, 1985.

National Crisis Prevention Institute. Nonviolent crisis intervention, Brookfield, Wis., 1988. The Institute.

Rosen JN: The concept of "acting in." In Abt LE and Weissman SL, editors: Acting out, ed 2, Northvale, N.J., 1987, Jason Aronson, Inc.

Segal SP, et al: Civil commitment in the psychiatric emergency room, Arch Gen Psychiatry 45:753, 1988.

Simmel G: Conflict and the web of group affiliations, Glencoe, Ill., 1955, The Free Press (originally published in 1908).

Smith P: Empirically based models for viewing the dynamics of violence. In Babich K, editor: Assessing patient violence in the health care setting, Boulder, Colo., 1981, Western Interstate Commission for Higher Education.

Sonkin DJ: Clairvoyance vs. common sense: therapist's duty to warn and protect, Victims Violence 1:7, 1986.

Steinmetz SK: The cycle of violence: assertive, aggressive and abusive family interaction, New York, 1977, Praeger.

Straus MA: A general systems theory approach to a theory of violence between family members, Soc Sci Information, 105, June, 1973.

Tanke ED and Yesavage JA: Characteristics of patients who do and do not provide visible cues of potential violence, Am J Psychiatry 142:1409, 1985.

Tardiff K: The use of medication for assaultive patients, Hosp Community Psychiatry 33:307, 1982.

Turpin JP: The violent patient: a strategy for management and diagnosis. Hosp Community Psychiatry 34:1, 1983.

Williams R: The trusting heart: type As, take note: ambition won't kill you; it's hostility that can be fatal. New Age J 6(May-June):26, 1989.

Zuckerman M: Sensation seeking and psychopathology. In Hare R and Schalling D, editors: Psychopathic behavior: approaches to research, London, 1978, John Wiley.

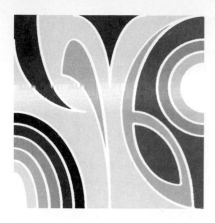

## CHAPTER 8

# Working with Groups of Patients

LEARNING OBJECTIVES

After reading this chapter you should be able to

- Outline the basic goals of group therapy.
- Describe specific therapeutic benefits of groups.
- Identify the major purpose of each type of group.
- Explain the value of coleadership of groups.
- Recognize physical factors important for group functioning.
- Identify intervention strategies for specific group situations.

Working with groups of patients is an integral component of both inpatient and outpatient psychiatric care. Nursing has 24-hour accountability for patient care on the inpatient psychiatric unit. This responsibility dictates economical use of nursing personnel. Hence, working with groups of patients addresses manpower concerns while providing a proven therapeutic intervention. Not surprisingly, "nurses are the most frequent leaders of group work on psychiatric wards" (Affonso, 1985).

Groups can be effective on short-stay units. Patients with mental illnesses face problems in their daily living like anyone else "but with an additional burden of doing so with symptoms of mental illness" (Maxmen, 1984). Even though mental illness interferes with the way patients are able to cope with their problems, conflicts, and interpersonal relationships, patients have the capacity to learn how to cope and negotiate life's problems. Groups deal with current issues and stresses that the patient will face on discharge. Patients gain awareness and knowledge about their behaviors and how those behaviors impede communication and coping. They become aware of alternatives that help them make better decisions and choices.

On inpatient units, numerous educational and skill-development groups are led by nurses. Nurses also lead groups for patients' families, to teach them about mental illness and to help them cope with a mentally ill member.

This chapter is dedicated to answering two questions:

1. Given a patient population that has serious interpersonal and cognitive disturbances, how does group work benefit the individual?
2. What can the nurse realistically expect to accomplish through informal and formal group work with patients?

Since inpatient groups typically have short-term, goal-oriented sessions and are composed of acutely ill patients, nurses need relevant information for developing group strategies. Benefits of groups, types of groups, and group leadership are addressed to provide this information. Because working effectively with groups of patients is so inextricably related to milieu management, the nurse is encouraged to read this chapter and Chapter 16 concurrently.

## BENEFITS OF GROUPS

Following are some of the benefits that patients receive from any group experience:

- Patients gain knowledge about how their maladaptive interpersonal communication behaviors interfere with their ability to develop interpersonal relationships. More specifically, patients learn how their behaviors interfere with or prevent them from forming the relationships they desire (Van Servellen, 1983; Yalom, 1983).
- Patients gain acceptance, reassurance, and support from their peers and the group leader.
- Patients gain feelings of hopefulness and a sense of power regarding their ability to help themselves and each other.
- Patients are provided with the opportunity to test out new behaviors with others during their hospitalization.

- Patients can share their feelings, problems, concerns, and ideas with others in a safe and structured environment.
- Patient strengths that can enhance self-esteem are affirmed and built upon.
- Patients experience a sense of importance and an increased sense of worth.

These benefits may occur at different times for individual patients and in different group situations. Each group, depending on its goal or purpose, may focus on one particular outcome. For example, an activity group may focus on acceptance so that, no matter what the patient paints, he will be accepted and praised for his work.

### Therapeutic factors

Dr. Irvin Yalom has described eleven "therapeutic factors" that help patients in any therapeutic group (see Box 8-1). Yalom initially described them as "curative factors"

---

**Box 8-1**
YALOM'S THERAPEUTIC FACTORS

- **Instillation of hope:** Patients receive hope from observing others who have benefited from the group experience.
- **Universality:** Patients experience relief in knowing that they are not alone and unique but that others experience similar problems, feelings, and concerns.
- **Imparting of information:** Patients learn or are provided with information about areas related to their needs.
- **Altruism:** Patients experience themselves as being helpful or useful to others.
- **Corrective recapitulation of primary family group:** Patients review previous dysfunctional family patterns and learn that those past patterns can be changed to effectively meet their present needs.
- **Development of socializing techniques:** Patients are taught appropriate social skills.

- **Imitative behavior:** Patients selectively model healthy behaviors of the leader and other group members.
- **Catharsis:** Patients not only are allowed to express feelings but learn how to express them appropriately.
- **Existential factors:** Patients share feelings about "ultimate concerns" of existence, like death or isolation, and learn to accept that there exists a limit to their control of these issues.
- **Cohesiveness:** Patients experience feelings of being accepted, valued, and part of a group experience.
- **Interpersonal learning:** Patients learn how their behaviors affect others and try out more appropriate ways of relating in the supportive atmosphere of the group.

but later relabeled them. He stated that "different groups accent different clusters of these therapeutic factors and that different patients in the same group may make use of very different factors" (Yalom, 1983). Thus patients experience certain factors or benefits, depending on the type of group that they participate in as well as on what the patients as individuals deem to be beneficial and important to themselves. The meaning of these therapeutic factors and their significance to patients are important for nurses to understand. If nurses understand that groups benefit patients, they will be more likely to initiate, lead, and participate in informal and formal groups.

Research studies have been conducted to determine which therapeutic factors operate in groups. One study found that patients who benefited from groups rated all curative factors more highly than did patients who thought that they did not benefit. "It may be that it is the individual's presence in a group, with an opportunity to reconnect socially and to talk over experiences, that is most important to patients" (Kahn et al., 1986). Nurses, then, are in a prime position to facilitate therapeutic encounters with patients informally as well as on a more formal basis. Nurses constantly communicate to patients that interactions with them are "valued as important and meaningful to the individual sharing them" (Affonso, 1985). Nurses do not make therapeutic factors happen but facilitate their development and occurrence for patients.

## TYPES OF GROUPS

Making the inpatient group a positive, beneficial experience for patients is of primary importance (Yalom, 1983). Patients need to feel they have gained something for themselves during their hospitalization. A positive inpatient group experience will favorably predispose the patient to seek treatment on an outpatient basis.

Numerous types of groups can be offered in both the inpatient and the outpatient setting: support, activity, education or problem solving, insight without reconstruction, and personality reconstruction (Van Servellen, 1983). Self-help or special-problem groups and multiple-family or couple groups also exist.

### Support groups

The very nature of nursing implies support. Nurses support patients in their daily therapeutic interactions. Supporting patients means accepting, empathizing, and showing concern while listening and talking with them. Nurses focus on responding to patients' needs. The nurses' presence, interest, and encouragement facilitate expression of patients' feelings and concerns. Nurses are then instrumental in helping patients cope with their feelings and situations. Support is used by nurses in many types of group situations.

The support group is a maintenance group. Its purpose is to reinforce or maintain existing patient strengths and behaviors instead of confronting or changing behaviors or defenses. Patients in a support group can be acutely or chronically ill. They may need much reassurance and emotional support during their hospitalization. These patients also need to reduce their anxiety to mild or moderate levels.

The reality-orientation group is a support group frequently found in an inpatient setting. Patients exhibiting confusion and short attention spans due to psychopath-ology benefit from this type of group. Nurses must provide an atmosphere of safety and security, since these patients often feel overwhelmed, anxious, alone, uncomfortable, and isolated. The reality-orientation group can assist patients with decreasing iso-lation and increasing self-esteem. Focusing on the here and now provides a frame-work with structure, social support, and reality testing. Nurses as leaders of these groups facilitate orientation to time, person, and place, rules and routine of the unit, and behavioral expectations, including some limit setting. Being valued, respected, and important as human beings are feelings these patients may not have experienced recently.

## Activity groups

Activity groups use a variety of techniques to facilitate patient communication and interaction (Van Servellen, 1983). For example, some groups may use art or music to motivate patients to interact and also to promote socialization. Withdrawn, de-pressed, and regressed patients benefit from these groups because they have ex-perienced isolation and lack interpersonal relationships. The general goals of these groups are to help patients increase their self-esteem, their openness, and the expres-sion of their feelings and to decrease isolation. When interpersonal communication increases, focus on the activity per se decreases. The activity is a vehicle or means to facilitate self-expression and patient interaction.

*Recreation* is a form of activity therapy used in most psychiatric settings. Ther-apeutic recreation can occur as informal Ping-Pong and card games, structured softball, basketball, or volleyball games, and as trips outside the hospital to bowl, or attend sports events, and so on. Recreation or play activities provide patients with the opportunity for fun and for feeling good (Jack, 1987). It lends balance to their daily schedule and helps in treating the whole patient.

Nurses can use a recreational activity as a foothold for establishing a therapeutic relationship with patients or as a platform for therapeutic encounters with patients who are frightened, withdrawn, or reluctant to participate. Some patients view games as being nonthreatening and are able to tolerate informal interactions during a game of pool, Ping-Pong, or softball. Patients who play games with each other experience predictability, security, order, success they can see and feel, and acceptance by a group (Jack, 1987). Nurses can be role models of healthy behaviors for patients if they can display a sense of humor while engaging in therapeutic recreation. The familiar axiom of "laughter is the best medicine" helps patients discharge tension and anxiety. A structured exercise group can also help relieve tension. It can be scheduled in the morning to help patients feel better physically as they start their day and to give them a sense of accomplishment and participation. It is beneficial for hyperactive patients because it channels their energy constructively within a specific framework.

*Creative expression* is another type of activity group. In some settings creative expression is part of occupational therapy or arts and crafts. Patients participate in ceramics, woodworking, and other projects. Even though patients work on individual projects, isolation is decreased because they are in a group setting. They achieve a sense of accomplishment by finishing their projects, express feelings through their work, and receive positive feedback for their efforts.

On the inpatient unit, nurses can initiate and plan with groups a variety of activities of daily living, such as grooming, cooking, money management, and laundry. Patients often share paintings or drawings with nurses. Communication of feeling through an art form can lead to the verbalization of feelings. Because nurses focus on accepting and understanding patients, sharing of intense inner feelings can occur.

Some settings may employ art therapists for the purpose of conducting art therapy groups. Art therapists are trained to "be in tune, in a feeling way, with patients' needs and psychic processes" (Lubell, 1983). Art therapists are able to recognize and interpret symbols and clues in art work that are valuable in assessing patients. Art therapy can help patients to create and to communicate what they are unable to verbalize or to admit to themselves.

Dance therapy fosters patients' ability to help themselves and the ability to communicate with others (Klein, 1983). It is an active process in which patients develop body awareness (Klein, 1983). Music is chosen to create a therapeutic environment and is based on patients' needs. Some inpatient units provide patients with a piano or even a music room with stereo equipment of some type. Nurses can organize sing-a-long or music groups with patients to facilitate expression of feelings, cohesiveness, socialization, and an increase in self-esteem.

Books and magazines are creative vehicles nurses can use in group settings to help patients cope with their feelings. Books, chosen for their literary as well as therapeutic value, are placed on inpatient units. Nurses can direct patients to books on a particular topic based on the patients' needs (for example, books that might facilitate therapeutic communication and resolution of such issues as grief, divorce, and abuse).

Poetry therapy "stresses emotional response and affect over intellectual or substantive content" (Morrison, 1986). Group activity centered on writing poems fosters creativity and expression of feelings. Writing poetry provides patients "with an opportunity for creative search of self" (Houlding and Holland, 1988). Poetry groups offer nurses the opportunity to gain further insights into patients and their concerns.

Pet therapy or the use of animals as a therapeutic resource can improve the mental and physical health of patients. A cat or dog provides unconditional acceptance and companionship. It also promotes feelings of caring and responsibility on the part of its caretaker. Animals such as rabbits and guinea pigs are kept in inpatient psychiatric settings to promote communication, socialization, and participation in their care. Stroking and talking to animals promotes a sense of well-being and pleasure. The presence of pets in the milieu can be therapeutic to patients of all ages.

### Medication groups

Nurses working in the inpatient setting continuously dispense medications, answer questions, and intervene with patients about their concerns and complaints regarding side effects. In the course of inpatient hospitalization before discharge most patients attend a medication group led by a nurse. The nurse explains types of medication, dosages, therapeutic effects, and side effects.

In the outpatient setting, nurses typically lead groups for patients who are taking intramuscular long-acting psychotropic medications such as fluphenazine (Prolixin) or haloperidol (Haldol). Patients taking these medications usually have chronic mental illness, with problems of medication compliance. The primary goal of these groups is to improve adherence to medication regimens, "which is a critical factor in preventing decompensation and promoting stability in the chronically mentally ill" (Cassino et al., 1987). Additional goals focus on providing a regular opportunity for socialization and problem solving for the patients meeting in the group (Selander and Miller, 1985). Nurses are able to assess the patients' symptoms and side effects, teach, and support in addition to administering medication. For some patients, this group may be their only social outing or opportunity to interact with others. Outpatient medication groups "reduce recidivism rates of its members in number of hospitalizations, in total length of hospitalizations, and in length of each hospitalization" (Selander and Miller, 1985). Information about specific drugs is discussed in Unit Three.

## Problem-solving groups

Nurses in therapeutic encounters with patients help them to solve problems based on immediate needs. Nurses also facilitate problem solving in many types of group situations. Specific group issues may center on ward issues, conflict resolution, job concerns, and discharge planning. A structured problem-solving group aims to have patients identify and define current problems, discuss possible alternatives, choose a particular solution, and try to enact the solution outside the group setting (Pekala et al., 1985). Nurses use their interpersonal skills together with the problem-solving process to facilitate patients' progress. The steps of problem solving entail recognizing, defining, and describing a current problem; developing and considering alternate solutions and their effects; and deciding on an alternate method of behaving and trying it. The alternate method must be evaluated to determine whether it worked. If it did not, another method will be tried and the process continued.

## Stress-management groups

Everyone experiences stress; yet each person deals with stress in a unique manner. Inpatients on psychiatric units "either had not developed adequate coping strategies to handle the stress, or they had come to a point in their life where their coping strategies were no longer sufficient in handling their present situations" (Hoover and Parnell, 1984). Helping patients to cope with stress can be accomplished in stress-management groups where nurses use their knowledge about stress theory to facilitate adaptive coping behaviors with patients. Nurses can combine didactic material (e.g., life-style balance and management and discussion of stress-related problems) and relaxation training in group sessions (Griffin et al., 1985). Nurses are incapable of modifying or removing stressors from patients' lives, but they can certainly teach adaptive coping skills to help patients toward better health.

## Social skills groups

Social skills groups focus on realistic, day-to-day patients needs in response to the isolation, loneliness, rejection, and low self-esteem felt by patients. Social skills training may deal with meeting new people, initiating conversation, going on a job interview, shopping, or negotiating return of a purchase. "The goal of group social skills training is to help patients learn, practice, and develop the skills necessary to effectively interact with others" (Plante, 1989). (See Chapter 16.)

### Insight without reconstruction

"Small groups where patients are given the opportunity to talk to each other about themselves, their problems, and their relationships with each" (Erickson, 1981) are different from problem-solving groups. Problem solving about postdischarge living arrangements is concrete, with specific options and solutions. Although insight groups may focus on the "here and now," the emphasis is on communication and interpersonal issues leading to emotional integration and intellectual insight (Van Servellen, 1983). Patients' problems are discussed to facilitate knowledge and understanding of how individuals affect and are affected by others. Patients can learn new reactions and behaviors, once they understand the "why" of underlying feelings and discover new ways of interacting and behaving.

### Personality-reconstruction groups

Long-term group personality-reconstruction therapy is not appropriate on short-term inpatient units. These groups are conducted on an outpatient basis, usually by persons with extensive training and education in psychotherapy. The origins of problems are thoroughly reviewed for each person in the group. Patients are expected to give up their defense mechanisms and to change behaviors after gaining an understanding of the origins of their problems (Van Servellen, 1983). These groups are psychoanalytically oriented and meet for lengthy periods.

### Self-help or special problems groups

**Psychodrama.**  Psychodrama is described by Moreno as a psychotherapeutic group that focuses on self-awareness and interpersonal learning (Moreno, 1983). Psychodrama can be scheduled as a separate group for inpatients, or its methods can be used in other groups. This group is usually conducted by a psychodramatist or director who has received specialized training in this therapeutic method. In psychodrama a patient or protagonist acts out his own role in an interaction or a situation as if it were presently occurring. Other patients and staff members assume the roles of auxiliary egos to enact other roles needed in the drama. The role of alter ego is assumed by an individual to voice the thoughts and feelings of the protagonist. The other patients or audience lends support to the protagonist. Psychodrama plays or scripts can be used by the director. Moreno has structured each session to include the warm-up, the action or drama, and the postaction or discussion. The director uses the discussion to promote interpersonal learning. He leads the group members through discussion of feelings and identification of problems. Psychodrama sessions can be draining for patients, especially the protagonist, because of the strong feelings elicited during the drama.

**Sociodrama.**  In psychodrama an individualized conflict unique to the individual is developed. Sociodrama is a form of psychodrama that emphasizes the social roles of people. For example, a sociodrama could focus on aspects of the role of being a mother. A woman, dissatisfied with a particular interaction that occurred with her teenage son over limit setting is asked to assume the social role of mother. The interaction with her son is unique to her social role as mother and is the particular aspect of communication the group would concentrate on for that session. Reenactment of the specific interaction between mother and son would be played out. The group works on alternate ways for the mother to communicate. The alternative is then acted out in the safe environment of the group. The use of sociodrama gives patients the opportunity to participate in role playing, decision making, and feedback. Insight and confidence are facilitated in acting out or role-playing solutions to interpersonal relationships and communication.

**Problem-centered groups.**  Numerous groups focus on helping persons with special problems (for example, child abuse, anorexia and bulimia, and diabetes). These groups are homogeneous, meaning that all group members share the same problem. Members feel accepted and understood by the group and therefore are freer to share their concerns and to ask questions. Information or education is shared together with personal feelings and difficulties. Members assist each other with helpful strategies. They do not feel alone or isolated but learn that others with the same problem or need are coping effectively. Nurses who lead special problem groups have an interest in and additional knowledge and skills for working with that specific problem area and that specific type of patient (Van Servellen, 1983).

**Traditional self-help groups.**  Traditional self-help groups are homogeneous, like the problem-centered groups, but are not professionally organized and led. Self-help groups are organized and led by group members who share the same problem. They believe that only one who has or has had the problem can truly help the other person. It is estimated that 12 million persons participate in about 500,000 self-help groups (Hurley, 1988). In some groups, such as Alcoholics Anonymous, individual 24-hour support is available to group members if requested. Members of these groups understand each other's life-styles and needs and help each other with problem-solving and coping with stress. Members also confront each other about "alcoholic" behaviors. Professionals may be invited for a specific purpose, such as providing an educational program. Nurses may be asked to serve as consultants. Since they commonly refer individuals to self-help groups, nurses need to be knowledgeable about the self-help groups in their area. Interested individuals can call their local mental health organization for information.

## GROUP LEADERSHIP

Group leadership functions range from the informal to the formal. The inpatient psychiatric nurse may engage in spontaneous and informal interactions with a group of patients in a card game or participate formally in a planned and structured group session in a special setting. An informal card game provides the nurse with an opportunity for therapeutic interpersonal interaction, socialization, and role-modeling behavior. Another example might be responding to medication questions that come up in small informal groups. By providing drug education, the nurse reinforces compliance with medication and may alleviate anxiety or concerns. Such informal, spontaneous interventions with groups of patients occur repeatedly during the course of a day on an inpatient unit.

Although degrees of formality and types of patient vary, the nurse invariably uses group leadership skills to meet patient needs in the therapeutic milieu. As managers and providers of patient care (24 hours a day), nurses are the most frequent initiators of therapeutic group interactions with patients (Affonso, 1985). Consequently, nurses need to understand general principles of group interaction that have clinical applications.

Nurses on inpatient units need to be aware of factors influencing the clinical setting. Short-stay inpatient hospitalization affects group work in many ways. Short hospitalizations create a rapid turnover of patients in groups. It is unrealistic to think that a high level of trust and cohesion will develop in a group in which patients continuously leave and others join. Patients will have an assortment of illnesses and will be seriously ill. The nature of the therapeutic milieu dictates that most patients are expected to participate in groups. "Nurses can present the message that patients with problems can give, as well as receive, help" (Erickson, 1981). Nurses will need to quickly assess how soon patients can enter groups and which patients cannot tolerate a group at all.

Confidentiality must be explained to group participants; that is, they must understand that what is said or takes place in the group must stay in the group. However, what is stated in group sessions may be shared with staff members or the treatment team since they are all responsible for patient care. Of course, information shared in the group should not leave the unit and the hospital. Charting patient progress in the group is an important task.

## Coleadership

An important factor to consider about group leadership is that nurses have days off and may rotate shifts. Therefore, the presence of a coleader can lend consistency to the group and directly support the structure and purpose of the group. Coleaders can complement each other and learn from each other. They share responsibility for the group. If the group is large, charting and communicating information to other staff members can be expedited. In addition, one leader may observe something in group that the other nurse may not see. Coleadership provides active modeling of how to relate to others, mutual respect, and collaboration (Van Servellen, 1983).

## The physical setting

Physical arrangements are important for group leaders to consider in creating an atmosphere conducive to group work. Finding adequate space or a private room is often difficult, but it is important to ensure privacy for patients as well as a quiet atmosphere. Adequate lighting, temperature, seating, and equipment also contribute to successful group function. Forming a circle of chairs allows patients to see each other and states to patients that they are expected to relate to the leaders and to each other. At times, chairs in rows may be appropriate for a didactic group. A blackboard or a dry marked board may be necessary.

# Formal groups

Nurse leaders must be active, structured, and empathetic. Because of time con-straints, leaders cannot afford to be nondirective or to allow the group to be free floating. The formal group should meet for about an hour. The leader succinctly states the purpose at the beginning of the group session. Most of the session is spent on the work to be accomplished. Patients generally prefer leaders who provide the group "with a clear sense of the basic group task and direction and focus the group's attention on work" (Yalom, 1983). The final 5 to 10 minutes is used to summarize and close the session. The summary should focus on positives and include what the patients have learned or gained from the group. The leader should give positive feedback to the group on how well they have done during the session.

Patients should be expected to arrive at the group session on time. On some units the group leader will gather the group of patients and walk with them to the session. No smoking or refreshments are permitted during group sessions. Patients should remain for the entire group session if possible. Permission may be given to pace or to leave the room and return when the patient is able to. Inability to sit still for a period of time may be due to anxiety or to drug side effects (e.g., akathisia). The decision to exclude patients from the group should be made carefully. The nurse may exclude patients who are acutely manic, disoriented, or too psychotic to benefit from group therapy or who will disrupt the group. Patients who are hostile and verbally threatening are also not appropriate candidates for group therapy.

## Interventions

Basic interventions for groups are based on facilitative communication techniques (see Chapter 5). Nurses use these skills with patients individually and in groups. Nurses who are able to facilitate group interactions on a therapeutic level will enable patients to share feelings and problems. Some basic communication skills useful for nurse leaders are found in Table 8-1. These skills are not unique to the group setting but are based on skills nurses use on a daily basis. These general interventions are therapeutic, regardless of the type of group. The use of positive statements also helps patients decrease their anxiety and increase their comfort (Pekala et al., 1985). For example, a patient may be attempting to use a particular assertiveness skill and goes off on a tangent. The nurse can say, "You have done well, Mr. J. When you gave us the example of saying to your boss, 'I need to talk with you about my work schedule,' you used an excellent example of 'I' statements." The nurse chooses to repeat the portion of Mr. J.'s statement that was realistic and a correct example of an "I" statement for emphasis and clarity. As a result the patient feels a sense of accomplishment and increased self-esteem.

*Gatekeeping* functions are also within the nurse's repertoire. They serve to involve all the patients in the group by limiting domineering patients and allowing others to contribute (Pekala et al., 1985). For example, the nurse can say, "Miss B., you are doing well in contributing to our session today, but I would like to hear what others are thinking about at this time." This intervention can forestall mono-polization of the group by a particular patient without putting her down and gives others the opportunity to express themselves. The other patients in the group may

**TABLE 8-1**  Communication skills: eliciting, qualifying, and clarifying communication

| Techniques of the leader(s) | Group member response | Outcome |
| --- | --- | --- |
| 1. **Giving information:** "My purpose in offering this group experience is . . ." | **Further validates** his assumptions: "How is this going to happen?" | Leader(s) and member(s) enter into a dialogue in which member(s) get more information to make decisions and build trust in group experience. |
| 2. **Seeking clarification:** "Did you say you were upset with John because he said that?" | **May try to restate** his thoughts or feelings: "Yes, I guess I was upset." | Member becomes aware that he was not clear and learns to identify thoughts and feelings more precisely, at the same time taking responsibility for them. |
| 3. **Encouraging description and exploration** (delving further into communication or experiences): "How did you feel when Joann said that to you?" | **Elaborates** on his message: "I was angry." | Member deals in greater depth with an experience in the group and again takes responsibility for his reactions. (This example also places events in time or sequence, lending further perspective to group events.) |
| 4. **Presenting reality:** "Would other members think Joann was unstable if they interviewed her for a job? You don't appear shaky to me." | **Listens and considers** other possibilities. | Member compares perception of self with others' perceptions of him. |
| 5. **Seeking consensual validation** (seeking mutual understanding of what is being communicated): "Did I understand you to say that you feel better now than you did last week?" | **Further clarification:** "Well, yes, I'm better than last week but not as good as I'd like to be." | Group and leader(s) learn how member views his progress and in which way they should receive his evaluation of himself. |
| 6. **Focusing** (identifying a single topic to concentrate on): "Maybe we could identify one problem you have and talk more about that." | **Channels thinking:** Members may think of the most puzzling problem they have. | Group and leader(s) identify specific topics they can resolve before the meeting ends. They increase their understanding of one problem before jumping to others. |

From Van Servellen G: Group and family therapy, St. Louis, 1983, The C.V. Mosby Co.

**TABLE 8-1** Communication skills: eliciting, qualifying, and clarifying communication—cont'd

| Techniques of the leader(s) | Group member response | Outcome |
|---|---|---|
| 7. **Encouraging comparison** (asking members to compare and contrast their experiences with others in the group): "How did the rest of the group handle this problem?" | **Group members share their experiences** as they relate to the topic. | Leader(s) and members gain greater insight into their commonalities and differences and learn from one another alternative ways of responding to problems. |
| 8. **Making observations:** "You look more comfortable now, John, than you did at the beginning of the meeting." or "The group has been silent for the last 5 minutes." | **Group members have something to respond to:** "I feel more at ease now." or "I think we are quiet because we are bored." | Group members and leader(s) place attention on significant events and can elaborate on their meanings. |
| 9. **Giving recognition or acknowledging:** "John, you are new to the group. Perhaps we can introduce ourselves." | **Feels acknowledged and included:** "Yes, I'm John, and I came here because ..." | Members view specific instances as important, and the leaders reinforce the behavior or event they choose to notice, in this case, the desire to come to group. |
| 10. **Accepting** (not necessarily agreeing with but receiving communication with openness): "Yes, I hear you say that you don't know if you want to be in the group or not." | **Feels heard and understood** without fear or attack. | Members learn that even "nonacceptable" attitudes can be talked about, and perhaps any thought is not so horrible that they cannot share it. |
| 11. **Encouraging evaluation** (asking the group as a whole or individual members to judge their experiences): "When Marilyn gives you support do you feel better?" or "How did we do in helping Joann with her problem?" | **Members reflect** on progress made: "Not exactly, because I don't know if I can trust her to be honest." or "It was hard, I'd like to know from her." | The criteria for success become clearer to members, and new directions may be formulated as a result of the discussion. |
| 12. **Summarizing** (encapsulating in a few sentences what has occurred): "The group discussed several issues and problems today—they were ..." | **Members recall** significant points and close off consideration of new or extraneous topics. | Members and leader(s) place events in perspective, identifying salient points of a group session. Such a summary can lead to a better understanding of group process. |

be unable to handle this patient or may be too afraid. If the group leader cannot control the patient or is afraid, the integrity of the group is compromised. The uninvolved patient presents another challenge to the nurse leader. The patient may be quiet because he is anxious or afraid. As patients become more comfortable in the group, their ability to participate verbally increases (Van Servellen, 1983). Chronic schizophrenics find it difficult and threatening to relate in group sessions. The nurse needs to start at the level of the learner (Frost, 1970). The nurse can say, "It is hard to talk about ourselves in group, but I know that everyone here has something to share that can help someone else." The nurse recognizes that patients are mistrustful and anxious but relates the message that each individual is important and capable of helping another. The *hostile patient's* hostility may mask underlying anger toward himself, fear, or unresolved anger toward others. To help this patient appropriately verbalize what his anger is all about, the nurse can say, "Mrs. R., you sound angry today. What happened?" Or "Tell us about it." The nurse directly confronts the patient in a supportive manner and attempts to help the patient deal with her feelings. Allowing nonverbal or verbal hostility to continue jeopardizes the progress of the group session. Unchecked hostility causes discomfort and uneasiness and impairs the ability of other patients to attend to the group's work. A patient may also mistakenly misinterpret the anger as being meant for him. These group interventions will help the nurse develop as a group leader. However, patients quickly recognize the group leaders' empathy, understanding, and respect for each patient as caring behaviors. Even though some patients make only minimal progress toward their individual treatment goals, they can increase their feelings of worth as human beings by interacting with the nurse who possesses these traits.

## KEY CONCEPTS

1. The psychiatric nurse interacts and intervenes with patients in informal groups as well as in formal, planned, and structured sessions.
2. As group leader, the nurse facilitates patient groups by focusing on words and behaviors.
3. Patients benefit from group experiences by gaining acceptance, hopefulness, and support from others. Through mutual sharing of feelings and problems, patients learn how their communication and behaviors interfere with relationships. Their strengths are reinforced and built upon.
4. Regardless of the purpose of the group, the patient needs help to determine personal outcomes.
5. Various types of groups exist in inpatient and outpatient settings to benefit the acutely and chronically ill. Typical groups are support, remotivation, education and problem-solving, insight, and self-help groups.
6. Nurses use facilitative communication techniques and role-modeling behaviors in their role as group leaders.
7. The nurse leader intervenes therapeutically with monopolizing, uninvolved, and hostile patients.

**REFERENCES**

Affonso DD: Therapeutic support during inpatient group therapy, J Psychosoc Nurs 23(11):21, 1985.

Cassino T, et al.: The prolixin brunch, J Psychosoc Nurs 25(10):15, 1987.

Cohen L: Bibbliotherapy, J Psychosoc Nurs 26(8):7, 1988.

Davidhizar R and McBride A: Teaching the client with schizophrenia about medication, Patient Educ Couns 7:137, 1985.

Davis J and Juhasz A: The Human/Companion animal bond: how nurses can use this therapeutic resource, Nurs Health Care 5:497, 1984.

Erickson R: Small-group psychotherapy with patients on a short-stay ward: an opportunity for innovation, Hosp Community Psychiatry 32:269, 1981.

Frost B: The active leader in group therapy for chronic schizophrenics, Perspect Psychiatr Care 8:(6)268, 1970.

Griffin W, Ling I, and Staley D: Stress management groups, J Psychosoc Nurs 23(10):31, 1985.

Harter L: Multi-family meetings on the psychiatric unit, J Psychosoc Nurs 26(8):18, 1988.

Hoover R and Parnell P: An inpatient educational group on stress and coping, J Psychosoc Nurs 22(6):17, 1984.

Houlding S and Holland P: Contributions of a poetry writing group to the treatment of severely disturbed psychiatric inpatients, Clin Soc Work J 16(2):194, 1988.

Hurley D: Getting help from helping, Psychol Today, p 63, January, 1988.

Jack L: Using play in psychiatric rehabilitation, J Psychosoc Nurs 25(7):17, 1987.

Kahn E, Webster P, and Storck M: Brief reports curative factors in two types of inpatient psychotherapy groups, Int J Group Psychother 36(4):580, 1986.

Keltner NL: Psychotherapeutic management: a model for nursing practice, Perspect Psychiatr Care 23(4):125, 1985.

Kelly H and Philbin M: Sociodrama: an action oriented laboratory for teaching interpersonal relationship skills, Perspect Psychiatr Care 6(3):110, 1968.

Klein V: Dance therapy. In Kaplan H and Sadock B, editors: Comprehensive group psychotherapy, ed 2, Baltimore, 1983, Williams & Wilkins, pp 184-188.

Kneisl C: Increasing interpersonal understanding through sociodrama, Perspect Psychiatr Care 6(3):104, 1968.

Lubell D: Art therapy in groups. In Kaplan H and Sadock B, editors: Comprehensive group psychotherapy, ed 2, Baltimore, Williams & Wilkins, 1983, pp 177-183.

Manderino M and Bzdek V: Social skill building with chronic patients, J Psychosoc Nurs 25(9):18, 1987.

Maxmen J: Helping patients survive theories: the practice of an educative model, Int J Group Psychother 34(3):355, 1984.

Moreno Z: Psychodrama. In Kaplan H and Sadock B, editors: Comprehensive group psychotherapy, ed. 2, Baltimore, Williams & Wilkins, 1983, pp 158-166.

Morrison M: Poetry as therapy, Curr Psychiatr Ther 23:59-66, 1986.

Pekala R, Siegel J, and Farrar D: The problem-solving support group: structured group therapy with psychiatric inpatients, Int J Group Psychother 35:391, 1985.

Plante T: Social skills training, a program to help schizophrenic clients cope, J Psychosoc Nurs 27(3):7, 1989.

Rusakoff L and Oldham J: Group psychotherapy on a short-term treatment unit: an application of object relations theory, Int J Group Psychother 34(3):339, 1984.

Selander J and Miller W: Prolixin group, J Psychosoc Nurs 23(11):16, 1985.

Toufexis A: Furry and feathery therapists, Time, p 74, March 30, 1987.

Van Servellen G: Group and family therapy, St. Louis, 1983, The CV Mosby Co.

Yalom I: Inpatient group psychotherapy, New York, 1983, Basic Books, Inc.

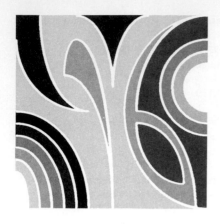

## CHAPTER 9

# Psychiatric Liaison/Consultant Nursing

VEDA MARIE BOYER AND JANET C. KIRSCH

LEARNING OBJECTIVES
After reading this chapter you should be able to

- Describe the roles of the nurse consultant.
- Describe the types of consultation.
- Identify the phases of consultation.
- Recognize the steps in implementing the consultant role.

Today's health care environment is significantly affected by both external forces and internal forces. The *external forces* include rapid technological advances, competition, and the multiple demands of certifying agencies. Among the *internal forces* are budget constraints, commitment to quality, maintenance of high staff morale, and shrinking resources. These demands often call for the use of a consultant, especially in the following situations:

1. When internal resources are lacking for completion of a project.
2. When the factors contributing to inefficiency in an area are unclear.
3. When a major organizational change is desired (Lancour, 1987).

Such an environment can benefit from the skills of the psychiatric nurse consultant. Consultation or liaison nursing is an area of expanded practice in psychiatric nursing that has evolved over the last two decades. Consultation has been defined as an interaction between two professionals—a specialist in a particular field (the consultant) and a person having difficulty with a work-related problem (the consultee) (Davis, 1983). This chapter gives an overview of this nursing consultation process. It compares and then consolidates the roles of the liaison nurse and the nurse consultant, describing various types of consultation, phases of consultation, and implementation of the consultant role.

## PSYCHIATRIC LIAISON NURSE

The liaison nurse is a psychiatric nurse engaged in the consultative process with an emphasis on psychosomatic illness and the psychosocial needs of patients in a general or nonpsychiatric setting. Initially, the liaison nurse was involved in the assessment, planning, intervention, and evaluation of the mental health aspects of a patient's care and served as a link between the patient and others. The need for the liaison nurse evolved from the stress associated with illness.

Today the role of the liaison nurse has expanded to include not only the needs of patients and their families but also those of individual staff members, staff members as a group, and organizations as a whole. The liaison nurse may work in a general hospital or in a number of other nonpsychiatric settings. Naturally, the liaison nurse in an outpatient setting will be involved in activities different from those encountered in an inpatient critical care setting. The liaison role is ongoing and informal, and it may be initiated by either consultant or consultee (Davis, 1983). The liaison role may be the primary responsibility or only one of the responsibilities of a nurse working on a psychiatric unit within a general hospital. The nurse for whom this is a primary role generally expands the liaison nurse's patient-focused concerns to include staff and organizational issues.

## PSYCHIATRIC CONSULTANT NURSE

The nursing consultant is responsible for many of the same activities as the liaison nurse, but consultation differs in that it is sporadic (as needed) and formal and is initiated by the consultee (Davis, 1983). In addition, staff-development content (for example, stress management, conflict, change, and psychosocial issues) is commonly addressed by a consultant. The nurse from an inpatient psychiatric unit may serve sporadically as a nurse consultant to the nonpsychiatric area on request.

The literature often uses the terms *psychiatric liaison nurse* and *psychiatric nurse consultant* interchangeably. In this chapter the term *psychiatric nurse consultant* will be used to refer to both liaison and consultant roles.

## KEY FACTORS IN THE CONSULTATION PROCESS

Several factors are key to the role of the successful consultant (Davis, 1983; Lehman, 1987):

- That she be in a staff rather than a supervisory position to facilitate open communication (it may be difficult to be frank with the boss) and to remove any appearance of coercion for acceptance of solutions she proposes.
- That the professionals with whom the consultant nurse works accept the recommendations of their own free will.
- That the focus be professional (having to do with problems encountered in the work setting) and not personal.
- That the consultee remain ultimately responsible for the patient.
- That the consultant join the consultee in a partnership for problem solving in a professional-peer relationship rather than one of superior-subordinate.

## QUALIFICATIONS

The knowledge base of the psychiatric nurse consultant must include a thorough understanding of psychiatric nursing theory and clinical experience. In addition, she must understand the formal and informal structure of the organization. For example, the informal leaders of a work group may exert considerable influence and should not be ignored. Doing so could doom the consultation process. Those psychiatric nurses who are creative and who want to learn will function best in the unstructured role of consultant.

## THE CONSULTATION FOCUS

In the role of consultant, the nurse uses her expertise to provide three main types of consultation: patient-focused, consultee-focused, and system or organization-focused. Consultee-focused consultation can be further broken down into staff, intragroup (within a group), and intergroup (among two or more groups). In all types of consultation the interventions may be direct or indirect. The types of consultation are described in Table 9-1.

### Patient-focused activities

With patient-focused activities the consultant may intervene with the patient or family (direct) or may work through the professionals already involved (indirect) in the patient's care. Usually patient-focused requests are for assistance with difficult and complex psychosocial problems, such as psychosomatic illnesses, behavior problems, ineffective coping, death and dying, and grief. Consultations may be nurse to nurse or may extend to the multidisciplinary team (see Table 9-1).

**TABLE 9-1**　Types of consultation

| Type | Focus | Purpose | Primarily responsible to | Example |
|------|-------|---------|--------------------------|---------|
| Patient-direct | Consultant works with patient, patient's family, patient's environment, patient's community | To actively intervene with mental health needs of the patient, such as death and dying, anger, change in body image, grief, and loss | Patient family | Patient who has undergone a mastectomy and is dealing with a change in body image |
| Patient-indirect | Consultant works with patient caregiver | To facilitate interventions by patient caregiver | Caregiver | Helping caregiver respond to family members who are dealing with the impending death of a patient in critical care |
| Consultee: staff-direct | Consultant works with staff member | To deal with mental health needs of staff member, such as adjustment to new role, stress of workload, multiple patient deaths | Staff member | Staff member who is considering leaving nursing because of workload demands |
| Consultee: staff-indirect | Consultant works with manager regarding a staff member | To facilitate interventions by manager for a professional staff member's growth and to help manager work with other staff in relation to the problem staff member. | Manager | Assisting a staff member to confront a peer (problem staff member) who does not assume her share of the workload |

*Continued.*

**TABLE 9-1**   Types of consultation—cont'd

| Type | Focus | Purpose | Primarily responsible to | Example |
|---|---|---|---|---|
| Consultee: intragroup-direct | Consultant works directly with a group of staff members on their issues | To actively intervene in mental health and group dynamics issues of a group of staff members | Group of staff members | Group discussion with staff members who are dealing with the death of a long-term patient |
| Consultee: intragroup-indirect | Consultant works with a group of staff members to learn process for dealing with their own issues | To help a staff group learn to deal with the group's mental health and group-dynamics concerns | Group of staff members | Working with group of staff members to define group norms and role definitions |
| Consultee: intergroup-direct | Consultant works directly with two or more groups in relation to communication, collaboration, and conflict resolution | To actively intervene with two or more groups to develop or change patterns of communication, collaboration, or conflict resolution | Two or more groups | Physicians desire research; nurses desire clearly written research protocols |
| Consultee: intergroup-indirect | Consultant works with two or more groups to develop a process for dealing with their own communication, collaboration, and conflict resolution | To facilitate two or more groups in the implementation of patterns of relating that promote the development of goals, plans, and programs beyond the dynamics of the group | Two or more groups | Establishing a framework for communication for development of standards of care |

**TABLE 9-1** Types of consultation—cont'd

| Type | Focus | Purpose | Primarily responsible to | Example |
|------|-------|---------|--------------------------|---------|
| Organizational or system-direct | Consultant works directly with administrators and managers on an administrative or organizational problem | To actively intervene in assessment, diagnosis, and change of organizational behavior | Administrator manager | Provision of interventions needed for turnover problem |
| Organizational or system-indirect | Consultant assists administrators and managers to develop proactive processes and programs to facilitate a mentally healthy organizational climate | To facilitate administrators and managers in the process of program development based on perceived mental health needs of employees | Administrator manager | Employee assistance programs, stress-management programs |

## Consultee-focused activities

The role of the consultant in consultee-focused activities often involves interpersonal conflict between individuals or groups. The consultee can be an individual, a work group, or two or more groups. The consultant may provide assistance with the nonproductive staff member who is causing dissatisfaction among the rest of the staff or the staff member who uses ineffective communication skills. Often in such situations the consultant works with the nurse manager, who then intervenes with the staff member. In direct interaction with staff members, mental health concerns that interfere with the work role may be the focus. In consultee-focused activities the consultant may work with intragroup problems (e.g., within the day shift) or intergroup relations (e.g., between day shift and evening shift). In intergroup or intragroup activities, conflicts are often between nurses, nurses and administrators, or nurses and other disciplines. In the nonpsychiatric areas of the hospital, conflict most often arises when the severity of patient illness increases. Heightened staff stress also causes conflict (Fife, 1983) (Table 9-1). The current changing health care environment has increased the need for consultee-focused consultation of all three types. Major issues that affect health care today are presented in Box 9-1. The first four issues were identified by White (1988).

### Box 9-1
### MAJOR ISSUES AFFECTING HEALTH CARE

1. Critically short staffing
2. Coping with rapid change, including turnover in leadership
3. Depersonalization of complex systems
4. Interpersonal conflict
5. Communication breakdown
6. Rising number of acutely ill inpatients
7. Competency challenges of new technology
8. Ethical issues
9. Reduced resources and increased compliance criteria for accreditation and certification

### System- or organization-focused activities

The third category of consultation has a system or organization focus. Requests for assistance come from organizational and managerial leadership. Common problems are difficulties with communication, interpersonal relationships, and decision making (Fife, 1983). The type of consultation chosen depends on the needs of the consultees. Each model entails an assessment of the organization's structure, roles, and inter- action patterns. Interviews are a part of the organizational assessment.

Two specific types of system or organization-focused activity that have received particular attention over the last few years are formalized stress-management and employee-assistance programs. Such programs are usually offered for all staff mem- bers and include such aspects as educational seminars, career counseling, psycho- logical counseling, and physical fitness and wellness programs. Seminars are often related to stress management, prevention of job burnout, relaxation techniques, and time management (Table 9-2). The psychiatric nurse has a great deal to offer in such programs and often plays a leadership role in their development and imple- mentation.

### PHASES OF CONSULTATION

With any of the types of consultation the process begins with a request for assistance with a work-related problem. The consultant not only must possess the ability to do the job but also, and even more important, must have interpersonal skills to gain the trust and respect of those making the request and those with whom she will be working (Lancour, 1987). The consultation-consultee working relationship consists of six phases that parallel the nursing process (Lippett and Lippett, 1978; Fife, 1983; Lancour, 1987):

1. Entry and formulation of an agreement
2. Assessment and diagnosis

**TABLE 9-2** Focused consultation content

| Focus | Issues and concerns |
|---|---|
| Patient | Noncompliance |
| | Behavioral concerns |
| |   Self-injury |
| |   Assaultive |
| |   Withdrawn |
| |   Clinging |
| |   Depressed |
| | Response to chronic pain |
| | Response to chronic illness |
| | Death and dying |
| | Communicable diseases: Hepatitis B, AIDS, Herpes |
| | Interpersonal relationships |
| |   Patient and family |
| |   Family and family |
| |   Patient and staff |
| |   Family and staff |
| | Transplantation |
| |   Donor availability |
| |   Donor-recipient dynamics |
| |   Transplantation process and phases |
| | Developmental issues |
| |   Learning abilities |
| |   Developmental tasks and needs |
| | Dealing with life-sustaining technology |
| | Education of patient regarding the psychosocial aspects of his illness |
| | Stress management |
| | Psychosomatic illnesses |
| | Continued treatment of psychiatric illnesses in a nonpsychiatric hospital setting |
| Staff | Care planning for patients having the issues or concerns mentioned in patient-focused consultation |
| | Time management |
| | Team building |
| | Stress management |
| | Conflict management |
| | Group dynamics |
| | Using a psychoeducational approach to care |
| | Assertiveness |
| | Negotiation |
| | Empowerment through problem solving |
| | Mental health standards of care and practice |
| | Creation of a climate for excellence |
| System | Issues or concerns mentioned in staff-focused section |
| | Retention and recruitment |
| | Stress management for employees |
| | Employee assistance program |
| | Substance abuse education |
| | Policy and procedure formulation (mental health components) |
| | Organizational dynamics of a climate for excellence |
| | Dealing with planning for change |
| | Consumer-driven care and marketing strategies |

3. Goal setting and development of an action plan
4. Implementation of the action plan
5. Evaluation of outcomes
6. Disengagement and termination by the consultant

## Entry and formulation of agreement

During entry and formulation of an agreement a clear and concise definition of the desired outcome is developed. This includes the establishment of mutual consent between consultant and consultee(s). The consultant nurse must have access to people and information, the commitment of people's time, and the opportunity to be innovative. The agreement usually includes contact person, time frame, activities, involved individuals, and the process for ongoing progress reports (Lancour, 1987).

## Assessment

The second phase is that of assessment. The assessment includes (1) the consultee's perception of the problem, (2) the problem as perceived by others, (3) specific approaches that have been attempted and their outcomes, and (4) identification and evaluation of desired but realistic outcomes (Fife, 1983).

## Goal setting and development of an action plan

The third phase is that of goal setting and development of an action plan. The plan should be practical, mutually agreeable, and realistic as well as tailored to the situation. Recommended actions should be actions that are within the control of the consultee to improve the situation and to which the consultee is favorable (Lancour, 1987).

## Implementation

Implementation can often be accomplished by the consultee independently. Further support and validation from the psychiatric nurse should be available if needed (Fife, 1983).

## Evaluation

Evaluation includes an assessment of the degree to which the desired outcomes were achieved. It may be done immediately on completion of the action plan, or it may have built-in follow-up as time elapses. Included in the evaluation is self-appraisal by the psychiatric nurse.

## Disengagement and termination

The final phase is disengagement of the psychiatric nurse and termination of her services. This process has naturally occurred during the phases of implementation and evaluation and includes assessment by consultant and consultee regarding the steps of the actual consultation process. Periodic visits or telephone calls may occur as part of the termination process (Lancour, 1987).

## ADDITIONAL ROLES OF THE PSYCHIATRIC NURSE AS CONSULTANT

In conjunction with the consultation process and as a part of the consultant role, the psychiatric nurse plays the roles of educator, therapist facilitator, and researcher.

### Educator

As educator the nurse may be involved in both formal and informal teaching activities. A major goal of the consultation process is behavioral change that enables the individual or group(s) to perform more effectively in the future. The psychiatric nurse is involved in direct patient-education activities, such as the teaching of relaxation techniques, coping strategies, and communication skills. In addition, teaching occurs as the psychiatric nurse participates in patient care rounds throughout the hospital, attends care conferences and Kardex rounds, and participates in formal workshops. Indeed, learning needs that can best be met through planned learning experiences are often identified in the process of consultation. Workshops in assertiveness, communication skills, group process, concepts related to behavioral problems, grief and grieving, and death and dying are ones the psychiatric nurse is uniquely qualified to present.

### Therapist and facilitator

As therapist and facilitator the psychiatric nurse assists individuals and groups to use more effective coping and assists in the prevention and treatment of crises arising out of stress situations. With an individual staff member the psychiatric nurse might assist in the development of a stress-management plan. Such interventions as routine exercise, good nutrition, planning time with friends, journal writing, and routine vacations would be developed. When workload is excessive and staff conflict develops, the psychiatric nurse might assist the group to formulate a set of work-group norms to use in such situations.

### Researcher

Finally, the psychiatric nurse incorporates the role of researcher into the consultant role. Through her use of research, other professionals see firsthand how research can be applied to daily work activities. Second, the consultant encourages staff to test approaches to these problems, using scientific methods (Fife, 1983). For instance, nurses might test the effectiveness of relaxation techniques for preoperative patients in the attempt to reduce anxiety before surgery.

In summary, the psychiatric nurse consultant can be an important asset in the nonpsychiatric areas of a hospital setting. Other professionals, such as social workers, psychologists, psychiatrists, and chaplains, have been used in similar consultant roles; however, the psychiatric nurse, according to Fife (1983), is a more effective choice for two reasons. First, as a nurse, she understands the very real limits of patient care and the stressors nurses often experience. Second, a bond exists in the nurse-to-nurse consultant-consultee relationship. The expertise of the psychiatric nurse contributes to quality patient care, professional development, and retention of staff.

## IMPLEMENTATION OF THE CONSULTANT ROLE

Exciting opportunities await nurses in today's health care environment. Changes in funding, human resource availability, health care demands, consumer awareness, and standards-driven practice require a new approach to meeting health care outcomes. Old barriers to cooperative ventures are dissolving. There is an increased awareness of the need to share information and depend on one another's expertise. The competitive stance of being all things to all people is being replaced by the realization that quality outcomes can best be accomplished through the coordinated efforts of many experts. New partnerships that reflect a win-win philosophy are enlarging old territorial boundaries. No longer can disciplines, units, departments, services, or systems function under the fallacy that they are self contained. Survival and viability depend on doing what one does best, recognizing one's limitations, entering into a partnership with others who can effectively compensate for one's limitations, and collectively producing a service or product that meets the complex needs of today's health care consumer.

### The preconsultation experience

Once a nurse has chosen psychiatric nursing as a specialty and has fine-tuned the skills needed to competently and confidently carry out this role in a psychiatric setting, the consultation potential expands. Having clearly defined (1) what kind of problems one would be capable of solving (given one's theory- and skills-based experiences), (2) the people or groups needful of this expertise, and (3) specifically what one would offer each potential consultee, the nurse is prepared to offer her expertise to others within the health care system.

The first step in becoming known as a consultant will hardly seem like consultation at all. Since this does not meet the classic definition of consultation it can be described as a preconsultation experience. In the world of business it would be known as "marketing strategy" while health care providers might call it a "therapeutic intervention." In other words, although the nurse has the expertise to solve a problem or enhance the well-being of a person, group, or system, the person, group, or system is unaware of that ability. Furthermore, the potential consultees may even be unaware of the need at all. Once the need is articulated, the nurse can offer to help the consultees meet the need.

Being oblivious to a need is not uncommon in health care organizations. For example, many persons in today's health care system are unconsciously suffering from three major ills: isolation, change-related organizational chaos, and an imbalance of demands and resources. As a result, health care providers become victims of overcommitment, sensory overload, priority diffusion, and burnout. In a general health care setting or hospital, the consultant can assist health care professionals in coping with these issues.

The challenge of marketing for the nurse is to first visualize, then accept, the role of "helper" to the hospital staff. When a problem is observed, she should objectively assess it and then cautiously and respectfully intervene. Although it is not an easy task to remain therapeutic in the midst of conflict or chaos, if one is, the outcome is threefold:

1. People respond positively when their needs are addressed.
2. People share their positive experience with others.
3. The informal, preconsultation experience generates a more formal process of consultation.

The consultant begins receiving consultation requests for assistance in dealing with difficult patients, helping staff members cope with the emotional aspects of their job, providing input to staff development regarding psychosocial nursing orientation content, coping with change, conflict management, and, it is hoped, in developing a nurse-to-nurse system-wide consultation system.

## The process of consultation

Once the psychiatric nurse has been established as a consultant, it is her responsibility to live within the guidelines established by the organization. If no such guidelines exist, it is important to establish guidelines for each consultation process. It is also necessary to have a clear understanding of the terms listed in Box 9-2.

There are specific responsibilities inherent in the roles of consultant and consultee (Box 9-3). These responsibilities must be clearly defined and agreed upon before the consultation process can begin.

## The setting

Consultation may be held in the consultant's office or on the consultee's unit. The former provides more privacy for the consultee. The latter provides the consultant with more information about the consultee's environmental assets, liabilities, and current work situation.

## Relational aspects

As a consultant the nurse is entering a system that has functioned without "outside" assistance or that may have had unpleasant experiences with outside assistance in the past. She must be sensitive to the relationship aspects of this role. Developing a relationship from the start helps decrease resistance and increases the potential for cooperative collaboration.

Building a relationship begins with the establishment of mutual respect. As a consultant the nurse must be clear that the consultee has knowledge and skills related to his clinical area of expertise, staffing patterns, unit norms, and so on that are essential. Conversely, the consultant has expertise in areas that are important to the consultee. By acknowledging the consultee's value and uniqueness and suggesting collaboration rather than a prescriptive approach to the problem, the consultant can forestall many territorial and authority-based conflicts. The basic assumption becomes that both parties are competent in specific professional areas.

When one is engaged in patient-focused consultation, it is important to remain focused on patient issues. The consultant needs to be aware of the consultee's limitations and to work within those limitations. The purpose is not to change them. Emphasis should be on available strengths and resources, with recommendations based accordingly. Typical issues and concerns for each level of focus are found in Table 9-2.

**Box 9-2**
# DEFINITIONS

Begin with a clear understanding of each of the following:

1. *Consultant:* a resource with expertise in defined areas, who is sought out for advice or assistance.
2. *Consultee:* an individual, group, or system seeking advice or assistance.
3. *Consultation:* an interaction between a consultant and a consultee, which clearly defines consultee needs, consultant abilities, and responsibilities for both parties, including time, place, and fee factors.
4. *Focus of consultation*
   a. *Patient centered:* focused on direct patient assessment and recommendations and on how the consultant and consultee should proceed. It answers the questions, What are the mental health concerns? What may be going on with this patient? What needs to be done?
   b. *Consultee (staff) centered:* focused on improving individual-staff or group-staff functioning in areas of knowledge deficit, skill deficit, self-confidence, objectivity, conflict management, motivation, or problem solving. There may be concerns within one group (intragroup) or among two or more groups of staff (intergroup).
   c. *Organization or system centered:* focused on developing new programs, improving existing ones, or evaluating and making recommendations about current system-based concerns.
5. *Degree of psychiatric nurse participation*
   a. *Direct consultation:* the consultant actively does the assessment, plan, intervention, and evaluation of outcomes. She assumes responsibility and accountability for the process and outcomes.
   b. *Indirect consultation:* the consultant facilitates the consultee's efforts to assess, plan, intervene, and evaluate. The consultee remains responsible and accountable for the process and outcomes and the consultant for responsibly carrying out the process of consultation.

Expectations about who will document what, confidentiality, care plan interventions, and who has decision-making responsibility regarding the mental health needs of the patient must be agreed on by the health care team.

There are many opportunities for psychiatric nurse consultants in today's health care market. Staff, health care systems, and hospitalized individuals with mental health needs can benefit from their skillful intervention. Nurses well grounded in psychiatric nursing concepts are prepared to provide this important service.

### Box 9-3
## RESPONSIBILITIES OF THE CONSULTEE AND CONSULTANT

### Consultee responsibilities

- Identifies (in writing) the need for which she would like assistance
- Collaborates about the need for consultation assistance with appropriate clinical, administrative, or managerial individuals and receives approval for consultation
- Identifies who should be involved in the consultation
- If applicable, addresses fees or negotiates payment
- Sets up the time and place for the initial and follow-up sessions
- Takes action regarding the consultant's recommendations
- Is free to accept, reject, or modify the consultant's advice
- Evaluates the outcomes of the actions

### Consultant responsibilities

- Makes sure that the consultation process and responsibilities are clearly defined and agreeable
- Assesses whether her expertise matches the consultee's need or request
- Clarifies and assesses the stated need
- Facilitates the diagnosis of or diagnoses the problem or situation
- Facilitates the formulation of recommendations requiring patient, staff, or system actions
- Facilitates or carries out the recommendations
- Follows up on the consultee's response to the recommendations
- Provides a written summary of the consultation process
- Evaluates the process of consultation with the consultee

## KEY CONCEPTS

1. Because of internal and external forces, a need for psychiatric-mental health consultation has developed.
2. Traditionally the liaison consultant psychiatric nurse was engaged in the consultation process with an emphasis on psychosomatic and psychosocial needs of patients in a general nonpsychiatric population.
3. The role of the liaison consultant nurse today has expanded to include not only the patient but his family and unit staff as well.
4. The psychiatric nurse consultant provides three main types of consultation: (a) patient-focused, (b) consultee-focused, (c) system/organization focused.

5. Patient-focused consultation includes (a) patient-direct, working with the patient, or (b) patient-indirect, working with the patient's nurse.

6. Consultee-focused consultation includes (a) staff direct, working with a staff member, (b) staff-indirect, working with a staff member's manager, (c) intra-group-direct, working with a group of staff members on a problem, (d) intragroup-indirect, working with a group of staff members to develop a process for solving group problems, (e) intergroup-direct, working with two or more groups on a problem, (f) intergroup-indirect, working with two or more groups to develop a process for solving the groups' problems.

7. System/consultation-focused consultation includes (a) system/organizational-direct, working with administrators and managers on a problem, or (b) system/organization-indirect, working with administrators and managers to develop a process for solving system/organization problems.

8. The consultation process is composed of several phases that parallel the nursing process.

## REFERENCES

Beisser A with Green R: Mental health consultation and education, Palo Alto, 1972, National Press Books.

Caplan G: The theory and practice of mental health consultation, New York, 1970, Basic Books, Inc.

Davis DS: Psychiatric mental health nursing consultation in the general hospital: liaison nursing. In Adams C and Macione A, editors: Handbook of psychiatric mental health nursing, Bethany, Conn., 1983, Fleshner Publishing Company, pp 375-389.

Fife B: The challenge of the medical setting for the clinical specialist in psychiatric nursing, J Psychosoc Nurs Ment Health Serv 21:8, 1983.

Kohnke MF: The case for consultation in nursing: designs for professional practice, New York, 1978, Wiley Medical Publication.

Lancour J: Choosing and using a consultant. In Lewis AM and Spicer JG, editors: Human resource management handbook, Rockville, Md., 1987, Aspen Publishers, pp 99-111.

Lehman F: Liaison nursing: a model for nursing practice. In Stuart G and Sundeen S, editors: Principles and practice of psychiatric nursing, St. Louis, 1987, The CV Mosby Co, pp 784-800.

Lippett G and Lippett R: The consulting process in action, San Diego, 1978, University Association, Inc.

Robinson L: Psychiatric consultation liaison nursing and psychiatric consultation liaison doctoring: similarities and differences, Arch Psychiatr Nurs 1:73, 1987.

White CL: The psychiatric clinical specialist as mental health consultant, Nurs Management 19:80, 1988.

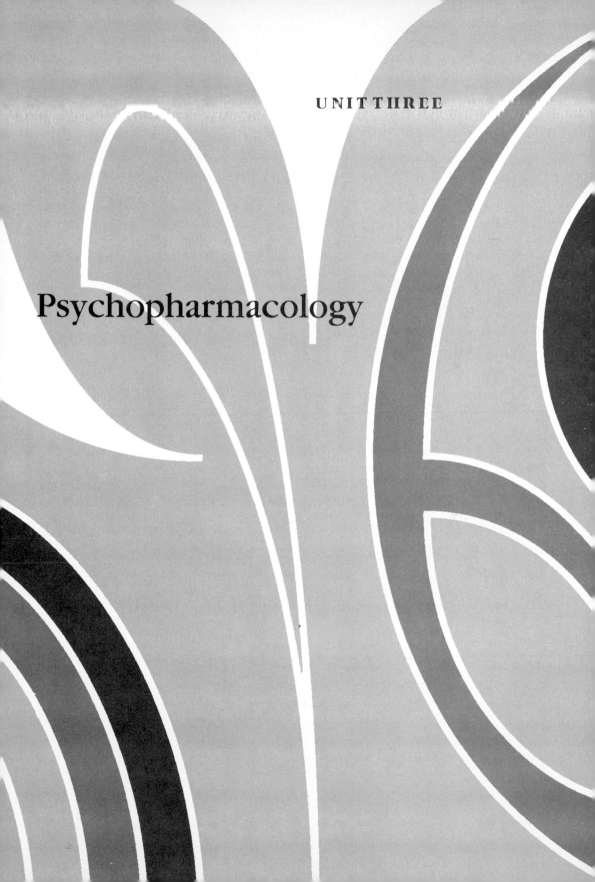

# Psychopharmacology

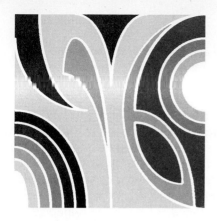

## CHAPTER 10

# Introduction to Psychotropic Drugs

LEARNING OBJECTIVES

After reading this chapter you should be able to

- State some benefits of patient teaching concerning medications.
- Describe the steps in the production of neurotransmitters.
- State the function of neurotransmitters.
- Describe how neurotransmitters are inactivated.
- State the function of the blood-brain barriers.
- Identify the chemical property that is most important in determining the ease with which a drug will cross the barrier.
- Articulate the importance for the psychiatric nurse of understanding the blood-brain barrier.

The second component of the *psychotherapeutic management* model is psychopharmacology. Psychopharmacology is an important dimension in psychotherapeutic management, albeit drugs are not always indicated. The treatment effectiveness of antipsychotic, antidepressant, and antimanic drugs is not questioned, as these drugs have enabled millions of persons to live more satisfying lives. Least-restrictive alternative, a concept that captures the community mental health effort to allow individuals to live their lives in an unrestrictive atmosphere, has evolved as a result of the impact of these drugs. Since nursing provides 24-hour care, the nurse is in an advantageous position to assess drug side effects, evaluate desired effects, and apply preventive care to reduce potential problems. In addition, the nurse most often makes decisions concerning p.r.n. medications. Nearly one half of all orders for antipsychotic drugs are written p.r.n. (Blair, 1990). The nurse, therefore, needs to understand key dimensions of psychotropic drug use. Each chapter in Unit III provides a discussion of pharmacologic effects (desired effects); absorption, distribution, and administration; side effects (undesired effects); and drug interactions. Equally important, a discussion of nursing implications emphasizes nursing intervention related to therapeutic versus toxic drug levels, side effects, interactions, and patient teaching.

To understand psychopharmacology, as opposed to memorizing facts, the reader must understand two concepts—neurotransmitters and the blood-brain barrier. An overview of these two important concepts is given in this chapter and should be studied before one reads about specific psychotropic drugs.

## PATIENT TEACHING

The importance of patient teaching cannot be overemphasized. Gellar (1982) found that only 8% of psychiatric inpatients knew the name, dosage schedule, and desired effect of any drug they were receiving. Although a risk is involved in discussing certain aspects of psychotropic drug use with patients because of the propensity for anxiety in the psychiatric population, nurses have a professional responsibility to do so. Of course, good professional judgment is important. For instance, one should teach the patient about what is visible and can be felt and emphasize regular checkups and tests. Brown and coworkers (1987) found side effects actually decreased as psychiatric patients were given instructions relating to those undesired effects. Patient teaching enables the patient to be an adult participant in his care and can decrease undesirable effects. Noncompliance, the failure to take medication as prescribed, can be reduced by effective patient teaching within the context of a meaningful nurse-patient relationship.

## NEUROTRANSMITTERS

Nerve cells or neurons are the basic unit of the nervous system. Nerve cells are designed to receive and give information. Dendrites are the projections from the neuron that receive information and transmit it to the cell body. Axons send information from the nerve cell to the dendrites of other neurons. Axons of one cell are separated from the dendrites of another by a microscopic space known as a synapse. Figure 10-1 depicts the relationship between neurotransmitters and neurons.

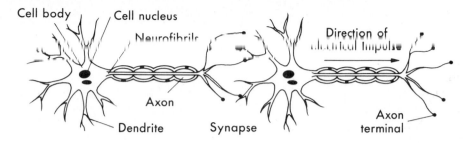

Cell body     Cell nucleus

Neurofibrils

Direction of
electrical impulse

Axon

Dendrite        Synapse

Axon
terminal

PRESYNAPTIC NEURON            POSTSYNAPTIC NEURON

**FIGURE 10-1** Neurotransmitter precursors produced in the cell body are carried by neurofibrils to axon terminals, where neurotransmitters are synthesized. An electrical impulse traveling from the cell body down the axon to the terminals causes release of transmitter into the space called the synapse. *(From Brown RP and Mann JJ: A clinical perspective on the role of neurotransmitters in mental disorders, Hosp Community Psychiatry 36(2):142, 1985).*

Information, in the form of an electrochemical excitation, is communicated between cells in a specific manner. An electrochemical impulse runs from the cell body through the axon to the presynaptic terminal. Neurotransmitters are stimulated and released from the presynaptic terminal into the synaptic cleft and combine with the postsynaptic receptors on the dendrites of the neuron, evoking a neuronal response. Neurotransmitters are synthesized from natural precursors in the body. These precursors are extracted from the bloodstream and are synthesized in the cell into neurotransmitters. Neurotransmitters are stored in storage vesicles in the presynaptic terminals of the cell. There are many kinds of neurotransmitter (perhaps only 5% have been identified), and they combine with specific receptors. For instance, norepinephrine, a neurotransmitter, will combine only with a norepinephrine receptor. Once norepinephrine electrochemically stimulates the norepinephrine receptor, information is transmitted from the dendritic outgrowth to the cell body, which in turn communicates to the next neuron and so on. Once the neurotransmitter is in the synaptic cleft, it can continue to stimulate the postsynaptic receptor until it (the neurotransmitter) is inactivated. Neurotransmitters are inactivated in two ways: (1) they are metabolized by enzymes or (2) they are taken back into the presynaptic storage vesicles (referred to as reuptake). Knowledge of this inactivation process has facilitated the evolution of psychopharmacology.

Psychotropic drugs, drugs that affect the central nervous system (CNS), can affect neurotransmitters in several ways (Fig. 10-2):

- The *release* of a neurotransmitter can be affected. Some drugs cause the release of stored neurotransmitters. Amantadine (Symmetrel), an antiparkinsonism drug, causes the release of the neurotransmitter dopamine.
- Psychotropic drugs can combine with a receptor and *block* the "natural"

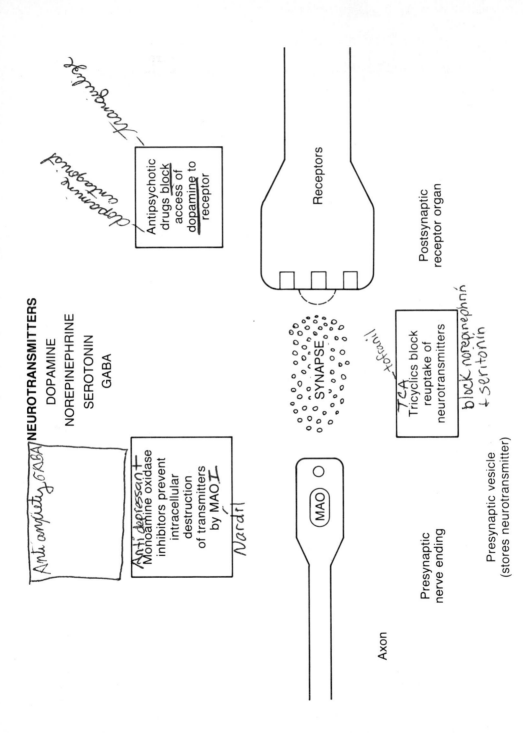

**NEUROTRANSMITTERS**

DOPAMINE

NOREPINEPHRINE

SEROTONIN

GABA

Anti anxiety GABA

Antipsychotic drugs block access of dopamine to receptor

thorazine

dopamine antagonist

Antidepressant
Monoamine oxidase inhibitors prevent intracellular destruction of transmitters by MAO I

Nardil

Receptors

Postsynaptic receptor organ

TCA
Tricyclics block reuptake of neurotransmitters

block norepinephrine + seritonin

tofranil

SYNAPSE

MAO

Presynaptic nerve ending

Axon

Presynaptic vesicle
(stores neurotransmitter)

**FIGURE 10-2**  Neurotransmission at the synapse. *(From Stuart G and Sundeen S: Principles and practice of psychiatric nursing, ed. 4, St. Louis, 1991, Mosby-Year Book Inc.)*

neurotransmitter from combining with it. Antipsychotic drugs such as chlorpromazine (Thorazine) block dopamine receptors.

■ Psychotropic drugs can affect the response of a receptor to a neurotransmitter.
■ Psychotropic drugs can *terminate the inactivation* of neurotransmitters. Tricyclic antidepressants block the reuptake of neurotransmitters, and antidepressants of another class, the monoamine oxidase inhibitors, block the enzymatic reduction of neurotransmitters (Brown and Mann, 1985).

## BLOOD-BRAIN BARRIER

The second concept, the blood-brain barrier, is also important if one is to understand psychotropic drug activity. Goldstein and Betz (1986) provided an excellent review of this topic in *Scientific American.* Life depends on homeostasis or balance. The brain, more than other organs of the body, requires a constant internal milieu. Whereas other parts of the body experience fluctuations in body chemistry, even small changes in the brain produce serious problems. The brain is protected from fluctuations by the blood-brain barrier. This barrier regulates the amount and the speed with which substances in the blood enter the brain. Water, carbon dioxide, and oxygen readily cross the barrier, but other substances are excluded from the brain.

The blood-brain barrier has two dimensions: an anatomical dimension and a physiological dimension. The structure of the capillaries that supply blood to the brain, the anatomical dimension, prevents many molecules from "slipping" through. The physiological dimension is a transport system that recognizes certain molecules and transports them into the brain. The discussion of transport systems is beyond the scope of this book. However, the reader is again directed to the work of Goldstein and Betz (1986).

Of the chemical properties that determine whether a molecule will pass through the blood-brain barrier, lipid solubility is the most important. Highly lipid-soluble substances pass the blood-brain barrier with relative ease. Highly water-soluble substances penetrate this barrier slowly and in insignificant amounts. Nicotine, ethanol, heroin, caffeine, diazepam (Valium), and levodopa are examples of highly lipid-soluble substances. Penicillin, dopamine, epinephrine, and potassium are not highly lipid soluble and do not penetrate the blood-brain barrier well. This is clinically significant because only drugs that can pass through this barrier in significant amounts are effective in treating a disorder in the brain (psychiatric or medical).

Certain non-lipid-soluble substances, such as glucose, the brain's primary energy source, and essential amino acids, which are needed for the synthesis of neurotransmitters, are required for normal brain function. Special transport systems carry these essential substances across the blood-brain barrier.

The importance of understanding the blood-brain barrier for the psychiatric nurse can be illustrated by several examples. If, for instance, penicillin were the only antibiotic available (which was true at one time), large doses would be needed because this water-soluble drug does not pass the blood-brain barrier well. When large doses of penicillin are given to get some penicillin into the brain, most of the penicillin is affecting the rest of the body. In the case of penicillin this does not cause alarm because it has relatively few adverse effects. On the other hand, dopamine (and many other drugs), which is used to treat parkinsonism (a dopamine-deficiency disease), has many adverse affects on the body. The dose needed to adequately affect the brain (a central effect) is so large that it would have serious adverse effects on the rest of the body (i.e., cardiac stimulation, a peripheral effect). Understanding the blood-brain barrier helps the nurse accurately conceptualize drug therapy. It also provides a base for understanding the highly lipid-soluble substances.

## KEY CONCEPTS

1. Psychotropic drugs have enabled millions of persons to live satisfying lives in a "least-restrictive environment."
2. Nurses assess for drug side effects, evaluate desired effects, and make decisions about p.r.n. medications, so it is important for nurses to understand general principles of psychopharmacology and to have specific knowledge concerning frequently used psychotropic drugs.
3. Patient teaching can decrease the incidence of side effects.
4. Neurotransmitters, neurochemical substances in the brain, evoke a neuronal response.
5. Neurotransmitters are synthesized from natural precursors in the body and are stored in storage vesicles in the presynaptic terminals of the neuron.
6. Since both neurotransmitter deficiency (e.g., depression) and excess (e.g., schizophrenia) are related to mental disorders, many psychotropic drugs are designed to increase or decrease the bioavailability of a specific neurotransmitter.
7. The blood-barrier protects the brain from the physiological fluctuations experienced by the rest of the body and regulates the amount and speed with which substances in the blood enter the brain.
8. Highly lipid-soluble drugs, such as ethanol, heroin, and diazepam (Valium), pass the blood-brain barrier with ease.
9. Only drugs that pass the blood-brain barrier can affect the central nervous system and consequently can be useful in the treatment of mental disorders.

### REFERENCES

Blair DT: Risk management for extrapyramidal symptoms, Quality Assurance Rev Bull 17:116, 1990.

Brown CS, Wright RG, and Christen DB: Association between type of medication instructions and patient's knowledge, side effects, and compliance. Hosp Community Psychiatry 36:141, 1985.

Brown RP and Mann JJ: A clinical perspective in the role of neurotransmitters in mental disorders. Hosp Community Psychiatry 36:141, 1985.

Geller JL: State hospital patients and their medications: do they know what they take. Am J Psychiatry 139:611, 1982.

Goldstein GW, Betz AL: The blood-brain barrier, Sci Am 255:74, 1986.

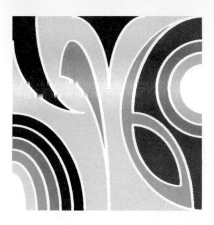

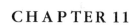

## CHAPTER 11

# Antiparkinsonism Drugs

LEARNING OBJECTIVES

After reading this chapter you should be able to

- Explain the concepts of neurotransmitters in relationship to parkinsonism.
- Describe differences among classes of drugs used in treating parkinsonism.
- Discuss side effects of antiparkinsonism drugs.
- Identify toxic versus therapeutic levels of antiparkinsonism drugs.
- Describe potential interactions with antiparkinsonism drugs.
- Discuss implications for patient teaching about antiparkinsonism drugs.

## PARKINSONISM

Parkinsonism is a progressive, chronic, degenerative disease involving the area of the brain called the extrapyramidal system, specifically the substantia nigra, which is the dopamine-generating portion of the brain. Through the balance of two neurotransmitters—dopamine and acetylcholine—the extrapyramidal system controls posture, balance, walking, and other movements. The three primary symptoms of parkinsonism are tremor, bradykinesia, and rigidity. Hosts of secondary symptoms are also quite common. Tremors, also referred to as rest tremors, are quite common (about 75 percent of parkinsonism patients have tremors). Historically, the terms *paralysis agitans* and *shaking palsy* were also used to identify parkinsonism. The *tremors* can usually be detected in one arm or hand when the person is at rest. Tremors are more amenable to treatment than some other symptoms. *Bradykinesia*, a generalized motor slowing, also manifests as mask facies (the face movements slow down) and decreased associated movements, for example, arm swings. Movements are difficult to initiate, slow, and difficult to stop. *Rigidity,* commonly referred to as cogwheel or lead pipe rigidity, makes movement and normal responses difficult. Other symptoms include postural difficulties, a gait disorder characterized by slow shuffling steps, and orthostatic hypotension. Falls can be a serious consequence. Finally, changes in mental status, such as depression and dementia, are not uncommon.

Secondary symptoms are caused by primary symptoms. Dysphagia, or difficulty in swallowing, creates difficulty with eating and can cause excessive accumulation of saliva and hence drooling (sialorrhea). Weight loss and choking are two more important considerations of dysphagia. Bradykinesia and rigidity combine to impair respiratory, bladder, and bowel function, compromising breathing and urinary function and causing involuntary elimination.

Idiopathic parkinsonism (cause unknown) is referred to as Parkinson's disease. (The cause, however, appears to be an age-related degeneration of the extrapyramidal system, usually occurring after the age of 40.) Known causes of parkinsonism (Box 11-1) not related to age are prescription drugs, such as antipsychotic agents and reserpine, brain injury, and environmental toxins, such as carbon monoxide and manganese. A contaminant of some street drugs can produce parkinsonism also.

## NEUROTRANSMITTERS

A balance between acetylcholine and dopamine is required for normal movements. Dopamine serves as an inhibitory neurotransmitter, and acetylcholine as an excitatory neurotransmitter. Imbalance can occur in three ways:

1. The brain may produce less dopamine, as occurs with degeneration of the substantia nigra.
2. Neuronal dopamine can be depleted chemically, for example, with reserpine.
3. Dopamine can be blocked at the postsynaptic receptor, as is done by the antipsychotic drugs.

When this imbalance occurs, motor neurons experience a continual "switched on" effect without the switching off needed for normal movement. Fig. 11-1 illustrates normal and imbalanced states of parkinsonism.

**Box 11-1**
## CAUSES OF PARKINSONISM

Parkinson's disease (idiopathic)          Brain injury
Prescriptive drugs                        Environmental toxins
  Antipsychotic drugs            Carbon monoxide
  Reserpine                       Manganese

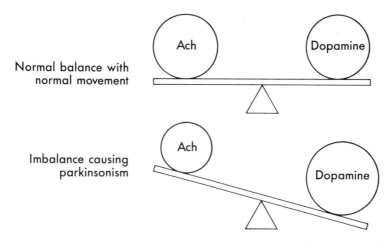

**FIGURE 11-1** Normal and imbalanced states of acetylcholine and dopamine (parkinsonism).

Drug treatment of parkinsonism is aimed at rebalancing the neurotransmitters acetylcholine and dopamine. Balance is accomplished in three ways:

1. Drugs are used to increase the level of dopamine (dopaminergic agents).
2. Drugs are used to decrease the level of acetylcholine (anticholinergic agents).
3. A combination of these two drugs is used to increase dopamine and decrease acetylcholine simultaneously (dopamine agents plus anticholinergic agents). Box 11-2 lists selected antiparkinsonism drugs.

## DOPAMINERGIC AGENTS

If parkinsonism is caused by a deficiency in dopamine, it would seem reasonable to give dopamine. However, because dopamine does not pass the blood-brain barrier easily, the large amounts that must be given to achieve therapeutic levels in the brain would produce serious adverse effects. Therefore dopaminergic agents, which

**Box 11-2**
## ANTIPARKINSONISM DRUGS

**DOPAMINERGIC DRUGS (increase dopamine availability)**

Dopamine precursor
  Levodopa (Dopar, Larodopa)
  Carbidopa-levodopa (Sinemet)
Dopamine releaser
  Amantadine (Symmetrel)
Dopamine receptor agonist
  Bromocriptine (Parlodel)
  Pergolide (Permax)
Dopamine-metabolism inhibitor
  Selegiline (Eldepryl)

**ANTICHOLINERGIC DRUGS (decrease acetylcholine availability)**

Trihexyphenidyl (Artane)
Benztropine (Cogentin)
Biperiden (Akineton)
Diphenhydramine (Benadryl)
Ethopropazine (Parsidol)
Procyclidine (Kemadrin)

cross the blood-brain barrier easily and increase dopamine levels in the brain, were developed to treat this condition. They fall into four categories:

1. Dopamine precursors, for example, levodopa and carbidopa-levodopa (Sinemet)
2. Dopamine releasers, for example, amantadine, which releases the small amounts of dopamine remaining in the dopaminergic neurons in the brain
3. Dopamine agonists, for example, bromocriptine, which mimics dopamine at the postsynaptic receptors in the brain
4. Dopamine metabolism inhibitors, for example, selegiline, which apparently blocks the metabolism of dopamine

## Dopamine precursors (levodopa, carbidopa-levodopa)

The *desired effect* of dopamine precursors is to increase central nervous system (CNS) levels of dopamine. Dopamine precursors include levodopa and a fixed-ratio combination of carbidopa and levodopa (Sinemet) and are used to treat all forms and stages of parkinsonism except drug-induced parkinsonism.

Levodopa (Dopar, Larodopa) is chemically identical to dopa, which is synthesized in the brain from phenylalanine and tyrosine, amino acids found in standard diets. Dopamine is in turn synthesized from dopa, and norepinephrine from dopamine. Norepinephrine deficiency is thought to cause depression and could explain the depression often associated with parkinsonism. (See Chapter 20 for a discussion of the role of norepinephrine in depression.) When levodopa is given alone, about 90% of it is metabolized to dopamine in the gut by the enzyme dopa decarboxylase before it reaches the bloodstream. Since dopamine does not pass the blood-brain barrier well, only about 10% of the levodopa administered reaches the brain. Dopamine is a potent cardiovascular stimulant used to treat acute heart failure. The large doses of levodopa needed to achieve adequate CNS dopamine levels produce dangerously high levels of dopamine in the peripheral nervous system (PNS). Therefore levodopa is seldom given alone in the treatment of parkinsonism. (See Table 11-1 for drug dosages.)

Levodopa is most frequently given in combination with carbidopa in fixed ratios. The trade name for this combination is Sinemet. Carbidopa is added to levodopa because it inhibits dopa decarboxylase. In other words, carbidopa blocks the metabolizing effect of dopa decarboxylase on levodopa, thus allowing levodopa to enter the bloodstream and travel to the brain, where it easily crosses the blood-brain barrier.

The fixed carbidopa-levodopa ratios, in milligrams, are 10/100, 25/100, and 25/250. The usual starting dose is one Sinemet 25/100 tablet three times a day. A tablet every day or every other day may be added up to six 25/100 tablets. Peripheral dopa decarboxylase is saturated with 70 to 100 mg of carbidopa a day. The lowest dose that produces significant improvement should be used, and tablets of different strengths can be used to optimize the daily dose for each patient. If a patient is being converted from levodopa alone to a carbidopa-levodopa combination, 8 hours should elapse between the last levodopa dose and the Sinemet. Otherwise a sudden increase in the dopamine levels in the PNS could occur.

## Dopamine releaser (amantadine)

Amantadine (Symmetrel) is a dopamine releaser. It releases the dopamine still available in the otherwise dopamine-depleted dopaminergic neurons. It is also thought to inhibit the reuptake of dopamine.

Amantadine was first used as an antiviral drug; however, its application as an antiparkinsonism drug has been established, even in the treatment of drug-induced parkinsonism (unlike levodopa). Since it has an anticholinergic aspect, amantadine is often used initially in the treatment of parkinsonism. It is effective in about 50% of patients for up to 6 months. However, patients with more than a mild form of the disease usually need levodopa.

Amantadine is also used adjunctively in the treatment of more severe forms of parkinsonism because its effectiveness as a "releaser" can be enhanced by levodopa; that is, there is more dopamine available to release. The usual dose of amantadine is 100 mg twice a day when used alone. When amantadine is combined with levodopa, the levodopa dosage should be reduced. Since amantadine is excreted

**TABLE 11-1** Dosages for selected antiparkinsonism drugs*

### DOPAMINERGIC DRUGS

| | |
|---|---|
| Levodopa (Dopar, Larodopa) | *Starting dose:* 0.5-1 g/d in divided doses |
| | *Increase:* Up to 0.75 g/d q 3-7 d |
| | *Maximum dose:* 8 g/d |
| Carbidopa-levodopa (Sinemet) | *Starting dose:* 1 Sinemet 25/100 mg tablet t.i.d. or 1 Sinemet 10/100 mg t.i.d. or q.i.d. |
| | *Increase:* By 1 tablet daily or every other day. |
| | *Maximum dose:* 6 Sinemet 25/100 mg tablets per day; 8 Sinemet 10/100 mg tablets per day. |
| Amantadine (Symmetrel) | *Starting dose:* 100 mg b.i.d. |
| | *Maximum dose:* 200 mg b.i.d. (with close supervision) |
| Bromocriptine (Parlodel) | *Starting dose:* 1.25 mg b.i.d. |
| (levodopa dose usually | *Increase:* By 2.5 mg/d q 14-28 d |
| remains constant) | *Maximum dose:* 100 mg/d |
| Selegiline (Eldepryl) | *Starting dose:* 5 mg at breakfast and lunch |
| Pergolide (Permax) | *Starting dose:* 0.05 mg/d in 3 divided doses |
| | *Increase:* By 0.1 or 0.15 mg/d every third day for the next 12 days, then by 0.25 mg/d every third day until optimal dosage |
| | *Maximum dose:* Usually 3 mg/d |

### ANTICHOLINERGIC DRUGS

| | |
|---|---|
| Trihexyphenidyl (Artane) | *Starting dose:* 1 to 2 mg/d |
| | *Increase:* By 2 mg/d q 3-5 d |
| | *Maximum dose:* 6-10 mg/d |
| | For drug-induced EPS usual dose range 5-15 mg/d |
| Benztropine (Cogentin) | *Starting dose:* 0.5-1 mg, h.s. |
| | *Maximum dose:* 4-6 mg/d |
| | *For EPS:* 1-4 mg, 1 or 2 times per day, p.o. or IM |
| | *For acute dystonic reactions:* 1-2 mg IM, then 1-2 mg, p.o. b.i.d. |
| Biperiden (Akineton) | *Starting dose:* 2 mg t.i.d. or q.i.d. |
| | *For EPS:* 2 mg 1-3 times per day |
| Ethopropazine (Parsidol) | *Starting dose:* 50 mg 1 or 2 times per day |
| | *Maximum dose:* 600 mg/d |

*Dosages for adults.

entirely by the kidneys, a reduced dosage is indicated for persons with renal impairment.

## Dopamine agonists (bromocriptine, pergolide)

Bromocriptine (Parlodel), a dopamine agonist, directly stimulates dopaminergic postsynaptic receptors, thus producing a dopamine-like effect. Technically, it does not add dopamine to the extrapyramidal system. It adds a dopamine substitute. Bromocriptine is used to treat endocrine disorders as well as all forms of parkinsonism. It inhibits prolactin secretion.

Bromocriptine is used alone and adjunctively with levodopa when high doses of that drug are required. It is particularly beneficial for patients who are no longer responding to levodopa. Bromocriptine has been used successfully in neuroleptic malignant syndrome, a dopamine-related condition caused by antipsychotic drugs.

Since side effects can be severe (i.e., extreme confusion, hypotension), bromocriptine is started at a very low dose and is increased slowly.

Pergolide (Permax), another dopamine agonist, is 10 to 1000 times more potent than bromocriptine on a milligram per milligram basis. It is used adjunctively with carbidopa-levodopa.

## Dopamine-metabolism inhibitor (selegiline)

A new drug that seems to hold great promise in the fight against parkinsonism in the early stages of the disease is selegiline (Eldepryl). It is used adjunctively with carbidopa-levodopa (Calesnick, 1990). Evidence reported by Tetrud and Langston (1989) suggests that selegiline is effective in delaying the need for levodopa by slowing the progression of parkinsonism. They report that disease progression was slowed by 40% to 83% in the group of patients in their study who were given selegiline. Selegiline is a monoamine oxidase B inhibitor, which may work by decreasing the metabolism of dopamine by monoamine oxidase B (Tetrud and Langston, 1989). A dose of 5 mg twice a day almost completely inhibits brain monoamine oxidase B.

## Side effects (undesired effects) of dopaminergic agents

Dopaminergic agents share not only similar therapeutic effects but also similar side effects (see Table 11-2). These drugs produce both CNS and PNS adverse effects. Side effects of levodopa and amantadine tend to be dose-related and reversible.

**CNS side effects.** Undesired CNS effects include nausea and vomiting, ataxia, hand tremors, insomnia, nightmares, anxiety, psychosis, and agitation. Choreiform movements may also be a side effect. Choreiform movements are rapid, irregular, involuntary movements like those seen in patients with Huntington's chorea. Two of these side effects will be more fully explained because an understanding of them helps in a broader understanding of neurotransmitters. Nausea and vomiting are side effects of the increased amounts of dopamine stimulating the chemoreceptor trigger zone. Compazine, technically an antipsychotic, is a drug commonly used to treat nausea and vomiting. Antipsychotic drugs block dopamine receptors; that is, they are dopamine antagonists. Psychosis is thought to be related to increased levels of dopamine; therefore dopaminergics could theoretically cause psychotic symptoms. The dopaminergics do increase dopamine levels, and some persons experience symptoms of psychosis, such as hallucinations. Antipsychotic drugs (see Chapter 10) are effective in treating psychosis because they block dopamine. Understanding antiparkinsonism drugs helps in the understanding of antipsychotic drugs.

**PNS and other peripheral side effects.** PNS effects include hypotension due to peripheral vasodilation and tachycardia due to the direct effect of dopamine (and its metabolites: norepinephrine and epinephrine) on cardiac muscle. Tachycardia can also be caused by reflex cardiac stimulation related to the aforementioned hypotension. Dry mouth, constipation, and urinary hesistancy and retention are other

**TABLE 11-2** Side effects and nursing interventions for major dopaminergics

| Drug* | Side effects | Interventions |
|---|---|---|
| L,A,B | CNS side effects (headaches, dizziness, weakness, confusion, hallucinations, delusions) | Treat headaches, dizziness, and weakness symptomatically. Cognitive and perceptual disturbances may require a reduced dosage or switching to another drug. |
| L | Coughing, hoarseness, breathing problems | Observe closely, particularly patients with a history of asthma or emphysema. |
| B | Shortness of breath | Advise to avoid strenuous activities. |
| L,A,B | Nausea, vomiting | Give with meals. |
| L | Dysphagia (difficulty swallowing) | Dysphagia can cause choking and makes eating difficult. Monitor size of portions. Modify diet as indicated. |
| L,A | Blurred vision | Caution about driving. |
| L | Mydriasis | Since mydriasis could cause serious problems in cases of undiagnosed narrow-angle glaucoma, have patient report eye pain immediately. |
| L | Choreiform movements (dystonia, ataxia) | Dosage may need to be reduced. Contact physician. |
| L,A,B | Hypotension | Advise patient to rise slowly and not to stand in one place too long. |

*L = levodopa; A = amantadine; B = bromocriptine.

PNS effects. Existing narrow-angle glaucoma (these drugs dilate the pupil), cardiovascular disease, or pulmonary, renal, hepatic, or endocrine problems could be intensified.

**Drug-specific effects.** The dopaminergic drugs levodopa, carbidopa-levodopa, amantadine, and bromocriptine also have specific effects that should be mentioned. Long-term use of levodopa and carbidopa-levodopa is associated with "end-of-dose failure," the "on-off phenomenon," and "secondary levodopa failure." The end-of-dose failure occurs when symptoms start appearing before the next dose is due. Giving smaller, more frequent doses helps for a while. The on-off phenomenon describes the inconsistency of these drugs in controlling symptoms. The patient may be free of symptoms, only to suddenly experience symptoms for a period of time. Secondary levodopa failure describes the loss of effectiveness of levodopa. This usually occurs after 2 to 5 years of treatment. All these problems might theoretically be resolved with higher doses; however, higher doses can have serious side effects, for example, cardiac stimulation. Adverse as well as therapeutic responses occur more rapidly with caribidopa-levodopa than with levodopa alone. CNS effects of amantadine include confusion, depression, and psychotic symptoms, particularly hallucinations. Amantadine also lowers seizure threshold, so patients with epilepsy may experience convulsions. Peripherally, amantadine can cause skin to become mottled and purple (livedo reticularis). Bromocriptine can cause serious hypotension and shortness of breath and lowers serum prolactin levels.

## Interactions with dopaminergic drugs

Since side effects of dopaminergic drugs include hypotension and cardiac stimulation, drugs that lower blood pressure (antihypertensives) and drugs that stimulate the heart (sympathomimetics) are potentiated by dopaminergics. Of particular concern to the psychiatric nurse is the patient with parkinsonism who is depressed (remember, there is a neurochemical relationship between parkinsonism and depression) and is being treated with both antidepressants and antiparkinsonism agents. Monoamine oxidase inhibitors (MAOIs) (see Chapter 13) have a potential for serious interactive effects when given with dopaminergic drugs. MAOIs cause an accumulation of norepinephrine in adrenergic nerve endings, which can be released by dopamine and cause a serious hypertensive crisis. On the other hand, drugs that block dopamine, such as the antipsychotic drugs, can hinder or neutralize the effects of the antiparkinsonism drugs.

Vitamin $B_6$ (pyridoxine)–containing foods (e.g., avocados, lentils, lima beans) should not be given with levodopa, because this vitamin enhances dopa decarboxylase activity and opposes the action of carbidopa. This has the two-fold effect of decreasing CNS levels of dopamine and increasing PNS levels. Both situations have undesirable consequences.

Amantadine has one major drug interaction: it enhances the anticholinergic effects of atropinelike drugs.

Bromocriptine increases the action of antihypertensive agents. The effectiveness of bromocriptine is compromised by antipsychotic drugs, reserpine, and methyldopa. With oral contraceptives, it may cause amenorrhea.

## Nursing implications for dopaminergic drugs

**Therapeutic versus toxic dosage levels.** Levodopa is usually given in an initial dose of 0.5 to 1.0 g daily (see Table 11-1). The usual optimal dose should not exceed 8 g per day. The usual maximum carbidopa-levodopa dose is six of the 25/100 mg tablets. When an overdose occurs, gastric lavage and other supportive measures should be instituted. Pyridoxine, which ordinarily should be avoided, may help decrease the antiparkinsonism actions of levodopa, but it does not reverse the action of carbidopa-levodopa. The usual starting dose of amantadine is 100 mg twice daily. Patients can receive up to 400 mg per day but should be closely supervised. There is no antidote for overdose; however, physostigmine given intravenously has been effective in reducing CNS toxicity. Fluids should be forced and, if necessary, given intravenously. Supportive measures should be used, and monitoring of blood pressure, temperature, pulse, and respirations is essential. Bromocriptine is usually given in a dose of 1.25 mg twice daily, and the dose of levodopa given is maintained. There is no antidote for overdose, so the bromocriptine should be stopped and supportive treatment instituted.

**Use in pregnancy and lactation.** Levodopa and amantadine should be used cautiously during pregnancy. Amantadine is contraindicated during lactation. Bromocriptine is contraindicated during pregnancy. It is prescribed for female infertility.

**Side effects.** The nurse should advise patients about the side effects most likely to occur and should monitor for subjective or objective signs of improvement (see Table 11-2). The physician should be notified if the side effects are severe or do not diminish with time. Four points are worth reemphasis:

1. Taking the drugs with food will usually reduce gastrointestinal irritation; however, high-protein foods will interfere with levodopa absorption.
2. Patients experiencing light-headedness should be advised to sit up and stand slowly and to support themselves. Patients with parkinsonism may need assistance in walking. Elastic stockings may reduce orthostatic hypotension. A number of factors may make driving hazardous, for example, light-headedness, blurred vision, unresolved tremor, and confusion. Patients should be advised to be cautious until the effect is known.
3. Mental status should be evaluated periodically to monitor for development (or worsening) of psychosis or depression.
4. Female patients should be warned to avoid conception while they are taking bromocriptine.

**Interactions.** The nurse should advise the patient with parkinsonism to report all current drug use. Some drug combinations should be avoided if possible. The nurse can recommend Larobec for those patients taking levodopa who want to take vitamins.

Patients taking amantadine, particularly elderly persons, should be advised that it intensifies the anticholinergic effect of over-the-counter drugs. Since amantadine is the dopaminergic drug most commonly prescribed for drug-induced parkinsonism, it is worth noting that high-potency antipsychotic drugs (e.g., haloperidol) have few anticholinergic properties.

**Patient teaching.** Patients and their families should be taught the side effects of the dopaminergic agents. The nurse must use judgment when discussing potential side effects so as not to cause alarm. Typically, the nurse teaches these persons about side effects they can see and feel while encouraging regular checkups. Patients and families should be advised about the following:

- That symptomatic relief usually takes 3 weeks to several months with levodopa and 2 months with bromocriptine
- That drugs should be taken exactly as prescribed and not stopped abruptly, because a parkinsonian crisis could occur
- That urine and sweat may be darker with levodopa
- That vitamin $B_6$-containing foods should be avoided when levodopa is taken
- That any sudden eye pain should be reported immediately, as this may indicate an acute glaucoma attack.

## ANTICHOLINERGIC AGENTS

Another way to restore the dopamine-acetylcholine balance is to decrease the availability of acetylcholine. The CNS-affecting anticholinergic drugs do that very thing and are useful in the early stages of parkinsonism. These drugs are used to treat drug-induced parkinsonism as well as parkinsonism from other causes. In fact, anticholinergic drugs are used more often than dopaminergics in the treatment of parkinsonism. They are also used as adjuncts to the dopaminergics as the parkinsonism progresses. When these drugs are given concomitantly, lower doses of each can be used, theoretically resulting in fewer side effects. All anticholinergic drugs that act on the CNS and that are discussed in this chapter are similar to the prototype of the class, trihexyphenidyl hydrochloride (Artane). Trihexyphenidyl will be discussed and the others mentioned when specific differences warrant.

## Pharmacologic effects (desired effects)

Trihexyphenidyl and the related anticholinergic drugs act primarily by inhibiting acetylcholine, thus preventing its stimulation of the cholinergic excitatory pathways. They may also inhibit reuptake of dopamine. Of course, both these effects contribute to restoration of the acetylcholine-dopamine balance. Trihexyphenidyl is effective alone or in combination with dopaminergic agents in the treatment of parkinsonism, but it is used alone in the treatment of parkinsonism induced by antipsychotic drugs.

**Treating parkinsonism.** The initial dose of trihexyphenidyl is 1 to 2 mg; this is increased by 2 mg every 3 to 5 days to a total daily dose of 6 to 10 mg. When trihexyphenidyl is given in combination with levodopa, the same initial dose is used, but the higher range typically is not reached. The levodopa dosage also is significantly less than when it is used alone.

**Treating drug-induced extrapyramidal symptoms (EPS).** Antipsychotic drugs block dopamine receptors, frequently causing EPS. Many of the symptoms associated with "naturally" occurring parkinsonism—that is, tremors, rigidity, and bradykinesia—are present in drug-induced parkinsonism, along with such related symptoms as akathisia, dystonic reactions, and dyskinesias. These symptoms contribute to the discomfort, anxiety, and frustration of this already troubled population. Patients taking antipsychotic drugs can experience a gradual or sudden onset of symptoms. As an illustration of how suddenly these side effects can occur, the following clinical anecdote is provided.

> A 25-year-old Hispanic woman who was taking an antipsychotic drug (haloperidol) started experiencing psychomotor slowing as she walked down a hallway. Before she reached the end of the hall she required assistance. Within 2 minutes of sitting down, she experienced oculogyric crisis, a state in which the neck becomes rigidly hyperextended and the eyes roll upward in a fixed stare. Her breathing became labored because of the position of her neck, and she was frightened. Since she was also delusional, one cannot imagine what this frightening side effect of her medication represented to her. Benztropine (Cogentin), 5 mg, was given intramuscularly. She responded in 15 minutes.

When trihexyphenidyl is used to treat the EPS caused by antipsychotic drugs, 1 mg is given initially with 1 mg added every few hours until the reaction has been controlled. The usual dosage is 5 to 15 mg per day. The crisis situation described in the preceding paragraph obviously required a less conservative approach. Trihexyphenidyl does not act rapidly enough to control oculogyric crises or other severe dystonic reactions.

## Side effects (undesired effects)

As with the dopaminergic drugs, the anticholinergic drugs have both CNS and PNS side effects (see Table 11-3). These effects are similar to those of atropine. CNS effects include confusion, agitation, dizziness, drowsiness, and disturbances in behavior. The cholinergic system is implicated in memory and learning, and anticholinergic drugs affect this system also.

PNS anticholinergic effects, such as dry mouth, blurred vision, nausea, and nervousness, occur in 30% to 50% of these patients. Constipation, a problem for parkinsonism patients because of rigidity, can be worsened by the anticholinergics. Urinary hesitance and retention, decreased sweating, tachycardia, and mydriasis are other PNS effects. Interestingly, the dry mouth and decreased sweating may be welcomed by parkinsonism patients who drool or perspire excessively.

## Interactions with nonparkinsonism anticholinergic drugs

The anticholinergic response is intensified when anticholinergics are administered with drugs that have similar effects. Drugs considered in this textbook, such as amantadine (a dopaminergic antiparkinsonism drug), chlorpromazine (an antipsychotic drug), and MAOIs (antidepressant drugs), intensify anticholinergic symptoms when they are taken with the anticholinergic antiparkinsonism drugs. An additive effect is also found with antihistamines and antiarrhythmic drugs. Sedative effects are intensified by CNS depressants. Finally, antacids and antidiarrheal drugs decrease the absorption of these anticholinergic drugs.

## Nursing implication for anticholinergic drugs
### Therapeutic versus toxic dosage levels
*Therapeutic ranges.* The therapeutic range for trihexyphenidyl is 6 to 10 mg a day for parkinsonism and 5 to 15 mg a day for drug-induced EPS (see Table 11-1). Overdose may result in CNS hyperstimulation (confusion, excitement, hyperpyrexia, agitation, disorientation, delirium, hallucinations) or CNS depression (drowsiness, sedation, coma). The atropine-like effects previously mentioned intensify. The cardiovascular, the urinary, and the gastrointestinal systems are particularly involved. The eye is also affected. High fevers are due to the CNS effects of trihexyphenidyl and its ability to decrease sweating.

*Intervention for toxic levels.* Gastric lavage is the preferred treatment if the patient is conscious. A short-acting barbiturate (e.g., thiopental) may be ordered by the physician if CNS stimulation occurs, but the nurse and the physician must be aware that stimulation may be preceding CNS depression. Supportive care is important and may require maintenance of an airway and mechanical assistance with breathing. Hyperthermia should be monitored (rectal temperature), and assessment for signs of convulsions, which may follow high fevers, should be made. Hyperthermia can be controlled with tepid baths or other nursing measures.

**TABLE 11-3** Side effects and nursing intervention for anticholinergics

| Side effects | Appropriate nursing intervention |
|---|---|
| Dry mouth | Provide sugarless hard candy and chewing gum, frequent rinses |
| Nasal congestion | Over-the-counter nasal decongestant if approved by physician |
| Urinary hesitation | Running water, privacy, warm water over perineum |
| Urinary retention | Catheterize for residual, fluids, encourage frequent voiding |
| Blurred vision, photophobia | Reassurance, normal vision typically returns in a few weeks, wear sunglasses, caution about driving |
| Constipation | Laxatives as ordered, diet with roughage |
| Mydriasis | See levodopa |
| Orthostatic hypotension | Request patient to get out of bed slowly, to then sit on the edge of the bed a short while, and rise slowly |
| Sedation | Help the patient get up early and then get the day started |
| Decreased sweating | This can lead to fever; take temperature; if fever occurs, reduce body temperature (e.g., sponge baths) |

*Use in pregnancy.* Anticholinergics should be used cautiously during pregnancy. Theoretically, these drugs will decrease milk flow during lactation.

**Side effects.** Numerous annoying side effects are associated with trihexyphenidyl and related drugs (Table 11-3). The nurse has several nondrug alternatives to help the patient. Sucking on sugarless hard candies, taking frequent sips of water, or chewing sugarless gum can help to moisten a dry mouth. Constipation can be alleviated by drinking adequate amounts of water (2500 to 3000 ml per day) and maintaining a high-fiber diet. Urinary hesitancy is best dealt with by voiding when the urge occurs, by running water over the perineum, or by just listening to running water. Taking medications with meals reduces nausea. Patients experiencing increased body temperatures should be advised to limit strenuous exercise and to dress appropriately in warm weather. Blurred vision is troublesome and may necessitate a discontinuance of certain high-risk activities, such as driving. However, the nurse should reassure the patient that tolerance to this effect usually develops in a short time.

**Interactions with anticholinergic drugs.** The nurse should alert the patient to over-the-counter drugs and other prescription drugs that will intensify the atropinelike effects of trihexyphenidyl and the related centrally acting anticholinergics. Antihistamines, commonly a component of cold remedies, will add to the anticholinergic effects. Alcohol and other depressants can increase drowsiness and should be avoided if possible. Over-the-counter antacids should not be taken unless ordered by the physician. Complications can be modified by giving antacids or antidiarrheals 1 to 2 hours before trihexyphenidyl is taken.

**Patient teaching.**  In addition to teaching appropriate information about side effects, the nurse should also emphasize certain points. The patient and family should be advised of the following:

- Not to discontinue these drugs abruptly. Tapering off over a 1-week period is advised.
- To avoid driving or other hazardous activity until tolerance occurs and drowsiness and blurred vision diminish.
- To avoid over-the-counter medications, such as cough and cold preparations, that have anticholinergic or antihistaminic properties; also to avoid alcohol, which will add to CNS depression, and antacids, which will interfere with absorption of anticholinergics.

### Related centrally acting anticholinergic drugs

**Benztropine (Cogentin).**  Benztropine is used to treat all forms of parkinsonism, including drug-induced extrapyramidal symptoms (EPS). Since benztropine is from a different chemical class than trihexyphenidyl, it may be more effective in some patients. It is usually given orally with an initial dose of 1 to 2 mg a day. It can be given intramuscularly (1 to 2 mg) for noncompliant psychotic patients and intramuscularly or intravenously (5 mg) for frightening dystonic reactions. Benztropine causes greater and longer-lasting sedation than trihexyphenidyl; when given at bedtime, this may be a desirable effect.

**Biperiden (Akineton).**  Biperiden is used adjunctively in all forms of parkinsonism, including drug-induced EPS. It is similar to trihexyphenidyl and should be effective if trihexyphenidyl is effective. Typically, 2 mg three to four times daily is used for all forms of parkinsonism, except drug-induced EPS, for which 2 mg one to three times daily is given. For acute symptoms, 2 mg is given intramuscularly or intravenously every half-hour as needed (up to 8 mg in 24 hours).

**Diphenhydramine (Benadryl).**  Diphenhydramine, the prototype antihistamine, can be effective for most types of parkinsonism. The usual dose is 25 to 50 mg three to four times daily. It can cause considerable sedation in some persons and little in others.

**Ethopropazine (Parsidol).**  Ethopropazine is a phenothiazine derivative. This is interesting because phenothiazines are generally antipsychotics, and antipsychotics tend to make parkinsonism worse. The initial dose is 50 mg orally once or twice a day. Maintenance dosages range from 100 to 600 mg per day.

**Procyclidine (Kemadrin).**  Procyclidine is used for all forms of parkinsonism, including drug-induced EPS. It is found to be most effective for the symptomatic treatment of rigidity and sialorrhea (excessive salivation). It may increase tremors. The usual starting dose is 2.5 mg orally three times daily and can be increased to 5 mg three or four times a day (after meals and at bedtime). If procyclidine is replacing another anticholinergic drug, it should be started at a lower dose and the other drug gradually decreased.

## KEY CONCEPTS

1. Parkinsonism is related to a degeneration in the dopamine-generating portion of the brain called the substantia nigra.
2. In order for a person to have normal muscle activity, a balance between dopamine and acetycholine is required; consequently, a dopamine deficiency is responsible for symptoms of parkinsonism.
3. There are three primary symptoms associated with parkinsonism: tremors, brady-kinesia, and rigidity.
4. Secondary symptoms of parkinsonism (i.e., difficult swallowing, respiratory problems, constipation) are caused by primary symptoms.
5. Drug treatment of parkinsonism is based on reestablishment of a balance between dopamine and acetycholine.
6. There are three basic approaches to reestablishing this balance: (a) by using do-paminergic drugs to increase dopamine levels, (b) by using anticholingergic drugs to decrease acetycholine levels, or (c) a combination of the other two approaches.
7. There are four types of dopaminergic drug: (a) dopamine precursors, (b) dopamine releasers, (c) dopamine agonists, (d) dopamine metabolism inhibitors.
8. Dopamine precursors, such as levodopa (Dopar) and carbidopa-levodopa (Sinemet), work by putting new dopamine into the system.
9. The dopamine releaser amantadine (Symmetrel) works by enhancing the release of existing dopamine and also, perhaps, by inhibiting the reuptake of dopamine.
10. Bromocriptine (Parlodel), a dopamine agonist, directly stimulates dopaminergic postsynaptic receptors.
11. The dopamine metabolism inhibitor selegiline (Eldepryl) blocks the metabolism of dopamine.
12. Major anticholinergic-antiparkinsonism drugs include trihexyphenidyl (Artane) and benztropine (Cogentin).
13. Anticholinergic drugs are also used to treat drug-induced extrapyramidal symptoms caused by antipsychotic drugs.

## REFERENCES

Calesnick B: Selegiline for Parkinson's disease, Am Fam Phys 41:589, 1990.

Garrett E: Parkinsonism: forgotten considerations in medical treatment and nursing care, J Neurosurg Nurs 14:1318, 1982.

Glassman R and Salzman C: Interactions between psychotropic and other drugs: an update, Hosp Community Psychiatry 38:236, 1987.

Keltner NL: Antiparkinson drugs. In Shlafer M and Marieb E, editors: The nurse, pharmacology, and drug therapy, Menlo Park, Calif., 1989, Addison-Wesley.

Knoben JE and Anderson PO: Handbook of clinical drug data, Hamilton, Ill., 1983, Drug Intelligence Publications, Inc.

Lannon MC, et al: Comprehensive care of the patient with Parkinson's disease, J Neurosci Nurs, 18:121, 1986.

Tetrud JW and Langston JW: The effect of deprenyl (Selegiline) on the natural history of Parkinson's disease, Science 245:519, 1989.

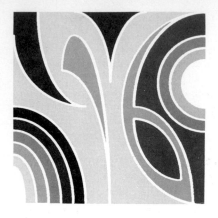

## CHAPTER 12

# Antipsychotic Drugs

LEARNING OBJECTIVES

After reading this chapter you should be able to

- Describe the concept of neurotransmitters in relationship to psychosis.
- Describe differences among classes of antipsychotic drugs.
- Discuss the side effects of antipsychotic drugs.
- Identify therapeutic versus toxic levels of antipsychotic drugs.
- Describe potential interactions of antipsychotic drugs.
- Discuss implications for patient teaching about antipsychotic drugs.

Antipsychotic drugs are used to treat the symptoms of psychosis and various other manifestations of mental illness. Chronic mental illness, specifically schizophrenia and symptoms of florid psychosis, and acute agitation in manic or disturbed patients are the major targets of these drugs (Overall et al., 1989). Other uses will be acknowledged briefly later in the chapter.

## History of antipsychotic drugs

In the late 1940s a pharmaceutical company developed a cold remedy that caused mild sedation, potentiated the effects of analgesics, and calmed anxious surgery patients. Further studies led to the discovery of a derivative, chlorpromazine, that effectively reduced psychotic symptoms in psychiatric patients.

Before the introduction and acceptance of chlorpromazine and the many related drugs, hundreds of thousands of patients with severe psychiatric disturbances were hospitalized under sometimes poor conditions and were isolated, physically restrained, and occasionally subjected to psychosurgery (lobotomy). These treatments rarely restored the patient to a state that enabled him to function productively or to interact in a reasonably normal way with others.

Although all the hopes for antipsychotic drugs have not been realized, these drugs have had dramatic impact on psychiatric care. With their use by the psychiatric community, most of the early and ineffective treatments were abandoned, and long-term hospitalizations fell from more than ½ million patients in 1955 (before the widespread use of antipsychotic drugs) to about 120,000 in the mid-1980s (Fig. 12-1). Antipsychotic drug use in public hospitals began in about 1954. Most patients who previously would have been hospitalized are living and functioning well in their homes and jobs because of antipsychotic drug treatment. On the other hand, many previously hospitalized patients are now part of the vast homeless population; this indicates that psychopharmacological treatment alone is not enough.

The drugs discussed in this chapter are generally called antipsychotic agents, but they have also been referred to as major tranquilizers, ataractics (drugs that produce calmness or serenity), or neuroleptics (since they can produce neurological symptoms).

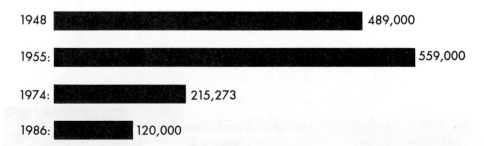

1948  489,000

1955:  559,000

1974:  215,273

1986:  120,000

**FIGURE 12-1** Mental patients hospitalized in public hospitals in the years surrounding the discovery of antipsychotic drugs.

**Box 12-1**
## ANTIPSYCHOTIC DRUGS

Phenothiazines
  Aliphatic phenothiazines    *low potency*
    Chlorpromazine (Thorazine)*
    Promazine (Sparine)
    Triflupromazine (Vesprin)
  Piperidine phenothiazines
    Mesoridazine (Serentil)
    Thioridazine (Mellaril)†
  Piperazine phenothiazines
    Fluphenazine (Prolixin, Permitil)†
    Perphenazine (Trilafon)
    Trifluoperazine (Stelazine)†

Butyrophenones    *-high potency*
    Haloperidol (Haldol)†
  Thioxanthenes
    Chlorprothixene (Taractan)
    Thiothixene (Navane)†
  Dibenzoxazepine
    Loxapine (Loxitane)†
  Dihydroindolone
    Molindone (Moban)†
  Dibenzodiazepine
    Clozapine (Clozaril)

* First antipsychotic discovered and the one by which the potency of others is measured.

† Most commonly prescribed.

## Classification systems - *chemical class, potency*

Antipsychotic drugs are generally classified in two ways. The first and most accurate classification system is based on chemical class (see Box 12-1). These drugs have diverse chemical properties, even though they all effectively reduce various psychiatric symptoms. For instance, because of these chemical class differences the type, intensity, and frequency of side effects vary among these drugs (see Table 12-1). *Therefore, when a drug is "not working," the switch should be to a drug of a different class.*

The second means of classifying antipsychotic drugs is based on potency. This is admittedly a less "scientific" approach but has gathered support because of its clinical utility. Essentially, some drugs require much higher dosages to achieve like clinical results (see Table 12-1). For instance, about 100 mg of chlorpromazine (Thorazine) is required to achieve the same clinical effect as 2 mg of haloperidol (Haldol). Drugs that are one to four times as potent as chlorpromazine are designated as low potency and those 20 or more times as potent, as high potency (Gomez and Gomez, 1990). Accordingly, chlorpromazine is referred to as a low-potency antipsychotic drug and haloperidol as a high-potency one. Clinically, it appears that low-potency antipsychotic drugs produce more frequent and more intense anticholinergic side effects and that high-potency antipsychotic drugs produce more frequent and more intense extrapyramidal symptoms (EPS) (see Table 12-1).

## Neurochemical theory of schizophrenia

Although various theories of schizophrenia exist (see Chapter 19) and are vigorously debated, the neurochemical theory affords the best explanation for the effectiveness of antipsychotic agents. The neurochemical theory states that schizophrenia and psychotic symptoms (e.g., hallucinations and delusions) are caused by increased levels of dopamine in the limbic system of the brain. Since antipsychotic drugs are dopamine blockers, it follows that their effectiveness can be attributed to this do-pamine-blocking activity. Furthermore, this theory of schizophrenia is supported by clinical observations and clinical research, which demonstrates that high doses of levodopa and amphetamines can produce schizophrenic symptoms.

## Pharmacological effects (desired effects)

Chlorpromazine and the other antipsychotic drugs are used primarily to treat psychiatric disorders, specifically schizophrenia and chronic mental illness. Well-designed, vigorous clinical research has produced impressive evidence of their effectiveness. Not all patients respond, but the many who do have the potential to live their lives unencumbered by the oppressive symptoms of psychosis. Chlorpromazine, the first of these drugs developed and the prototype antipsychotic agent, will be discussed extensively, with a more condensed discussion of the other drugs.

Psychosis is a phenomenon of brain activity. Therefore a drug that affects psychosis acts primarily in the central nervous system (CNS). Tolerance to an antipsychotic effect is not common. Peripheral nervous system (PNS) effects will be discussed under the side effects (undesired effects) section.

**CNS effects.** CNS effects include sedation, emotional quieting, and psychomotor slowing, which explains why at one time these drugs were generally referred to as major tranquilizers. This emotional quieting enables the patient to take advantage of other forms of therapeutic intervention, for example, the therapeutic nurse-patient relationship and the therapeutic milieu.

Other CNS effects include a sedating quality that decreases insomnia, a frequent complaint of psychotic persons. Whether it is the sedating effect itself or the "freeing" from disturbing thoughts (or a combination of the two) that aids sleep is not precisely known. Not all antipsychotic drugs are particularly sedating. High-potency drugs are less sedating than the low-potency drugs. For example, haloperidol (Haldol) and fluphenazine (Prolixin) are not particularly sedating and yet are quite effective. The conclusion to be drawn from this is that the effectiveness of antipsychotic agents results from more than "just" their tranquilizing qualities.

**Psychiatric symptoms modified by antipsychotic drugs.** Patients are given antipsychotic drugs because other people note their behavior to be "crazy" (objective symptoms) or because these individuals are experiencing psychotic symptoms (subjective symptoms) and request help. Antipsychotic drugs are most effective in treating what have been called the positive symptoms of schizophrenia (see Chapter 19). Positive symptoms include hallucinations and delusions. Symptoms less responsive to antipsychotic drugs (or negative symptoms) include symptoms developed over an extended period of time such as flattened affect, verbal paucity, and

**TABLE 12-1**  Antipsychotic drugs

| Antipsychotic agent | Approximate equivalent oral dose (mg) | Adult daily dosage range (mg) | Sedation |
|---|---|---|---|
| Phenothiazines | | | |
|   Aliphatic phenothiazines | | | |
|     Chlorpromazine (Thorazine) | 100 | 30-800 | + + + |
|     Promazine (Sparine) | 200 | 40-1200 | + + |
|     Triflupromazine (Vesprin) | 25 | 60-150 | + + + |
|   Pirperidine phenothiazines | | | |
|     Mesoridazine (Serentil) | 50 | 30-400 | + + + |
|     Thioridazine (Mellaril) | 100 | 150-800 | + + + |
|   Piperazine phenothiazines | | | |
|     Fluphenazine (Prolixin, Permitil) | 2 | 0.5-40 | + |
|     Perphenazine (Trilafon) | 10 | 12-64 | + |
|     Trifluoperazine (Stelazine) | 5 | 2-40 | + |
| Butyrophenone | | | |
|   Haloperidol (Haldol) | 2 | 1-15 | + |
| Thioxanthenes | | | |
|   Chlorprothixene (Taractan) | 100 | 75-600 | + + + |
|   Thiothixene (Navane) | 4 | 8-30 | + |
| Dibenzoxazepine | | | |
|   Loxapine (Loxitane) | 15 | 20-250 | + + |
| Dihydroindolone | | | |
|   Molindone (Moban) | 10 | 15-225 | + |
| Dibenzodiazepine | | | |
|   Clozapine (Clozaril) | 50 | 300-900 | + + + |

Incidence of side effects: + + + = high; + + = moderate; + = low.

*Wysowski DK and Baum C: Antipsychotic drug use in the United States, 1976-1985, Arch Gen Psychiatry 46:929, 1989.

Adapted from Olin BR, editor: Drug facts and comparisons, St. Louis, JB Lippincott, 1990, p. 265.

lack of drive or goal-directed activity. Improvement in objective and subjective or positive and negative symptoms is the yardstick by which progress is gauged. Psychotic symptoms associated with mania and organic brain syndrome also may respond to antipsychotic drugs.

*Altered perception.* As a rule of thumb, the more bizarre the behavior of a person experiencing psychotic symptoms, the more likely that an antipsychotic drug will be beneficial. Hallucinations and illusions are reduced with these drugs. Even when the symptoms are not fully eradicated, antipsychotic drugs may enable the person to understand that hallucinations and illusions are not real. This is indicative of therapeutic gain.

*Alterations of thought.* With antipsychotic drugs, reasoning improves, ambivalence decreases, and delusions decrease. Since clouded reasoning, ambivalence, and delusional thoughts are frustrating and at times frightening, antipsychotic agents can free the patient for better communication with others.

| Extrapyramidal symptoms | Anticholinergic effects | Orthostatic hypotension | Therapeutic plasma concentration (ng/ml) | Relative market share (rank)* |
|---|---|---|---|---|
| + + | + + | + + + | 30-500 | 12% (3) |
| + + | + + + | + + | | 0.7% (10) |
| + + | + + + | + + | | 0.5% (14) |
| + | + + + | + + | | 1.5% (9) |
| + | + + + | + + + | | 31.2% (1) |
| + + + | + | + | 0.13-2.8 | 5.6% (6) |
| + + + | + | + | 0.8-1.2 | 4.2% (7) |
| + + + | + | + | | 8.7% (4) |
| + + + | + | + | 5-20 | 24.2% (2) |
| + + | + + | + + | | 0.5% (12) |
| + + + | + | + | 2-57 | 8.2% (5) |
| + + + | + | + + | | 1.9% (8) |
| + + + | + | + | | 0.6% (11) |
| + | + + + | + + + | | Too new |

*Alterations of activity.* Often persons with schizophrenia are hyperactive because of their internal turmoil and perhaps their neurochemical state. Antipsychotic drugs slow psychomotor activity. Low-potency drugs such as chlorpromazine (Thorazine) are sedating and may be used for agitated and combative persons.

*Altered consciousness.* Mental clouding and confusion are anxiety-producing symptoms associated with psychosis. Some mental health professionals believe these disorders are the most disabling. Antipsychotic drugs are effective in decreasing confusion and clouding.

*Altered interpersonal relationships.* Schizophrenic patients often have a history of asociality and withdrawal and have few, if any, close personal relationships (this includes ambivalent relationships with family members). The schizophrenic person invests little in his appearance and is not particularly careful about his behavior. Introspection and self-focused speech combine to produce ineffective communication patterns, which reinforce his isolation. These behaviors also keep other people away. In the give-and-take of society the schizophrenic has little to give and thus is basically unattractive to most people socially. Antipsychotic drugs enable the patient to become less self-focused and to divert his attention away from himself and toward others. His socially damaging introspectiveness may be due to the considerable energy he must expend to maintain some degree of equilibrium in the face of the psychological turmoil previously discussed. This parallels how most of us give less attention to our appearance or behavior when we are ill. Antipsychotic drugs reduce the inner turmoil, freeing psychic energy for normal interpersonal relationships and for the therapeutic nurse-patient relationship.

*Alterations of affect.* Affective disorders alone are not treated with antipsychotic drugs, but affective flattening, inappropriateness, and lability are affective symptoms sometimes associated with schizophrenia that often respond to antipsychotic drugs.

**Other uses of antipsychotic drugs.** The site of neuronal control of nausea and vomiting is the chemoreceptor trigger zone (CTZ), which is well supplied with dopaminergic receptors. When these receptors are stimulated with dopamine, nausea and vomiting occur. Since antipsychotic drugs block dopamine, most phenothiazines are effective antiemetics. Prochlorperazine (Compazine) is prescribed primarily for its antiemetic quality.

Antipsychotic drugs also block PNS muscarinic acetylcholine receptors and α-adrenergic receptors, which makes them responsible for some distressing side effects associated with these drugs.

### Absorption, distribution, administration

Chlorpromazine enters the CNS rapidly. A tranquilizing effect occurs within 60 minutes of an oral dose and within 10 minutes of an intramuscular dose. In some persons, however, the actual antipsychotic effect may not be realized for several weeks to several months. Chlorpromazine accumulates in fatty tissue and is released slowly from these sites. Traces of metabolites of this drug are found in the urine months after therapy has stopped. This also may explain why patients who abruptly stop taking this medication continue to experience an antipsychotic effect for awhile; that is, the chlorpromazine continues to be released from fatty storage sites after being discontinued. This slow release from fatty stores may also account for noncompliance, since the patient who stops taking this medication does not experience an immediate return of symptoms.

Because most of the chlorpromazine given binds to plasma proteins (95% to 98%), which can cross the blood-brain barrier only in negligible amounts, only a fraction of the drug ingested accounts for its effect. Understandably, chlorpromazine has a more potent effect on older persons because of their decreased protein-binding capabilities. Chlorpromazine is metabolized in the liver and has a half-life of 30 hours. Impaired hepatic function will extend its half-life and therefore its effect.

Although many antipsychotic drugs are available, there is little to document that one is more effective than another. Some patients, however, respond to chlorpromazine, for example, and some respond to haloperidol. Therefore the choice of which antipsychotic drug to prescribe is usually based on the physician's preference and experience, the likelihood that a certain drug will be helpful (e.g., on the basis of the patient's previous response to a certain drug), and an educated guess about the chance of drug-induced side effects. Because of nurses' prolonged contact with inpatients and periodic contact with outpatients, few psychiatric professionals have a better opportunity to assess both desired and undesired responses that help identify the best drug for a particular patient. Additionally, since nearly one half of all orders for antipsychotic medications are written as p.r.n. orders and since nurses typically make the decision about p.r.n. medications, nurses have added reason to evaluate the response to these drugs (Blair, 1990).

Most antipsychotic drugs are available in oral and parenteral forms. Oral administration is the preferred route for a variety of reasons, not the least of which is that people generally prefer this route. Tablets, however, have consistently created a problem because they are so easy to "cheek." "Cheeking" occurs when a person places the tablet to one side of his mouth and only acts as if he is swallowing it. An estimated 46% of patients—both inpatient and outpatient—take less of these medications than is ordered (Blair, 1990). Noncompliance is thought to be the single most important cause of symptom exacerbation and rehospitalization. Psychiatric patients may not want to take their medication for several reasons, including the admission of illness that taking medication may imply, paranoid fears of poisoning, or unpleasant reactions or side effects. Many inpatient units must use liquid forms of these drugs to counteract noncompliant tendencies. Liquids or concentrates usually have an unpleasant taste and should be diluted. Two issues related to "cheeking" or noncompliance with which the nurse must be concerned are decompensation and hoarding. It should be emphasized that it is not humane to allow a person to continue along in a psychotic state.

For severely disturbed patients, chlorpromazine 25 mg t.i.d. is usually ordered to start and is increased every 1 or 2 days by 20 to 50 mg, up to about 400 mg per day. The usual daily dose ranges from 30 to 800 mg.

Another form of administration is the parenteral route. Parenteral drugs are usually used to treat acutely disturbed persons or patients who represent significant compliance risks (see Table 12-2). Both haloperidol and fluphenazine are available

**TABLE 12-2**   Parenteral antipsychotic drug use

| Drug | Parenteral administration (IM) |
| --- | --- |
| **ACUTE AGITATION** | |
| Chlorpromazine (Thorazine) | Initially 25 mg, repeated in 1 h as needed; switch to oral dose as soon as possible |
| Haloperidol (Haldol) | Initially 2-5 mg, repeated every 1-8 h as needed |
| **LONG-TERM MAINTENANCE OR NONCOMPLIANT BEHAVIOR** | |
| Fluphenazine decanoate* (Prolixin decanoate) | Initially 12.5-25 mg, repeated q 2-4 wk |
| Haloperidol decanoate* (Haldol decanoate) | Initially 10-15 times oral dose of haloperidol; usually maintenance dose of 50-100 mg q 4 wk |

*Long-acting antipsychotics.

in long-acting injectable forms that require injection as seldom as once per month or at longer intervals. These long-acting injections are particularly beneficial in community outpatient clinics. Middlemiss and Beeber (1989) describe a Z-track injection technique to decrease skin irritation. Other antipsychotics available in parenteral form are

- Chloroprothixene (Taractan)
- Loxapine (Loxitane)
- Mesoridazine (Serentil)
- Perphenazine (Trilafon)
- Thiothixene (Navane)
- Trifluoperazine (Stelazine)

When a patient is not responding to antipsychotic drug therapy, the nurse's assessment of the patient may be quite helpful to the prescribing physician. Three principles should be kept in mind whenever one is assessing a patient's response and the possibility of changing drugs:

1. If the patient is not taking the original drug as ordered, it is impossible to evaluate its potential therapeutic value. If it is at all possible, the nurse should establish whether the patient is compliant.
2. The drug currently being used should be given a fair trial. Daily therapy for 3 to 6 weeks or more may be needed before a drug's effectiveness (or ineffectiveness) can be ascertained. The emphasis on short hospital stays may make evaluation more difficult.
3. If a change of medication is indicated, the new agent should be taken from a different chemical class (or subclass of the phenothiazines) in order for the patient to profit from inherent differences between classes. Drugs within a class or subclass act similarly and offer no therapeutic advantage.

### Side effects (undesired effects)

The antipsychotic drugs produce numerous side effects because of PNS and CNS actions (see Table 12-1). Side effects due to PNS autonomic blocking (i.e., anticholinergic, antiadrenergic) actions are more likely to be caused by low-potency forms, such as chlorpromazine. CNS extrapyramidal symptoms are more likely to be caused by high-potency drugs, such as haloperidol. The latter effects are more devastating.

**PNS effects.** PNS anticholinergic effects—dry mouth, blurred vision, and photophobia—are common and can often be managed with nondrug interventions. Mydriasis can cause an increase in intraocular pressure, which can aggravate glaucoma. Other relatively common anticholinergic effects are constipation and urinary hesitance. Patients with a history of glaucoma or prostatic hypertrophy are not ordinarily placed on these drugs. Tachycardia is another PNS effect, and persons with cardiovascular disease should be carefully evaluated before being given these drugs. Sudden death related to arrhythmias and decreased cardiac output has been caused by antipsychotic drugs. Thioridazine (Mellaril) has been implicated in more cases of sudden death than any of the other drugs.

Hypotension is the major antiadrenergic effect of antipsychotic drugs. It occurs most often in the elderly (Gomez and Gomez, 1990). Hypotension often occurs when the individual stands or changes positions suddenly (orthostatic hypotension). Thus precautions against falls must be instituted. Besides falling, hypotension causes a reflex tachycardia that can, in turn, cause general cardiovascular inefficiency. Antipsychotic drugs are usually not prescribed for persons with severe hypotension, heart failure, or a history of arrhythmias.

**CNS extrapyramidal symptoms (EPS).** It is estimated that up to 75% of all patients receiving antipsychotic medications have EPS (Blair, 1990). Abnormal voluntary movement disorders develop because of drug-induced imbalances between two major neurotransmitters, dopamine and acetylcholine, in portions of the brain. This imbalance seems to be caused more often by high-potency antipsychotic drugs such as haloperidol. EPS can be grouped as follows: akathisia, dystonias, dyskinesias, akinesias, drug-induced parkinsonism, and neuroleptic malignant syndrome. Tardive dyskinesia, a late-appearing dyskinesia, is one of the most serious and least treatable of all the EPS.

*Akathisia.* Akathisia, an almost unbearable need to move, is an unpleasant subjective and objective response to antipsychotic drugs. It is the most common EPS (about 50% of all EPS) and probably accounts for more noncompliant behavior than the other side effects. Some clinicians believe most patients receiving antipsychotic drugs suffer from akathisia. It was first described in 1911, long before antipsychotic drugs were available, which suggests that other variables may contribute to this distressing side effect. *Subjectively,* the patient often feels jittery or uneasy. He may report a lot of "nervous energy." *Objectively,* the patient is restless and cannot sit still, even during group activities. Unfortunately, restlessness and verbal reflections of subjective anguish can be misinterpreted as a worsening of the psychotic process. *If additional antipsychotic drug is given because of this misinterpretation, the patient will suffer much more.* Nurses must be aware of drug-induced akathisias. Akathisia usually responds to anticholinergic drugs, such as trihexyphenidyl.

*Dystonias.* Dystonic reactions may cause rigidity in muscles that control posture, gait, or ocular movement. In oculogyric crisis the eyes roll back, which is very frightening. Torticollis, another dystonic reaction, is a contracted state of the cervical muscles, producing torsion on the neck. A laryngeal-pharyngeal dystonia, which is associated with gagging, cyanosis, respiratory distress, and asphyxia (particularly in young men), is life threatening. All these frightening conditions respond to intramuscular anticholinergic antiparkinsonism drugs.

*Akinesia.* Akinesia refers to an absence of movement. More often a state of bradykinesia, or a slowing of movement, exists. Movement is difficult to initiate and difficult to maintain. The patient lacks spontaneity in movement and speech. Paradoxically, these same symptoms (for different reasons) are common in schizophrenia, the focus of treatment. Historically, it has not been uncommon for nurses to mistake bizarre postures caused by EPS for exacerbation of schizophrenic symptoms. The dilemma is real. If a manifestation of schizophrenia is occurring, then more medication may be indicated. If it is an EPS, more medication will worsen the symptoms.

***Drug-induced parkinsonism.*** Antipsychotic drugs can produce the constellation of symptoms peculiar to parkinsonism: tremors, rigidity, and bradykinesia are possible consequences of antipsychotic drug therapy. Antipsychotic drugs can intensify existing "naturally occurring" parkinsonism, so they are seldom prescribed for persons with this condition.

***Dyskinesias and tardive dyskinesia.*** *Dyskinesia* refers to abnormal voluntary skeletal muscle movements, which usually produce a jerky motion. Treatment with any antipsychotic drug involves the risk of tardive dyskinesia, which is one of the most serious EPS. The term *tardive* means late-appearing. Typically, tardive dyskinesia appears after months or years of drug usage. It can appear sooner, however. Although the other EPS are caused by a dopamine deficiency much like that in parkinsonism, tardive dyskinesia is thought to be caused by a hypersensitivity to dopamine and a cholinergic deficit. Therefore, although anticholinergic antiparkinsonism drugs (e.g., Artane, Cogentin) are beneficial for the other EPS, they may mask tardive dyskinesia and thus exacerbate it. Tardive dyskinesia affects about 15% to 25% of the patients treated with antipsychotic drugs.

Tardive dyskinesia usually affects the muscles of the mouth and face. Signs of tardive dyskinesia include lip smacking, grinding of the teeth, rolling or protrusion of the tongue, tics, and diaphragmatic movements, which may impair breathing. These involuntary movements are generally coordinated, fluctuate in severity, and disappear during sleep. Patients with tardive dyskinesia are three times as likely to have an impaired gag reflex.

Since tardive dyskinesia is considered to be irreversible (except in the early stages), the physician should be notified if it is suspected. The abnormal involuntary movement scale (AIMS) (see Appendix G) provides a handy vehicle for assessing tardive dyskinesia. The dopamine agonist bromocriptine (Parlodel) has been found effective in treating this side effect.

***Neuroleptic malignant syndrome.*** A final side effect worthy of discussion is the neuroleptic malignant syndrome (NMS). NMS is an underdiagnosed adverse response to antipsychotic drugs (Keltner and McIntyre, 1985). It occurs in as many as 1% (some research estimates run as high as 2.4%) of patients taking antipsychotic drugs; of this number 14% to 30% may die (Hooper et al., 1989). It also occurs most often when high-potency antipsychotic drugs are prescribed. It is not related to toxic drug levels and may occur after only a few doses. It shares some symptoms with other EPS. It is manifested by muscular rigidity, tremors, impaired ventilations, muteness, altered consciousness, and autonomic hyperactivity. Perhaps the cardinal symptom is high body temperature. Temperatures as high as $42.2°$ C ($108°$ F) have been reported.

**Other side effects.** Other side effects that can occur in patients taking antipsychotic drugs include hyperglycemia, jaundice, blood dyscrasias, susceptibility to hyperthermia, blue-gray skin rash, sun-sensitive skin (sunburn), nasal congestion, wheezing, galactorrhea (seepage from breast), gynecomastia (enlarged breast in either sex), impaired ejaculation, and amenorrhea. A non-EPS CNS effect is memory loss. Since the cholinergic system is implicated in memory and learning, anticholinergic antiparkinsonism drugs and low-potency antipsychotic drugs could play a role in this cognitive symptom. A new antipsychotic, clozapine (Clozaril), causes agranulocytosis in 1% of the persons who take it (Barrett et al., 1990). Thirty-five percent of those in whom agranulocytosis developed in 1986 died (see discussion of clozapine at end of this chapter.)

### Guidelines for minimizing EPS

1. Antipsychotic drugs should not be used for nonapproved indications; that is, they should not be used, for example, to treat anxiety.
2. The dose for certain groups should be limited. Older persons, for instance, are especially susceptible to hypotension and tardive dyskinesia.
3. As with all drugs, but especially because there seems to be a dose-EPS relationship, the lowest effective dose of an antipsychotic drug should be given. Since these drugs are metabolized primarily in the liver, persons with reduced liver function due to old age or liver disease should be given comparatively lower doses.
4. Drug holidays, brief periods when the patient is taken off drugs, can decrease side effects without jeopardizing the therapeutic value of the drug.
5. After 1 year of continuous antipsychotic drug therapy the patient should be gradually weaned from the drug. This will allow the treatment team to evaluate the current need for the drug and will also help in the detection of an emerging tardive dyskinesia.

## Interactions with other drugs

See discussion of Interactions under Nursing Implications.

## Nursing implications

**Therapeutic versus toxic levels.** Overdoses of antipsychotic drugs are seldom fatal. Symptoms of overdose include severe CNS depression (somnolence to coma), hypotension, and other EPS. Restlessness or agitation, convulsions (antipsychotic drugs lower the seizure threshold), hyperthermia, increased anticholinergic symptoms, and arrhythmias are other indicators of an overdose. Treatment is mostly supportive: gastric lavage to empty the stomach, amphetamine for severe CNS depression (although a risk of seizure is incurred), and antiparkinsonism drugs for severe EPS. Norepinephrine or phenylephrine can be used for severe hypotension.

**Use in pregnancy.** Although the risks to the fetus are statistically low, exposure to antipsychotic drugs during the first trimester is still to be avoided. During the remainder of the pregnancy, tapering to the lowest possible dose is desirable. If possible, antipsychotic drugs should be discontinued to reduce the risk of transient neonatal toxicity (Cohen, 1989).

**Side effects.** PNS anticholinergic and antiadrenergic effects of antipsychotic drugs are troublesome but are not always as serious or as disturbing to the patient as the CNS extrapyramidal symptoms (EPS). Nurses are often the first psychiatric professionals to observe these side effects. There are several specific interventions the nurse can provide to ameliorate the side effect or to prevent serious consequences (see Box 12-2).

### Box 12-2
## SIDE EFFECTS OF ANTIPSYCHOTIC DRUGS AND APPROPRIATE NURSING INTERVENTIONS

**PNS EFFECTS**

- *Constipation:* Encourage high dietary fiber and increased water intake; give laxatives as ordered.
- *Dry mouth:* Advise patient to take sips of water frequently; provide sugarless hard candies, sugarless gum, and mouth rinses.
- *Nasal congestion:* Give over-the-counter nasal decongestant if approved by physician.
- *Blurred vision:* Advise the patient to avoid tasks that are potentially dangerous. Reassure the patient that normal vision typically returns in a few weeks as tolerance to this side effect develops.
- *Mydriasis:* Advise patient to report eye pain immediately.
- *Photophobia:* Advise the patient to wear sunglasses out-of-doors.
- *Photosensitivity:* Advise use of sun screen and appropriate clothing.
- *Hypotension or orthostatic hypotension:* Ask the patient to get out of his bed or chair slowly. He should sit on the side of the bed for 1 full minute

while dangling his feet, then slowly rise. If hypotension is a problem, take blood pressure before each dose is given. Observe to see whether a change to another antipsychotic agent is indicated.
- *Tachycardia:* This is usually a reflex to hypotension. If intervention for hypotension (above) is effective, reflex tachycardia should decrease.
- *Urinary retention:* Encourage frequent voiding and voiding whenever the urge is present. Catheterize for residual fluids. Ask the patient to monitor urine output and report to the nurse. Older men with benign prostatic hypertrophy are particularly susceptible to this problem.
- *Urinary hesitation:* Provide privacy, run water in the sink, or run warm water over the perineum.
- *Sedation:* Help the patient get up early and get the day started.
- *Weight gain:* Help the patient order an appropriate diet; diet pills should not be taken.

**Interactions.** Antipsychotic drugs compromise and are compromised by many other drugs. Since these drug-drug interactions can be serious, it is important for the nurse to, first, know potential offending agents and, second, advise the family and patient accordingly. CNS depressants, such as alcohol, antihistamines, antianxiety drugs, antidepressants, barbiturates, meperidine, and morphine, have additive effects that can cause profound CNS depression. The nurse should review prescriptions for this possible inadvertent combination and should advise the patient to avoid both alcohol and certain over-the-counter medications.

**Box 12-2**
# SIDE EFFECTS OF ANTIPSYCHOTIC DRUGS AND APPROPRIATE NURSING INTERVENTIONS—cont'd

## CNS EFFECTS

- *Akathisia:* Be patient and reassure the patient who is "jittery" that you understand his need to move and that appropriate drug interventions can help differentiate akathisia and agitation. Since akathisia is the chief cause of noncompliance with antipsychotic regimens, switching to a different antipsychotic drug class may be necessary to achieve compliance.
- *Dystonias:* If severe reactions such as oculogyric crisis or torticollis occur, give prn antiparkinsonism drug (e.g., Cogentin) or antihistamine (e.g., Benadryl) immediately and offer reassurance. More than likely an intramuscular order will not have been written, so call the physician at once to obtain the order. For less severe dystonias, notify the physician in the event that an order for an antiparkinsonism drug is warranted.
- *Drug-induced parkinsonism:* Assess for the three major parkinsonism symptoms—tremors, rigidity, bradykinesia—and report to physician. An-

tiparkinsonism drugs will probably be ordered.
- *Tardive dyskinesia:* Assess for signs by using the AIMS test (Appendix G). Drug holidays may help prevent tardive dyskinesia. Since antiparkinsonism drugs may mask tardive dyskinesia, their use should be reviewed (question use of more than 90 days' duration), particularly indiscriminant prophylactic use. However, young men taking large doses of high-potency antipsychotic drugs (e.g., haloperidol) are one group in which prophylactic use of antiparkinsonism drugs may be more prudent than not using them (American Psychiatric Association Task Force on Tardive Dyskinesia, 1980).
- *Neuroleptic malignant syndrome:* Be alert for this potentially fatal side effect. *Routinely* take temperatures and encourage adequate water intake among all patients on antipsychotic drugs and *routinely* assess for rigidity, tremor, and so on.

Since antacids decrease absorption of antipsychotic drugs, the nurse should give these agents 1 to 2 hours after an oral antipsychotic drug has been given.

The nurse should be aware of other drugs that interact adversely with the antipsychotic drugs (see Box 12-3).

**Patient teaching.** Patient teaching is an important dimension of the nursing care of patients who are taking antipsychotic drugs. The nurse should use discretion in selecting the content of patient teaching sessions because some patients have a tendency to become anxious about potential side effects. The nurse should focus

**Box 12-3**
## ADVERSE ANTIPSYCHOTIC–OTHER DRUG INTERACTIONS

- Amphetamines: Decrease antipsychotic effect.
- Anticholinergic antiparkinsonism drugs: Increase anticholinergic effect.
- Diazoxide: Can cause severe hyperglycemia.
- Dopaminergic antiparkinsonism drugs: Antagonize the antipsychotic effect.
- Guanethidine: Its control of hypertension is decreased.
- Insulin, oral hypoglycemics: Their control of diabetes is weakened.
- Lithium: Decreases antipsychotic effect; may cause neurotoxicity when combined with haloperidol; lithium toxicity may be masked by antiemetic effect of antipsychotic drugs.
- Beta-adrenergic blocking agents (propranolol): Effect of either or both drugs increased.

on symptoms that can be seen or felt. Some patient education issues have been discussed throughout this chapter. Those not previously mentioned follow. The patient and family should be taught the following:

- To avoid hot tubs, hot showers, and hot tub baths since hypotension may occur, causing falls
- To avoid abrupt withdrawal, because EPS can occur
- To utilize a sunscreen to prevent sunburn
- To take the drug as prescribed (Noncompliance is the leading cause of symptom exacerbation.)
- To report sore throat, malaise, fever, or bleeding immediately (Such signs may indicate a blood dyscrasia.)
- To dress appropriately in hot weather and to drink plenty of water to avoid heat stroke

### Selected related drugs by chemical class

**Other phenothiazines.**  The phenothiazines are divided into three subclasses: the aliphatics, the piperidines, and the piperazines.

***Aliphatics: chlorpromazine, promazine, triflupromazine.***  Chlorpromazine is a member of the aliphatic subclass. The other two drugs, *promazine* (Sparine) and *triflupromazine* (Vesprin), are seldom ordered.

***Piperidines: thioridazine, mesoridazine.***  Thioridazine (Mellaril) is almost as old as chlorpromazine, and is the largest-selling antipsychotic in the United States (Wysowski and Baum, 1989). It is frequently ordered, and some patients tend to respond to it better than to other drugs. Thioridazine is also used for the short-term treatment of marked depression accompanied by anxiety in adult patients and for agitation, anxiety, depressed mood, tension, sleep disturbances, fears, and other symptoms in geriatric patients. In children with severe behavioral problems marked by combativeness, thioridazine has been therapeutic. Thioridazine has a maximum upper limit of 800 mg per day because of the possibility of pigmentary retinopathy. Mesoridazine (Serentil) is not prescribed as often as is thioridazine.

**Piperazines: fluphenazine, trifluoperazine, perphenazine.** The two most often prescribed piperazines are fluphenazine and trifluoperazine. Fluphenazine, a high-potency antipsychotic, is available in a long-acting form. Fluphenazine decanoate (Prolixin decanoate), the long-acting form, is beneficial for patients who do not comply with a daily oral medication regimen. This injection can be given every 2 to 4 weeks. Fluphenazine hydrochloride (Prolixin, Permitil) has a "regular" duration and is available in tablet, concentrate, and "regular-acting" parenteral forms. There are restrictions for diluting the concentrate; it should not be mixed with tea, apple juice, or caffeine (e.g., coffee, colas).

Trifluoperazine (Stelazine) is prescribed relatively often. It is available in tablets, concentrate, and for parenteral use and is indicated for excessive anxiety, tension, and agitation, as well as for psychotic manifestations. Dosage information for both fluphenazine and trifluoperazine are found in Table 12-1.

Perphenazine (Trilafon) is often used with antidepressants for patients who are both psychotic and depressed. It can be given separately or is available in a fixed-dose combination with amitriptyline (Elavil). The fixed-dose combination of perphenazine-amitriptyline is called Triavil.

**Butyrophenone: haloperidol.** Haloperidol (Haldol) is from the butyrophenone chemical class of antipsychotic drugs. It is a high-potency drug (2 mg of haloperidol is equivalent to 100 mg of chlorpromazine) and tends to cause more EPS and fewer anticholinergic side effects than do the low-potency drugs. It is the most prescribed antipsychotic and is used extensively in the elderly (because of fewer anticholinergic effects) and in pediatric psychiatry. Haloperidol is also used for Gilles de la Tourette's disease, which is characterized by facial grimaces, tics, purposeless movements of the upper body, shoulder, and arms, coprolalia (frequent extreme profanity), and echolalia (repetition of words spoken to patient).

Haloperidol decanoate is a long-acting form and can be given at 2- to 4-week (or longer) intervals. It is particularly beneficial for persons who struggle with compliance.

**Thioxanthenes: chlorprothixene and thiothixene.** Chlorprothixene (Taractan) and thiothixene (Navane) have different potencies. Chlorprothixene is similar to chlorpromazine or the aliphatic phenothiazines in potency. Thiothixene is twenty times as potent as chlorpromazine (see Table 12-1), or more like the piperazine phenothiazines. Thiothixene is prescribed relatively often. Thiothixene exhibits rather weak anticholinergic properties but relatively powerful EPS (see Table 12-1).

**Dibenzoxazepine: loxapine.** Loxapine (Loxitane) is available in capsule, concentrate, and parenteral forms. The concentrate is unpleasant and should be diluted with orange or grapefruit juice shortly before administration. Specific EPS have been reported frequently (in approximately 20% of patients), particularly during the first few days of treatment. Specific EPS include akathisia and parkinsonism symptoms—tremors, rigidity, sialorrhea, and masked facies. A reduction of the loxapine plus the administration of an antiparkinsonism drug will usually control these manifestations.

**Dihydroindolone: molindone.** Molindone (Moban) is about 10 times as potent as chlorpromazine (see Table 12-1) and is used exclusively for the treatment of psychosis. Some studies indicate that molindone may be the ideal antipsychotic because it produces fewer overall side effects. It is available only for oral administration and has several unique properties. It provokes heavy menstruation in previously amenorrheal women and contains calcium ions that can interfere with the absorption of tetracycline antibiotics or phenytoin (Dilantin).

**Dibenzodiazepine: clozapine.** Clozapine (Clozaril) is the first new antipsychotic agent to be introduced in the United States in 20 years. Although clozapine has been used in Europe and China for the treatment of schizophrenia for some time, it was not approved in the United States until 1990 because of the seriousness of its side effect, agranulocytosis. A study made in 1986 revealed that about 1% of the patients who take clozapine develop agranulocytosis and that, of these, 35% die.

Clozapine has proven successful in helping patients who have not been helped by chlorpromazine (Thorazine) and haloperidol (Haldol). Remarkable case studies of patients who have not responded to other treatment strategies but who have responded to clozapine have encouraged mental health professionals (Barrett et al., 1990).

Because of the potential for life-threatening agranulocytosis, patients will not receive clozapine through a pharmacy but will, instead, have weekly home visits from a nurse or a technologist. Each week a blood sample will be drawn and tested for agranulocytosis. Patients can receive only a 1-week supply of clozapine. Because dispensing clozapine is so labor and technology intensive, it is expensive, costing about $9000 per year. In comparison, the cost of AZT, the anti-AIDS drug, runs about $8000 per year.

## KEY CONCEPTS

1. The dopamine hypothesis of schizophrenia states that schizophrenia is caused by an excessive level of dopamine in the brain.
2. Antipsychotic drugs block dopamine receptors, reducing the effect of excessive availability of dopamine in the brain.
3. Antipsychotic drugs are classified in two ways: (a) on the basis of chemical class and (2) on the basis of potency.
4. Desired effects of antipsychotic drugs include sedation, emotional quieting, psychomotor slowing, and the alleviation of major symptoms of schizophrenia (i.e., alterations in perceptions, thoughts, consciousness, interpersonal relationships, and affect).
5. Anticholinergic side effects (e.g., dry mouth, blurred vision, constipation) and extrapyramidal symptoms (EPS), including akathisia, dystonic reactions, aki-

nesia, drug-induced parkinsonism, and tardive dyskinesia, are the major categories of side effects associated with antipsychotic drugs.

6. High-potency antipsychotic drugs, such as haloperidol (Haldol) and fluphenazine (Prolixin), tend to cause more EPS and low-potency antipsychotic drugs, such as chlorpromazine (Thorazine) and thioridazine (Mellaril), tend to cause more anticholinergic side effects.

7. Neuroleptic malignant syndrome (NMS) is a serious adverse effect of antipsychotic drugs (primarily high-potency drugs); it has a morbidity rate of 1% to 2% and a mortality rate of 20% to 30%.

8. Overdosages with antipsychotic drugs are seldom fatal.

9. Antipsychotic drugs interact with other CNS depressants, such as alcohol, meperidine (Demerol), and morphine, thereby increasing CNS depression.

10. Patient teaching should focus on the recognition of side effects and the avoidance of CNS depressants.

11. The nurse should routinely assess for NMS by taking the patient's temperature and evaluating for rigidity and/or tremors.

## REFERENCES

American Psychiatric Association Task Force on Tardive Dyskinesia: The task force on late neurological effects of antipsychotic drugs: tardive dyskinesia: summary of a task force report of the American Psychiatric Society. Am J Psychiatry 137:1163, 1980.

Barret N, Ormiston S, and Molyneux V: Clozapine: a new drug for schizophrenia, J Psychosoc Nurs 28:24, 1990.

Blair DT: Risk management for extrapyramidal symptoms, Quality Assurance Rev Bull 17:116, 1990.

Cohen LS: Psychopharmacology: psychotropic drug use in pregnancy, Hosp Community Psychiatry 40:566, 1989.

Gomez GE and Gomez EA: The special concerns of neuroleptic use in the elderly, J Psychosoc Nurs 28:7, 1990.

Harris E: Antipsychotic medication, Am J Nurs 81:1316, 1981.

Hooper JF, Herren CK, and Goldwasser H: Neuroleptic malignant syndrome, J Psychosoc Nurs 27:13, 1989.

Keltner NL: Antipsychotic drugs. In Shlafer M and Marieb E, editors: The nurse, pharmacology, and drug therapy, Menlo Park, Calif., 1989, Addison-Wesley.

Keltner NL and McIntyre CW: Neuroleptic malignant syndrome: J Neurosurg Nurs 17:362, 1985.

Middlemiss MA and Beeber ZS: Depot antipsychotics, J Psychosoc Nurs 27:36, 1989.

Overall JE, et al: Justifying neuroleptic drug treatment, Hosp Community Psychiatry 40:749, 1989.

Richelson E: Neuroleptic affinities for human brain receptors and their use in predicting adverse effects, J Clin Psychiatry 45:331, 1984.

Wysowski DK and Baum C: Antipsychotic drug use in the United States, 1976-1985, Arch Gen Psychiatry 46:929, 1989.

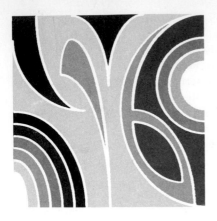

## CHAPTER 13

# Antidepressant and Antimanic Drugs

LEARNING OBJECTIVES
After reading this chapter you should be able to

- Understand concepts of neurotransmitters in relationship to depression and mania.
- Describe differences among classes of antidepressant and antimanic drugs.
- Discuss side effects of the antidepressant and antimanic drugs.
- Identify therapeutic vs toxic drug levels.
- Describe potential interactions of antidepressant and antimanic drugs.
- Discuss implications for patient teaching for antidepressant and antimanic drugs.

Antidepressant and antimanic drugs are used in the treatment of mood disorders. In conceptualizing a "mood continuum," one would place depression (or dysphoria) on one end and elation (euphoria or mania) on the other. Although these extremes in emotions are seemingly opposite, they are related phenomena. This chapter will focus on the two major psychopharmacological classes of drugs used to treat mood disorders, the *antidepressants* and the *antimanic* drugs (Box 13-1). A complete discussion of *mood disorders* is found in Chapter 20.

## ■ Antidepressants

The treatment of depression was revolutionized in the late 1950s when tricyclic antidepressant drugs were first introduced. In the first research report Kuhn (1958), referring to imipramine (Tofranil), stated that the patients "again became interested in things, are able to enjoy themselves, despondency gives way to a desire to undertake something, despair gives place to renewed hope in the future." Subsequent vigorous clinical research over the years has consistently underscored the efficacy of these drugs in the treatment of depression.

Although a number of theories concerning the cause of depression have been propounded, the efficacy of antidepressants is best understood from a neurochemical

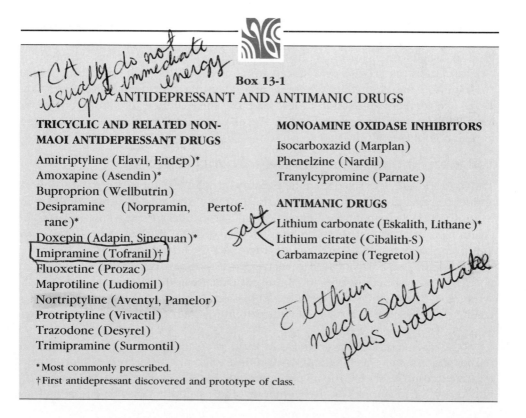

*TCA usually do not give immediate energy*

**Box 13-1**

**ANTIDEPRESSANT AND ANTIMANIC DRUGS**

**TRICYCLIC AND RELATED NON-MAOI ANTIDEPRESSANT DRUGS**

Amitriptyline (Elavil, Endep)*
Amoxapine (Asendin)*
Buproprion (Wellbutrin)
Desipramine (Norpramin, Pertofrane)*
Doxepin (Adapin, Sinequan)*
Imipramine (Tofranil)†
Fluoxetine (Prozac)
Maprotiline (Ludiomil)
Nortriptyline (Aventyl, Pamelor)
Protriptyline (Vivactil)
Trazodone (Desyrel)
Trimipramine (Surmontil)

**MONOAMINE OXIDASE INHIBITORS**

Isocarboxazid (Marplan)
Phenelzine (Nardil)
Tranylcypromine (Parnate)

**ANTIMANIC DRUGS**

*salt*

Lithium carbonate (Eskalith, Lithane)*
Lithium citrate (Cibalith-S)
Carbamazepine (Tegretol)

*c̄ lithium need a salt intake plus water*

*Most commonly prescribed.
†First antidepressant discovered and prototype of class.

perspective. According to the neurochemical theory, endogenous depression (depression that is not a reaction to loss) is caused by an imbalance or decreased availability of certain neurotransmitters or biogenic amines. Specifically, deficiencies of norepinephrine, serotonin, and possibly dopamine cause depression according to this view. Psychopharmacological treatment is based on restoration of normal levels of these neurotransmitters through drugs in one of three ways (Brown and Mann, 1985):

1. By blocking neurotransmitter reuptake into nerve endings (tricyclic antidepressants [TCAs] block neurotransmitter reuptake)
2. By inhibiting neurotransmitter breakdown by monoamine oxidase (monoamine oxidase inhibitors [MAOIs] inhibit enzymatic action on neurotransmitters)
3. Possibly by reducing the stimulation of β-adrenergic receptors (which seem to be involved in depression) by norepinephrine (effect of both TCAs and MAOIs).

Much more is known about the first two views of drug efficacy. However, the third hypothesis is supported by the fact that some antidepressants (e.g., trazodone) do not significantly inhibit neurotransmitter reuptake but effectively treat depression.

The two major classes of antidepressants are (1) TCAs and several related non-MAOI drugs and (2) MAOIs. In this chapter when the term *antidepressant* is used, it usually refers to the TCAs and the related non-MAOI drugs. Monoamine oxidase inhibitors are always referred to as MAOIs. Classification of these drugs commonly is based on their ability to inhibit reuptake of neurotransmitters (the TCAs and related non-MAOI drugs) and on their ability to inhibit enzymatic metabolism of neurotransmitters (MAOIs). These two classes cause serious reactions if combined.

## TRICYCLIC AND RELATED NON-MAOI ANTIDEPRESSANTS

The term *tricyclic* is derived from the chemical structure of these drugs (i.e., tricyclic antidepressants contain three hydrocarbon rings). The related drugs inhibit neurotransmitter uptake but have different chemical structures; for example, maprotiline (Ludiomil) has four hydrocarbon rings (a tetracyclic). Most of these drugs share important properties with imipramine, the first TCA introduced.

Antidepressants are not used for all types of depression. When they are indicated, however, approximately 85% of those patients treated experience remission of symptoms. These drugs do not cure depression, but long-term use has been successful. Most relapse is associated with patient-initiated tapering off or discontinuance.

TCAs are usually the first choice in antidepressant therapy because of the potential serious side effects of MAOIs. MAOIs are usually the second choice. A third treatment approach, electroconvulsive therapy (ECT), is discussed in Chapter 27. Obviously, various forms of psychotherapy and psychotherapeutic interaction are always indicated. TCAs produce both central nervous system (CNS) effects (increasing neurotransmitter availability) and undesired peripheral nervous system (PNS) effects (anticholinergic responses).

## Pharmacological effects (desired effects)

Theoretically, the serum level of biogenic amines in the depressed person is so low it renders him incapable of achieving a normal mood. TCAs alleviate the symptoms of depression by blocking the reuptake of released neurotransmitters (amines)—norepinephrine, serotonin, and dopamine—back into the nerve endings from which they were released. Since neurotransmitter activity is terminated by reuptake, this blocking causes greater neurotransmitter availability and thus prolongs their stimulating action. Paradoxically, clinical studies have shown that this specific effect occurs quickly; yet there is a lag period of 2 to 4 weeks before an antidepressant effect is experienced. Exactly what this means is not clear; however, it seems to indicate that more than neurotransmitter availability is involved in depression.

Some TCAs block norepinephrine reuptake, and others block serotonin reuptake. Theoretically, the physician could order available laboratory tests to determine which neurotransmitter was deficient. A metabolite of norepinephrine, MHPG (3-methoxy-r-hydroxyphenylglycol), is found in the urine; a metabolite of serotonin, 5-HIAA (5-hydroxyindoleacetic acid), is found in the spinal fluid. Although possible, these tests are seldom ordered. Drugs that increase the availability of norepinephrine are termed *secondary amines* and include amoxapine (Asendin), desipramine (Norpramin), and protriptyline (Vivactil). Drugs that increase serotonin availability are called *tertiary amines* and include imipramine (Tofranil), amitriptyline (Elavil, Endep), and doxepin (Sinequan). Trimipramine (Surmontil), a tertiary amine, and nortriptyline (Aventyl, Pamelor), a secondary amine, do not potentiate neurotransmitters as strongly as others in this group.

Sedation is another effect. Since insomnia and agitation are experienced by depressed persons, sedation is often welcome. Tolerance to this sedation usually develops. Another positive side effect is an improved appetite. Anorexia is often a symptom of depression, so appetite stimulation is significant. Whether this is due to a central antihistaminic effect (which some researchers suspect) or to improved mood is not clear.

In summary, TCAs are thought to treat depression by increasing the availability of specific neurotransmitters. In addition to this desired effect, TCAs often produce sedation and improve appetite.

TCAs are not prescribed only for depression. Recommended uses include treatment of anxiety associated with depression, alcoholism, and neurotic disorders. TCAs have been successfully used in the treatment of panic attacks and other phobic anxieties. A desired PNS effect of imipramine, urinary hesitancy, is used in treating childhood enuresis (bedwetting).

## Absorption, distribution, administration

The TCAs are absorbed well from the gastrointestinal tract and are usually given orally. Imipramine and amitriptyline are available in parenteral forms. TCAs are metabolized in the liver, and some metabolites have antidepressant effects (desipramine is a metabolite of impramine; nortriptyline, a metabolite of amitriptyline).

Peak plasma concentrations are reached in 3 to 4 hours. TCAs are water soluble and are highly bound to plasma proteins (imipramine 90% to 95%). Their effects are due to a small fraction of free drug, so even a small increase in free drug is potentially serious. Persons with diminished liver function (e.g., the elderly, the young, alcoholics), with decreased plasma protein levels (the elderly), and with decreased total body water (the elderly) are at special risk of elevated serum levels.

As is true with the antipsychotic drugs, TCAs seem to be equally effective. Imipramine, the first antidepressant, is as effective as any of the newer drugs. Newer antidepressants, such as amoxapine (Asendin), maprotiline (Ludiomil), and trazodone (Desyrel), have been heralded as having faster onset of actions but clinical trials have been inconclusive. Bupropion (Wellbutrin), fluoxetine (Prozac) and other new antidepressants, are said to have fewer side effects than the older TCAs. The ability of a drug to potentiate a specific neurotransmitter and the type, severity, and numbers of side effects it engenders are the primary considerations in selection of these drugs (see Table 13-1).

### Side effects (undesired effects)

Patients taking TCAs experience both PNS and CNS undesired side effects.

**PNS side effects.** Anticholinergic effects on the peripheral autonomic nervous system are the major side effects. Dry mouth is common but not dangerous. Visual disturbances include blurred vision, tearing, and photosensitivity due to mydriasis. These symptoms, too, are more annoying than dangerous. (However, mydriatic action can precipitate an acute attack of glaucoma.)

Other anticholinergic side effects include slowing of the gastrointestinal tract, leading to constipation, and slowing of bladder function, which leads to hesitancy or retention. The elderly are most susceptible to these side effects, and elderly men with benign prostatic hypertrophy are at special risk of bladder problems. Anhidrosis (decreased sweating) impairs body cooling. Anticholinergic effects on the cardiovascular system are common enough to warrant serious consideration. Tachycardias, orthostatic hypotension, reflex tachycardia, and arrhythmias can lead to myocardial infarction and heart block. Patients with a history of heart problems must be carefully evaluated and closely monitored. Doxepin (Sinequan) and fluoxetine (Prozac) are reported to produce fewer cardiovascular side effects.

**CNS side effects.** A number of CNS effects have been reported. Sedation is common and can be helpful since insomnia is a frequent symptom of depression. Less pleasant CNS effects include confusion, disorientation, delusions, agitation, hallucinations, and lowering of the seizure threshold. These psychiatric side effects are probably due to a CNS anticholinergic effect and may be found in as many as 5% to 15% of patients treated with TCAs (Meador-Woodruff, 1990). These usually occur when serum TCA levels are elevated (see Table 13-1). Other potential CNS effects include anxiety, insomnia, nightmares, ataxia, and tremors. Some patients report nightmares so terrifying that they avoid sleep, even though they are sleep deprived. (One licensed vocational nurse purposely worked the night shift and limited her sleeping to a few fitful hours per day because of nightmares. Her physical state so deteriorated that it compounded her depression. She became acutely suicidal, partially because of her compromised physical state.)

**Suicide.** A paradoxical effect of antidepressants is their ability to energize suicidal patients. Suicide among depressed persons is not uncommon. Often depressed persons, although "suicidal," are too depressed to act on their ideas. As the antidepressants succeed and the depression lifts, the patient may have the energy to act on his suicidal thoughts. Suicidally depressed persons warrant special nursing consideration after antidepressant therapy is initiated.

### Interactions

Several serious drug interactions occur with TCAs. Such interactions are (1) CNS depression, (2) cardiovascular and hypertensive effects, and (3) additive anticholinergic effects. In addition, other problematic interactions occur.

**CNS depression.** Increased CNS depression may occur when TCAs are taken with such CNS depressants as alcohol, anticonvulsants, antipsychotics, benzodiazepines (e.g., Valium), sedatives, and some antihypertensives (e.g., beta blockers, clonidine, reserpine).

**Cardiovascular and hypertensive effects.** Cardiovascular arrhythmias or hypertension can occur when sympathomimetic drugs are given with TCAs. Since TCAs block the reuptake of norepinephrine, drugs with sympathomimetic agents will cause an increase in norepinephrine in the synaptic cleft. Interactants to avoid include norepinephrine, dopamine, ephedrine, and phenylpropanolamine (found in many over-the-counter stimulants). MAOIs, the other class of antidepressants, must be completely avoided. Severe reactions, including high fever, seizures, and a fatal hypertensive crisis, can occur. MAOIs are usually not prescribed unless TCAs have failed. When changing to MAOIs, the patient must be off TCAs for 14 days before the new drug is given. In addition, TCAs block the release of several antihypertensives from presynaptic cells, thus compromising their effectiveness.

**Additive anticholinergic effects.** Additive anticholinergic effects can occur when TCAs are given with other anticholinergic drugs, including antipsychotic drugs, atropine, scopolamine, anticholinergic antiparkinsonism drugs, and antihistamines. This is particularly true in elderly patients. All the PNS autonomic effects and CNS anticholinergic effects mentioned earlier can be compounded.

**Other interactions.** Two other significant interactants are guanethidine and methylphenidate (Ritalin). Guanethidine is blocked, thus eliminating its antihypertensive effect. Methylphenidate blocks imipramine and desipramine metabolism, thus increasing serum levels of those drugs.

### Nursing implications

**Therapeutic vs toxic blood levels.** TCAs do not produce euphoria and are not addicting, so their potential for abuse is not great. However, overdose is a real issue. TCA overdose accounts for 25% to 50% of all hospital admissions for overdose (Harsch and Holt, 1988). The difference between a therapeutic dose and a lethal dose is small. Just 10 to 30 times the daily dose can be fatal. For this reason, it is not uncommon for outpatients to be restricted to a 7-day supply if suicide is a risk.

**TABLE 13-1** Tricyclics and related non-MAOI antidepressants

| Drug | Usual daily adult dosage range (mg) | Half-life (hours) | Therapeutic plasma levels (ng/ml) | Neurotransmitter effect* | | Relative frequency of side effect* | | | |
|---|---|---|---|---|---|---|---|---|---|
| | | | | Serotonin | Norepinephrine | Sedation | Anticholinergic | Antianxiety | Orthostatic hypotension |
| Amitriptyline (Elavil, En-dep) | S = 25 t.i.d. M = 40-100 h.s. | 31-46 | 110-250 | 4× | 2× | 4× | 4× | 5× | 2× |
| Amoxapine (Asendin) | S = 50 bid or t.i.d. M = 200-300 h.s. | 8 | 200-500 | 2× | 3× | 2× | 3× | 2× | × |
| Bupropion (Wellbutrin) | S = 100 b.i.d. M = 100 t.i.d. | 8-24 | — | +/0 | +/0 | 2× | 2× | — | × |
| Desipramine (Norpramin, Pertofrane) | S = 25 t.i.d. M = 100-200 h.s. | 12-24 | 125-300 | 2× | 4× | × | × | × | × |
| Doxepin (Adapin, Sinequan) | S = 25 t.i.d. M = 75-150 h.s. | 8-24 | 100-200 | 2× | × | 3× | 2× | 3× | 2× |

| | Drug / Dosing (mg) | | | | | | | | |
|---|---|---|---|---|---|---|---|---|---|
| Fluoxetine (Prozac) | S = 20 in AM<br>M = 20-40/d (AM and noon) | 7-9 d | — | 5× | × | ×/0 | × | † | × |
| Imipramine (Tofranil) | S = 100-150/d<br>M = 50-150 h.s. | 11-25 | 200-350 | 4× | 2× | 2× | 2× | 2× | 3× |
| Maprotiline (Ludiomil) | S = 75/d<br>M = 75-150/d | 21-25 | 200-300 | 0/+ | 3× | 2× | 2× | 3× | × |
| Nortriptyline (Aventyl, Pamelor) | S = 25 t.i.d. or q.i.d.<br>M = 75-150/d | 18-44 | 50-150 | 3× | 2× | 2× | 2× | × | × |
| Protriptyline (Vivactil) | S = 15-40/d<br>M = 20-40/d | 67-89 | 100-200 | 2× | 4× | × | 3× | 0 | × |
| Trazodone (Desyrel) | S = 50 t.i.d.<br>M = 150-400/d | 4-9 | 800-1600 | 3× | 0 | 2× | × | 4× | 2× |
| Trimipramine (Surmontil) | S = 75 mg/d<br>M = 50-150 h.s. | 7-30 | 180 | + | + | 3× | 2× | 3× | 2× |

S = to start; M = maintenance; × = relative intensity of effect; 0 = none; — = not known

*Based on manufacturer information.

†Fluoxetine can cause nervousness.

Adopted from Olin BR: Drug facts and comparisons, St Louis, 1990, JB Lippincott. p. 262.

### Box 13-2
## NURSING INTERVENTIONS FOR TCA OVERDOSE

- Monitor blood pressure, heart rate and rhythm, and respirations.
- Maintain patent airway.
- ECG is recommended.
- Induce vomiting or gastric lavage with activated charcoal to prevent further drug absorption (for up to 24 hours).
- The antidote for severe TCA poisoning (anticholinergic toxicity) is physostigmine (Antilirium), an acetylcholinesterase inhibitor (inhibits the breakdown of acetylcholine).

Toxic blood levels may result in sedation, ataxia, agitation, stupor, coma, respiratory depression, and convulsions. Exaggeration of side effects previously mentioned can also occur. Cardiovascular reactions can occur suddenly and cause acute heart failure. On the other hand, cardiovascular reactions can be "delayed," that is, occur after "recovery" from depression. For these reasons, all antidepressant overdoses should be considered serious, and the patient should be admitted to a hospital for monitoring. It should be noted, however, that some studies suggest that imipramine also has antiarrhythmic properties. Imipramine arrhythmic and antiarrhythmic properties underscore the need for more knowledge about TCAs.

The nurse should be aware of several assessment and intervention strategies when a toxic level of TCAs is suspected (see Box 13-2).

**Use in pregnancy.**  Depressive symptoms, such as loss of appetite, can interfere with fetal development by preventing adequate fetal weight gain. During pregnancy TCAs with low anticholinergic effects (such as nortriptyline and desipramine) are preferred to those with high anticholinergic effects. The TCAs need to be tapered off before delivery to avoid transient perinatal toxicity (Cohen, 1989).

**Side effects.**  Selected side effects and appropriate nursing interventions are listed in Box 13-3.

**Interactions.**  The nurse should be aware of the interactants mentioned in Table 13-3 and Box 13-4. As a general rule, persons taking TCAs should avoid certain categories of drugs:

- Drugs that have anticholinergic properties (e.g., anticholinergic antiparkinsonism drugs)
- Drugs that depress the CNS (e.g., alcohol)
- Drugs that stimulate the CNS (e.g., sympathomimetics such as phenylpropanolamine)
- MAOIs (Patients receiving TCAs and MAOIs concurrently should be kept under close supervision. Deaths have been reported from this combination.)

**Box 13-3**
## SIDE EFFECTS AND NURSING INTERVENTIONS FOR TCAs

**PNS EFFECTS**

- *Dry mouth:* Advise frequent sips of water, hard candies, sugarless gum.
- *Mydriasis:* Advise wearing of sunglasses outdoors.
- *Diminished lacrimation:* Suggest artificial tears.
- *Blurred vision:* Caution about driving and potential for falls. The patient should remove objects in the house that might be tripped over (e.g., throw rugs, small tables).
- *Eye pain:* Advise patient to report eye pain immediately, as it may indicate an acute glaucoma attack. All elderly persons should be screened for glaucoma before treatment with TCAs is initiated.
- *Urinary hesitancy/retention:* Monitor fluid intake. Patient should be told to avoid putting off urinating. Running water or pouring water over the perineum can stimulate urination. Catheterization may be needed.
- *Constipation:* Monitor fluid and food intake. Urge patient to heed the urge to defecate. A high-fiber diet and large amounts of water (2500 to 3000 ml per day) are helpful.
- *Anhidrosis:* Decreased sweating can lead to increased body temperature. Adequate fluids, appropriate clothing, and sensible exercise should be stressed.
- *Cardiovascular effects:* TCAs are contraindicated during the recovery phase of myocardial infarction.
- *Orthostatic hypotension:* Advise patient to assume sitting position on side of bed, to wait and dangle feet for one full minute, then to rise slowly. Patients should not stand in one position too long and should avoid hot showers and tub baths. The elderly may require assistance at these times.

**CNS EFFECTS**

- *Sedation:* Caution patient about driving.
- *Delirium or mania:* Discontinue the drug and call the physician.
- *Suicidal patients:* Observe patients closely since TCAs may increase energy for suicide.

A history of hypersensitivity to TCAs precludes their use. Since TCAs lower the seizure threshold, concomitant electroconvulsive therapy (ECT) must be carefully considered.

**Patient teaching.** The nurse should discuss side effects and several important principles with the patient and his family:

- A "lag period" of 2 to 4 weeks occurs before full therapeutic effects are experienced.
- Certain interactants must be avoided, including over-the-counter preparations. (See Interactions discussion.)

- Abrupt discontinuation can cause nausea, headache, and malaise.
- Eye pain must be reported immediately.

### Related antidepressant drugs

**Imipramine.** Imipramine (Tofranil) is the oldest of the TCAs. It has relatively high anticholinergic and sedative effects. None of the newer antidepressants have proved to be more effective. Imipramine pamoate (Tofranil PM) is available in a single bedtime dose for adults.

**Amitriptyline.** Amitriptyline (Elavil, Endep) is prescribed often. It potentiates serotonin. It has the most anticholinergic and antianxiety effects and is one of the most sedating. Because of its sedating quality, it is often prescribed in one dose at bedtime. Amitriptyline is available in parenteral form and in a fixed-dose combination with the antipsychotic perphenazine. The trade name for this combination antidepressant-antipsychotic drug is Triavil.

**Amoxapine.** Amoxapine (Asendin), a newer drug, is not a tricyclic antidepressant. It is a metabolite of the antipsychotic drug loxapine and blocks dopamine receptors. It potentiates norepinephrine. Its manufacturer claims amoxapine has a faster onset of action, but clinical trials are inconclusive in this regard. Extrapyramidal reactions have been reported and are no doubt related to the dopamine-blocking property.

**Bupropion.** Bupropion (Wellbutrin) is a relatively new antidepressant and is not a TCA or an MAOI. Clinical tests indicate that orthostatic hypotension, cardiovascular conduction problems, anticholinergic effects, and daytime sedation are minimal compared to other antidepressants. On the other hand, agitation is not uncommon. Bupropion is contraindicated for patients with seizure disorders or a prior diagnosis of bulimia or anorexia, and it should not be given in combination with MAOIs.

**Desipramine.** Desipramine (Norpramin, Pertofrane) is a widely used TCA that potentiates norepinephrine. It is a naturally occurring metabolite of imipramine. Some clinicians believe it to be the drug of choice for the depressed elderly patient known to be sensitive to anticholinergic side effects (the elderly with narrow-angle glaucoma or prostatic hypertrophy) because it has the lowest incidence of anticholinergic effects. It is also less sedating.

***Doxepin.*** Doxepin (Adapin, Sinequan) is a widely used TCA that potentiates serotonin. It is sedating and has anticholinergic activity and relatively high antianxiety effects. It is used often for patients with a history of cardiac problems because it has fewer cardiovascular effects.

***Fluoxetine.*** Fluoxetine (Prozac) is a new antidepressant that potentiates serotonin. It has a half-life of 7 to 9 days, so it is often given on a once-per-day basis and can be given on a schedule of three times per week. It should be given before noon because of its ability to cause sleep disturbances. In a premarketing study 4% of the patients developed a rash that required discontinuation of the drug. There is also a risk of weight loss in already thin persons. Fluoxetine is the most frequently prescribed antidepressant. It costs about $1.50 per tablet, more than 10 times the cost of other antidepressants (Monroe, 1990). If fluoxetine is not tolerated, the patient must wait 5 weeks before starting another antidepressant.

*Maprotiline.* Maprotiline (Ludiomil), a newer antidepressant, is not a TCA but a tetracyclic. It potentiates norepinephrine. It has relatively mild anticholinergic effects and is sedating. Dosage increases are generally made slowly.

*Nortriptyline.* Nortriptyline (Aventyl, Pamelor), a TCA, is preferred for persons with a history of an unfavorable response to antidepressants because it has fewer sedative and anticholinergic effects than most other TCAs. It is a metabolite of amitriptyline.

*Protriptyline.* Protriptyline (Vivactil) is different from other TCAs in that it does not sedate but stimulates. It may produce a greater incidence of tachycardia and cardiovascular problems. Since some depressed patients experience hypersomnia instead of insomnia, protriptyline may enable those persons to reduce their amount of sleep.

*Trazodone.* Trazodone (Desyrel) is not a TCA. It potentiates serotonin. It is prescribed often because it has almost no anticholinergic effects and little cardiac effect. Trazodone's absorption is increased by 20% if it is taken right after a light meal. One unusual adverse reaction to this drug is priapism, prolonged penile erection. Surgical intervention has been required in a significant percentage of affected men. If priapism occurs, the nurse should stop the medication and notify the physician.

*Trimipramine.* Trimipramine (Surmontil) is a TCA that *theoretically* potentiates serotonin; however, this has not been established. It is quite sedating and has moderate anticholinergic effects.

## Investigational antidepressants

Antidepressants currently under investigation include sertraline, paroxetine, fluvoxamine (like fluoxetine but better tolerated and has a shorter half-life), and ventafexine, which has a more rapid onset than fluoxetine.

## MONOAMINE OXIDASE INHIBITORS (MAOIs)

Monoamine oxidase inhibitors (MAOIs), the other class of antidepressants, are usually administered to hospitalized patients or to persons who can be closely supervised. These drugs are almost always prescribed after several TCAs have been tried and failed, although an argument can be made that MAOIs are particularly effective in treating atypical depression (hypersomnia, excessive eating). This second-class status reflects the seriousness of the adverse reactions to these drugs. Although many expert clinicians believe this "fear" of MAO inhibitors is unwarranted, a reluctance to use them seems to be the norm.

## Pharmacologic effects (desired effects)

MAOIs block monoamine oxidase, the major enzyme involved in the metabolic decomposition and thus inactivation of norepinephrine, serotonin, and dopamine. This increases levels of these neurotransmitters in the PNS as well as in the CNS. According to the neurochemical theory of depression, depressed persons have less than "normal" amounts of these neurotransmitters available. MAOIs help achieve the "normal" amount by slowing the deactivation of these amines. This is in contrast to the TCAs, which help achieve the "normal" amount by preventing the reuptake

**TABLE 13-2**   Monoamine oxidase inhibitors

| Drug | Usual daily dose (mg) | Comments* |
|---|---|---|
| Isocarboxazid (Marplan) | S = 30/d<br>M = 10-20/d | Mildly stimulating |
| Phenelzine (Nardil) | S = 15 t.i.d., then increase to 60-90/d<br>M = 15/d | Most sedating; preferred MAOI |
| Tranylcypromine (Parnate) | S = 10 in morning<br>10 in afternoon<br>M = 10, 1-2 times per day | Most stimulating |

S = start; M = maintenance.
*Comments adapted from Knoben and Anderson, 1983, p. 483.

of amines by the neurons. It takes 10 days to 4 weeks for the antidepressant effect of MAOIs to occur; but, as with the TCAs, the physiological action (the inhibition of monoamine oxidase) occurs right away. This suggests that factors other than low levels of specific neurotransmitters are involved in depression.

In the PNS the slowed release of norepinephrine causes decreased heart rate, decreased vasoconstriction, and hypotension. MAOIs also inhibit monoamine oxidase in the liver, which leads to elevated levels of other drugs that are normally metabolized in the liver by monoamine oxidase.

## Absorption, distribution, administration

MAOIs are well absorbed from the gastrointestinal tract and are given orally. They are metabolized in the liver. Table 13-2 presents usual dosages for these drugs.

## Side effects (undesired effects)

MAOIs cause CNS, cardiovascular, and anticholinergic side effects. Serious, life-threatening reactions can occur when MAOIs interact with certain drugs or foods (see Interactions discussion).

Because MAOIs increase the availability of biogenic amines in the brain, CNS hyperstimulation has occurred, causing agitation, acute anxiety attacks, restlessness, insomnia, and euphoria. In persons thought to have quiescent schizophrenia (an unrecognized, latent form) full schizophrenic episodes have erupted. Hypomania (less than full mania) is a more common effect.

Hypotension is a common cardiovascular effect. Pargyline, an MAOI, is used not as an antidepressant but as an antihypertensive. The slowdown in the release of norepinephrine is the cause. Unlike the effect of TCAs, a reflex tachycardia does not occur because the slowed release of norepinephrine is also experienced by other adrenergic nerves, and the heart does not reflexively speed up. Hypotension combined with failure of a compensatory increased heart rate can lead to heart failure.

MAOIs can cause anticholinergic effects, such as dry mouth, blurred vision, urinary hesitancy, and constipation. Hepatic and hematological dysfunctions can occur and, although rare, are potentially serious. Blood counts and liver function should be obtained before therapy begins.

## Interactions

MAOIs have a number of serious interactions. Potentially lethal interactants include both drugs (Table 13-3) and foods (Box 13-4).

**Drug-drug interactions.** The nurse should be aware of several types of drug interaction:

- Those that cause *hypertension* (including *hypertensive crisis*)
- Those that cause severe *anticholinergic responses*
- Those that can cause profound *CNS depression.*

Sympathomimetic drugs are classified as direct-acting, indirect-acting, and mixed-acting (having both direct and indirect properties). Indirect-acting and mixed-acting sympathomimetics cause serious and sometimes fatal hypertension. Direct-acting sympathomimetics act by adding new norepinephrine to the body, whereas indirect-acting sympathomimetics release existing norepinephrine from the neuron. Since MAOIs increase the amount of stored norepinephrine in the PNS, the potential for indirect-acting and mixed-acting sympathomimetics to release relatively large amounts of norepinephrine makes the avoidance of these interacting drugs crucial. Evan small amounts can trigger a hypertensive crisis. Typical indirect-acting and mixed-acting sympathomimetics include amphetamines, cocaine, methylphenidate (Ritalin), dopamine, mephentermine, and ephedrine, Over-the-counter weight-loss and stimulant products contain phenylephrine, phenylpropanolamine, and pseudoephedrine, which are mixed or indirect-acting sympathomimetics. Direct-acting sympathomimetics such as norepinephrine, epinephrine, and isoproterenol *theoretically* should not trigger the release of existing norepinephrine. Finally, MAOIs should not be given in combination with TCAs except in unusually refractory cases.

The initial symptoms of hypertensive crisis are palpitation, tightness in the chest, stiff neck, and a throbbing, radiating headache. Very high blood pressure with elevation of heart rate is common. Cardiovascular consequences have included myocardial infarction, cerebral hemorrhage, myocardial ischemia, and arrhythmias. Diaphoresis and pupillary dilation are also prominent signs.

Anticholinergic effects can be severe if other anticholinergic drugs are given with MAOIs. Typical anticholinergic side effects can be reviewed in the discussion of TCA side effects.

Finally, since MAOIs "inhibit" monoamine oxidase in the liver, some drugs, particularly CNS depressants, are not metabolized there, creating serum levels high enough to seriously depress the CNS. Meperidine (Demerol) is specifically contraindicated. A marked potentiation of these drugs can occur. Hypotensive drugs are also potentiated by MAOIs.

**Food-drug interactions.** Food-drug interactions center around the amino acid tyramine, a precursor to dopamine, norepinephrine, and epinephrine. Tyramine is found in many foods commonly consumed in the North American diet (Box 13-4). Aged cheese, bananas, salami, and coffee are a few tyramine-containing foods that must be avoided by the patient. In fact, all high-protein foods that have undergone protein breakdown by aging, fermentation, pickling, or smoking should be avoided. Hypertension and hypertensive crisis can develop from this food-drug combination.

**TABLE 13-3** Drugs to avoid while taking MAOIs

| Drugs | Interaction |
|---|---|
| Anticholinergic drugs | Compound anticholinergic response |
| Anesthetics (general) | Deepen CNS depression |
| Antihypertensives (diuretics, β- blockers, hydralazine) | Cause hypotension |
| CNS depressants | Intensify CNS depression |
| Guanethidine, methyldopa, reserpine | Produce severe hypertension |
| Sympathomimetics (mixed and indirect acting): amphetamines, methylphenidate, dopamine, phenylpropanolamine (in many over-the-counter hayfever, cold, diet medications) | Precipitate hypertensive crisis, cardiac stimulation, arrhythmias, cerebrovascular hemorrhage |
| Sympathomimetics (direct-acting): epinephrine, norepinephrine, isoproterenol; less likely to cause problems | Same as above but theoretically should not produce as severe a reaction |
| Tricyclic antidepressants | Same as above |

*[handwritten: ✳ Marplan ✳ Nardil ✳ Parnate]*

*[handwritten: fermented or overripe]*

**Box 13-4**

**TYRAMINE-RICH FOODS TO AVOID WHILE TAKING MAOIs**

*[handwritten: Combined foods]*

Alcoholic beverages
  Beer and ale
  Chianti and sherry wine
Dairy products
  Cheese: cheddar, blue, brie, mozzarella  *[handwritten: any aged cheese]*
  Sour cream
  Yogurt
Fruits and vegetables
  Avocados
  Bananas
  Fava beans
  Canned figs
  *[handwritten: lima beans, Kidney beans, split peas]*

Meats
  Bologna
  Chicken liver
  Fish, dried
  Liver
  Meat tenderizer
  Pickled herring
  Salami
  Sausage
Other foods
  Caffeinated coffee, colas, tea (large amounts)
  Chocolate
  Licorice
  Soy sauce  *[handwritten: (hoisin sauce)]*
  Yeast
  *[handwritten: Caviar]*

*[handwritten: avoided ✱ 2 wks before + 2 wks after beginning drugs (MAOI)]*

## Nursing implications

**Therapeutic vs toxic drug levels.** An intensification of the effects already discussed occurs with overdose. A lethal dose of MAOIs is only 6 to 10 times the daily dose (see Table 13-2 for typical dosages). Careful monitoring during the time medications are passed out is important. "Cheeking" and hoarding of these drugs could be disastrous. If MAOI overdose is suspected, the nurse should know the following:

- Emesis and gastric lavage may be helpful if performed early.
- Monitoring of vital signs is important.
- External cooling is warranted if high fevers occur.
- Hypotension should be treated in the standard manner.

**Use in pregnancy.** MAOIs should be given during pregnancy only if the anticipated benefit justifies the potential risks to the fetus.

**Side effects.** The nurse should be familiar with the common side effects of MAOIs and the appropriate nursing interventions (see Box 13-5).

**Interactions (and contraindications).** It is important for the nurse to understand that drug-drug and food-drug interactions are serious and potentially fatal. The nurse should know the following:

- Sympathomimetic drugs should not be combined with MAOIs.
- Tyramine-containing foods must not be ingested by the patient who is taking MAOIs.

### Box 13-5
### SIDE EFFECTS AND NURSING INTERVENTIONS FOR MAOIs

- *CNS hyperstimulation*: Reassure the patient. Assess for developing psychosis, hypomania, or seizures. If symptoms warrant, withhold the drug and notify the physician.
- *Hypotension*: Monitor blood pressure frequently and intervene to prevent falls and injuries; having patient lie down may help return blood pressure to normal.
- *Anticholinergic effects*: See TCA side effects for appropriate nursing interventions.
- *Hepatic and hematological dysfunction*: Blood counts and liver function tests should be performed. If dysfunction is apparent, MAOI should be discontinued.

- MAOIs are contraindicated in patients
  - With a history of stroke or cardiovascular disease
  - With a pheochromocytoma, a tumor that secretes pressor substances
  - Undergoing elective surgery (because of the hypotensive potential of combined MAOIs and anesthesia)
- MAOIs should not be given in combination with
  - Other MAOIs
  - TCAs
  - Meperidine (Demerol)
- Hypertensive crisis is a major concern. If it occurs the nurse should
  - Discontinue MAOIs and contact the physician
  - Know that therapy to reduce the blood pressure is warranted and know that phentolamine (Regitine) 5 mg intravenously is the appropriate drug
  - Manage fever by external cooling
  - Institute supportive nursing care as indicated

**Patient teaching.** The nurse must be persistent in teaching the patient and family about MAOIs and their side effects. Although most of these drugs will be administered in a closely supervised setting, teaching responsibilities remain. Since patients taking an MAOI can experience serious reactions to certain other drugs and foods, the nurse must convey this information clearly. However, she must understand the concept of balance. If the nurse says too much she runs the risk of discouraging and frightening the patient. If teaching is inadequate, the patient could die. Obviously, for this class of drugs one must err on the side of teaching too much. The nurse should teach the patient and his family the following:

- Therapeutic effects are achieved within 10 days to 4 weeks.
- Driving must be avoided if the patient is drowsy.
- Certain over-the-counter drugs should be avoided, and all physicians, not just the psychiatrist, should be aware the patient is taking an MAOI.
- High-tyramine foods should be avoided.
- Headaches, palpitations, and stiff neck should be reported immediately.

## Related MAOIs

Three MAOIs are used in the treatment of depression.

**Isocarboxazid.** Isocarboxazid (Marplan) is considered to be the least effective MAO inhibitor. A clinical response may not be noticed for 4 weeks or longer after therapy has begun. It is mildly stimulating.

**Phenelzine.** Phenelzine (Nardil) has been found to be most effective in depressed persons who are clinically characterized as "atypical." It is considered the most effective MAOI and is the most sedative. A clinical response is experienced in about 4 weeks.

**Tranylcypromine.** Tranylcypromine (Parnate) seems most effective for severe reactive or endogenous depression. A clinical effect is experienced in about

10 days, sooner than in the other MAOIs. It is the most stimulating. Tranylcypromine is contraindicated in patients over 60 years of age.

**Moclobemide.** Moclobemide is under investigation. It is a quickly reversible MAOI.

# ■ Antimanic Drugs

## LITHIUM

Lithium, a naturally occurring element, is not much different from sodium. The differences, however are significant enough to make lithium useful in the treatment of manic depression. Lithium was discovered in 1817 by Arfwedson, who named it after the Greek word for stone. Lithium was touted as a cure for epilepsy, gout, and other problems. In the 1940s lithium was used as a salt substitute for cardiac patients in the United States. It was removed from the market after some of these persons died of lithium toxicity. In 1949 an Australian, John Cade, reported that his research showed lithium to be helpful in the treatment of manic depression. Lithium was not made available in the United States for this purpose until 1970. It is now used for the treatment and prophylaxis of the manic phase of manic-depressive illness. There is also a growing body of clinical research that supports its use as an anti-depressant.

## Pharmacological effects (desired effects)

Although precisely how lithium achieves its normalizing effect on mania is not known, it is thought that the lithium ion substitutes for the sodium ion in neurons, thereby compromising the ability of the neurons to release, inactivate, and respond to neurotransmitters.

## Absorption, distribution, administration

Lithium is well absorbed from the gastrointestinal tract. It is given orally in tablets, capsules, or concentrate. Peak blood levels are reached in 1 to 3 hours. More than 95% of the amount ingested is excreted by the kidneys. It is not metabolized. The plasma half-life of lithium is about 24 hours. Renal disease lengthens the half-life, necessitating reduction in dosage.

Absorption and excretion of lithium are closely linked to those of sodium. If dietary sodium intake increases, it is likely that plasma lithium levels will drop as lithium is excreted more rapidly. Conversely, if sodium in the diet decreases or if sodium is lost in ways other than through the kidney (e.g., sweating, diarrhea), lithium levels will increase. Since a therapeutic serum level of lithium is not much lower than a toxic serum level, such considerations are significant. Diet and activity levels should not change abruptly.

Lithium primarily is manufactured in 300 mg capsules and tablets. A 450 mg, sustained-release capsule is available also. Lithium is effective in 80% of the cases; however, it takes 1 to 2 weeks to achieve a clinical response. Lithium dosage is based on both the clinical response and serum lithium levels. The typical dose for acute mania is 600 mg three times per day, which usually produces a serum level of 1.0 to 1.5 mmol/L. Desirable *maintenance blood levels* are 0.6 to 1.2 mmol/L and can be maintained on 900 to 1200 mg per day. Blood levels over 1.5 mmol/L can be toxic.

## Side effects (undesired effects)

Lithium's side effects are linked to serum blood levels. Blood levels over 1.5 mmol/L can be considered toxic. Common side effects are nausea, dry mouth, diarrhea, and thirst. Drowsiness, mild hand tremor, polyuria, weight gain, a bloated feeling, sleeplessness, and light-headedness are other relatively common side effects. These effects occur at therapeutic levels but usually cease after the sixth week. On the other hand, these same side effects will increase in severity at toxic serum levels.

Side effects unrelated to serum levels include weight gain, a metallic taste, headache, edema of the hands and ankles, and pruritus. Lithium, even in therapeutic levels, can affect thyroid gland function. Some patients may require thyroid hormone. Lithium may impair the mental or physical abilities required for driving.

Usually lithium therapy is contraindicated in persons with renal disease and requires close supervision of these patients should it be necessary. Lithium is also generally contraindicated in persons with cardiovascular disease. Lithium may harm the fetus also. Adverse reactions to toxic blood levels are discussed below.

## Interactions

Familiarity with the drugs that can elevate lithium serum levels is essential. Diuretics (except acetazolamide) decrease lithium excretion and thereby elevate serum lithium levels. Indomethacin and possibly other nonsteroidal antiinflammatory drugs increase serum lithium levels by reducing renal elimination of lithium. Switching to a low-salt diet will also elevate serum lithium levels.

Some drugs decrease serum lithium levels and pose the problem of inadequate treatment and symptom exacerbation. Drugs decrease serum levels in one of two ways: by increasing lithium excretion or by decreasing lithium absorption. Drugs that increase lithium excretion include acetazolamide (Diamox), caffeine, and alcohol.

It is not uncommon for lithium and antipsychotic drugs to be combined. Antipsychotics are ordered with lithium because of lithium's clinical response time of 1 to 2 weeks. Antipsychotic agents are prescribed to produce a neuroleptic effect until the lithium produces a clinical response. A potential problem with this combination is that the antiemetic properties of the antipsychotic will mask early signs of lithium toxicity—nausea and vomiting. A second concern centers on the specific combination of lithium and haloperidol. Some studies report a significantly higher percentage of neurotoxicity with this combination.

Lithium also prolongs the paralyzing effect of neuromuscular blocking agents given before surgery and ECT. Apnea and oxygen deprivation can be avoided if appropriate steps (e.g., extra oxygenation) are taken.

## Nursing implications

**Therapeutic versus toxic drug levels.** *Therapeutic* serum lithium levels are 0.6 to 1.2 mmol/L. At serum levels above 1.5 mmol/L adverse reactions can occur. Typically, the higher the serum levels, the more severe the reaction. Mild to moderate toxic reactions occur at levels from 1.5 to 2.5 mmol/L, and moderate to severe reactions at 2.0 to 2.5 mmol/L. Diarrhea, vomiting, drowsiness, muscular weakness, and lack of coordination can be early signs of lithium toxicity. At higher levels ataxia, giddiness, tinnitus, blurred vision, and large output of dilute urine may be seen. At serum levels above 3 mmol/L multiple organs and organ systems may be involved, leading to coma and death (Sugarman, 1984). Interestingly, serum levels as high as 10 mmol/L have been survived. Serum levels should be monitored and not allowed to exceed 2 mmol/L.

There is no antidote for lithium poisoning. Discontinuing the drug may be enough when supportive nursing care is available. Gastric lavage has been used successfully. Parenteral normal saline solution (1 to 2 L) infused over 6 hours may provide enough volume to prevent hypovolemia and restore blood pressure and enough sodium to counteract lithium's neural effects and enhance renal excretion for serum levels below 2.5 mmol/L. For severe lithium poisoning, forced diuresis may be needed. If so, mannitol may be used. Acetazolamide, which alkalinizes the urine, may be given to increase lithium excretion even more. Finally, in some severe cases, hemodialysis has been found helpful.

**Use in pregnancy.** Cessation of lithium during pregnancy is suggested because of its relationship to Ebstein's malformation if it is used in the first trimester. If antimania treatment is essential in the first trimester, carbamazepine may be beneficial. When lithium is prescribed in the second and third trimesters, dosages should be reduced as much as 50% before delivery because of possible neonatal toxicity from high maternal serum levels of lithium (Cohen, 1989).

**Side effects.** Because lithium has a narrow therapeutic index, serum lithium levels should be determined frequently. Daily levels are not uncommon in some acute treatment units. Once the patient is stabilized, monthly serum level determinations are usually adequate. Blood levels are usually drawn before the first dose in the morning (usually 8 to 12 hours after the last dose). However, the nurse should not rely on laboratory tests alone and should continue clinical evaluation of the patient (see Box 13-6).

**Interactions.** The nurse should help the patient understand the basic mechanisms affecting serum lithium levels. Drug interactions that increase or decrease serum levels should be reviewed. The nurse must impress upon all patients the necessity for alerting all other health care providers to their lithium treatment, even though some persons may be reluctant to do so.

**Patient teaching.** The nurse should teach the patient and his family the following:

- The symptoms of minor toxicity, which include vomiting, diarrhea, drowsiness, muscular weakness, and lack of coordination

**Box 13-6**
## NURSING INTERVENTIONS FOR PATIENTS TAKING LITHIUM

- Prepare the patient for expected side effects in a non-anxious manner.
- Discuss which side effects should subside (nausea, dry mouth, diarrhea, thirst, mild hand tremor, weight gain, bloatedness, insomnia, lightheadedness).
- Identify the side effects that require immediate notification of the physician (e.g., vomiting, severe tremor, sedation, muscle weakness, vertigo).
- Suggest taking lithium with meals to reduce nausea.
- Suggest drinking 10 to 12 8 oz (240 ml) glasses of water per day to reduce thirst and maintain normal fluid balance.
- Advise patient to elevate feet to relieve ankle edema.
- Advise patient to maintain a consistent dietary sodium intake but to increase sodium if there is a major increase in perspiration.

- The symptoms of major toxicity, which include giddiness, tinnitus, blurred vision, and dilute urine
- The side effects associated with lithium and when to notify the physician
- To avoid conception since lithium may harm the fetus
- To avoid driving until the patient is stablized on the lithium

See Box 13-7 for Patient Guidelines for Taking Lithium (Keltner and Huff, in press).

### CARBAMAZEPINE

Carbamazepine (Tegretol) is an alternative treatment for manic episodes if lithium is ineffective or is contraindicated, for example, because of pregnancy. Although it is an effective anticonvulsant, it is chemically related to the tricyclic antidepressants. Patients with rapidly cycling manic depressive episodes may respond to carbamazepine. Carbamazepine may at times be given in combination with lithium.

### KEY CONCEPTS

1. According to the neurochemical theory, depression is a result of a decreased availability of norepinephrine, serotonin, and possibly dopamine in the brain.
2. There are two major classes of antidepressants: (a) tricyclic antidepressants (TCAs) and (b) monoamine oxidase inhibitors (MAOIs).
3. TCAs block the reuptake of these neurotransmitters back into the nerve ending, thereby increasing their availability.
4. MAOIs slow the breakdown of these neurotransmitters by inhibiting the enzyme

**Box 13-7**

## PATIENT GUIDELINES FOR TAKING LITHIUM

To achieve a therapeutic effect and prevent lithium toxicity, patients taking lithium should be advised of the following:

1. Lithium must be taken on a regular basis, preferably at the same time daily. If a patient is taking lithium, for example, on a three-times-daily schedule, and forgets a dose, he should wait until the next scheduled time to take the lithium but should not take twice the amount at that time, since lithium toxicity could occur.
2. When lithium treatment is initiated, mild side effects, such as a fine hand tremor, increased thirst and urination, nausea, anorexia, and diarrhea or constipation, may develop. Most of the mild side effects are transient and do not represent lithium toxicity. Also, in some patients taking lithium, some foods such as celery and butter fat will have an unappealing taste.
3. Serious side effects of lithium that will necessitate its discontinuance include vomiting, extreme hand tremor, sedation, muscle weakness, and vertigo. The prescribing physician should be notified immediately if any of these occur.
4. Lithium and sodium compete for elimination from the body through the kidneys. An increase in salt intake will increase lithium elimination, and a decrease in salt intake will decrease lithium elimination. Thus it is important that the patient maintain a balanced diet and salt intake. If the patient wishes to alter his diet, he should first consult with the prescribing physician.
5. Various situations can require an adjustment in the amount of lithium administered to a patient, for example, the addition of a new medication to the patient's drug regimen, a new diet, or an illness with fever or excessive sweating.
6. Blood for determination of lithium levels should be drawn in the morning approximately 8 to 14 hours after the last dose was taken.

monoamine oxidase, thereby increasing the availability of these neurotransmitters.

5. Common side effects of TCAs are associated with their anticholinergic properties (dry mouth, blurred vision, constipation, tachycardia).
6. Since TCAs have a narrow therapeutic index, amounts not much greater than therapeutic dosages can be fatal (10 to 30 times the daily dose can be fatal) and TCA overdoses account for 25% to 50% of all hospital admissions for overdoses.

7. Patients should be taught about the "lag time" of 2 to 4 weeks that it takes for a full therapeutic effect to be experienced with TCAs.
8. MAOIs can cause central (stimulation), cardiovascular (hypotension), and anticholinergic side effects.
9. MAOIs interact with several tyramine-containing foods (aged cheese, bananas, salami, etc) and indirect and mixed-acting sympathomimetic drugs (amphetamines, methylphenidate [Ritalin]) to cause hypertensive crisis.
10. MAOIs have a lag time of 10 days to 4 weeks.
11. Lithium is the drug of choice for the manic phase of bipolar illness.
12. Clinically therapeutic serum levels are 0.6 mmol/L to 1.2 mmol/L, but at higher serum levels serious to even fatal reactions occur.
13. Common side effects of lithium include nausea, dry mouth, diarrhea, thirst, and a fine hand tremor.
14. Lithium has a narrow therapeutic index and a lag time of 7 to 10 days.

**REFERENCES**

Brown RP and Mann JJ. A clinical perspective of the role of neurotransmitters in mental disorders, Hosp Community Psychiatry 36:141, 1985.

Cohen LS: Psychotropic drug use in pregnancy, Hosp Community Psychiatry 40:566, 1989.

Harsch HH and Holt RE: Use of antidepressants in attempted suicide, Hosp Community Psychiatry 39:990, 1988.

Keltner NL and Huff MR: A manic depressive mutual support group, Perspect Psychiatr Care (in press).

Knoben JE and Anderson PO: Handbook of clinical drug data, Hamilton, Ill., 1983, Drug Intelligence Publications, Inc.

Kuhn R: Treatment of depressive states with G22355 (imipramine hydrochloride), Am J Psychiatry 115:459, 1958.

Meador-Woodruff JH: Psychiatric side effects of tricyclic antidepressants, Hosp Community Psychiatry 41:84, 1990.

Monroe LR: New weapons in the assault on depression, Los Angeles Times, Jan. 2, 1990, p. E1, 4.

Sugarman JR: Management of lithium intoxication: Fam Pract 18:237, 1984.

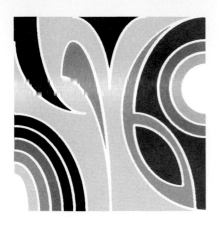

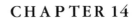

CHAPTER 14

# Antianxiety Drugs and Anticonvulsants

LEARNING OBJECTIVES

After reading this chapter you should be able to

- Describe differences among classes of antianxiety and anticonvulsant drugs.
- Discuss the side effects of antianxiety and anticonvulsant drugs.
- Identify therapeutic and toxic levels of the antianxiety and anticonvulsant drugs.
- Describe potential interactions of the antianxiety and anticonvulsant drugs.
- Discuss the implications for patient teaching for the antianxiety and anticonvulsant drugs.

**Box 14-1**
## ANTIANXIETY AGENTS

| **Benzodiazepines** | **Other antianxiety drugs** |
|---|---|
| Alprazolam (Xanax) | Buspirone (Buspar) |
| Chlordiazepoxide (Librium) | Propranolol (Inderal) |
| Clorazepate (Tranxene) | |
| Diazepam (Valium) | |
| Lorazepam (Ativan) | |
| Oxazepam (Serax) | |

## ■ Antianxiety Drugs

*Antianxiety agents,* sometimes referred to as *anxiolytics* and formerly called *minor tranquilizers,* are widely used by both psychiatric and general medicine patients (Box 14-1). They are used regularly by some persons with chronic anxiety and for time-limited periods by persons going through crisis. Antianxiety agents are commonly used to decrease presurgery "jitters." Recent evidence also suggests their effectiveness as antipanic agents (Lydiard et al., 1988). These drugs are used to treat anxiety, a subjective experience that can be objectively assessed. The anxious person feels excessively alert, is easily startled, moves constantly and is restless, talks too much, visually scans his environment, has tremors, and may have dilated pupils. The benzodiazepines are the drugs used most often to treat anxiety (Lydiard et al., 1988). However, they should not usually be taken for the stresses of everyday living. They have no therapeutic value in the treatment of psychosis but may be effective in treating the anxiety that is often associated with neuroleptic dose reduction (Garcia et al., 1990).

### Pharmacological effect (desired effect)

Antianxiety agents depress the reticular activating system of the central nervous system (CNS). Because the reticular activating system is depressed, incoming stimuli are muted and produce less reaction. This effect is probably achieved by the potentiation of gamma-aminobutyric acid (GABA), an inhibitory neurotransmitter. Hyperalertness and environmental scanning are defensive reactions. As the antianxiety agent "decreases" environmental input, there is a general relaxing of the guardedness of the anxious posture. The drugs can cause several levels of CNS depression, progressing from sedation to anesthesia. Antianxiety drugs do this by sedating the patient and depressing the inhibitory neurons affecting arousal. The latter effect causes a state of disinhibition or loosening of inner impediments to conduct. Disinhibition results in feelings of euphoria and excitement, which can result in poor

**TABLE 14-1**　Antianxiety agents: adult dosage, speed of onset, half-life, and elderly dosage

| Drug | Adult dosage range (mg/d) | Speed of onset (p.o) | Elimination half-life (h) | Elderly dosage (mg) |
|---|---|---|---|---|
| Alprazolam (Xanax) | 0.75-4 | Intermediate | 12-16 | 0.25 b.i.d. or t.i.d. |
| Chlordiazepoxide (Librium) | 15-100 | Intermediate | 5-30 | 5 b.i.d. to q.i.d. |
| Clorazepate (Tranxene) | 15-60 | Fast | 30-100 | 7.5-15 in 2 doses |
| Diazepam (Valium) | 4-40 | Very fast | 20-80 | 2-2.5 q.d. or b.i.d. |
| Lorazepam (Ativan) | 2-4 | Intermediate | 10-20 | 1-2 in divided doses |
| Oxazepam (Serax) | 30-120 | Intermediate to slow | 5-20 | 10 t.i.d. |
| Buspirone (Buspar) | 20-30 | Intermediate | 2-8 | Up to 15 q.d. |

Adapted from Olin BR: Drug facts and comparisons, St Louis, 1990, JB Lippincott, p 261A.

judgment because natural restraints are depressed. Because of these "desired effects" antianxiety drugs have become drugs of abuse (Schedule IV; see Appendix J). Benzodiazepines account for approximately 15% of all prescriptions, and, in one study of 1200 medical patients, 82% of psychotropic drugs ordered were benzodiazepines (Smith et al., 1986).

### Absorption, distribution, administration

The benzodiazepines are metabolized by the liver and excreted in the urine. The active metabolites can exert an effect for up to 10 days. Onset of effect is usually relatively fast; diazepam (Valium) is effective within 1 hour. Drugs that interfere with liver metabolism (e.g., alcohol) dangerously compound the effect of benzodiazepines. Benzodiazepines can be given orally and parenterally. Parenteral diazepam is the drug of choice for controlling status epilepticus. Table 14-1 presents the usual adult dosage information, speed of onset after oral administration, elimination half-life, and typical dosage for elderly persons.

### Side effects (undesired effects)

Commonly, CNS side effects are manifested. CNS effects include drowsiness, fatigue, and ataxia. A certain mental impairment and slowing of reflexes also occur. Less frequently confusion, depression, and headache may be present. PNS effects include occasional constipation, double vision, hypotension, incontinence, and urinary retention. Benzodiazepines can exacerbate narrow-angle glaucoma.

Beyond these undesired effects are the triple problems of dependence, withdrawal, and tolerance (needing more drug to achieve the same result) (Beeber, 1989). Dependence can be defined as a state in which the body functions "normally" when a drug is present. The body, in turn, functions "abnormally" when the drug is not present. When the drug is withdrawn from the benzodiazepine-dependent person, he experiences such symptoms as agitation, tremor, irritability, insomnia, vomiting, sweating, and even convulsions. Abrupt withdrawal from benzodiazepines can have serious effects, i.e. convulsions; thus gradual tapering in dosage is important. Withdrawal probably creates a situation in which the function of the GABA-binding sites is compromised, thus reducing GABA-induced inhibition (Rapport and Covington, 1989). Tolerance to side effects develops quickly. Older persons with impaired liver or renal function and debilitated persons experience more side effects and should consequently receive less of the drug (see Table 14-1).

## Interactions

The benzodiazepines, CNS depressants, interact *additively* with other CNS depressants. Alcohol, TCAs, MAOIs, opiates, antipsychotics, and antihistamines increase the sedative effects of benzodiazepines.

## Nursing implications

**Therapeutic vs toxic drug levels.** The benzodiazepines taken alone are relatively safe drugs. Overdoses hundreds of times higher than a therapeutic dose have been reported without death resulting. However, if benzodiazepines are combined with other drugs, such as alcohol, effects can easily be fatal. Signs and symptoms of overdose include somnolence, confusion, coma, diminished reflexes, and hypotension. Effective treatment begins with emptying the stomach by induced vomiting and gastric lavage followed by activated charcoal. The nurse should monitor blood pressure, pulse, and respirations and provide supportive care as indicated. Hypotension can be combined with a potent sympathomimetic amine such as metaraminol (Aramine).

**Use in pregnancy.** The association of benzodiazepine use and fetal abnormalities is not supported in recent studies (Cohen, 1989). However, if the drug cannot be discontinued without exacerbation of symptoms, tapering to the lowest possible dose is desirable, even before conception.

**Side effects.** The most common side effects are related to mental alertness. The patient should be cautioned about driving or operating hazardous machinery. Tolerance to most side effects quickly develops. Blood pressure of inpatients should be monitored routinely, and a drop of 20 mm Hg (systolic) on standing warrants withholding the drug and notifying the physician. Other side effects and nursing interventions are listed in Box 14-2.

The nurse should evaluate for therapeutic response. The evaluation should include anxiety level, sleep patterns, mental alertness, drowsiness, and physical dependency.

**Interactions.** The benzodiazepines interact with a number of CNS depressants. The nurse should explain this carefully to the patient who is taking benzodiazepines.

**Box 14-2**

## SIDE EFFECTS AND NURSING INTERVENTIONS FOR BENZODIAZEPINES

- Dry mouth: Advise rinsing mouth with water often, eating sugarless hard candies and chewing sugarless gum.
- Ataxia: Provide assistance with ambulation.
- Dizziness, drowsiness: Assist with ambulation and with getting in and out of bed. Caution about driving.

Since a high percentage of psychiatric patients abuse drugs (Carey, 1989), the potential for deadly combinations is real. It is also probable that these persons will develop a cross-tolerance to hepatic metabolized drugs. For instance, persons who develop a tolerance to alcohol will have an increased tolerance to diazepam but not when alcohol and diazepam are taken together. It is not uncommon to hear the "experienced diazepam taker" speak with disdain about typical dosages; for example, "10 mg of Valium doesn't even touch me!" The nurse should remind these patients that if they mix diazepam with alcohol they could die.

**Patient teaching.** Benzodiazepines have tremendous potential for abuse. Consequently, it is important to teach the patient and his family something about these drugs. The nurse should instruct the patient and the family as follows:

- Benzodiazepines are not for the minor stresses of everyday life.
- Over-the-counter drugs may potentiate the actions of benzodiazepines.
- Driving should be avoided until tolerance develops.
- Alcohol and other CNS depressants do not mix with the benzodiazepines.
- Hypersensitivity to one benzodiazepine may mean hypersensitivity to another.
- These drugs should not be stopped abruptly.

### THE BENZODIAZEPINES

**Diazepam.** Diazepam (Valium) is an often prescribed antianxiety agent. It has multiple uses related to its CNS-depressing effect. Besides anxiety disorders and short-term relief of symptoms of anxiety, diazepam is used preoperatively to relieve presurgery "jitters," for skeletal muscle spasms (e.g., lower back pain), as the drug of choice for status epilepticus, and as an adjunct for endoscopic procedures. In addition, diazepam may be useful for symptomatic relief of alcohol withdrawal.

**Alprazolam.** Alprazolam (Xanax) is particularly useful for anxiety associated with depression. It is being studied clinically for use in a variety of conditions, including depression, marked agitation associated with severe depression and panic attacks.

**Chlordiazepoxide.** Chlordiazepoxide (Librium) is prescribed for anxiety disorders, for the relief of the symptoms of anxiety, and for acute alcohol withdrawal. It is absorbed well orally.

**Clorazepate.** Clorazepate (Tranxene) is used to treat anxiety, acute alcohol withdrawal, and adjunctively in the treatment of partial seizures.

**Lorazepam.** Lorazepam (Ativan) is used to treat anxiety disorders. It is available for oral and parenteral administration. The metabolites of lorazepam are inactive, so the effects of this drug do not persist. Patients with impaired liver function can handle this drug better than they can other benzodiazepines. There is some evidence that lorazepam impairs learning.

**Oxazepam.** Oxazepam (Serax) is similar to lorazepam in that its metabolite is inactive. Thus the drug is effective for a relatively short time (24 hours) and is suitable for persons with liver disorders or for the elderly.

## OTHER ANTIANXIETY AGENTS

**Buspirone.** Buspirone (Buspar) is not a benzodiazepine. There is considerable interest in this drug because no cross tolerance with sedatives or alcohol has been demonstrated and because there is no evidence that it creates dependence (i.e., causes withdrawal symptoms). It does not depress the CNS. It is purported to have no abuse potential and is not a controlled substance. Buspirone must be administered for 1 to 2 weeks before a significant effect occurs. It has a half-life of 2 to 8 hours, so it is usually given three times a day (Lydiard et al., 1988). Side effects include dizziness, nausea, headache, nervousness, lightheadedness, and excitement.

**Propranolol.** Propranolol (Inderal) is a β-blocker that effectively interrupts the physiological responses of anxiety. It is less effective than the benzodiazepines but is relatively safe and has little abuse potential. Most side effects are transient and mild. However, bradycardia, lightheadedness, and heart block can occur.

**Tricyclic antidepressants.** Imipramine (Tofranil) in doses over 150 mg per day has proven to be effective for panic anxiety attacks (Beeber, 1989). Desipramine at higher doses and for longer trial periods has also proven effective. Clomipramine (Anafranil), a relatively new TCA, has been found effective in the treatment of obsessive-compulsive disorders. Treatment starts at 25 mg per day and may gradually be increased to a maximum of 250 mg per day.

# ■ Anticonvulsants

Anticonvulsants are used in the treatment of seizure disorders (Box 14-3), of which epilepsy is the most common. Seizure disorders are not uncommon among psychiatric patients; nor is it unusual for seizures to occur on a psychiatric unit. McKenna et al. (1985) report that 7% of patients with epilepsy have persistent psychosis. Although many clinicians may disagree with this finding, anticonvulsants merit brief mention in a psychiatric nursing textbook. The student should note that there are many variants of epilepsy and that each has its own treatment approach. A discussion of epilepsy is beyond the scope of this book, and only drugs used in the treatment of tonic-clonic seizures (grand mal), psychomotor seizures, and status epilepticus

---

**Box 14-3**
SELECTED ANTICONVULSANTS

- Hydantoins: phenytoin (Dilantin)
- Long-acting barbiturates: phenobarbital (Luminal)
- Benzodiazepines: diazepam (Valium)

---

(successive grand mal seizures without interruption, a life-threatening phenomenon) will be discussed.

Anticonvulsants suppress the start of seizures (abnormal brain electrical activity) or reduce the spread of seizures to other areas of the brain. The four major chemical classes of anticonvulsants are the hydantoins, long-acting barbiturates, succinimides, and benzodiazepines. There are other anticonvulsants that do not fit into these chemical classes. The hydantoins and long-acting barbiturates are used in the treatment of tonic-clonic seizures, and diazepam, a benzodiazepine, is the drug of choice for status epilepticus. Since succinimides are used primarily for absence (petit mal) seizures, they will not be discussed in this book. One drug from the hydantoin group and one from the long-acting barbiturates will be discussed, as well as diazepam. For a more comprehensive treatment of this complex subject the reader is directed to a pharmacology textbook.

## HYDANTOIN ANTICONVULSANTS

Phenytoin (Dilantin) is the most widely used hydantoin. It is used in the treatment of both tonic-clonic and complex partial seizures. In addition, if diazepam is not available, phenytoin is a second-choice drug for status epilepticus.

### Pharmacological effect (desired effect)

Phenytoin inhibits the spread of abnormal brain electrical activity by normalizing abnormal fluxes of sodium across the nerve cell membrane during or after depolarization, which stabilizes a state of hyperexcitability.

### Absorption, distribution, administration

Phenytoin is absorbed from the gut after oral administration. Peak serum levels are reached within 2 hours (with promptly absorbed form). The therapeutic serum level is 10 to 20 µg/ml. The average half-life is 22 hours, so 4 to 7 days of drug use is required before a steady-state blood level is reached. Parenteral administration poses absorption problems. Phenytoin given intramuscularly is poorly and inconsistently absorbed, necessitating a 50% increase in the dosage to achieve comparable serum levels when changing from an oral form. Obviously, when a change from the

**TABLE 14-2** Anticonvulsants

| Drug | Therapeutic serum levels (µg/ml) | Toxic serum levels (µg/ml) | Usual dosage | Seizure type |
|------|----------------------------------|----------------------------|--------------|--------------|
| Phenytoin (Dilantin) | 10-20 | >20 | Adults: 100-200 mg t.i.d. or q.i.d. p.o. | Grand mal, psychomotor |
| Phenobarbitol (Luminal) | 10-30 | >40 | Adults: 50-100 mg b.i.d. or t.i.d. p.o. | Grand mal, psychomotor |
| Diazepam (Valium) | | | Adults: 5-10 mg IM or IV (preferred); repeat every 10-15 min, if needed, up to a total dose of 30 mg given as slow injection | Status epilepti-cus |

intramuscular to the oral form is made, the dosage must be reduced by the same margin (Table 14-2).

Phenytoin is metabolized in the liver and excreted in the urine. The nurse should not substitute one "brand" of phenytoin for another because phenytoin preparations from different manufacturers can vary by 10% to 90% in their bio-availability.

### Side effects (undesired effects)

Side effects to phenytoin usually involve the CNS. Sluggishness, ataxia, nystagmus, confusion, and slurred speech are relatively common. Less common effects are dizziness, insomnia, nervousness, and fatigue. Gastrointestinal responses, such as nausea, vomiting, and constipation, occur in many patients. Persons who practice poor oral hygiene are subject to gingival hyperplasia. Often oral surgery is required to cut back the excessive tissue and to reestablish a normal gum line. Blood dyscrasias, such as suppression of the immune system, thrombocytopenia, and anemia, are adverse reactions.

Effects that may be particularly troublesome to women include excessive growth of body hair, enlargement of the lips, and acne. Osteomalacia caused or aggravated by phenytoin's interference with vitamin D metabolism can lead to chronic and debilitating skeletal problems. Phenytoin can cause birth defects (cleft lip, cleft palate), so its use during pregnancy must be weighed against the risk of fetal damage.

### Interactions

Many drugs will increase or decrease phenytoin serum levels, and phenytoin will compromise or compound the effects of many drugs.

*Drugs that increase serum phenytoin levels* typically do so by inhibiting phenytoin metabolism or by displacing phenytoin from plasma protein. They include alcohol (acute ingestion only), allopurinol, aspirin, chlorpromazine and most other antipsychotics, dicumarol, diazepam, disulfiram, and methylphenidate.

Drugs that decrease serum phenytoin levels do so typically by stimulating phenytoin metabolism or by inhibiting absorption. They include chronic alcohol use (causing the liver to speed up metabolism), antacids, folic acid, and some CNS depressants.

Phenytoin increases the effects of oral anticoagulants, antihypertensives, propranolol, and thyroid hormone. Phenytoin inhibits the effects of corticosteroids, dicumarol, oral contraceptives, quinidine, and vitamin D because it enhances the rate of their metabolism in the liver.

## LONG-ACTING BARBITURATES

Phenobarbital (Luminal) is the prototype barbiturate used as an anticonvulsant. Mephobarbital (Mebaral), metharbital (Gemonil), and primidone (Mysoline) are related barbiturates. Their only approved long-term use is as anticonvulsants.

### Pharmacological effects (desired effects)

Phenobarbital has traditionally served as a sedative. At lower doses it has proved to be effective as an anticonvulsant. Phenobarbital alters neuron physiology and inhibits nerve transmission to the cerebral cortex. Like other anticonvulsants, phenobarbital suppresses the start and spread of seizure stimuli in the brain.

### Absorption, distribution, administration

Phenobarbital is usually given orally. The therapeutic serum level is between 10 and 30 µg/ml and can be achieved with normal adult dosage. The steady state is reached within 16 to 21 days, with an average half-life of 80 hours. The half-life is reduced over time because phenobarbital speeds its own metabolism in the liver. It is excreted by the kidneys. Parenteral (intravenous) phenobarbital is used to treat status epilepticus and other serious seizure forms when diazepam (Valium) is not effective or is not available.

### Side effects (undesired effects)

Common side effects of phenobarbital include sedation, general CNS depression, nausea and vomiting, and stimulation of vitamin D metabolism (leading to vitamin D deficiency and osteomalacia). Hypoventilation and bradycardia can also occur. Phenobarbital should be used with caution in persons with hepatic damage or nephritis.

### Interactions

Drugs that depress the CNS are the chief interactants with phenobarbital. Since many CNS depressants (including the barbiturates) stimulate hepatic drug-metabolizing enzymes, a quickening of the metabolic process occurs. However, faster metabolism occurs only when the drug is given alone. When two CNS depressants are combined (e.g., phenobarbital and alcohol), one is metabolized more quickly and the other is metabolized much more slowly. The slowly metabolized drug accounts for severe CNS depression.

Phenobarbital combined with furosemide (Lasix) can cause severe orthostatic hypotension.

## BENZODIAZEPINE ANTICONVULSANTS

**Diazepam.** Diazepam (Valium) has already been discussed as an antianxiety agent. It is also the drug of choice for status epilepticus. It is effective about 95% of the time when used to stop this life-threatening seizure. A single parenteral dose of 5 to 10 mg will stop most seizures within 5 minutes. Nonetheless, seizures may return in 10 to 15 minutes, at which time diazepam may be repeated or, as is more commonly the case, phenytoin is given parenterally. Side effects and drug interactions are described in the discussion of antianxiety drugs, pages 231 and 232.

### Nursing Implications

Specific nursing implications for diazepam are found in the discussion of antianxiety drugs, page 232.

#### Therapeutic vs toxic drug levels

*Phenytoin.* There is no universal antidote for anticonvulsants; nor is there a specific antidote for any one anticonvulsant. However, treatment for overdoses is similar. Anticonvulsant overdose is a medical emergency that requires knowledgeable treatment. A toxic effect of phenytoin occurs at serum levels above 20 $\mu$g/ml. Serum levels above 100 $\mu$g/ml are lethal. Toxicity causes nystagmus, ataxia, tremor, and slurred speech.

*Phenobarbital.* Serum phenobarbital levels over 40 $\mu$g/ml are toxic. A tolerance to many barbiturate effects develops with chronic use, but a tolerance to anticonvulsant effects does not develop. So, while an increased amount of barbiturate may be needed for sedation, an increase is not required for continued anticonvulsant activity. Tolerance does not develop to lethal levels either. At toxic levels respiratory and CNS depression, tachycardia, hypotension, hypothermia, and coma can occur. In cases of severe overdose, apnea, circulatory collapse, respiratory arrest, and death have been reported. Treatment for overdose consists of maintaining a patent airway and assistance with ventilation and oxygenation if needed. Gastric lavage can be used to empty the stomach. Monitoring of vital signs and fluid balance is important. If renal function remains normal, forced diuresis and alkalinizing the urine help eliminate the phenobarbital.

#### Use in pregnancy.
Both phenytoin and phenobarbital have been implicated in congenital defects. Their use must be carefully weighed against potential danger to the fetus.

#### Side effects

*Phenytoin.* Patients experiencing dizziness and ataxia should be instructed to rise slowly and should be cautioned against driving a car. Upset stomach and other gastrointestinal problems can be decreased by taking the drug with meals. The nurse should continually assess for blood dyscrasias. Fever, sore throat, general malaise, bleeding, bruising, and pallor may indicate a hematological problem.

*Phenobarbital.* The patient should be cautioned about operating hazardous machinery if he is experiencing drowsiness. The nurse should be aware of results of blood studies and liver function tests during treatment. She should evaluate mood, sensorium, and memory as well as respiratory depression to ascertain adverse reactions.

### Interactions

*Phenytoin.* The nurse must be aware of the potential for drug interactions and should provide a list of interactants and discuss them with the patient and his family.

*Phenobarbital.* Drugs that depress the CNS are the chief interactants with phenobarbital, so the patient who requires phenobarbital in conjunction with another CNS depressant should be carefully observed by physicians and nurses. The nurse should explain as clearly as possible to both the patient and his family the physiological rationale for avoiding the mixing of phenobarbital with alcohol, for example. The patient should be assessed continuously for CNS depression.

**Patient teaching.** The nurse should teach the patient and his family about all dimensions of drug use, including action, dose, route, and when to notify the physician. Specifically, the patient should be instructed to do the following:

- Report side effects and adverse reactions.
- Avoid driving while sedated or drowsy.
- Practice good oral hygiene, particularly if taking phenytoin.
- Avoid interactants, particularly alcohol.

## KEY CONCEPTS

1. Antianxiety drugs (the benzodiazepines are by far the most common type) are used (a) to treat persons with chronic anxiety, (b) for time-limited periods in persons going through crisis, (c) for presurgery jitters, and (d) in the treatment of panic disorders.
2. Antianxiety drugs work by depressing the CNS, particularly the reticular activating system, thus muting incoming stimuli.
3. Antianxiety drugs, the most commonly prescribed class of psychotropic drug, have a high abuse potential and cause dependence (there is a withdrawal syndrome). Discontinuance should be gradual (tapered).
4. Side effects include drowsiness, fatigue, ataxia, and other peripheral and central effects; however, tolerance to side effects does occur.
5. Benzodiazepines are relatively safe drugs if taken alone, but they can be deadly if mixed with other CNS depressants (i.e., alcohol).
6. Anticonvulsants are used to treat seizure disorders by suppressing abnormal brain electrical activity or by reducing the spread of seizures to other areas of the brain.
7. There are four major classes of anticonvulsant: (a) hydantoins, (b) long-acting barbiturates, (c) benzodiazepines, and (d) succinimides, as well as other anticonvulsants that do not fit into these chemical classes. Only the first three classes are discussed in this chapter.

8. Phenytoin (Dilantin) is a commonly used *hydantoin* for the treatment of grand mal and psychomotor seizures. Side effects include sluggishness, ataxia, nystagmus, confusion, and slurred speech. The therapeutic serum level is 10 to 20 $\mu$g/ml and the half-life is 22 hours.

9. Phenobarbital (Luminal) is the prototype *long-acting barbiturate* and is used in the treatment of grand mal and psychomotor seizures. Side effects include sedation, general CNS depression, nausea and vomiting, and stimulation of vitamin D metabolism. The therapeutic serum level is 10 to 30 $\mu$g/ml and the average half-life is 80 hours.

10. Diazepam (Valium), a *benzodiazepine,* is the drug of choice in the treatment of status epilepticus.

## REFERENCES

Beeber LS: Treatment of anxiety, J Psychosoc Nurs 27:42, 1989.

Carey KB: Emerging treatment guidelines for mentally ill chemical abusers, Hosp Community Psychiatry 40:341, 349, 1989.

Cohen LS: Psychotropic drug use in pregnancy, Hosp Community Psychiatry 40:566, 1989.

Garcia RI et al: Use of lorazepam for increased anxiety after neuroleptic dose reduction, Hosp Community Psychiatry 41:197, 1990.

Lydiard RB, Roy-Byrne PP, and Ballinger JC: Recent advances in the psychopharmacological treatment of anxiety disorders. Hosp Community Psychiatry 39:1157, 1988.

McKenna PJ, Kane JM, and Parrish K: Psychotic syndromes in epilepsy, Am J Psychiatry 142:895, 1985.

Rapport DJ and Covington EC: Motor phenomena in benzodiazepine withdrawal, Hosp Community Psychiatry 40:1277, 1989.

Smith AR, et al: Trends in psychotropic prescribing practice and general medical patients, Postgrad Med J 62:637, 1986.

# Milieu Management

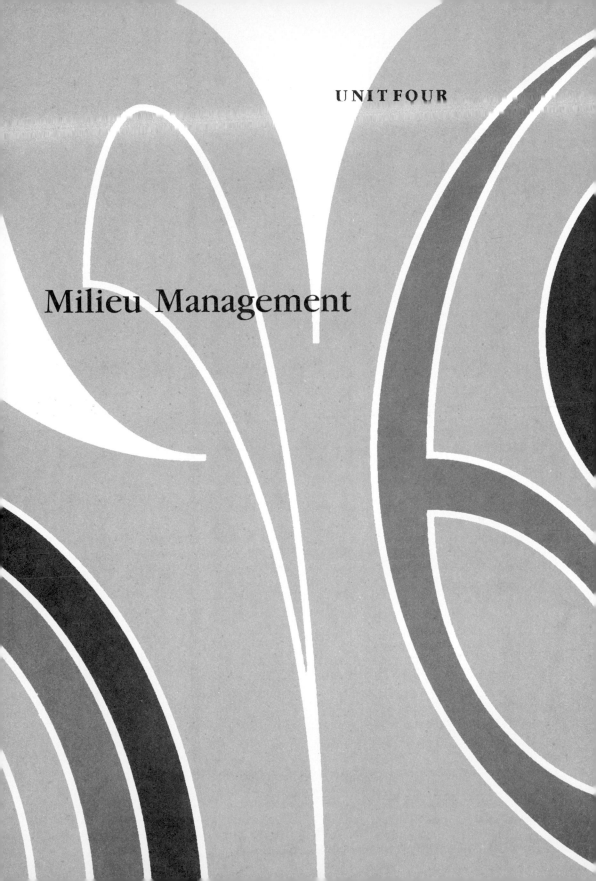

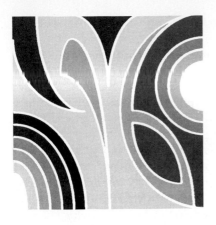

## CHAPTER 15

# Introduction to Milieu Management

LEARNING OBJECTIVES

After reading this chapter you should be able to

- Define and describe the therapeutic milieu.
- Describe the goal of milieu management in the care of psychiatric patients.
- Identify the elements of the therapeutic milieu.

The purpose of a psychiatric inpatient unit is to help patients recognize and recover from the psychiatric problems that led to their hospitalization. If an hour once or twice a week with an outpatient therapist is sufficient to accomplish those same goals, then financial considerations alone would dictate that outpatient care be used. For many persons hospitalization is preferable or required. These persons can best recover from their psychiatric problems when all aspects of the environment are focused on their recovery. In such an environment there is no "down time" or wasted time. All the resources of the environment are harnessed to provide optimal psychiatric care for the patient. The terms *therapeutic milieu* and *therapeutic environment* are used to describe such an atmosphere. Providing a therapeutic environment is a fundamental psychiatric nursing activity (Benfer, 1980; ANA, 1976).

Because nurses are the prime shapers and molders of the therapeutic environment, it is critical that they understand the importance of milieu management. They provide 24-hour, around-the-clock care in the inpatient setting. They are with the patient at all times. No other professionals spend nearly as many hours in contact with patients as nurses do. Nurses are the managers of the inpatient milieu.

To the degree that nursing staff members are trained and motivated to deliver care, the inpatient climate consistently reflects the unit's philosophy of care. Stated another way, the most promising psychiatric model of inpatient therapy cannot overcome a poorly trained and poorly motivated nursing staff. The nursing staff members are "representatives" of the unit's model of care, once the psychiatrist and the head nurse are off duty for the day (5 PM until 8 AM weekdays and weekends). In fact, the real test of the unit's philosophy does not occur during a 9 AM team meeting but at 11 PM when a single staff member interacts with a single patient. The term "representatives" is used advisedly, for in a well-functioning therapeutic environment the nurses are not really representatives at all. They are equal partners in the development and implementation of the philosophy of care. They *are* "the model of care." They are not behaving as a supervisor wants them to behave but are simply living out their professional commitment to treatment.

Wilmer (1981) labels environments in psychiatric facilities much like a journalist might label political groups. He refers to them as left, right, and center. He views the first two as distortions of what should be. Environments to the left are characterized by permissiveness and an antiprofessional stance. Unit staff members work too hard at identifying with their patients. Identification may take the form of using a lot of foul language, being "hip," males wearing long hair and earrings, and so on. Unit leaders have closed minds to new approaches, suggesting their approach is the only path to mental health. The right-leaning environments tend to follow one theoretical model blindly without flexibility, thus helping the staff gain comfort in their work environment. Wilmer's most interesting comment is that right-leaning milieus have staffs with high morale amid dismal results. The challenge for psychiatric nurses is to develop a balanced therapeutic environment.

The psychiatric environments in the center are characterized by their emphasis on the here and now and by their recognition of a need for flexibility.

## THERAPEUTIC MILIEU

Milieu management is the purposeful use of all interpersonal and environmental forces to enhance mental health. Talbot and Miller (1966) said: "An ideal psychiatric hospital is not merely a sanctuary, a cotton-padded milieu that emphasizes the fragility, the incompetence, the helplessness, the bizarreness of patients. It is a sane society when it permits the optimal use of the intact ego capacities through its social organization, its social supports, and its community values."

Traditionally, the hospital has been the only setting thought appropriate for milieu concerns. Today psychiatric nurses in other settings expend therapeutic energies in developing a "therapeutic environment." Historically, the term *therapeutic milieu* conveyed a broad conceptual approach in which all aspects of the environment were channeled to provide a therapeutic environment for the patient. "At its root is the idea that variables in the interaction between person and environment affect behavior" (Emrich, 1989). The milieu could be therapeutic in and of itself (e.g., "milieu therapy" [Jones, 1953]) and could be developed in many settings. The *therapeutic community,* on the other hand, was a concept restricted to the inpatient setting in which a patient-led government established and "enforced" community rules. Over the years the distinction between terms has all but disappeared, and they are now often used synonymously. *Milieu management* is a descriptive term that implies the need for purposeful activity by the nursing staff to develop a *therapeutic environment.*

Florence Nightingale was first to recognize nursing's responsibility for creating and controlling the patients' milieu (Emrich, 1989). Psychiatric nursing, in the inpatient setting, has 24-hour responsibility for patient care. No other discipline provides this on-site, around-the-clock care. Patients and nurses alike benefit from the recognition of the value of a therapeutic environment. Patients benefit because the use of *all* resources (interpersonal interactions, psychotropic drugs, and environment) helps staff members maintain a consistent focus on and involvement with the recipients of care, the patients. Nurses benefit because attention and value are brought to a dimension of psychiatric care that is decidedly nursing.

June Mellow (1986), an important figure in psychiatric nursing, has said about the milieu: "Certainly nurses, as the chief inhabitants of its terrain, have not emphasized enough its great therapeutic potential, perhaps because so much of the experiential medium is comprised of what are considered mundane activities associated with women's sphere of work—feeding, bathing, dressing, granting privileges, teaching, comforting, scolding, joking, socializing, counseling. Yet it is the often unstructured, unpredictable flow of these activities, compared with the more structured world of verbal therapy, that can be transposed and shaped into a therapeutic modality." As Kahn and White (1989) noted "[nursing] staff exert a powerful therapeutic effect through their moment-to-moment interactions with the patient." Mellow calls for nurses to recognize the significance of the environment they, and they alone, manage, the significance of milieu management.

## HISTORICAL OVERVIEW

Historically, custodial care was the norm in inpatient settings. Custodial care does not necessarily mean cruel care or neglected care. Custodial care refers to a mind-set in which the nurse's responsibilities are focused exclusively on safety and physical needs. Often even these basic goals were not reached. In "better" (usually private) institutions, custodial care took place 23 hours of the day, and then for one brief, precious hour the patient was ushered into the presence of the therapist. Less than 5% of the day was spent in a therapeutic situation. After World War II several individuals began to be concerned about this "waste." It began to be recognized that institutionalization was pathological in itself, causing apathy, lack of interest, and an unwillingness to leave. Stanton and Schwartz (1954) noted the discrepancy between "what could be and what was" in the hospital. They believed a better yield from hospitalization could be realized if therapeutic mileage could be gained from all dimensions of care. The most notable figure of this time was Maxwell Jones. Jones (1953) wrote a landmark book, *The Therapeutic Community: A New Treatment Method In Psychiatry,* in which he described the benefits of an environment that was therapeutic in and of itself. He proposed that patients become involved in decision making, that group meetings be held, that patients participate in planning ward events, and that patients practice self-regulation. As milieu therapy began to evolve, the therapeutic benefits of a multidisciplinary staff in the rehabilitation process became recognized (Gutheil, 1985). Nurses, in particular, assumed more "therapeutic territory" as their importance to the therapeutic environment became apparent. As nurses became full partners in the therapeutic efforts (in the early 1960s) they gave up their white uniforms (Pinsker and Vingiano, 1988). This bond of humanity described by Jones, that is, we are all just people who need to wear clothes, was mined for its therapeutic value.

Just as the therapeutic environment was being seriously considered as a legitimate psychiatric modality, other forces converged to direct energies away from milieu therapy. Psychopharmacology, concern for patients' rights, and reactions to institutional care culminated in the community mental health movement. These forces worked against a basic underpinning of milieu therapy—hospital care for the patient. As Gutheil (1985) pointed out, proponents of psychopharmacology viewed hospitalization as a time when patients could be "held still" long enough to be stabilized on medication. If anything beyond stabilization took place, "well and good," but it was not necessary. Community mental health advocates viewed the inpatient staff as psychiatric evangelists in business to "convert" inpatients to outpatients as fast as possible. The pendulum is swinging back. Hospitalization and particularly the effective use of the milieu (therapeutic environment) are being looked at closely again.

## GOAL OF MILIEU MANAGEMENT

The goal of milieu management is to organize all interpersonal and environmental forces to develop an atmosphere that facilitates patient growth, rehabilitation, and restoration. Major responsibility for overall direction belongs to the head nurse and the head of psychiatry. Ultimately, however, the effectiveness of milieu therapy can be judged by its effectiveness during times other than Monday through Friday, "9 to 5." All nursing staff members are responsible for understanding and maintaining the therapeutic environment.

Nurses must be active in the therapeutic environment. Patients will be no more active than the nurses (Kahn and White, 1989). Nurses must be available to patients. They must be flexible and willing to help patients develop problem-solving skills and coping mechanisms to deal with problems (Leibenluft and Goldberg, 1987). Gunderson (1978) identified three essential features of the therapeutic environment:

1. Distribution of responsibility and decision making
2. High levels of interaction between patients and staff
3. Clarity of the role and leadership of the program

Milieu management achieves these characteristics by establishing community meetings, activity groups, social skills groups, physical exercise programs, psychoeducational programs, transition groups, and work programs. In addition, the therapeutic community is enhanced by staff groups in which milieu status is reviewed and ongoing training occurs.

## ELEMENTS OF THE EFFECTIVE MILIEU

For the milieu to be effectively managed, five environmental elements must be present: unit structure, unit norms, limit setting, balance, and unit modification.

*Unit structure* can be identified as the physical environment, the unit regulations, and the daily schedule of classes and groups (Emrich, 1989). It is provided by establishing community meetings, activity groups, social skills groups, physical exercise programs, psychoeducational programs, transition groups, and work programs. Groups, both formal and informal, in which patients share problems and triumphs are also part of the therapeutic environment. Structure also denotes the design of the unit. Space, areas for socializing, and areas for privacy are required. Telephones must be available and visiting rooms appropriate. Since seclusion rooms are often necessary, their design, location, and furnishings must maintain both safety and dignity. Furnishings, the color of the walls, and so on all communicate something to patients and staff. While reviewing "structure" in Chapter 16, the reader should ask the question: "What is it about a given dimension of unit structure that makes it therapeutic?"

*Unit norms* are those aspects of a unit that pervade the setting. For instance, violent behavior might be expected on one unit, but on another unit it is not. Norms of nonviolence, physical and emotional security, personal control (e.g., taking or not taking a psychotropic drug may not be negotiable, but the dosage schedule may be), openness, giving and receiving feedback, respect for the patient, privacy, acceptance, independence, and individual responsibility build a climate of universality or shared experience.

*Limit setting* is important on the unit and is related to unit norms. Limits should be set on acting-out behavior, such as self-destructive acts, physical aggressiveness, lack of compliance, use of alcohol or illicit drugs, use of over-the-counter drugs, and elopement. If patients are likely to engage in any of these behaviors, it is important to discuss them in an anticipatory fashion rather than to wait until after the fact (Leibenluft and Goldberg, 1987).

*Balance* is also an important concept, but it is more difficult to describe and does not lend itself to a concrete list of do's and don'ts. Balance is the process of gradually allowing independent behaviors in a dependent environment. Independence is gained gradually because too much independence may overwhelm the patient. An example or two will best illustrate this point. In the case of the self-destructive patient the nurse attempts to balance the patient's (and the nurse's) need for safety (a dependency-creating approach) with the patient's need for control over his life or independence (Assay, 1985). A seemingly different example is the patient who is very religious. The nurse may have to balance the patient's right to religious expression with the patient's need for treatment. A not uncommon situation occurs when a patient refuses medication on religious grounds, even though he is frankly psychotic. Is this refusal a true representation of religious beliefs, or is it a psychotic manifestation?

Balance is an important concept because it forces the nurse to articulate what opposing forces are at work. The skillful use of balance comes with understanding of ethical concerns, legal issues, and psychopathology.

Through *unit modification* the nurse can facilitate the development of a therapeutic environment and communicate patient worth. Physical arrangement, safety issues, and orientation features, when addressed, can create an atmosphere in which patients are enabled to maximize their strengths.

Together, unit structure, unit norms, limit setting, balance, and unit modification are tools the psychiatric nurse uses to manage the milieu. In an environment where all resources are used, every verbal interaction becomes significant because it is part of a larger process developed to facilitate mental health and personal growth. Each individual reaction is important but finds even greater meaning within the construct of psychotherapeutic management in the well-managed milieu.

## ROLES OF PSYCHOTHERAPEUTIC MANAGER

In managing the milieu, nurses serve in multiple roles. They work with patients individually, lead groups, participate in community meetings, coordinate medical care (with physicians), dispense routine medications and make decisions concerning p.r.n. medications, make discharge arrangements, and work with families. In addition, they provide leadership in interdisciplinary team meetings and are the professionals who most often implement team decisions (Keltner, 1985).

## KEY CONCEPTS

1. Milieu management is the purposeful use of all interpersonal and environmental forces to enhance the mental health of psychiatric patients through the development of a therapeutic environment.
2. Since nursing, in the inpatient setting, has 24-hour accountability for patient care, nurses have the major responsibility for molding the therapeutic environment.
3. Historically, nurses provided only custodial care, but after World War II Maxwell Jones (1953) and others conceptualized an environment in which all aspects of the psychiatric patient's day would be used to promote mental health.
4. Nurses and nursing gained more influence over the patient's care as the result of this emphasis. However, just as milieu therapy was gaining acceptance as a viable treatment form, other forces converged and changed the locus of psychiatric treatment from a therapeutic inpatient setting to a community mental health setting.
5. Today, hospitalization and the effective use of milieu management are being reconsidered as psychiatric nursing leaders look for more effective ways to treat persons with mental disorders.
6. The goal of milieu management is to organize all interpersonal and environmental forces so as to develop an atmosphere that is conducive to patient growth, rehabilitation, and restoration.
7. Three essential features of the therapeutic environment are (a) distribution of responsibility and decision making, (b) high levels of interaction between patients and staff, and (c) clarity of the role and leadership of the program (Gunderson, 1978).
8. The effectively managed milieu is composed of five elements: (a) unit structure, (b) unit norms, (c) limit setting (d) balance, and (e) unit modification.

### REFERENCES

American Nurses' Association, Division of Psychiatric and Mental Health Nursing Practice: Statement on psychiatric and mental health nursing practice, Kansas City, 1976, The Association.

Assey JL: The suicide prevention contract, Perspect Psychiatr Care 23:99, 1985.

Benfer B: Defining the role and function of the psychiatric nurse as a member of the team, Perspect Psychiatr Care 18:166, 1980.

Emrich K: Helping or hurting? Interacting in the psychiatric milieu, J Psychosoc Nurs 27:26, 1989.

Gunderson JG: Defining the therapeutic processes in psychiatric milieus, Psychiatry 41: 327, 1978.

Gutheil T: The therapeutic milieu: changing themes and theories, Hosp Community Psychiatry 36: 1279, 1985.

Jones M: The therapeutic community: a new approach in psychiatry, New York, 1953, Basic Books.

Kahn EM and White EM: Adapting milieu approaches to acute inpatient care for schizophrenia patients, Hosp Community Psychiatry 40:609, 1989.

Keltner NL: Psychotherapeutic management: a model for nursing practice, Perspect Psychiatr Care 23:125, 1985.

Leibenluft E and Goldberg RL: Guidelines for short-term inpatient psychotherapy, Hosp Community Psychiatry 38:38, 1987.

Mellow J: A personal perspective of nursing therapy, Hosp Community Psychiatry 37:182, 1986.

Pinsker H and Vingiano W: A study of whether uniforms help patients recognize nurses, Hosp Community Psychiatry 39:78, 1988.

Stanton A and Schwartz M: The mental hospital, New York, 1954, Basic Books.

Talbot E and Miller SC: The struggle to create a sane society in the psychiatric hospital, Psychiatry 29:165, 1966.

Wilmer HA: Defining and understanding the therapeutic community, Hosp Community Psychiatry 32:95, 1981.

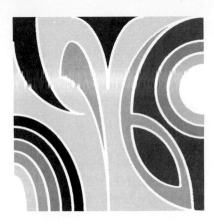

## CHAPTER 16

# Developing the Therapeutic Environment

LEARNING OBJECTIVES

After reading this chapter you should be able to

- Understand the implications for JCAH guidelines for a therapeutic environment.
- Describe the various approaches to developing unit structure.
- Describe the various dimensions of unit norms.
- Describe common themes on psychiatric units involving limit setting.
- Understand the competing issues involved in balance.
- Identify important measures in unit modification.

Nursing has the unique expertise required to develop the therapeutic environment and is in an advantageous position to influence the patient's environment. "The interpersonal environment in which a patient lives may be therapeutic or non-therapeutic depending almost entirely on the interest and ability of the [nursing] staff" (Kyes and Hofling, 1974). Since patients are incapable of not interacting with their environment, the nurse has the potential to shape the environment to cause that "inevitable interaction" to be therapeutic.

In Chapter 15 milieu building was presented as a process of establishing unit structure, unit norms, limit setting, balance, and unit modification. These, in turn, are derived from unit philosophy and objectives. Those concepts will be developed in this chapter. First, however, a review of the Joint Commission on Accreditation of Hospitals (JCAH) criteria for a therapeutic environment is presented. JCAH has developed a comprehensive list of environmental requirements that serve as a guide to psychiatric nurses. The extensiveness of the JCAH criteria underscores the importance of milieu management (Box 16-1).

Superimposed on these basic environmental considerations are the establishment of structure, unit norms, limit setting, balance, and unit modification.

## UNIT STRUCTURE

Unit structure is the framework around which the therapeutic community, therapeutic milieu, or therapeutic environment revolves and takes direction. The goal is not to make a perfect environment but to develop a nurturing setting that can contain and soothe aggression, frustration, deprivation, disappointment, and loss (Kahn and White, 1989). If all resources in the patient's environment are to be used for achieving this goal, a strategy or structure must be developed to use those resources therapeutically. To enhance the therapeutic environment and add structure and direction to the treatment program, the psychiatric nurse and other treatment team members may add community meetings, activity groups, social skills groups, physical exercise programs, psychoeducational programs for patients and families, transition groups, and work groups.

**Community meetings.** The community meeting is a common group found on units with a therapeutic environment. The community is a large group, typically consisting of all patients in the treatment setting, staff, and students. It incorporates both small-group dynamics and large-group characteristics. The community meeting can be run by a staff of patient officers (patient government) or by the treatment staff. During community meetings new patients are welcomed, unit rules are reviewed, patient government leaders (if appropriate) are identified, staff members are identified, and general announcements about the day's activities are made. For newly admitted, disturbed persons, this businesslike atmosphere can seem threatening; for example, "these people act like 'business as usual' and my life is coming apart. This is crazy!" But the dominant opposite theme has more lasting impact; for example, "people with problems are not acting 'crazy.' They are influencing the treatment setting. They are acting rational." The latter message comforts and encourages on several levels and communicates the ability to get on with the business of life.                    *Text continued on page 257.*

**Box 16-1**

## JCAH CRITERIA FOR A THERAPEUTIC ENVIRONMENT

1. The facility establishes an environment that enchances the positive self-image of patients and preserves their human dignity.
2. The grounds of the facility have adequate space for the facility to carry out its stated goals.
    2.1 When patient needs or facility goals involve outdoor activities, areas appropriate to the ages and clinical needs of the patients are provided.
3. The facility is accessible to handicapped individuals or the facility has written policies and procedures that describe how the handicapped can gain access to the facility for necessary services.
4. Waiting or reception areas are comfortable, and their design, location, and furnishings accommodate the characteristics of patients and visitors, the anticipated waiting time, the need for privacy and/or support from staff, and the goals of the facility.
    4.1 Appropriate staff are available in waiting or reception areas to address the needs of patients and visitors.
    4.2 Rest rooms are available for patients and visitors.
    4.3 A telephone is available for private conversations.
    4.4 An adequate number of drinking units are accessible at appropriate heights.
        4.4.1 If drinking units employ cups, only single-use, disposable cups are used.
5. Facilities that do not have emergency medical care resources have first-aid kits available in appropriate places.
    5.1 All supervisory staff are familiar with the locations, content, and use of the first-aid kits.
6. Programs providing partial-hospital or 24-hour care services provide an environment appropriate to the needs of patients.
    6.1 The design, structure, furnishings, and lighting of the patient environment promote clear perceptions of people and functions.
    6.2 When appropriate, lighting is controlled by patients.
    6.3 Where possible, the environment provides views of the outdoors.
    6.4 Areas that are used primarily by patients have windows or skylights.
    6.5 Appropriate types of mirrors that distort as little as possible are placed at reasonable heights in appropriate places to aid in grooming and to enhance patients' self-awareness.
    6.6 Clocks and calendars are provided in at least major-use areas to promote awareness of time and season.

From Joint Commission on Accreditation of Hospitals: Consolidated Standards Manual for Child, Adolescent, and Adult Psychiatric, Alcoholism, and Drug Abuse Facilities and Facilities Serving the Mentally Retarded/Developmentally Disabled, 1987, pp. 177-182.

*Continued.*

**Box 16-1**

## JCAH CRITERIA FOR A THERAPEUTIC ENVIRONMENT—cont'd

7. Ventilation contributes to the habitability of the environment.
   7.1 Direct outside air ventilation is provided to each patient's room by air-conditioning or operable windows.
   7.2 Ventilation is sufficient to remove undesirable odors.
8. All areas and surfaces shall be free of undesirable odors.
9. Door locks and other structural restraints are used minimally.
   9.1 The use of door locks or closed sections is approved by the professional staff and the governing body.
10. The facility has written policies and procedures to facilitate staff-patient interaction, particularly when structural barriers in the therapeutic environment separate staff from patients.
    10.1 Staff respect a patient's right to privacy by knocking on the door of the patient's room before entering.
11. Areas with the following characteristics are available to meet the needs of patients:
    11.1 Areas that accommodate a full range of social activities, from two-person conversations to group activities.
    11.2 Attractively furnished areas in which a patient can be alone, when appropriate.
    11.3 Attractively furnished areas for private conversations with other patients, family members, or friends.
12. Appropriate furnishings and equipment are available.
    12.1 Furnishings are clean and in good repair.
    12.2 Furnishings are appropriate to the ages and physical conditions of the patients.
    12.3 All furnishings, equipment, and appliances are maintained in good operating order.
    12.4 Broken furnishings and equipment are repaired promptly.
13. Dining areas are comfortable, attractive, and conducive to pleasant living.
    13.1 Dining arrangements are based on a logical plan that meets the needs of the patients and the requirements of the facility.
    13.2 Dining tables seat small groups of patients, unless other arrangements are justified on the basis of patient needs.
    13.3 When staff members do not eat with the patients, the dining rooms are adequately supervised and staffed to provide assistance to patients when needed and to assure that each patient receives an adequate amount and variety of food.
14. Sleeping areas have doors for privacy.
    14.1 In rooms containing more than four patients, privacy is provided by partitioning or the placement of furniture.
    14.2 The number of patients in a room is appropriate to the goals of the facility and to the ages, developmental levels, and clinical needs of the patients.

Box 16-1

## JCAH CRITERIA FOR A THERAPEUTIC ENVIRONMENT—cont'd

14.3 Except when clinically justified in writing on the basis of program requirements, no more than eight patients sleep in a room.

14.4 Sleeping areas are assigned on the basis of the patient's need for group support, privacy, or independence.

    14.4.1 Patients who need extra sleep, whose sleep is easily disturbed, or who need greater privacy because of age, emotional disturbance, or adjustment problems are assigned to bedrooms in which no more than two persons sleep.

15. Areas are provided for personal hygiene.

15.1 The areas for personal hygiene provide privacy.

15.2 Bathrooms and toilets have partitions and doors.

15.3 Toilets have seats.

16. Good standards of personal hygiene and grooming are taught and maintained, particularly in regard to bathing, brushing teeth, caring for hair and nails, and using the toilet.

16.1 Patients have the personal help needed to perform these activities and, when indicated, to assume responsibility for self-care.

16.2 Incontinent patients are cleaned and/or bathed immediately upon voiding or soiling, with due regard for privacy.

16.3 The services of a barber and/or beautician are available to patients either in the facility or in the community.

17. Articles for grooming and personal hygiene that are appropriate to the patient's age, developmental level, and clinical status are readily available in a space reserved near the patient's sleeping area.

17.1 If clinically indicated, a patient's personal articles may be kept under lock and key by staff.

18. Ample closet and drawer space are provided for storing personal property and property provided for patients' use.

18.1 Lockable storage space is provided.

19. Patients are allowed to keep and display personal belongings and to add personal touches to the decoration of their rooms.

19.1 The facility has written rules to govern the appropriateness of such decorative display.

19.2 If access to potentially dangerous grooming aids or other personal articles is contraindicated for clinical reasons, a member of the professional staff explains to the patient the conditions under which the articles may be used.

    19.2.1 The clinical rationale for these conditions is documented in the patient record.

19.3 If hanging of pictures on walls and similar activities are privileges to be earned for treatment purposes, a member of the professional staff explains to the patient the conditions under which the privileges may be granted.

    19.3.1 The treatment and granting of privileges are documented in the patient record.

*Continued.*

**Box 16-1**

## JCAH CRITERIA FOR A THERAPEUTIC ENVIRONMENT—cont'd

20. Patients are encouraged to take responsibility for maintaining their own living quarters and day-to-day housekeeping activities of the program, as appropriate to their clinical status.
    - 20.1 Such responsibilities are clearly defined in writing, and staff assistance and equipment are provided as needed.
    - 20.2 Descriptions of such responsibilities are included in the patient's orientation program.
    - 20.3 Documentation that these responsibilities have been incorporated in the patient's treatment plan is provided.
21. Patients are allowed to wear their own clothing.
    - 21.1 If clothing is provided by the program, it is appropriate and is not dehumanizing.
    - 21.2 Training and help in the selection and proper care of clothing are available as appropriate.
    - 21.3 Clothing is suited to the climate.
    - 21.4 Clothing is becoming, in good repair, of proper size, and similar to the clothing worn by patients' peers in the community.
    - 21.5 An adequate amount of clothing is available to permit laundering, cleaning, and repair.
22. A laundry room is accessible so patients may wash their clothing.
23. The use and location of noise-producing equipment and appliances, such as television sets, radios, and record players, do not interfere with other therapeutic activities.
24. A place and equipment are provided for table games and individual hobbies.
    - 24.1 Toys, equipment, and games are stored on shelves that are accessible to patients as appropriate.
25. Books, magazines, and arts and crafts materials are available in accordance with patients' recreational, cultural, and educational backgrounds and needs.
26. The facility formulates its own policy regarding the availability and care of pets and other animals, consistent with the goals of the facility and the requirements of good health and sanitation.
27. Depending on the size of the program, facilities are available for serving snacks and preparing meals for special occasions and for recreational activities.
    - 27.1 The facilities permit patient participation.
28. Unless contraindicated for therapeutic reasons, the facility accommodates patients' need to be outdoors through the use of nearby parks and playgrounds, adjacent countryside, and facility grounds.
    - 28.1 Recreational facilities and equipment are available, consistent with patients' needs and the therapeutic program.
    - 28.2 Recreational equipment is maintained in working order.

Community meetings can also be used to plan such activities as unit picnics or social get-togethers. Patient assignments, such as housekeeping chores, can be discussed, assigned, or evaluated. Such topics as preparing for life outside the hospital and gaining insight into the reason for hospitalization are appropriate for the community meeting (Arons, 1982). Finally, the community meeting provides a forum for exploring the problems of ward living. Conflicts between patients or between patients and staff are frequent concerns. Common patient-patient issues are conflicts over TV use (who controls what is viewed), conflicts between generations (e.g., the radio played too loudly), and conflicts over personal hygiene (e.g., someone is not bathing regularly). Patient-staff conflicts are more delicate, but in the effective community meeting they will be skillfully handled. Common conflicts between patients and staff include depersonalizing attitudes by some staff, rudeness by staff, or a change in nursing staff behavior once the day-shift nurses and other professionals leave. Balance, a concept to be discussed later, is required. The head nurse must balance the need to respond to patients' concerns (and all the therapeutic advantages coupled with doing so) with her need to support her staff. Community meetings are not forums to demonstrate the pathologic condition of patients or for students to impress their teachers with their knowledge and skill in group dynamics or patient care (Arons, 1982).

*Constitution.* A community constitution is a written document that provides the basis for the therapeutic community. The document presents definitions, objectives, meetings, responsibilities of elected patient officers, officer approval or removal procedures, and community response to infractions.

*Step system.* A step system is a process by which patients gain privileges and responsibilities. New patients and acutely disturbed patients are designated as ward status, the most restrictive level. Through various efforts carefully noted in the constitution, individual patients can "earn" privileges and responsibilities approaching discharge status. A step system serves to motivate patients and provides content for community meetings. Baenninger and Tang (1990) note that as budgetary constraints tighten and as patients' rights legislation reduces the number of privileges that can be withheld, "step" programs arc losing some of their therapeutic appeal.

**Activity groups.** There are many kinds of activity (remotivation) groups. Nurses may direct these groups, or the groups may be directed by occupational, recreational, or music therapists. The emphasis is on activity or doing something. The therapeutic payoff comes from the sense of accomplishment achieved by making an item (e.g., a wallet or a belt), the distraction from internal processes, and the socialization experience. As patients focus on matters outside themselves, fewer energies are used in self-defeating, morbid thinking. Structured socialization in a nonthreatening environment can be beneficial to psychiatric patients.

**Social skills groups.** Social skills groups, as might be expected, represent efforts to help psychiatric patients who are deficient in social skills learn, practice, and develop certain skills. Skills training might focus on appropriate dress, grooming, or table manners. More advanced efforts address appropriate social and interpersonal skills on a verbal level, for example, meeting new people, initiating conversations, and job interviewing. For instance, it is not uncommon for some persons to tell more about themselves than anyone needs or wants to know in just a matter of minutes after meeting someone. Such behavior tends to be self-defeating.

Practical living skills can be incorporated into this group also. Such skills as paying bills, shopping for groceries, house cleaning, and returning an item of purchase, are important social skills also.

*Approaches to social skill training.* Group sessions need to be structured, with each skill simply explained and demonstrated by the nurse leader. An opportunity for role playing is essential for learning. Plante (1989) lists 13 role playing scenarios:

1. How to start a conversation
2. How to keep a conversation going
3. How to end a conversation
4. How to say "no"
5. How to ask a favor
6. Giving and receiving compliments graciously
7. Making introductions
8. Interviews
9. Coping with shyness
10. How to tell a joke
11. Listening skills
12. Nonverbal social skills
13. How to ask someone for a date

The opportunity to try out beginning skills and make mistakes in a safe environment is also crucial for learning new skills. Each attempt by the patients to practice a particular behavior or skill must be acknowledged and praised during and outside the group session. Feedback helps the patient assess his social skill development. Specific skills may need to be taught and demonstrated in specific steps. For example, verbal skills and nonverbal behaviors may need to be taught and practiced separately and then combined after patients have learned both components.

**Physical exercise groups.** Physical health and mental health are linked. As patients become withdrawn and asocial, their motivation to exercise decreases. Exercise groups counter this tendency to a degree. If exercise were the key to mental health, then everyone would want to be a marathon runner. Such reasoning is invalid on the surface, and yet a certain level of fitness enhances a sense of mental well-being. Physical exercise can also distract from stressful thoughts, that is, by taking one's mind off oneself. Just as playing racquetball during his lunch hour serves the businessman as a distracting physical activity, exercise provides a similar benefit for the psychiatric patient.

**Psychoeducational programs.** Teaching psychiatric patients and their families about their illness is a relatively new therapeutic strategy. While "patient teaching" has been a focus for some time, the concept of psychoeducation has emerged just recently in the literature. Greenberg and associates (1988) state,

> The psychoeducational model is a systematic goal-directed, psychosocial technique that uses a collaborative approach in which clinicians, patients, and their families learn from each other. The goals of the process are to impart information and to enhance understanding of the illness, needed treatment resources, and supportive services; to acknowledge patients' and families' capacities and their right to know about the illness; and to create a more productive alliance between patients, families, and mental health professionals.

Glynn et al. (1990) found that families want information and help in coping with their family member's illness. Common themes in psychoeducational groups include the discussion of symptoms, both physical and psychosocial, and how those symptoms affect home life, work life, and social life. Theories of etiology—biological, psychosocial, and developmental—are discussed in understandable language. Treatment approaches, including pharmacological and psychological therapies, are reviewed. Side effects of medication are discussed candidly, and patients are encouraged to share their own experiences with side effects.

These efforts are based on empirical evidence that understanding mental illness helps the patient and family better cope with the illness (Lamb, 1976; Leff et al., 1982). Occasionally psychoeducational programs have taken a more rudimentary form. Psychiatric patients who have academic problems with basic arithmetic and reading are taught those skills. Although "three R's" education is not true psychoeducation, it can benefit the patient in a number of ways.

**Transition groups.** Aroian and Prater (1988) point out that newly hospitalized psychiatric patients experience both the crisis of the personal problem that brought them into the hospital and the crisis of being hospitalized. Transition groups can ease new patients into the unit structure and by doing so decrease anxiety and clarify unit expectations. Transition programs linked with existing community programs can facilitate successful outpatient treatment (McRae et al., 1990).

**Work groups.** Work is an adult activity that reinforces a person's sense of well-being (Palmer, 1989), but many psychiatric patients have experienced one work-related setback after another. Work groups can focus on the social skills needed to gain a job, work-defeating behaviors, and actual work skills (Barter et al., 1984).

*Skills related to gaining employment.* Often psychiatric patients lack the basic prerequisites to even be considered as candidates for a job. Getting to work on time, being presentable, and a history of reliability are basic to the job-seeking process. Group work, including role playing and videotaping, are helpful approaches for reinforcing social competencies.

*Work-defeating behaviors.* Poor work habits, poor self-confidence, lack of motivation, and a negative attitude toward work contribute to keeping psychiatric patients from gaining employment. In addition, some persons have few tangible skills to offer an employer.

*Developing work skills.* A meaningful work group activity focuses on the development of basic work skills. Orientation to the expectations of the workplace, sharing of positive work experiences, tips on getting along with coworkers, and job application and interviewing skills are all helpful if the patient anticipates returning to the workplace.

## UNIT NORMS

Norms can be defined as unit expectations or unit climate. Norms are related to rules and limit setting but are more abstract. Unit norms permeate the atmosphere. To illustrate, two examples will be used:

1. First, consider two persons in the same position in the same work setting who differ in their expectations of others. One expects people to treat her with respect; the other does not expect such treatment. It is not uncommon for each to be treated as they expect to be treated.
2. The second illustration is closer to the topic of psychotherapeutic management. Two psychiatric units may be different in the level of assaultive behavior they experience; yet both, as psychiatric units, seek to eliminate these aggressive behaviors. The difference may be the unit norms manifested by unit staff. Norms of nonviolence, physical and emotional security, personal control, openness, giving and receiving feedback, respect for the individual, privacy, acceptance, independence, and individual responsibility build a climate of universality or shared experience.

**Nonviolence.** A norm of nonviolence simply means that violence is neither expected nor accepted in the environment. Staff members are trained to defuse potentially violent situations and do not let their own need "not to back down" get in the way of the therapeutic goal. Levy and Hartocollis (1976) found that all female–staffed psychiatric units experienced less assaultive behavior than units staffed by both male and female personnel. They suggested that male staff members may have allowed their "male egos" to push situations to a crisis.

**Physical and emotional security.** The psychiatric unit should be a safe place physically and emotionally. Physical safety relates to the norm of nonviolence already addressed. It also relates to safe administration of medications and treatments (e.g., ECT). Emotional safety addresses the patient's need to feel accepted as he is. Many experienced psychiatric nurses can attest to the fact that disturbed patients occasionally will "calm down" almost immediately upon admission. This phenomenon is related to the asylum or sanctuary concept mentioned in Chapter 1. The fact the person knows he is "emotionally safe" is tranquilizing. The freedom to be "ill" is therapeutic.

**Personal control.** The norm of personal control simply underscores the human need to make decisions about oneself. To the degree one makes responsible decisions about himself, he is moving toward responsible adult behavior. In the inpatient environment many daily decisions come under the discretionary control of others, (for example, when to smoke, what to wear, and telephone use). As staff members are able to "give up" control, the patient is allowed to gain more control over his life. Menu choices are a good example of personal control that can be emphasized. Even actively psychotic persons can be helped to make these basic decisions. For others, even control over medications may be advisable (e.g., dosage schedule). The unit norm of personal control facilitates maturity and responsibility and defuses remnants of custodial mentality.

**Openness.** Openness means an atmosphere in which a free exchange of thoughts and feelings can occur without fear of mockery or retaliation. Feelings and thoughts need not be guarded for fear of emotional blackmail. However, as Gutheil (1985) points out, an overemphasis on self-disclosure can lead to regressive outpouring of psychotic material that is destructive to the patient. The nurse should monitor a *balanced* approach to openness.

**Feedback.** The process by which one person shares his perception of what another person has meant or how the speaker has affected other people is called feedback. Feedback enables us to better understand how others perceive us. It is exciting but risky. As patients are able to "hear and respond," they are moving toward responsible adult behaviors.

**Respect for the individual.** Respect is crucial. Without respect the environment mocks the individual. Even great clinical skill, in the absence of respect, is not adequate in psychiatric nursing. It is a form of elitism to provide care (i.e., medications) while not respecting the individual.

**Privacy.** Privacy is a measure of status. The wealthy have beautiful homes surrounded by acreage. The middle class have their 6-foot fences behind which they erect satellite dishes to bring the world to their living rooms. The poor live out in the open; that is, some of their private events are not very private, for example, domestic fights and relaxation (sitting outside on a busy street to "get some privacy"). Privacy on the psychiatric unit conveys respect for human dignity. Knocking before entering a room says something to the patient. Opening a door without knocking communicates disrespect.

**Acceptance.** Acceptance is the ability to start where the psychiatric patient is. An anxious person cannot attend to details; a person experiencing akathisia cannot sit down; persons who live on the street cannot stay clean. Acceptance of the individual recognizes these less than ideal states. The therapeutic task is to facilitate a decrease in anxiety, to administer p.r.n. benztropine for akathisia, and to help the street person get cleaned up.

**Independence.** Independence is related to personal control but is more far reaching. Psychiatric treatment facilities foster dependent behaviors. From telling patients when to eat and sleep (in the hospital) to telling them how to be healthy (all settings), these facilities, by definition, create dependency. As independent actions and thinking can be reinforced and supported, the patient can begin to test out his ideas. Independence is yet another mark of responsible adult behavior.

**Individual responsibility.** In the effective therapeutic environment patients are given responsibilities and are held accountable for fulfilling them. The step system, mentioned under "Unit Structure," is usually responsibility driven. As patients accept and handle greater responsibilities, they move upward through the step system.

■    ■    ■

These unit norms or unit expectations enhance the living environment of the psychiatric patient. The nursing staff must embrace these values in order for the norms to permeate the unit around the clock. The development and implementation of these unit norms are a major nursing responsibility.

## LIMIT SETTING

Limit setting is the art of clearly identifying acceptable and unacceptable behavior. There is a certain amount of conceptual overlap with unit structure and unit norms, but limit setting is distinct and warrants special mention. Limits should be clearly identified early to persons who are prone to "test the system." Self-destructive acts, acts of physical aggression (including offensive language and stealing), noncompliance with treatment plans, use of alcohol or illicit drugs, use of over-the-counter drugs, inappropriate sexual behavior, smoking, and elopement (running away) are examples of common behaviors requiring that limits be placed.

**Self-destructive acts.** It is important to communicate to the suicidal patient that self-destructive acts are not permitted and that staff members will do everything within their power to prevent such an act from occurring. Most units have "no harm" or "no self-injury" contracts that the patient is asked to sign. The patient agrees to contact the staff should he have an impulse to be self-destructive.

**Physical aggressiveness toward others.** Probably the greatest concern most students and nurses have about psychiatric nursing has to do with the potential for violence. Chapter 7 addresses this issue. Within the context of the therapeutic environment, physical aggressiveness (including offensive language) toward others is not allowed. This should be clearly stated, and a contract of nonviolence and appropriate conduct should be developed with this patient.

Theft is an ever present concern on psychiatric units, and when it occurs, it is often handled by patient government. One approach patient governments use is to close the unit until the missing item is returned. Although protests are predictable, the process is often successful, and much therapeutic dialogue transpires.

**Noncompliance.** Psychiatric patients are expected to follow the treatment program. The very nature of some disorders (e.g., paranoid thinking) and the type of admission (involuntary) work against this, but the expectation is still therapeutic. If an initial agreement can be reached, compliance may be maintained throughout treatment. Compliance to medication regimens is an ongoing problem. As many as 46% of psychiatric inpatients do not consistently take ordered medication. They may "cheek" the medication (that is, hide the pill in their cheek and only pretend to swallow it) and then spit it out or save it. To counter noncompliance tendencies, liquid medications are often the drug form of choice at the inpatient level, and long-acting depot injections the choice for outpatients.

**Alcohol and illicit drugs.** Use of alcohol and illicit drugs by psychiatric patients probably occurs often (Carey, 1989). Besides the obvious concern of engaging in countertherapeutic activity, drug interactions between psychotropic drugs and these mind-altering substances can be harmful. It is not uncommon for "friends" of the patient to take advantage of the privacy provided for patients to bring drugs in from the outside.

**Over-the-counter drugs.** Over-the-counter (OTC) drugs can have harmful interactions with psychotropic drugs. Only those OTC drugs approved by the staff should be permitted.

**Inappropriate sexual behaviors.** Limits must be set on sexual activity on the psychiatric unit to protect patients from uninformed decisions or unwanted sexual activity. As Coumos et al. (1990) have noted, "prevention of sexual activity within a state hospital is difficult, and preventing male homosexual activity in dormitories at night may be the most difficult of all." It is essential that criteria for acceptability be clearly presented so that nurses and patients understand the parameters of sexual behavior. In many states both heterosexual and homosexual activity between patients must be reported (Holbrook, 1989). While reporting may embarrass, it also protects.

**Smoking.** Smoking is more prevalent on psychiatric units than in other types of hospital units (Hughes et al., 1986). Since smoking is the leading cause of hospital fires and deaths related to fires, and is generally recognized to be unhealthy, some psychiatric units do not permit smoking (Resnick and Bosworth, 1989).

**Elopement.** Just as the suicidal or assaultive patient may be asked to sign a contract, the patient who is prone to run away can be asked to sign a contract that states he will notify the staff before leaving the hospital. Although reasons for elopement are numerous, there are two general causes:

1. The patient believes the treatment is not meeting his needs.
2. The person does not believe he needs treatment.

**Unit rules.** A concept closely related to limit setting is establishment of unit rules. Unit rules must be clearly communicated to patients. It is not uncommon for psychiatric units to have rules concerning such things as dress, appearance, group meetings, medication, visiting hours, and telephone use. For instance, if there is a dress standard, for example, no halter tops for women, patients should be told of it to avoid an embarrassing confrontation. Morrison (1987) has identified 18 rules on the psychiatric unit that nurses believe to be important. Nine of the rules are social, and nine are therapeutic (Box 16-2).

## BALANCE

The psychiatric patient is often in a position of dependency. The patient is asking other people to help him achieve mental health. With dependency, comfort is gained initially because the patient is handing over his problems to the staff to be fixed. Nurses also find comfort in this dependency arrangement because as they are able to "control the patient," there are fewer risks and patient dependency may meet a need they have to be "needed." But maintaining dependency is countertherapeutic, and nurses cannot "fix" the problem anyway. Regaining mental health is a process more analogous to recovery from a medical illness than it is to recovery from a surgical procedure. The nurse should foster independence, and as the patient progresses, he not only will become more independent but also may well resent vestiges of dependency. Balance is the careful negotiation of these competing phenomena. The patients' rights movement has exposed another dimension of balance. Nurses

## Box 16-2
## IMPORTANT UNIT RULES

### SOCIAL RULES

- Abides by unit rules regarding smoking and handling of matches.
- Listens attentively when others talk in meetings.
- Does not dress in a sexually revealing manner.
- Does not interrupt conversations.
- Uses telephone with consideration for others.
- Uses TV and stereo with consideration for others.
- Eats at designated places and times.
- Does not intrude into areas designated off-limits by staff.
- Abides by unit rules regarding visitors.

### THERAPEUTIC RULES

- Actively participates in setting therapeutic goals for self.
- Participates in family therapy and group conferences.
- Acknowledges the need for treatment.
- Accepts the need for hospitalization.
- Participates in individual therapy.
- Attends individual therapy as scheduled.
- Attends family or group therapy as scheduled.
- Seeks out staff to help control psychotic or illness-related behavior.
- Examines own progress realistically when considering changes in status.

From Morrison EF: Determining social and therapeutic rules for psychiatric inpatients, Hosp Community Psychiatry 38:994, 1987.

and physicians are continually balancing the patient's right to make his own decision against the staff's need to provide treatment that is effective and safe for all. To better illustrate these concepts a few relatively common dependency-independency (balance) examples follow:

**The suicidal patient.** The nurse must balance the patient's need for safety with the patient's need to regain control over his life (Assey, 1985). Should the patient be allowed to go to the bathroom alone? Or will he seek to take his life in the bathroom? To watch someone use the toilet is both unpleasant for the nurse and embarrassing for the patient.

> **Case study:** Mary T., a 29-year-old Hispanic woman, entered the bathroom. The nurse waited outside the door. After 3 to 4 minutes the nurse looked in. Maria was attempting to hang herself on a handrail next to the toilet.

**The religious patient.** A person may be a member of a religious body that prohibits the use of medication, and yet his psychosis requires psychopharmacological intervention. The nurse must balance his right to practice his religion and his need to be treated.

> **Case study:** Bill, a 44-year-old man, belongs to a Pentecostal group that does not "believe in" medication. The use of medication is construed as a lack of faith in God. He is actively psychotic, yet he, his wife, and his pastor do not want him to be given medication.

**The assaultive patient.** The violent person frightens patients and staff alike. The nurse must balance the need to protect others by secluding the assaultive patient with the patient's right to unencumbrance.

> **Case study:** A pregnant woman began hitting other patients. Since psychotropic drugs may harm the fetus, the nursing staff had to decide how to protect other patients (and protect the offending patient from retaliation) and yet not do anything that might compromise the pregnancy.

**The dangerous patient.** Sometimes dangerous patients tell nurses or their therapist about plans to hurt someone. The patient's right to confidentiality must be balanced with the potential victim's right to know about the threat. There is much discussion about this dilemma in psychiatry today (see Chapter 4). The Tarasoff case (1974) was a landmark legal decision, which states that psychiatric staff members have a duty to warn potential victims of danger from psychiatric patients. Nonetheless, judgment must be used because indiscriminate warnings do violate the patient's trust and may cause undue concern to the potential victim.

■     ■     ■

Balance is an important concept because it forces the nurse to articulate what competing interests are at work. The skillful use of balance comes with understanding of ethical concerns, legal issues, and psychopathology. To paraphrase Pellegrino (1987), "Nothing more exposes [a nurse's] ethics than the way he or she balances his or her own interests against those of the patient."

## UNIT MODIFICATION

Attention to the physical environment can make the treatment environment more effective. Physical arrangement of furniture, safety issues, and orientation strategies embedded within the environment can enhance other treatment modalities. Often the nurse manager is faced with making the best of a physical plant that was never intended to serve the special needs of a psychiatric population. Large corporations, on the other hand, design hospitals to maximize the environment's therapeutic potential.

**Physical environment.** Privacy and adequate room are of major importance in designing the psychiatric unit. Territoriality, proxemics, crowding, and density are persistent human themes that need to be addressed anticipatorily. Dayroom and dining room areas should be designed so that social, recreational, or occupational therapy events can be conducted with minimal conversion time.

Bedrooms should be attractive and private. The nurses' station (some units no longer have traditional nurses' stations) should offer an unobstructed view of the unit. Seclusion rooms are needed for persons who require seclusion or isolation, and safety is a primary concern. The bed in the seclusion room(s) should be bolted to the floor. No other furniture is warranted. An intercommunication system for audio contact is also a common feature in newer facilities.

In units without these architectural considerations, a number of environment-enhancing changes can contribute to the milieu. Color is important. Subtle hues are most commonly desired. Paintings, flowers, and pleasant furniture add to an overall impression of a unit norm of civility and caring. Games and cards should be available for socializing. Magazines and books should be set out for browsing. Furniture should be arranged in a way that encourages socializing. Long rows of chairs lined against the wall, besides being uninviting, discourage patient conversation. On the other hand, an arrangement of three or four facing chairs around a table encourage group seating and lends itself to informal group work.

**Safety.** Much of what has just been discussed relates to safety issues. In addition, bedrooms must be assigned so that privacy is protected and yet safety is ensured (the balance issue again). Small windows in the door are still common. They afford the nurse the opportunity to look in to see if all is well and yet protect the privacy of the patient. Doors to stairways are locked, as are doors to janitorial supplies and the medication room. Some hospitals install "break-away" closet rods and curtain rods to prevent patients from hanging themselves. Since fire remains a concern, advanced fire prevention and containment features are common in newer facilities.

**Orientation strategies.** Persons who are severely disturbed or who are organically impaired may not be able to navigate the hospital environment without environmental cues. Environmental cues include large orientation boards on which the date, time, and location of daily events are posted. This serves to keep the individual current. Other environmental orientation approaches include public address systems, clearly marked names (e.g., bathroom, bedrooms with name on the door), and color-coded facilities.

## KEY CONCEPTS

1. Since psychiatric patients are incapable of not interacting with their environment, the nurse has the potential to shape the environment in order to cause that inevitable interaction to be therapeutic.
2. The Joint Commission on Accreditation of Hospitals (JCAH) mandates that psy-

chiatric facilities invest resources in developing a therapeutic environment and has established detailed criteria for that environment (see Box 16.1)

3. The effectively managed milieu consists of five distinct elements. (a) unit structure, (b) unit norms, (c) limit setting, (d) balance, and (e) unit modification.

4. *Unit structure* provides the framework for the therapeutic environment and includes (a) community meetings, (b) activity groups, (c) social skills groups, (d) physical exercise groups, (e) psychoeducational programs, (f) transition groups, and (g) work groups.

5. *Unit norms* are the expectations of behavior that are communicated to the patient in both direct and indirect ways and includes norms of (a) nonviolence, (b) physical and emotional security, (c) openness, (d) feedback, (e) respect for the individual, (f) privacy, (g) acceptance, (h) independence, and (i) individual responsibility.

6. *Setting limits* is the skill of clearly identifying acceptable and unacceptable behavior, including clear communication about (a) self-destructive acts, (b) physical aggressiveness toward others, (c) personal control, (d) noncompliance with treatment plans, (e) use of alcohol and illicit drugs, (f) use of over-the-counter drugs, (g) sexual inappropriateness, (h) smoking, and (i) elopement.

7. *Balance* is the art of carefully negotiating the two competing phenomena of dependence and independence that are commonly found in the context of psychiatric nursing care.

8. *Unit modification* is the purposeful arrangement of the environment and includes attention to (a) the physical environment, (b) safety issues, and (c) orientation strategies.

## REFERENCES

Aroian K and Prater M: Transition entry groups: easing new patients' adjustment to psychiatric hospitalization, Hosp Community Psychiatry 39:312, 1988.

Arons BS: Effective use of community meetings in psychiatric treatment units, Hosp Community Psychiatry 33:480, 1982.

Assey JL: The suicide prevention contract, Perspect Psychiatr Care 23:99, 1985.

Baenninger LP and Tang W: Teaching chronic psychiatric inpatients to use differential attention to change each other's behaviors, Hosp Community Psychiatry, 41:425, 1990.

Barter JT, Queirolo JF, and Ekstrom SP: A psychoeducational approach to educating chronic mental patients for community living, Hosp Community Psychiatry 35:793, 1984.

Carey KB: Emerging treatment guidelines for mentally ill chemical abusers, Hosp Community Psychiatry 40:341, 349, 1989.

Cournos F et al: HIV infection in state hospitals: case reports and long-term management strategies, Hosp Community Psychiatry 41:163, 1990.

Glynn SM, Pugh R, and Rose G: Predictor of relatives' attendance at a state hospital workshop on schizophrenia. Hosp Community Psychiatry 41:67, 1990.

Greenberg L et al.: An interdisciplinary psychoeducation program for schizophrenia patients and their families in an acute care setting, Hosp Community Psychiatry 39:277, 1988.

Gutheil T: The therapeutic milieu: changing themes and theories, Hosp Community Psychiatry 36:1279, 1985.

Holbrook T: Policing sexuality in a modern state hospital, Hosp Community Psychiatry 40:65, 1989.

Hughes JR et al.: Prevalence of smoking among psychiatric outpatients, Am J Psychiatry 143:993, 1986.

Kahn EM and White EM: Adapting milieu approaches to acute inpatient care for schizophrenic patients, Hosp Community Psychiatry 40:609, 1989.

Kyes G and Hofling C: Basic psychiatric concepts in nursing, ed 3, Philadelphia, 1974, JB Lippincott Co, p 455.

Lamb HR: An educational model for teaching living skills to long-term patients, Hosp Community Psychiatry 27:875, 1976.

Leff HR et al: A controlled trial of social intervention in the families of schizophrenic patients, Br J Psychiatry 141:121, 1982.

Levy P and Hartocollis P: Nursing aides and patient violence, Am J Psychiatry 133:429, 1976.

McRae J et al: What happens to patients after five years of intensive care management stops? Hosp Community Psychiatry 41:175, 1990.

Palmer F: The place of work in psychiatric rehabilitation, Hosp Community Psychiatry 40:222, 1989.

Pellegrino E: Altruism, self-interest, and medical ethics, JAMA 258:1939, 1987.

Plante TG: Social skills training, J Psychosoc Nurs 27:7, 1989.

Resnick MP and Bosworth EE: A smoke-free psychiatric unit, Hosp Community Psychiatry 40:525, 1989.

*Tarasoff v Regents of the University of California,* 529, P2d, 553, 1974.

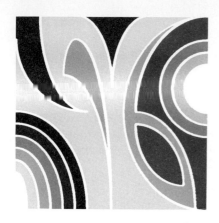

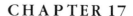

CHAPTER 17

# Roles of the Psychotherapeutic Manager and Other Members of the Psychiatric Team

LEARNING OBJECTIVES
After reading this chapter you should be able to

- Identify the multiple roles of the psychotherapeutic manager.
- Describe the responsibilities for each role of the psychotherapeutic manager.
- Describe the roles of other mental health professionals.

In managing the milieu nurses serve in multiple roles. They work with patients individually, lead groups, participate in community meetings, coordinate medical care (with the physician), dispense routine medications and make decisions concerning p.r.n. medications, participate in discharge planning and make discharge arrangements, work with families, provide leadership in interdisciplinary team meetings, and are the professionals who most often implement team decisions. These roles are a mix of clinical and administrative activities. As a composite, they define the role of the psychotherapeutic manager.

Many of these roles are discussed in other chapters. The purpose of this chapter is to discuss those roles not mentioned elsewhere. To do so, four broad categories will be addressed:

1. Working with other professional disciplines
2. Team-meeting leadership
3. Supervision and training of psychiatric technicians, student nurses, and aides
4. Consultation and patient assessment for and with other departments

## WORKING WITH OTHER PROFESSIONAL DISCIPLINES

One benefit of working in psychiatry is the opportunity to work collegially with other professionals. Psychiatrists, psychiatric social workers, psychologists, occupational therapists, and psychiatric nurses are all part of the treatment team. Discussions of treatment issues by the team lends itself to unique input from all disciplines. The nurse is able to share information with fellow team members on the basis of assessment data gathered in settings typically managed by the nursing staff.

Following are basic descriptions of the members of a multidisciplinary team.

**Psychiatrist.** Certification of a physician (M.D.) in psychiatry by the American Board of Psychiatry and Neurology requires a 3-year residency, 2 years of clinical practice, and completion of an examination. Psychiatrists are permitted to prescribe psychotropic medications.

**Psychologist.** The psychologist working in the mental health field is known as a clinical psychologist. This designation differentiates the clinical psychologist from varied nonpsychiatric roles other psychologists fill. The clinical psychologist has a doctorate (Ph.D.) in psychology. The psychologist is prepared to perform therapy, conduct research, and administer and interpret psychological tests. Many psychologists are behaviorally oriented and develop behavior-modification programs for the individual patient or for the entire milieu (see Chapter 26). "Most behavior therapy programs on adult psychiatric wards rely on privileges and concrete primary reinforcers, such as coffee, snacks, and cigarettes, which patients earn through secondary reinforcers, such as points, tokens and credits" (Baenninger and Tang, 1990).

**Psychiatric social worker.** The psychiatric social worker is prepared at the master's level (M.S.W.). Social workers are part of the treatment team, and their unique contributions are working with families and mobilizing community support systems. Psychiatric social workers often assume the role of primary therapist.

**Occupational therapist.** The occupational therapist (O.T.) uses arts and crafts to help psychiatric patients. Through accomplishment and distraction a therapeutic gain is achieved. Some occupational therapists teach self-help and employment skills.

## TEAM-MEETING LEADERSHIP

Nurses often assume or share leadership in team meetings. Other disciplines rely on the nursing service to provide an accurate report on patient status and to report on implementation or treatment team plans.

"The team meets routinely to discuss the patients' problems, progress, and needs during hospitalization" (Ambrose, 1989). During team meetings patients are discussed individually, and decisions regarding treatment are developed. In healthy team meetings each discipline recognizes and respects the contributions of other disciplines. At times there is an overlapping of disciplines. When the welfare of the patient is foremost, such distractions can be resolved. When disciplines have "turf wars," patient care is compromised.

If interdiscipline harmony contributes to the therapeutic environment, then it is important to seek such harmony. Interdiscipline relations are enhanced by respect, the desire to help, and understanding. When professionals respect each other, desire to help the patient, and understand the dynamics of interprofessional conflict (i.e., loss of turf, envy, professional jealousy, mistrust), interdiscipline harmony will result. When respect, the desire to help, and understanding are lacking, interprofessional conflict results and undermines the therapeutic environment.

## SUPERVISION AND TRAINING

An important dimension of psychotherapeutic management is the supervision and training of other members of the nursing staff. The nursing staff is composed of nurses, student nurses, psychiatric technicians, mental health workers, and psychiatric aides.

Supervision and training are almost inseparable components of managing the milieu. The nursing staff must strive to consistently represent the agreed-upon unit philosophy and conscientiously implement treatment plans. To do so, individual staff members require training. Supervision reinforces the unit leadership's commitment to these objectives and provides a focus for evaluation.

Training should focus on therapeutic communication (Unit II), position-appropriate understanding of psychopharmacology (Unit III), and maintenance of the therapeutic environment (Unit IV), all underscored by a position-appropriate understanding of psychopathology (Unit V). Other specialized issues can be taught as necessary (Units VI and VII contain some special issues in psychiatric nursing).

There are distinct groups among the generic category called nursing staff. Their roles overlap, but this potentially disharmonious situation is easily mitigated by good leadership.

**Other nurses.** Multiple entry levels into nursing confuse other professionals and have been the source of much conflict intraprofessionally. Academic psychiatric preparation may be anywhere from 3 to 10 weeks long; therefore novice psychiatric nurses require supervision and training from more experienced nurses. Student nurses gaining clinical experience on the psychiatric unit are also supervised and trained by unit nurses (albeit this may be done indirectly). It is important that students be given every opportunity to experience meaningful learning situations.

**Psychiatric technician.** Psychiatric technician is a licensed category of health care provider in some states. Typically, training takes 1 year. These persons are authorized to administer medications. In California some psychiatric technicians have risen through the ranks to become chief executive officers of large state hospitals.

**Mental health worker.** This category was established to more effectively meet the needs of persons from lower socioeconomic classes. Disadvantaged persons were recruited into these training programs, which vary from certificate programs to programs that lead to college degrees (associate and baccalaureate).

**Psychiatric aide.** Psychiatric aides require no previous training to be hired. They are taught on site. Psychiatric facilities have in-service departments to train psychiatric aides, but the general hospital psychiatric unit may have to provide its own training for these persons.

■    ■    ■

Supervision and training of all nursing staff members is a vital dimension of milieu management. The therapeutic environment depends on every member of the team to understand and enhance the principles described in Chapter 16.

## CONSULTATION AND PATIENT ASSESSMENT FOR OTHER DEPARTMENTS

Psychiatric nurses working in a general hospital psychiatric unit may be called upon to consult with other nursing departments. Providing consultation may involve formal or informal processes.

Typically, a "problem" or "disturbed" patient triggers the consultation; that is, a "problem" patient taxes the ability of the unit nursing staff to provide effective care. In the hope that the psychiatric nursing department can help, a consultation is requested. In some hospitals this is a relatively informal process. In many larger hospitals the role of psychiatric liaison or consultant nurse has developed to provide these services.

Consultation typically takes one of two forms. The psychiatric nurse may work with the "troubled" patient directly or may do so indirectly by working with the nurses requesting the consultation. "Problem" patients can be roughly grouped into those who have a history of diagnosable psychiatric disturbance and those who are experiencing a disturbance secondary to their current physical problem. The consulting psychiatric nurse uses the nursing process to develop an intervention strategy. Chapter 9 provides a thorough discussion of these concepts.

## KEY CONCEPTS

1.  Psychiatric nurses serve in multiple roles, including (a) working with patients individually, (b) leading groups of patients, (c) participating in community meetings, (d) coordinating medical care (with the physician), (e) dispensing routine medications and making decisions about p.r.n. medications, (f) participating in discharge planning and making discharge arrangements, (g) working with the families of patients, (h) providing leadership in interdisciplinary team meetings, and (i) implementing team decisions.

2. In this chapter four categories of roles are discussed: (a) working with other professional disciplines, (b) team meeting leadership, (c) supervising and training other nurses, psychiatric technicians, student nurses, and psychiatric aides, and (d) consultation and patient assessment for and with other departments.

3. The psychiatric nurse most frequently works with the following professionals: (a) psychiatrists, (b) psychiatric social workers, (c) psychologists, and (d) occupational therapists.

4. The psychiatric nurse usually assumes responsibility for *team-meeting leadership.* During the team meeting patients are discussed and decisions regarding treatment and discharge or disposition are developed.

5. The *supervision and training* of subordinates is an important function of the psychotherapeutic manager because milieu management is dependent on all members of the team being able to contribute. Training focuses on therapeutic communication, position-appropriate understanding of psychopharmacology, maintenance of the therapeutic environment, and position-appropriate understanding of psychopathology.

6. Psychiatric nurses are often called upon to fulfill the role of *consultant* to other departments within the hospital. The student is referred back to Chapter 9 for a full discussion of this role.

**REFERENCES**

Ambrose JA: Joining in: therapeutic groups for chronic patients, J Psychosoc Nurs 27:28, 1989.

Baenninger LP and Tang W: Teaching chronic psychiatric inpatients to use differential attention to change each other's behaviors, Hosp Community Psychiatry 41:425, 1990.

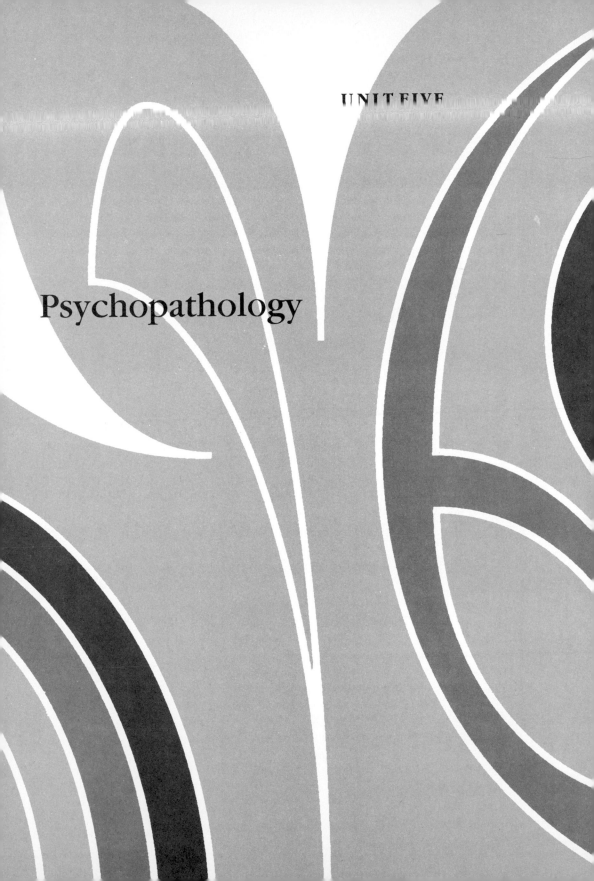

# Psychopathology

## CHAPTER 18

# Introduction to Psychopathology

LEARNING OBJECTIVES

After reading this chapter you should be able to

- List requirements for understanding psychopathology
- Name three diagnostic systems that fulfill these requirements.
- Give several guidelines applicable to all aspects of psychotherapeutic management.

According to a survey conducted by the National Institute of Mental Health (NIMH), at any given moment 29 million Americans have some type of mental disorder. Anxiety disorders are the most prevalent disorders, followed by mood disorders, substance abuse, and schizophrenia (about 1% of the population). (See Table 1-1.) Most of these persons (80%) do not seek professional help.

The incidence of psychopathology is high, and an understanding of psychopathology is considered basic to effective psychotherapeutic management of mental disorders by nurses (Keltner, 1985). To understand psychopathology, knowledge must be organized, operational definitions formed, and criteria for diagnosis developed. Several diagnostic systems have accomplished these tasks: the Feighner criteria (Feighner et al., 1972); the Research Diagnostic Criteria (RDC) (Spitzer et al., 1975), and the *Diagnostic and Statistical Manual of Mental Disorders* (American Psychiatric Association, 1952 [DSM-I], 1968, [DSM-II], 1980 [DSM-III], and 1987 [DSM-III-R]). The DSM-III-R, the lastest DSM version, is the diagnostic system most widely used in American psychiatric care, and for that reason is used in this unit to help convey important concepts related to each mental disorder discussed. In addition, each chapter presents a discussion of common behaviors, etiology, and psychotherapeutic management.

## BEHAVIOR

Patient behaviors are presented to help the student identify behavioral phenomena. Some behaviors can be observed directly (objective), whereas others must be reported by the patient (subjective). Knowledge of these signs and symptoms helps the nurse anticipate and plan appropriate interventions.

## ETIOLOGY

For many years psychiatric clinicians have typically fallen into one of two etiological camps, those who see mental disorders as arising from nature (organic, biological, genetic) and those who see mental disorders as arising from nurture (functional, environmental, due to early life experiences). Threads of the "nature vs nurture" argument (or the "organic vs functional" argument) are presented under Etiology; however, the overriding theme is the recognition of the unifying symptoms that point to the contributions of each etiological factor.

### PSYCHOTHERAPEUTIC MANAGEMENT

The psychotherapeutic management section of each chapter draws on the general intervention strategies presented in Units II to IV to develop appropriate interventions for each disorder. In addition, a case study and a related nursing care plan (see sample on opposite page) are presented for each disorder. The following rules provide relevant guidelines for all aspects of psychotherapeutic management:

- Provide support for the patient. By treating the patient with respect, dignity, and as an individual, the nurse helps the patient mobilize his strengths.
- Strengthen the patient's self-esteem. Treat the patient as an adult. Do not succumb to the temptation to patronize him.

## Nursing Care Plan

WEEKLY UPDATE: _____

NAME: _____  ADMISSION DATE: _____

DSM-III-R DIAGNOSIS: _____

*ASSESSMENT:*
**Areas of strength**: _____
_____
_____

**Problems**: _____
_____
_____

*DIAGNOSES*: _____
_____
_____

*PLANNING:*                               *Date met*
**Short-term goals**: _____   _____
_____   _____
_____   _____

**Long-term goals**: _____   _____
_____   _____
_____   _____

*IMPLEMENTATION/INTERVENTIONS:*
**Nurse-patient relationship**: _____
_____

**Psychopharmacology**: _____
_____

**Milieu management**: _____
_____
_____

*EVALUATION:* _____
_____

- Prevent failure or embarrassment. Do not involve the patient in situations in which he will fail or feel inadequate; for example, competitive games may be inappropriate for some patients. If the patient does something "crazy," like taking off all clothes, remove him from public view and assist him in putting on proper attire.
- Treat the patient as an individual. While the patient may be similar to previous patients on the unit, he is unique, and generalizations may damage the nurse-patient relationship.
- Provide reality testing. This rule applies to the patient who feels very anxious or unreal, as well as to the schizophrenic patient. Reinforce reality.
- Handle hostility therapeutically. Hostile themes are not uncommon on a psychiatric unit. The nurse who is intimidated and frightened by every occurrence will be defensive and may not be able to be therapeutic. The ability to be calm and matter-of-fact about unit norms and limits projects control of oneself and of the situation and is therapeutic.

## THE NURSES NEED TO UNDERSTAND PSYCHOPATHOLOGY

The psychiatric nurse can no more effectively plan and provide psychiatric care without an understanding of psychopathology than the medical-surgical nurse can plan and provide care without an understanding of pathophysiology. As self-evident as this statement may seem, not all psychiatric nurses agree. Some believe nurses need only focus on behavior; others have a knee-jerk reaction to anything "medical," going to elaborate extremes to avoid "medical terminology." The eschewing of a common language and a diagnostic system is not new. In the early days of modern psychiatry (1859) Heinrich Neuman stated that we ought "to throw overboard the whole business of classification. There is but one type of mental disturbance, and we call it insanity" (Lehman, 1980). The authors of this book obviously disagree, as we have included chapters on the following mental disorders: schizophrenia, mood disorders, anxiety, organic mental disorders, personality disorders, drug and alcohol abuse, and eating disorders.

## KEY CONCEPTS

1. According to a National Institute of Mental Health survey, 29 million Americans suffer from some type of mental disorder at any given time.
2. Anxiety disorders are the most common category of mental disorder, followed by mood disorders, substance abuse, and schizophrenia.
3. Understanding psychopathology is fundamental to effective psychotherapeutic management.
4. Several diagnostic systems have been developed to facilitate the understanding of mental disorders and inter- and intraprofessional communication.
5. The *Diagnostic and Statistical Manual,* third edition, revised (DSM-III-R, [APA, 1987]) is the diagnostic system most commonly used in American psychiatry.
6. Etiological explanations of mental disorders can be placed under one of two categories: biological (nature or organic causes) and psychological (nurture or functional causes).

## REFERENCES

American Psychiatric Association: Diagnostic and statistical manual of mental disorders, ed 3, revised (DSM-III-R), Washington, D.C., 1987, American Psychiatric Association.

Feighner JP et al: Diagnostic criteria for use in psychiatric research, Arch Gen Psychiatry 26:57, 1972.

Keltner NL: Psychotherapeutic management: a model for nursing practice, Perspect Psychiatr Care 23:125, 1985.

Lehman HE: Schizophrenia: history. In Kaplan HI et al, editors: Comprehensive textbook of psychiatry, Baltimore, 1980, Williams & Wilkins, p 1106.

Spitzer RL, Endicott J, and Robins E: Research diagnostic criteria, New York, 1975, New York State Psychiatric Institute, Biometrics Research.

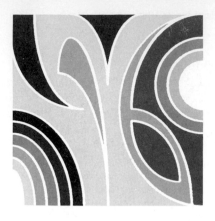

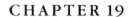

## CHAPTER 19

# Schizophrenia and Other Psychoses

LEARNING OBJECTIVES

After reading this chapter you should be able to

- Describe the major historical figures, events, and theories that have contributed to our present-day understanding of schizophrenia.
- Recognize DSM-III-R criteria and terminology for schizophrenia.
- Describe DSM-III-R subtypes and type I and type II subtypes.
- Recognize and describe objective and subjective symptoms of schizophrenia.
- Describe three theoretical biological explanations for schizophrenia.
- Describe two theoretical psychodynamic explanations for schizophrenia.
- Develop a nursing care plan for a person with schizophrenia.
- Evaluate the effectiveness of nursing interventions for schizophrenic patients.

# ■ Schizophrenia

*Schizophrenia* is a diagnostic term used by mental health professionals to describe a group of mental disturbances that feature withdrawal, affective problems, and interrupted thought processes. Persons with schizophrenia may appear dull and colorless, dependent and apathetic, and emotionally isolative. The cost in human suffering is incalculable; it is known that about 1% of the population will experience schizophrenia. Economic costs are in the tens of billions of dollars each year.

Morel was the first to give name to these psychiatric symptoms. In 1856, while treating an adolescent boy, he used the phrase *dementia praecox* (precocious senility) to describe the group of symptoms he observed. Kahlbaum (in 1868) and Hecker (in 1870) added to the lexicon with their diagnostic categories *catatonia* and *hebephrenia*, respectively. Kraepelin (1902) added the term *paranoia* and engaged in a rigorous study of what we now call schizophrenia. He found commonalities among these three mental disorders (catatonia, hebephrenia, and paranoia) and in 1896 labeled them *dementia praecox*. Kraepelin believed schizophrenia was the result of neuropathology and envisioned a progressive deteriorating course resulting in disabling mental impairment with little hope of recovery.

It was left to Bleuler (1950) in the early 1900s to coin the term *schizophrenia* in a book subtitled "the group of schizophrenias." Bleuler found that schizophrenia does not always follow a course of deterioration (so *dementia* was inappropriate), nor does it always occur early in life (*praecox* was inappropriate also). Bleuler broadened Kraepelin's concept by focusing on symptoms rather than on outcomes (Harding et al., 1987). Bleuler identified four primary symptoms that he believed were present in all persons with schizophrenia. All these symptoms begin with the letter "A," which has facilitated the memorization of these classic symptoms (Box 19-1).

Kraepelin, for instance, on finding someone who had "recovered," believed the person had never had schizophrenia. On the basis of Bleuler's wider grouping, pessimism eased, and some clinicians began to see improvements in their patients. Bleuler explored psychological explanations for schizophrenia, indicating the influence of Freud and other psychodynamic theorists; yet he never abandoned the

**Box 19-1**
### BLEULER'S FOUR A'S

Affective disturbances: inappropriate, blunted, or flattened affect
Autism: preoccupation with self without concern for external reality
Associative looseness: the stringing together of unrelated topics
Ambivalence: simultaneous opposite feelings

biological theory of Kraepelin. In recent years a resurgence of interest in biological research has resulted in renewed respect for Kraepelin's work. On the other hand, Bleuler's contributions have been viewed as a "softening of the diagnostic criteria," which has served to obscure the deteriorating course of the illness and has led to overdiagnosis, particularly in blacks and lower socioeconomic groups (Jones and Gray, 1986).

## DSM-III-R TERMINOLOGY AND CRITERIA

The DSM-III-R criteria for schizophrenia are found in Box 19-2. Since the inception of schizophrenia as a diagnostic entity, attempts have been made to divide it into homogeneous subtypes (Kendler et al., 1988). Early attempts at identifying ho-

### Box 19-2
### DSM-III-R DIAGNOSTIC CRITERIA FOR SCHIZOPHRENIA

A. Presence of characteristic psychotic symptoms in the active phase: either (1), (2), or (3) for at least one week (unless the symptoms are successfully treated):
   1. Two of the following:
      a. Delusions
      b. Prominent hallucinations (throughout the day for several days or several times a week for several weeks, each hallucinatory experience not being limited to a few brief moments).
      c. Incoherence or marked loosening of associations.
      d. Catatonic behavior.
      e. Flat or grossly inappropriate affect.
   2. Bizarre delusions (i.e., involving a phenomenon that the person's culture would regard as totally implausible, e.g., thought broadcasting, being controlled by a dead person).
   3. Prominent hallucinations [as defined in 1.b above] of a voice with content having no apparent relation to depression or elation, or a voice keeping up a running commentary on the person's behavior or thoughts, or two or more voices conversing with each other.
B. During the course of the disturbance, functioning in such areas as work, social relations, and self-care is markedly below the highest level achieved before onset of disturbance (or, when the onset is in childhood or adolescence, failure to achieve expected level of social development).
C. Schizoaffective disorder and mood disorder with psychotic features have been ruled out, i.e., if a major depressive or manic syndrome has ever been present during an active phase of the disturbance, the total duration of all episodes of a mood syndrome has been brief relative to the total duration of the active and residual phases of the disturbance.

## Box 19-2
### DSM-III-R DIAGNOSTIC CRITERIA FOR SCHIZOPHRENIA—cont'd

D. Continuous signs of the disturbance for at least six months. The six-month period must include an active phase (or at least one week or less if symptoms have been successfully treated) during which there were psychotic symptoms characteristic of schizophrenia (symptoms in A), with or without a prodromal or residual phase, as defined below.

*Prodromal phase:* A clear deterioration in functioning before the active phase of the disturbance that is not due to a disturbance in mood or to a psychoactive substance use disorder and that involves at least two of the symptoms listed below.

*Residual phase:* Following the active phase of the disturbance, persistence of at least two of the symptoms noted below, these not being due to a disturbance in mood or to a psychoactive substance use disorder.

*Prodromal or Residual Symptoms:*
1. Marked social isolation or withdrawal
2. Marked impairment in role functioning as wage-earner, student, or home-maker
3. Markedly peculiar behavior (e.g., collecting garbage, talking to self in public, hoarding food)
4. Marked impairment in personal hygiene and grooming
5. Blunted or inappropriate affect
6. Digressive, vague, overelaborate, or circumstantial speech, or poverty of speech, or poverty of content of speech
7. Odd beliefs or magical thinking, influencing behavior and inconsistent with cultural norms, e.g., superstitiousness, belief in clairvoyance, telepathy, "sixth sense," "others can feel my feelings," overvalued ideas, ideas of reference
8. Unusual perceptual experiences, e.g., recurrent illusions, sensing the presence of a force or person not actually present
9. Marked lack of initiative, interests, or energy

*Examples:* Six months of prodromal symptoms with one week of symptoms from A; no prodromal symptoms with six months of symptoms from A; no prodromal symptoms with one week of symptoms from A and six months of residual symptoms.

E. It cannot be established that an organic factor initiated and maintained the disturbance.

F. If there is a history of autistic disorder, the additional diagnosis of schizophrenia is made only if prominent delusions or hallucinations are also present.

**Box 19-3**
## DSM-III-R CRITERIA FOR SCHIZOPHRENIC SUBTYPES

### Catatonic type

1. Catatonic stupor (marked decrease in reactivity to the environment and/or reduction in spontaneous movements and activity) or mutism.
2. Catatonic negativism (an apparently motiveless resistance to all instructions or attempts to be moved).
3. Catatonic rigidity (maintenance of a rigid posture against efforts to be moved).
4. Catatonic excitement (excited motor activity, apparently purposeless, and not influenced by external stimuli).
5. Catatonic posturing (voluntary assumption of inappropriate or bizarre postures).

### Disorganized type

1. Incoherence, marked loosening of associations, or grossly disorganized behavior.
2. Flat or grossly inappropriate affect.
3. Does not meet the criteria for catatonic type.

### Paranoid type

1. Preoccupation with one or more systematized delusions or with frequent auditory hallucinations related to a single theme.
2. None of the following: incoherence, marked loosening of associations, flat grossly inappropriate affect, catatonic behavior, grossly disorganized behavior.

### Undifferentiated type

1. Prominent delusions, hallucinations, incoherence, or grossly disorganized behavior.
2. Does not meet the criteria for paranoid, catatonic, or disorganized type.

### Residual type

1. Absence of prominent delusions, hallucinations, incoherence, or grossly disorganized behavior.
2. Continuing evidence of the disturbance, as indicated by two or more of the residual symptoms listed in criterion D of schizophrenia (see Box 19-2).

Reprinted with permission from the *Diagnostic and Statistical Manual of Mental Disorders, Third Edition, Revised,* Copyright 1987 American Psychiatric Association.

**Box 19-4**
## SYMPTOMS AND PATHOANATOMY OF POSITIVE
## AND NEGATIVE SCHIZOPHRENIA

| **TYPE I** | **TYPE II** |
|---|---|
| **Positive symptoms** | **Negative symptoms** |

**TYPE I**

**Positive symptoms**

- Severe hallucinations
- Severe delusions
- Marked positive formal thought disorder
- Repeated instances of bizarre or delusional behavior
- Develops over a short period of time

**Pathoanatomy**

- Hyperdopaminergic process
- No structural changes

**TYPE II**

**Negative symptoms**

- Alogia
- Affective flattening
- Anhedonia
- Attentional impairment
- Avolition

**Pathoanatomy**

- Nondopaminergic process
- Structural changes:
  - Increased VBRs
  - Decreased CBF

mogeneous groups resulted in the subtypes catatonia, hebephrenia, and paranoia. Bleuler later added *simple* schizophrenia to the nomenclature. This early thinking is still reflected in official diagnostic classifications today (e.g., DSM-III-R). The DSM-III-R identifies five subtypes of schizophrenia: catatonic type, disorganized type, paranoid type, undifferentiated type, and residual type (Box 19-3).

The authors find more promising the subtyping approach advocated by current biologically oriented diagnosticians. Andreasen (1982a,b), Crow (1982), and others have developed two subtypes, positive and negative schizophrenia, based on well-designed research. Positive or type I schizophrenia has a different constellation of symptoms than does negative or type II schizophrenia (see Box 19-4). Type I is positive in the sense that symptoms are an embellishment of normal cognition and perception. The symptoms are "additional." Positive symptoms are believed to be caused by a subcortical dopaminergic process (too much dopamine) affecting cortical areas. Type II is labeled negative because symptoms are essentially an absence of what should be, that is, lack of affect, lack of energy, and so on. Type II is thought to be nondopaminergic and caused by cortical structural changes (e.g., cerebral atrophy), not unlike Alzheimer's disease. Pathoanatomy consistently mentioned in the literature is decreased cerebral blood flow (CBF), particularly in frontal areas, and increased ventricular brain ratios (VBRs). The basic differences between type I and type II are listed in Box 19-4.

According to biological theory, antipsychotic drugs (drugs that block dopamine receptors) are likely to be beneficial for positive schizophrenia, and since negative schizophrenia is a structural process and is not specifically related to excessive levels of dopamine, dopamine-blocking drugs (antipsychotics) have relatively less effect. Accordingly, the more flagrant the psychotic symptoms (as in positive schizophrenia), the greater the likelihood of a positive response to antipsychotics.

See Box 19-5 for a number of the terms a student must know to be able to

## Box 19-5
## SPECIAL TERMS

**ambivalence** simultaneous opposite feelings (for example, love and hate for a person). Often expressed as approach-avoidance behavior.

**anergia** absence of energy.

**anhedonia** the inability to experience pleasure.

**apathy** lack of feeling, concern, interest, or emotion.

**autism** preoccupation with self without concern for external reality. A self-made private world of the schizophrenic.

**avolition** lack of motivation.

**blocking** interruption of thoughts due to psychological factors.

**clanging associations** use of rhyming words.

**concrete thinking** the use of literal meaning without ability to consider abstract meaning (for example, "don't cry over spilt milk" might be interpreted as meaning "because the milk is dirty").

**delusions** fixed, false beliefs of importance to the individual that are resistant to reason or fact.

**double-bind** conflicting demands by significant individuals in patient's life. Cannot meet both demands so is doomed to failure.

**echolalia** repetition of words heard.

**hallucinations** a false sensory perception not related to external stimuli (for example, seeing things that are not there).

**ideas of reference** the belief that some events have a special meaning (for example, people laughing are perceived as laughing at the patient).

**illusion** misinterpretation of a real sensory stimuli.

**loose association** thinking characterized by speech in which ideas shift from one subject to another that is unrelated.

**neologism** a word or expression invented by the patient.

**paranoia** extreme suspiciousness of others and their actions.

**premorbid** a state before onset of the disorder.

**psychosis** the inability to recognize reality complicated by severe thought disorder and the inability to relate to others.

**religiosity** preocupation with religious ideas or content.

**withdrawal** behaviors designed to avoid interacting with others.

**word salad** randomized set of words without any logical connection.

understand "morning" report and to discuss schizophrenic patients with other professionals.

## BEHAVIOR

> My identity began to fragment and seemed to blend with my environment. Rather than just enjoying the wind, for instance, I thought I had merged with it. I had to stare at the sun to appreciate its warmth. Yet gradually I was able to see myself separate from those things. As I neared discharge, I began to feel some stirring of belief in myself. It was not until much later that I made a conscious effort to develop a sense of control, realizing that I had the power to decide what form my life would take and who I would be (Leete, 1987).

As with all mental disorders, patients come to the attention of mental health professionals in only one of two ways. Either subjective symptoms are so troubling that the person seeks relief through professional intervention or the person draws attention to himself through behavior that bothers, concerns, or frightens other people (objective signs), who in turn assist him in securing professional help. These categories are not as discrete as first glance might indicate. For instance, hallucinations, which are a subjective phenomenon, can easily cause objective signs that will catch the eye of others (e.g., responding to a hallucination). Nonetheless, dividing expressions of schizophrenia into subjective symptoms and objective signs is a rational and convenient approach to understanding this mental disorder.

The six major categories of disorder in schizophrenia (Box 19-6) are readily grouped into objective signs or subjective symptoms. *Altered social interaction* and *alterations of activity* are highly visible to others (objective signs), whereas *altered perception, alterations of thought, altered consciousness,* and *alterations of affect* are not so visible. The Psychiatric Mental Health Nursing Diagnosis (PND-I) for Clients with Schizophrenic Disorders provides more categories of disordered or altered behavior and is found in Box 19-7.

### Objective signs

**Altered social interactions.** Schizophrenic patients often have altered interpersonal relationships that become apparent when one is working with them. Altered social interactions take several forms. Often these problems develop over a long period of time, well before the schizophrenic illness is diagnosed, and become more pronounced as the illness progresses. As positive symptoms (Box 19-4) occur, the patient's inability to adequately relate to others becomes more acute.

Frequently the patient will become less concerned with his appearance and may not bathe without persistent prodding. Table manners and other social skills we all "require" in others may diminish to the point where the patient is disheveled, smelly, and disgusting while eating. These behaviors are related to introspection (autism) and extreme self-absorption. The patient is so focused on internal processes that his external social world collapses. Schizophrenia can diminish the energy (anergia) level, which also complicates social interactions.

Interpersonal communication becomes inadequate and may be inappropriate. Again, internal processes are at work. Hostility, a not uncommon theme, also dis-

**Box 19-6**

## MAJOR OBJECTIVE AND SUBJECTIVE BEHAVIORAL DISORDERS IN SCHIZOPHRENIA

**OBJECTIVE SIGNS**

**Altered social interactions**

- Decreased attention to appearance; social amenities related to introspection and autism
- Inadequate or inappropriate communication
- Hostility
- Withdrawal

**Alterations of activity**

- Psychomotor agitation
- Catatonia

**SUBJECTIVE SYMPTOMS**

**Altered perception**

- Hallucinations
- Illusions
- Paranoid thinking

**Alterations of rhought**

- Flight of ideas
- Retardation
- Blocking
- Autism
- Ambivalence
- Loose associations
- Delusions
- Poverty of speech

**Altered consciousness**

- Confusion
- Incoherent speech
- Clouding
- Sense of "going crazy"

**Alterations of affect**

- Inappropriate, blunted, flattened, or labile affect
- Apathy
- Ambivalence
- Overreaction
- Anhedonia

Box 19-7
## PSYCHIATRIC NURSING DIAGNOSES (PND-1) FOR PATIENTS WITH SCHIZOPHRENIC DISORDERS

| | |
|---|---|
| 05.01 | Altered communication processes |
| 06.04 | Altered sensory perceptions |
| 06.04.03 | Hallucinations |
| 06.01.02 | Hyperalertness |
| 02.07 | Altered thought content |
| 02.07.01 | Delusions |
| 04.02.02 | Anxiety |
| 05.02.02.02 | Bizarre behaviors |
| 05.02.02.04 | Disorganized behaviors |
| 02.08.04 | Thought insertion |
| 02.07.03 | Magical thinking |
| 05.05.02 | Social isolation/withdrawal |
| 08.01.03 | Loneliness |

A. O'Toole, M. Loomis. 1989. "Classifying Human Responses in Psychiatric-Mental Health Nursing," from *Classification Systems for Describing Nursing Practice: Working Papers,* pp. 20-30. Kansas City, MO: American Nurses Association. Reprinted with permission.

tances the patient from others. Finally, the schizophrenic patient withdraws, further compromising his ability to engage in meaningful social interactions.

**Alterations of activity.** The schizophrenic patient also displays alterations of activity. He may be too active (psychomotor agitation), that is, unable to sit still, and continuously pacing, or he may be inactive (catatonic). Both signs respond to antipsychotic drugs. However, the nurse must be careful in her nursing diagnosis because psychomotor agitation could be caused by akathisia (an extrapyramidal side effect [EPS]) and rigidity could be neuroleptic malignant syndrome (NMS) instead of catatonia. Both EPS and NMS are side effects of antipsychotic drugs. In other words, while it would be appropriate to administer a p.r.n. dose of haloperidol for psychomotor agitation or catatonia, it would only serve to intensify akathisia and could prove fatal for the patient with NMS.

### Subjective symptoms

Subjective symptoms are, by definition, experienced by the patient in a personal way. The patient could hide these symptoms from others. In fact, some clinicians advise patients who resist psychiatric care to "keep your symptoms to yourself, and no one will ever know." Presumably there are persons in society who are not reporting their subjective symptoms to anyone and are thus avoiding psychiatric intervention. For the most part, however, subjective symptoms of schizophrenia spill over into behavior that is noticeable to others. Subjective symptoms can be grouped into the four categories previously mentioned.

**Altered perception.** Altered perception includes hallucinations, illusions, and paranoid thinking.

Hallucinations are false sensory perceptions. They can be auditory, visual, olfactory, tactile, gustatory, or somatic (strange body sensations). Auditory hallucinations are the most common and often take the form of accusations ("you slut," "hey, queer") or commands. Visual hallucinations are not as common in schizophrenia. The nurse should suspect a toxic process (drugs, fever) if visual hallucinations are present. Historically, hallucinations have been regarded either as expressions of excess brain activity (i.e., hyperdopaminergic) or as an adaptive behavior; that is, hallucinations help the patient cope with unacceptable thoughts (Bick and Kinsbourne, 1987). The former view blends with biological theories, while the latter takes on the language of the psychodynamic theorists.

Some clinicians believe command hallucinations (an auditory command to do something) are associated with danger-related events (Yesavage, 1983), whereas others (Hellerstein et al., 1987) find that most commands are ignored. More than 50% of command hallucinations are of a suicidal nature.

Bick and Kinsbourne (1987) found auditory hallucinations can be terminated by having the patient open his mouth very wide. They believe auditory hallucinations are precipitated by subvocal speech, which the patient interprets as coming from an external source. Subvocalization is impossible with the mouth wide open. Interestingly enough, none of their patients expressed relief when they were able to control hallucinations. Bick and Kinsbourne suggest that this finding may support the adaptive function of hallucinations. Thus hallucinations should not be terminated unless new coping skills are available to handle the stress.

Illusions are misinterpretations of real external stimuli. For example, a tree might be mistaken for a threatening person.

Paranoid thinking is manifested by a persistent interpretation of the actions of others as threatening or demeaning. Paranoid themes can color delusions and hallucinations, as well as ordinary behavior of others. Paranoid thinking is "correctable" with facts, whereas paranoid delusions are not.

A final example of altered perception is based on an observation that the ability to perceptually adapt (or selectively attend) is altered in schizophrenic patients.

> **Case study:** A patient was looking out a seventh-floor window. As the nurse approached to look, she noticed the activity in the yard below and commented. The patient, however, could not visually get past the wire mesh screen and was looking only at it. He was unable to filter out what for most people would not be a distraction at all. The inability to filter out extraneous stimuli (selectively attend) is a perceptual problem for some patients.

**Alterations of thought.** Alterations of thought are common in schizophrenia and they too are disturbing and frightening at times. Antipsychotic drugs are beneficial. Often insomnia diminishes as these symptoms subside, indicating that insomnia is a secondary symptom. Common thought disorders include flight of ideas, retardation, blocking, autism, ambivalence, loose associations, delusions, and poverty of speech or content.

Flight of ideas is rapid, with fragmented movements from one unconnected topic to another stimulated by either external or internal processes. Related phenomena include clanging (rhyming) and punning.

Retardation is a slowing down of mental activity. The patient may state, "I just can't think."

Blocking is the interruption of a thought and the inability to recall it. This is very disturbing to the patient and at times frightening. Blocking may be caused by intrusions of hallucinations, delusions, or emotional factors.

Autism occurs when the patient is so introspective that he is distracted from external events. The patient is preoccupied with himself and is oblivious to the reality around him, which results in a personalized view of reality.

Ambivalence is a state of having two opposite strong feelings simultaneously. The patient may be both attracted and repelled by the same person, object, or goal. Ambivalence (love-hate) toward a domineering parent is not uncommon. Another common example is the simultaneous need for people and the fear of people, resulting in an ambivalence-caused immobilization. The schizophrenic patient may be immobilized by his ambivalence regarding a matter as simple as deciding whether to drink orange juice or apple juice for breakfast.

Loose association is the stringing together of unrelated topics with a vague connection (as opposed to flight of ideas, in which there is no connection). For example, the children's rhyme "Mary Had a Little Lamb" may lead to "Mary was the mother of Christ who was born in a manger. I hate to lie on straw. It makes my skin itch. Have you ever had poison ivy? I have." The patient may even leave out some of the phrases, for example, "Mary had a little lamb. I hate to lie on straw. Have you ever had poison ivy?" but be able to make the connections clear if asked.

Delusions are fixed, false beliefs and can take many forms also. Delusional content can include somatic, grandiose, religious, nihilistic, referential, and paranoid content. An example of each type follows:

- *Somatic delusions:* A patient, after medical tests confirmed otherwise, still believes that "I have cancer in my stomach."
- *Grandiose delusions:* A patient stated, "I am Jesus Christ."
- *Religious delusions:* A woman attempted to kill her children because she believed the devil wanted her to do so. "The Devil told me to kill my children."
- *Nihilistic delusions:* A patient stated, "I am dead," and in response to "If you are dead, how can you talk?" said, "I don't know, but I'm dead."
- *Delusions of reference:* "The TV is talking about me. They are making fun of me."
- *Delusions of influence:* "I can control her with my thoughts."
- *Paranoid delusions:* "They all think that I am a homosexual."

Related phenomena found in some patients are the schizophrenic beliefs that thoughts can be inserted by others, that others can "read my mind," and that "my thoughts are being broadcast so that everyone can hear."

**Altered consciousness.** Altered consciousness is perhaps the most troubling to patients but, fortunately, also the most responsive to antipsychotic drugs. Manifestations of altered consciousness include confusion, incoherent speech, clouding, and a sense of "going crazy." The last item, "going crazy," deserves special mention. Many students are surprised on entering a psychiatric unit to find patients are not "crazy." In fact, although by definition psychiatric patients are struggling with mental disorders, psychiatric units are not wild, bizarre environments. Patients readily differentiate between the "normal struggle" of dealing with their mental disorder and the feeling of "going crazy" (loss of control).

**Alterations of affect.** Alterations of affect are varied and include inappropriate, flattened, blunted, or labile affect; apathy; ambivalence; overreaction; and anhedonia. If one laughs upon hearing bad news, the affective response does not match the circumstances and is *inappropriate.* If the patient is unable to generate much affect and the response to the bad news is weakly appropriate, the affect is blunted. The inability to generate any affective response is referred to as flattened affect. This is related to *apathy,* the lack of concern or interest. Labile affect is a condition in which emotional tone changes quickly. A patient may be telling a happy story, only to start crying and then, as quickly, return to the happy disposition. The rapid changing of emotional tone is referred to as labile affect.

Ambivalence, discussed under "Alterations of Thought," is a condition in which the patient is immobilized by opposite feelings. The patient may not be able to decide whether to go to a group meeting and may literally get up to go, only to sit back down, get up, sit down, and so on.

Another alteration of affect is the tendency to overreact to events. An analogy is the small child who, when closing a car door, needs to put so much energy into the effort that the door slams shut, offending the ears of adults nearby. Because of physical limitations, the child has to push as hard as he can to overcome inertia. Because of emotional limitations, the schizophrenic patient has to overreact to normal events to overcome his mental and social inertia. And, like the child, he may wind up offending the sensitivities of those nearby.

Anhedonia is the inability to experience pleasure or happiness. Perhaps the anhedonic person is the most miserable person of all.

## ETIOLOGY

Many authorities suggest that multiple factors cause schizophrenia. They do not believe that any single theory satisfactorily explains this disorder. Explanations can be broadly categorized into biological or psychological (psychodynamic) causes. These two categories parallel the "nature vs nurture" debate and the "organic vs functional" dichotomy discussed in Chapter 18. Biological theories and psychodynamic theories will be discussed. The discussion will close with a vulnerability-stress model, an eclectic approach that seems to capture the major forces at work in the genesis of schizophrenia.

### Biological theories

Biological theorists take the position that schizophrenia is caused by anatomical or physiological abnormalities. Biological explanations include biochemical, neurostructural, and genetic theories. If these theories provide the *sole* explanation of schizophrenia, interventions outside the scope of biological therapies (psychotropic drugs, somatic therapies) would be of little help to these patients. Since other treatment forms are helpful, biological theories do not completely explain schizophrenia.

Some clinicians reject the use of biological therapies because they find the use of psychotropic drugs and somatic therapies to be inhumane. Also some clinicians lack the professional qualifications required to administer these treatments (only physicians and nurses are qualified to participate in the administration of biological therapies). On a positive note, biological theories minimize the "blaming" inherent in other explanations. Just as viewing alcoholism as an illness has helped clinicians, families, and patients get beyond the blaming and on to the treatment, so too biological theories can facilitate the treatment of schizophrenia. To illustrate, the diabetic or cardiac patient has to learn to cope with illness (e.g., change in lifestyle, threat of death) and the psychiatric patient has to learn to cope with the limitations of his illness.

**Biochemical theories.**  Biochemical theory can be traced to 1952, when Delay and Deniker reported the antipsychotic effects of chlorpromazine (see Chapter 12). Andreasen and Olson (1982a), Crow (1982), and others have postulated a biochemical process that accounts for the positive symptoms of schizophrenia. The prevailing biochemical explanation is referred to as the dopamine hypothesis. According to this hypothesis, excessive dopaminergic activity in cortical areas causes acute positive (type I) symptoms of schizophrenia (hallucinations, delusions, and thought disorders). Excessive dopamine could be a result of increased dopamine synthesis, increased dopamine release or turnover, or an increase in the number and activity of dopamine receptors (Brown and Mann, 1985).

Other biochemical explanations are not as convincing as the dopamine hypothesis. Elevated norepinephrine levels, lowered homovanillic acid levels, and activity of various neuromodulators (including opioid peptides, GABA, prostaglandins, acetylcholine, and histamine) have been implicated in the genesis of schizophrenia; yet research efforts have not consistently linked these altered biochemical states with schizophrenia.

**Neurostructural theories.**  The neurostructural theorists propose that schizophrenia, particularly negative or type II schizophrenia, is a result of pathoanatomy. The three specific neurostructural changes mentioned most often are increased ventricular brain ratios (VBRs), brain atrophy, and decreased cerebral blood flow (CBF). Computed tomography (CT), magnetic resonance imaging (MRI), regional cerebral blood flow (RCBF), positron emission tomography (PET), and brain electrical activity mapping (BEAM) are techniques used to develop images of the brain (Andreasen, 1988). CT and MRI provide images of brain structure (i.e., for VBRs and brain atrophy). PET, RCBF, and BEAM provide information on both brain structure and brain activity.

1. Computed tomography (CT): This is the most widely used x-ray method for imaging the living brain. It causes the patient no pain but does expose him to radiation.

2. Magnetic resonance imaging (MRI): MRI provides clearer and more complete pictures than a CT scan but is more expensive. In this procedure the patient is surrounded by a strong magnetic field through which are projected pulses of radio frequency irradiation that realign hydrogen atoms. The altered radio frequency caused by the realignment is converted into an image by a computer.
3. Regional cerebral brain flow (RCBF): In this technique the patient inhales radioactive xenon gas, which is absorbed in the blood. The radioactive elements can be traced, thus providing information on blood flow in the brain.
4. Positron emission tomography (PET): Glucose containing radioactive atoms is given to a patient, and a computerized image of brain activity can be developed. Since glucose is the primary source of body energy, the extent of metabolic activity in specific brain sites can be traced. PET technology is expensive.
5. Brain electrical activity mapping (BEAM): BEAM is an advanced form of electroencephalography.

*Ventricular brain ratios.*  The finding that a significant subgroup of persons with schizophrenia have enlarged ventricles according to CT scan was first reported by Johnstone et al. (1976). Persons with enlarged ventricles have a poorer prognosis and exhibit the negative symptoms (type II) noted by Crow (1982), Andreasen et al. (1982c, 1985), Rabins et al. (1987), and others. These persons also suffer from disabling mental impairment and have limited social abilities (Seidman et al., 1987).

*Brain atrophy.*  Anatomical pathology in subcortical areas has been confirmed in postmortem examination of individuals with type II schizophrenia. Limbic, diencephalic, hypothalamic structures, as well as the amygdala and the substantia nigra, have been found to have neuropathological changes. Persons with these changes also have lower cortical gray matter blood flow, particularly in the prefrontal cortex (Berman et al., 1987). Cognitive demands, such as organizing, planning for the future, learning from experience, problem solving, introspection, and critical judgments, are compromised (Berman et al., 1987).

*Cerebral blood flow.*  A significant subgroup of schizophrenics with negative symptoms also demonstrate decreased CBF and consequent lowered metabolic activity in the prefrontal cortex as noted by in vivo studies of CBF and glucose metabolism (Ingvar and Franzen, 1974; Berman et al., 1987).

**Genetic theories.**  Schizophrenic patients seem to inherit a predisposition to this disorder. Their relatives have a greater incidence of schizophrenia than chance alone would allow. When one parent is affected there is a 15% probability that the child will have schizophrenia. If both parents have schizophrenia, the probability of affected children rises to 35% (Rosen, 1978). However, this higher incidence alone does not adequately address the nature (genetics) vs nurture (upbringing) debate, because a mentally disordered parent may rear children so inadequately that the children are predisposed to schizophrenia on the basis of the parenting skills and not the biology of the parent.

To control the "nurture" variable, researchers have studied twins. Both monozygotic (identical) and dizygotic (fraternal) twins have been studied. Monozygotic twins have consistently reported a higher concordancy rate (meaning both twins do or do not have symptoms of schizophrenia). Concordancy rates as high as 58% have been reported. This is 50 times greater than the general population. These findings would seem to establish the genetic or nature basis of schizophrenia; however, there are still extraneous variables to account for. For instance, most monozygotic twins are dressed alike and are often misidentified; their upbringing is identical too. No wonder, some would argue, that they have a high concordancy rate. Unless the identical upbringing is controlled, one still cannot report with confidence the relative impact of nature and nurture. To control for the variable of environment, studies have been conducted in situations in which monozygotic twins have been separated since birth and reared apart from each other. Monozygotic concordancy rates remain significantly higher in these studies also.

**Other biological considerations.** In addition to the foregoing, a number of neurological abnormalities, such as motor coordination (balance, hopping, finger-thumb opposition) are found among persons with schizophrenia. Heinrichs and Buchanan (1988) report that these abnormalities are associated with alterations of thought found in schizophrenia.

## Psychodynamic theories of schizophrenia

Psychodynamic theories of schizophrenia focus on the individual's response(s) to life events. The common theme among these theories is the internal reaction to life stressors or conflicts. These etiological explanations include developmental and family theories.

**Developmental theories of schizophrenia.** During the early part of the twentieth century two men—Adolph Meyer and Sigmund Freud—held to the significance of developmental psychiatry. They believed that the seeds of mental health and illness are sown in childhood and that to understand the present-day functioning of a person it is important to understand his upbringing or development (Bowlby, 1988). Freud focused on mental processes, on the unconscious forces that influence the person. The primary difference between the two men was one's focus on fantasy (Freud) and the other's focus on real life events (Meyer). An extension of their arguments is that events in early life can cause problems as severe as schizophrenia. Freudian concepts, such as poor ego boundaries, fragile ego, ego disintegration, inadequate ego development, super-ego dominance, regressed or id behavior, love-hate (ambivalent) relationships, and arrested psychosexual developments are still used meaningfully in discussions of schizophrenia.

Two later developmental theorists whose work more directly explains schizophrenia are Erikson (1968) and Sullivan (1953). Erikson theorized an eight-stage model of human development. He saw the first step "trust or mistrust," as crucial to later interpersonal relationships. The child who is deprived of a nurturing, loving environment—who is neglected or rejected—is vulnerable to mental disturbances. Inadequate passage through this stage predisposes the child to mistrust, isolative behaviors, and other asocial behavior. Therapeutic intervention focuses on reestablishment of trust through consistent, anxiety-free relationships.

Sullivan, using different terms, expressed essentially the same ideas. The absence of warm, nurturing attention during the early years blocks the expression of those same effective responses in later years. Without this capacity, persons exhibit disordered social interactions, as well as other disturbances. The person learns to avoid interpersonal interactions because of their painfulness to him.

**Family theories of schizophrenia.** Family theories of schizophrenia are naturally linked to developmental theories. If early-life experiences are crucial in development, the argument is made, then the family—the environment in which most people grow up—is significant in the development of mental health or ill health. Lack of a loving, nurturing primary caregiver, inconsistent family behaviors, and faulty communication patterns are thought responsible for mental problems in later life. *Outdated theories* specifically tailored for the families of schizophrenics were the *schizophrenogenic mother theory* and the *double-bind theory.* The double-bind theory describes family practices in which the child is "damned if he does and damned if he doesn't." For example, the child who is expected to do well in school but is criticized for taking time away from his family to study is in a double bind. Geiser et al. (1988) have called the family theories the "blame theories" and described a concomitant bias toward families of schizophrenics; that is, they are viewed as causative agents, saboteurs of treatment, toxic influences, and as patients themselves, and sometimes they are treated with hostility and distrust. Since families bear the brunt of preprofessional and postprofessional care of these patients, it is important to work with families without alienating them.

### Vulnerability-stress model of schizophrenia

As stated above, no single etiological theory adequately answers the questions about the genesis of schizophrenia. The vulnerability-stress model appreciates the variety of forces that have an impact on some persons, causing schizophrenia, and in other cases causing the broader schizophrenia-spectrum problems of schizoaffective disorders and schizophrenia-related personality disorders.

This model recognizes that both biological and psychodynamic predispositions to schizophrenia, when coupled with stressful live events, can precipitate a schizophrenic process. According to this model a person with a predisposed vulnerability to schizophrenia may avoid serious mental disorder if he is protected from the stresses of life. On the other hand, other persons with similar vulnerability may succumb to schizophrenia if exposed to stressors. To illustrate, a wealthy person might be spared the brunt of some stressors because of his wealth, whereas a poor member of society, struggling to meet basic needs, finds confrontation with stressors a daily event. According to this model, the second person is more likely to display symptoms of schizophrenia.

### SPECIAL ISSUES RELATED TO SCHIZOPHRENIA

A number of special issues need to be clarified to help the student focus on the breadth of concerns involved in the psychiatric nursing care of the patient with schizophrenia.

**Families of schizophrenics.** Families, particularly mothers, have often been blamed for the problems of persons with schizophrenia. Although research substantiates the state of turmoil in these families, many clinicians argue that dysfunctional families are not the cause of schizophrenia but, rather, the result of having a family member with this illness. Nevertheless, once a family becomes dysfunctional there is a high probability that it will have a negative effect on the schizophrenic member.

Families of schizophrenics tend to have inappropriate family cohesion, and family members are emotionally overinvolved, hostile, and critical. These families are said to have a high expressed emotion (EE) index (Herz, 1987 de Cangas, 1990). Mothers of schizophrenic children are said to "smother instead of mother" and to be over-involved and overprotective. These families also demonstrate poor communication patterns. There is a tendency to be unclear, to lack focus, and to participate in incomplete communication. With education and therapy, families can diminish their negative impact on patients. Persons with schizophrenia, on the other hand, can be a disruptive influence on the family, particularly when they are noncompliant with prescribed medications. Although there is consensus that all the family character-istics described above are present, it should be noted that these families are studied after schizophrenia is identified, years after the family may have been disrupted by the illness.

Although the "blame" may be warranted in some situations, in most it is not. Blaming the family leads to a sense of alienation between the family and the treatment team. Families bear the brunt of care outside the hospital. Sixty-five percent of discharged psychiatric patients are sent home to live with their families (Kane, 1984). The family's stake in the patient's care is obvious. As Geiser et al. (1988) point out, families become the caregivers and must learn to deal with strange and frightening behaviors, such as apathy, poor personal hygiene, and violence. They add: "Family crises are emotionally draining experiences, and they may escalate into an event involving police or mental health crisis service staff." As time goes on, these families tend to become more and more isolated and to feel more and more frustrated, helpless, and hopeless, even if they care very much.

**Depression related to schizophrenia.** Twenty-five percent of the patients with schizophrenia experience a postpsychotic depression as the schizophrenic symptoms begin to subside (Weiss et al., 1989). This factor contributes to the high incidence of suicide (10% of persons with schizophrenia die by suicide) among these patients (Becker, 1988). There are three explanations for this phenomenon:

1. Depression is a natural part of schizophrenia but is masked during the acute phase of the illness.
2. Depression is a reaction to schizophrenia in the same way that depression is a reaction to physical illness.
3. The biological nature of the illness and the drugs used to treat it produce a depressive syndrome (Weiss et al., 1989). The relationship between schizo-phrenia and depression is underscored by the improvement in poorly func-tioning schizophrenic patients when they are treated with antidepressants (Mason et al., 1990).

**Relapse.** Both clinical opinion and research studies support the observation that many patients with schizophrenia experience relapse and remission of symptoms throughout their illness. Persons most likely to suffer relapse are those having frequent face-to-face contact with high-EE family members (Herz, 1984; de Cangas, 1990), those exposed to stressors, and those not given antipsychotic medications (or not taking them if they were prescribed). Herz (1984) has outlined five phases of relapse:

1. Overextension, a sense of being overwhelmed
2. Restricted consciousness, a stage of boredom and apathy
3. Disinhibition, the first psychotic stage
4. Psychotic disorganization
5. Psychotic resolution, marked by decreased anxiety and increased organization

A recovered patient with schizophrenia described her relapse as occurring in stages. She reported the following sequence:

> In the first stage, I feel just a bit estranged from myself... In the second stage, everything appears a bit clouded... In the third stage, I believe I am beginning to understand why terrible things are happening to me; others are causing it... In the fourth stage, I become chaotic and see, hear, and believe all manner of things. I no longer question my beliefs, but act on them (Lovejoy, 1984).

**Respite care.** Respite care is a treatment approach designed to decrease relapse or exacerbation of schizophrenic symptoms and to afford families relief from their caregiver responsibilities. Respite care programs (Geiser, 1988) provide "mini-hospitalizations" of a few days every 6 to 8 weeks to reinforce positive growth and to intervene in the early stages of relapse.

**Stress.** According to the vulnerability-stress model presented above, persons with schizophrenia are vulnerable to stress. The therapeutic mandate is to minimize the impact of stress on the vulnerable person. Two basic strategies are used, the reduction of real stress and the incorporation of healthy coping techniques in the patient's repertoire of daily living skills. Because of their economic and social status, many vulnerable persons face major stressors (e.g., those at the bottom rungs of society have more daily stress). Stated another way, those most vulnerable to stress have more stress to handle. Helping patients learn to identify and avoid stressful events is an important task for the psychiatric nurse.

**Drug abuse among schizophrenics.** A high percentage of schizophrenic persons abuse drugs. Miller and Tanenbaum (1989) found that 55% of the schizophrenic patients they studied abused drugs. Alcohol, marijuana, and cocaine accounted for 88% of the drugs abused. Drug abuse has a negative effect on the treatment program of these patients. Drug abuse may also account for the over-representation of schizophrenic persons in jail. Teplin (1990) found that 2.74% of the jail population sufferd from schizophrenia.

---

**PSYCHOTHERAPEUTIC MANAGEMENT**

> The schizophrenic is always fighting a battle within his brain. If his mind is not divided against itself, he is fighting against voices, imaginary people, hallucinations, or other terrifying symptoms. Most schizophrenics go on for years fighting and struggling alone without anyone to help make them stronger than their symptoms (Ruocchio, 1989).

Psychotherapeutic management is aimed at helping the patient become "stronger than his symptoms." The nursing interventions used in the treatment of the patient with schizophrenia flow from the appropriate development of the nursing care plan.

**PSYCHOTHERAPEUTIC NURSE-PATIENT RELATIONSHIP** The objective of this discussion is to provide specific principles of therapeutic communication for working with the patient with schizophrenia.

- The nurse should be calm when talking to the patient. Anxiety is contagious and is contraindicated when one is working with a patient with schizophrenia.
- The nurse should accept the patient as he is but not accept all behaviors. Acceptance increases self-worth.
- Keep promises. Dependability builds trust.
- Never reinforce hallucinations or delusions. The nurse cannot agree with a hallucination or a delusion. On the other hand, arguing is nonproductive and may make the perceptual disorder stronger. Simply state your perception of reality, voice doubt about the patient's perceptions, and move on to discuss "real" people or events.
- Provide reality testing.
- Reinforce reality.
- Orient the patient to time, person, and place. Orientation reinforces reality and builds on strengths.
- Do not touch the patient without warning. Patients who are paranoid may perceive a touch as a threat and strike out.
- Avoid whispering or laughing when the patient is unable to hear all the conversation. The suspicious patient will interpret these actions personally.
- Reinforce positive behaviors. Appropriate reinforcement leads to increased positive behaviors.
- Be consistent. Consistency increases trust.
- Be honest with the patient. Honesty increases trust.
- Avoid competitive activities for some patients. Competition is threatening and can lead to decreased self-esteem.
- Do not embarrass the patient. Persons with schizophrenia retain the ability to feel embarrassed and often avoid contacts for fear of being embarrassed.
- For withdrawn patients, start with one-to-one interactions with the nurse. Even in group situations, it is probably most therapeutic for interactions to be a series of nurse-to-patient rather than patient-to-patient interactions. Nurse-to-patient interactions are less threatening to the patient and can evolve into a wider circle of social interaction.
- Allow and encourage verbalization of feelings. The patient is helped if he can say what he thinks without the nurse's becoming defensive.

Following are more general principles for developing a therapeutic nurse-patient relationship, *with examples* of appropriate responses.

1. Do not argue about delusions. Arguing tends to reinforce the delusion and make the patient angry. Reflect reality and attempt to distract the patient in a matter-of-fact manner.

> *Patient:* The FBI and the Mafia are both after me. What am I going to do?
> *Nurse:* I know your thought seems real to you; however, it does not seem reasonable to me. Let's go into the dayroom and talk.

Proceed to talk about occupational therapy efforts (or some such topic), which will focus on the patient's real world.

2. Do not reinforce hallucinations. To do so minimizes the patient's condition.

> *Patient:* The voices are calling me terrible names. Can't you hear them?
> *Nurse:* I understand that you are hearing voices; however, I do not hear anything but your voice and mine.

3. If patient is acting odd and the nurse suspects he is hallucinating, she should ask the patient about it.

> *Patient behavior:* Looks around the room, eyes darting to corners of the room.
> *Nurse:* It looks like you might be listening to something. Are you hearing voices?

4. Help the patient identify stressors that might precipitate hallucinations or delusions. This effort might lead to identification and avoidance of triggering events.

> *Patient:* Nurse, I started hearing the voices last night right after I went to bed.
> *Nurse:* Tell me about your evening last night. There may be a link between something that happened and your hearing voices again.

5. Focus on real people and real events. This helps patients stay in touch with reality.

> *Patient:* I keep hearing the voices.
> *Nurse:* I understand, but I want to help you focus away from those voices. Let's go to the dayroom and talk.

Proceed to bring patient closer to reality by talking about his daily life.

6. Be diligent in attempting to understand the patient. It is always therapeutic to help the patient communicate what it is he wants to say.

> *Patient:* I could have been bitten. It was never a dog's day.
> *Nurse:* I am not sure what you are saying, but I want to understand. Are you talking about almost being hurt?

7. Attempt to balance between siding with inappropriate behavior and crushing a fragile ego.

> *Patient:* I hit Bill yesterday.
> *Nurse:* I know you got upset with him. Let's talk about what you can do differently next time you get upset that might work better.

## PSYCHOPHARMACOLOGY

Medication is invaluable in helping the schizophrenic feel better. I am grateful that I/If me it takes away some of the [illegible] a day intensity of visual distortions, nightmarish states one right after another, and "spacey" attacks (Ruocchio, 1989).

The student is encouraged to review Chapter 12, which provides a complete discussion of antipsychotic drugs, the drugs of choice for schizophrenia and other psychoses. Usual daily dosages are given in Table 12-1. See Box 12-2 for side effects and appropriate nursing interventions.

Schizophrenic patients need to take psychotropic drugs as prescribed. As many as 46% of inpatients and 60% of outpatient psychiatric patients do not comply with their medication regimen. See Box 19-8 for nursing interventions to help assure compliance.

Clozapine, a new antipsychotic drug, became available for use in 1990. Clinical studies indicate that clozapine can help previously treatment-resistant schizophrenic patients to dramatically improve (Green and Salzman, 1990).

### MILIEU MANAGEMENT

Intensely active, highly staffed units may be disruptively intense for schizophrenic patients, who more often benefit from decreased stimulation and a greater measure of solitude and clear role models (Simpson and May, 1982).

Milieu management is an important dimension of psychiatric nursing care of the schizophrenic patient. The reader is referred to Unit IV for a complete discussion of milieu management. General principles that specifically address the environment of the schizophrenic patient are considered on p.p. 304 to 306.

### Box 19-8
### NURSING INTERVENTIONS TO INCREASE COMPLIANCE

- Observe patient for side effects and intervene accordingly. Akathisia is a troubling side effect that patients cannot tolerate.
- When giving tablets or pills, make sure the patient does not "cheek" the medications (hide the medication in cheeks or mouth) to spit them out or hoard them for later.
- Teach the patient and his family about drugs including side effects, potential interactions, dosage schedule when discharged, and so on.
- Depot drugs (see Chapter 12) are effective for patients who do not comply with drug therapy.

### The disruptive patient

- Set limits on disruptive behavior.
- Decrease environmental stimuli. Place escalating patient in a low-stimulus environment.
- Frequently observe escalating patient in order to intervene. Intervention (e.g., medication) before acting out occurs protects the patient and others physically and prevents embarrassment for the patient later.
- Modify environment to minimize objects that can be used as weapons. Some units use furniture so heavy that it cannot be lifted by most persons.
- Be careful in stating what the staff will do if a patient acts out; however, follow through, once a violation occurs (e.g., "if you break the window, we will place you in restraints").
- When using restraints, provide for patient safety by evaluating status of hydration, nutrition, elimination, and circulation.

### The withdrawn patient

- Arrange nonthreatening activities that involve the patient in "doing something," for example, walking tour of park, leather work, painting.
- Arrange furniture in semicircle or around a table so that patients are "forced" to sit with someone. Interactions are permitted in this situation but should not be demanded. Sit with patient in silence if he cannot respond yet. Some will move a chair away anyway.
- Help the patient participate in decision making as appropriate (for example, selecting menu for next day's meals).
- Provide community meetings in which each patient is encouraged to respond in some way. Structured activities help (for example, taking turns reading a passage or rehearsing a "speech" to be given in another meeting).
- Provide nonthreatening socialization opportunities with the nurse on a one-to-one basis, with the goal of progressing to spontaneous patient-patient experiences.
- Reinforce appropriate grooming and hygiene (assist at first if needed).
- Provide remotivation and resocialization group experiences.
- Provide psychosocial rehabilitation, training in community living, and social and health care skills.

### The suspicious patient

- Be matter of fact in dealing with this person.
- Staff should not laugh or whisper around the patient unless the patient can hear what was said. Clarify if patient has misperceived what was said.
- Do not touch the suspicious patient without warning him. Avoid close physical contact.
- Be consistent in activities (for example, time, staff, approach to activity).
- If patient fears being poisoned, let him open a can of food and serve himself. Obviously this may be difficult to arrange in some hospital settings.

- Maintain eye contact.
- Do not "slip" medications into juices or foods without talking to the patient "Catching" the nurse in this act of doing this will undermine his sense of trust.

## The patient with impaired communication

- Provide opportunities for the patient to make simple decisions.
- Be patient and do not pressure to make sense.
- Do not place the patient in group activities that would cause frustration, damage self-esteem, or overtax his abilities.
- Provide opportunities for purposeful psychomotor activity (for example, painting, ceramic work, exercise, gross motor games).

## The patient with disordered perceptions

- Attempt to provide distracting activities.
- Discourage situations in which the patient talks to others about his disordered perception.
- Monitor TV selections. Some programs seem to cause more perceptual problems than others (for example, horror movies). If staff cannot censor, then be available to discuss and clarify afterward.
- Monitor for command hallucinations that may increase potential for dangerousness.
- Have staff available in dayroom so that patient can talk to real people about real people or real events.
- Paging systems may reinforce perceptual problems and should be eliminated if possible.

## The disorganized patient

- Remove patient to less stimulating environment.
- Provide calm environment; the staff should appear calm.
- Provide safe and relatively simple activities for the patient.
- Provide information boards with schedules and refer to them often so patient can begin to use this as an orienting function.
- Help protect patient's self-esteem by intervening if patient does something that is embarrassing (for example, patient's taking clothes off or becoming overtly sexual).
- Assist with grooming and hygiene.

## The patient with altered levels of activity

### *Hyperactivity*

- Allow the patient to stand or get up for a few minutes during group meetings.
- Provide safe environment and place to pace without bothering other patients inordinately.
- Encourage participation in activities or games that do not require fine motor skills or intense concentration.

## Case Study

Bill, a 25-year-old man, was brought to the hospital by police. He was in a downtown bus station preaching loudly. He stated in the emergency room that he had spoken to God and that God had told him to save San Francisco. He admitted to hearing both God and Satan arguing and was terrified at times. In talking with his family, it is discovered that Bill was a solid student until about a year ago. He began to struggle in school but continued to pass his coursework. He dropped out of school 3 months ago. His family believes his problem started when his girlfriend of 4 years broke off their engagement.

He began hearing voices a couple of weeks ago, according to his family, but the family lost contact with him until they were notified of this hospitalization. His family is committed to helping Bill. On admission to the unit, Bill is oriented to time, place, and person but states: "God has chosen me to be his special angel. I must save the sinners of San Francisco." Bill then stands up and turns his head rapidly from side to side. When asked, he says: "God and Satan are arguing about what I should do. Stop. I don't want to die. Save me." See Bill's nursing care plan on the opposite page.

### *Immobility*

- If patient is catatonic or immobile, provide nursing care to minimize circulatory problems or loss of muscle tone.
- Provide adequate diet, exercise, and rest.
- Maintain bowel and bladder function and intervene before problems arise.
- Observe patient to prevent victimization (physical and verbal) by others.

## ■ Other Psychotic Disorders

In addition to schzophrenia, there are several other psychotic disorders with which the student should be familiar. Interventions for these disorders are directed at prominent symptoms and are the same as the interventions used for those symptoms in persons with schizophrenia.

**Delusional (paranoid) disorder.** These persons manifest symptoms similar to those seen in the patient with schizophrenia. Substantial differences do exist and necessitate a diagnostic differentiation. The following symptoms differ delusional disorders from schizophrenic disorders:

- Delusions have a basis in reality
- Hallucinations are not dominant

Nursing Care Plan

WEEKLY UPDATE: ___6-21-90___

NAME: _____Bill Wilson_____    ADMISSION DATE: ___6-14-90___

DSM-III-R DIAGNOSIS: _____295.93 Schizophrenia: undifferentiated type_____

*ASSESSMENT:*
*Areas of strength:* past accomplishments; past good heterosexual IPRs; alert, oriented to time, place, person; acute symptoms respond to medications; family support.
*Problems:* religious hallucinations, religious delusions, thought disorder; broken engagement; dropped out of school.

*DIAGNOSES:* auditory hallucinations related to thought disturbance. Anxiety related to disturbed perceptions.

*PLANNING:*                                                          Date met
*Short-term goals:* Patient will voice freedom from hal-    _____
lucinations
   Patient will report lack of fear of others.              _____
   Patient will discuss feelings about loss of girlfriend.  _____
*Long-term goals:* Patient will verbalize need for medi-    _____
cation and counseling.
   Patient will make appointment for outpatient program     _____
assessment in mid-July.
   Patient will return to school in September.              _____

*IMPLEMENTATION/INTERVENTIONS:*
*Nurse-patient relationship:* do not reinforce hallucinations and delusions; voice doubt; encourage identification of strengths and accomplishments; encourage expression of feelings about broken engagement; discuss plans for immediate future.
*Psychopharmacology:* Haldol 5 mg t.i.d. p.o. (concentrate); Cogentin 1 mg p.r.n. for EPS.
*Milieu management:* provide distracting activities; monitor TV, particularly religious programming and movies with satanic themes; encourage participation in self-esteem group and anger management group.

*EVALUATION:* Patient responding to Haldol. Will see Ms. White, RN, CS, once a week as outpatient. Appt. 7-7-90 with R. Jones for education counseling.

## Case Study

A 40-year-old woman with a history of multiple admissions is admitted to the floor. Emma Rice was found wandering downtown incoherent and disheveled. During the assessment interview Emma is noted to have a flat affect and is withdrawn. She reports not seeing her family for 5 years and cannot remember when she last held a job. There is no history of hallucinatory or delusional thought content in this recent occurrence. The staff know Emma and know that during past admissions she has responded to chlorpromazine. On admission Emma says: "Let me go. Go on, onward, backwards. (pause) Emma hide, died." When asked where she lives she slowly responds: "Over there, somewhere, anywhere, nowhere." Emma's board and care operator knows her well and has indicated she is holding a bed for Emma. See the opposite page for Emma's nursing care plan.

- Behavior is relatively normal except in relation to this delusion
- Symptoms do not meet the criteria for schizophrenia

**Brief reactive psychosis.** Psychotic symptoms occur apparently in response to stressful life events. Symptoms do not last longer than 1 month, and a return to normal functioning occurs.

**Schizophreniform disorders.** Symptoms do not last longer than 6 months, and a return to normal functioning is possible. There are no visible precipitation stressors as in brief reactive psychosis.

**Schizoaffective disorders.** Schizophrenic symptoms are dominant but are accompanied by major depressive or manic symptoms.

**Induced psychotic disorders.** A psychotic state related to association with another psychotic person and evidenced by a marked delusional system.

**Atypical psychosis.** Psychotic symptoms that do not meet the criteria listed for other psychotic disorders.

### KEY CONCEPTS

1. The concept of schizophrenia has emerged over the past 100 years as a result of the contributions of early theorists such as Kraepelin and Bleuler and modern-day theorists such as Nancy Andreasen.
2. The DSM-III-R identifies five subtypes: catatonic, disorganized, paranoid, undifferentiated, and residual.
3. Bleuler contributed what he thought to be the four primary symptoms of schizophrenia: affective disturbances, loose associations, ambivalence, and autism (also known as "Bleuler's 4 A's").

Nursing Care Plan

WEEKLY UPDATE: _____7-7-90_____

NAME: _____Emma Rice_____          ADMISSION DATE: _____6-11-90_____

DSM-III-R DIAGNOSIS: _____295.12, Schizophrenia, disorganized type_____

### ASSESSMENT:
*Areas of strength:* Board and care operator knows Emma well and wants her back. Staff know and understand Emma.

*Problems:* Affective flattening, loose associations, withdrawn, chronic course of illness, no family support.

*DIAGNOSES:* Incoherent speech related to thought disturbance. Poor hygiene related to thought disturbance. Withdrawal related to lack of trust. Lack of housing related to chronic illness.

|  | Date met |
|---|---|
| **PLANNING:** | |
| *Short-term goals:* Patient will talk in coherent manner. | 6-30-90 |
| Patient will carry out ADLs. | 7-2-90 |
| Patient will participate in nonthreatening activities. | 6-17-90 |
| *Long-term goals:* Patient will maintain outpatient program. | |
| Patient will return to board and care. | Disc 7-9-90 |
| Patient will comply to medication regimen. | |

### IMPLEMENTATION/INTERVENTIONS:
*Nurse-patient relationship:* be patient; treat as adult; encourage hygiene and appropriate dress; reinforce positive social behaviors; start with one-to-one interactions with nurse and then encourage independent social behaviors.

*Psychopharmacology:* Chlorpromazine 150 mg t.i.d. p.o. (concentrate). May need long-acting form on discharge.

*Milieu management:* start pt in OT by end of week; invite pt to sit with staff and other pts; encourage to make decisions about meals or some other simple decisions; provide resocialization group experience and community living education.

*EVALUATION:* Pt stabilized on medications, will see Ms. Brown, RN, CS, once a week and will attend outpt resocialization group five times a week. Board and care operator will monitor drugs (single h.s. dose) and arrange transportation.

4. Andreasen (1982), Crow (1982), and others have conceptualized schizophrenia subtypes into two categories: type I (positive symptoms and very treatable with antipsychotic drugs) and type II (negative symptoms).

5. Objective signs of schizophrenia include alterations of social interactions and alterations of activity.

6. Subjective symptoms of schizophrenia include alterations of perception, thoughts, consciousness, and affect.

7. Etiological explanations are numerous and include both biological (dopamine hypothesis, pathoanatomy, and genetic theories) and psychodynamic theories (developmental theory, family theory).

8. The dopamine hypothesis, the view that schizophrenia is a result of increased bioavailability of dopamine in the brain, is a widely held theory of schizophrenia.

9. Antipsychotic drugs block dopamine receptors and relieve acute symptoms of schizophrenia.

10. Nursing interventions include therapeutic nurse-patient relationship (i.e., not reinforcing delusional statements), psychopharmacology (i.e., administering haloperidol 5 mg t.i.d. and evaluating for side effects), and milieu management (i.e., providing an emotionally safe environment), all supported by an understanding of psychopathology.

## REFERENCES

Andreasen NC and Olsen S: Negative vs positive schizophrenia, Arch Gen Psychiatry 39:789, 1982a.

Andreasen NC: Negative symptoms in schizophrenia, Arch Gen Psychiatry 39:784, 1982b.

Andreasen NC, Olsen S, Dennert JW, and Smith MR: Ventricular enlargement in schizophrenia: relationship to positive and negative symptoms, Am J Psychiatry 139:297, 1982c.

Andreasen NC: Positive vs negative schizophrenia: a critical evaluation, Schizophr Bull 11:380, 1985.

Andreasen NC: Brain imaging: applications in psychiatry, Science 239:1381, March 18, 1988.

Becker RE: Depression in schizophrenia, Hosp Community Psychiatry 39:1269, 1988.

Berman KF et al: A relationship between anatomical and psysiological brain pathology in schizophrenia: lateral cerebral ventricular size predicts cortical blood flow, Am J Psychiatry 144:1277, 1987.

Bick PA and Kinsbourne M: Auditory hallucinations and subvocal speech in schizophrenic patients, Am J Psychiatry 144:222, 1987.

Bleuler E: Dementia praecox or the group of schizophrenias (1908), translated by Zinkin J: New York, 1950, International University Press.

Bowlby J: Developmental psychiatry comes of age, Am J Psychiatry 145:1, 1988.

Brown RP and Mann JJ: A clinical perspective on the role of neurotransmitters in mental disorders, Hosp Community Psychiatry 36:141, 1985.

Cohen CI and Berk LA: Personal coping styles of schizophrenic outpatients, Hosp Community Psychiatry 36:407, 1985.

Crow TJ: Two dimensions of pathology in schizophrenia: dopaminergic and nondopaminergic, Psychopharmacol Bull 18:22, 1982.

Dean SR: Focus on schizophrenia: the role of RISE and the Dean award. Schizophr Bull 5:509, 1979.

de Cangas JPC: Exploring expressed emotion: does it contribute to chronic mental illness? J Psychosoc Nurs 28(2):31, 1990.

Erikson E: Childhood and society, New York, 1968, WW Norton, 1968.

Geiser R, Hoche L, and King J: Respite care for the mentally ill patients and their families, Hosp Community Psychiatry 39:291, 1988.

Green AI and Salzman C: Clozapine: benefits and risks, Hosp Community Psychiatry 41:379, 1990.

Harding CM, Zubin J, and Stauss JS: Chronicity in schizophrenia fact, partial fact, or artifact? Hosp Community Psychiatry 38:477, 1987.

Heinrichs DW and Buchanan RW: Significance and meaning of neurological signs in schizophrenia, Am J Psychiatry 145:11, 1988.

Hellerstein D, Frosch W, and Koenigsberg HW: The clinical significance of command hallucinations, Am J Psychiatry 144:219, 1987.

Herz MI: Recognizing and preventing relapse in patients with schizophrenia, Hosp Community Psychiatry 35:344, 1984.

Ingvar DH and Franzen G: Abnormalities of cerebral blood flow distribution in patients with chronic schizophrenia, Acta Psychiatr Scand 50:425, 1974.

Johnstone EC et al: Cerebral ventricular size and cognitive impairment in chronic schizophrenia, Lancet 2:924, 1976.

Jones BE and Gray BA: Problems in diagnosing schizophrenia and affective disorders among blacks, Hosp Community Psychiatry 37:61, 1986.

Kane C: The family's response to deinstitutionalization, J Psychosoc Nurs Mental Health Serv 22:19, 1984.

Kendler KS, Gruenberg AM, and Tsuang MT: A family study of the subtypes of schizophrenia, Am J Psychiatry 145:57, 1988.

Kraepelin E: Clinical Psychiatry: a textbook for students and physicians (translated by Defendorf AR), New York, 1902, Macmillan.

Leete E: The treatment of schizophrenia: a patient's perspective. Hosp Community Psychiatry 38:486, 1987.

Liberman RA et al: Social skills training for chronic mental patients, Hosp Community Psychiatry 36:396, 1985.

Lovejoy M: Recovery from schizophrenia: a personal odyssey, Hosp Community Psychiatry 35:809, 1984.

Mason SE, Gingerich S and Siris SG: Patient's and caregiver's adaptation to improvement in schizophrenia, Hosp Community Psychiatry 41:541, 1990.

Miller FT and Tanenbaum JD: Drug abuse in schizophrenia, Hosp Community Psychiatry 40:847, 1989.

Rabins P et al: Increased ventricle-to-brain ration in late-onset schizophrenia, Am J Psychiatry 144:1216, 1987.

Rosen H. A guide to clinical psychiatry, Coral Gables, Fla., 1978, Mnemosyne.

Ruocchio PJ: How psychotherapy can help the schizophrenic patient, Hosp Community Psychiatry 40:188, 1989.

Seidman LJ et al: Lateral ventricular size and social network differeniation in young, nonchronic schizophrenic patients, Am J Psychiatry 144:512, 1987.

Simpson G and May P: Schizophrenic disorders. In Greist J, Jefferson J, and Spitzer R, editors: Treatment of mental disorders, New York, 1982, Oxford University Press.

Sullivan HS: The interpersonal theory of psychiatry, New York, 1953, WW Norton.

Teplin LA: The prevalence of severe mental disorder among male urban jail detainees: comparison with the epidemiologic catchment area program, Am J Public Health 80:663, 1990.

Weiss KJ, Valdiserri EV and Dubin WR: Understanding depression in schizophrenia, Hosp Community Psychiatry 40:849, 1989.

Yagi G and Itoh H: Follow-up of 11 patients with potentially reversible tardive dyskinesia, Am J Psychiatry 144:1496, 1987.

Yesavage JA: Inpatient violence and the schizophrenic patient, Acta Psychiatr Scand 67:353, 1983.

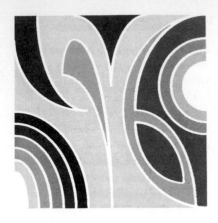

## CHAPTER 20

# Mood Disorders

LEARNING OBJECTIVES
After reading this chapter you should be able to

- Describe the historical classifications of depression.
- Recognize the DSM-III-R criteria and terminology for mood disorders.
- Compare and contrast the objective and subjective symptoms of a major depression and a manic episode.
- Describe the biological and psychodynamic explanations for mood disorders.
- Develop a nursing care plan for a person suffering from depression.
- Develop a nursing care plan for a person suffering from bipolar illness.
- Evaluate the effectiveness of nursing interventions for depressed and bipolar patients.

Everyone experiences the highs and lows of life. Mood disorders are characterized by exaggerations of that variability in mood. Being too high (mania,
euphoria) or too low (depression, dysthymia), or experiencing both extreme result in
intrapersonal and interpersonal anguish. However, because experiencing life's ups
and downs is normal, and indeed it would be unnatural not to do so, it is not always
clear where the dividing line between normal and abnormal or between healthy
and unhealthy should be drawn. For instance, each of us occasionally feels sadness
or guilt in response to some life event (e.g., loss of a loved one) or some wrong
we have done (e.g., lying on a job interview, cheating on a spouse). To have these
feelings is normal. Such experiences are intense but are typically self-limiting because
of coping and problem-solving skills we develop. The "depressed" person and others
in that person's life recognize the "normalness" of the response, and the person
eventually is able to "get on with life." In contrast, if the sadness or guilt goes on
too long, an imaginary line is crossed over at some point and a clinically significant
mood disorder exists. On the other hand, everyone feels elation from time to time
in response to life events. But again, inappropriate or excessive elation can cause
anguish and may require professional intervention.

Mood disorders are divided into bipolar disorders and depressive disorders. A
bipolar diagnosis indicates the presence of one or more manic or hypomanic episodes, usually accompanied by a history of depression. A depressive episode is
characterized by depression without a history of manic episodes. This chapter discusses both affective extremes (depression and mania). Familiarity with the terms
listed in Box 20-1 is required for an understanding of discussions dealing with mood
disorders.

## DEPRESSION

Everyone feels sad or guilty from time to time in response to the events of life. If
the sadness or guilt persists for too long, a diagnosable condition exists (see Box
20-2 for symptoms of depression). When depression occurs as a reaction to a life
event, historically such a condition has been referred to as reactive depression. Most
lay people and many nurses conceptualize all depression as being a reaction to some
life event (losses through death, shame, failure, etc.). In fact, not all depression is
related to a variant of loss but can occur seemingly independent of life events.
Because of this natural tendency to look for a "reason," many nurses become frustrated and even a little annoyed when the patient is without "a good reason" for
being depressed.

Depression has been with man since the beginning of existence. History contains
tales of commoner and king who experienced depression. In the Bible King Saul is
noted to have had deep bouts of depression that were soothed by the flute playing
of the shepherd boy David. Jeremiah was referred to as the weeping prophet. In
more modern times such noted statesmen as Abraham Lincoln and Winston Churchill
have recorded their struggles with deep depression. The effects of depression have
been felt politically as recently as the 1972 presidential election, when the press
discovered that a vice-presidential candidate had received electroconvulsive therapy
for depression. The disclosure caused his removal from the ticket.

Box 20-1

SPECIAL TERMS

**apathy** lack of feeling, absence of emotion, indifference, inability to be motivated, occasionally a mechanism for avoiding intense emotion.

**bipolar disorder** a disturbance in mood in which the symptoms of mania have occurred at least one time. An episode of depression may or may not have occurred.

**constant observation** continuous bedside or one-to-one staffing to prevent self-destructive behavior

**cortisol** a hormone formed in the adrenal cortex. The excretion of this hormone is suppressed in non-endogenously depressed and normal persons after injection of dexamethasone.

**cyclothymia** mood swings between hypomania (less severe than a manic episode) and depression (less severe than major depression).

**double depression** a patient with dysthymia who recovers from major depression only to still be dysthymic.

**depressive personality** a life-style or character disorder in which the person is chronically "down," is pessimistic, is a complainer, is unhappy with job, family, life position.

**dexamethasone suppression test (DST)** a diagnostic test for endogenous depression. A single injection of dexamethasone is given, followed by monitoring of urine or blood cortisol levels. In endogeously depressed persons cortisol levels do not fall.

**dysphoria** disquiet, restlessness, malaise.

**dysthymia** chronic depressed mood for at least 2 years. Not as severe as major depression.

**endogenous depression** produced within the person or caused by factors within the person as opposed to a reaction to some life stressor. Endogenous depression is thought to be related to neurotransmitter deficiency.

**ECT (electroconvulsive therapy)** a form of somatic therapy used in the treatment of depression that has proved refractory to other forms of therapy (see Chapter 27).

**euphoria** a subjective feeling of well-being characterized by confidence and assurance. Excessive, not normal.

**hypomania** a state of mania that is less severe than a manic episode. A mild form of mania.

**mania** a state of extreme excitement, euphoria, and accelerated mental and physical activity.

**MAOIs (monoamine oxidase inhibitors)** a major class of antidepressants. Generally, because of their potential for serious side effects, this class of drugs is used only after tricyclic antidepressants have proved ineffective.

**melancholia** a mental disorder characterized by extreme sadness and depression. This disorder usually occurs after the age of 45 years and is accompanied by vegetative symptoms.

**secondary depression** major depression related to a nonaffective disorder.

**TCAs (tricyclic antidepressants)** usually the first choice when antidepressants are indicated.

**vegetative symptoms** loss of appetite and weight (or the opposite), insomnia or loss of interest, anergia, guilt, decreased concentration, early morning awakening, and diurnal mood fluctuations that are worse in the morning.

## Box 20-2
## SYMPTOMS OF DEPRESSION

| Common symptoms | Other symptoms |
|---|---|
| Apathy | Fatigue |
| Sadness | Thoughts of death |
| Sleep disturbances (insomnia or | Decreased libido |
| hypersomnia) | Ruminations of inadequacy |
| Hopelessness | Psychomotor agitation |
| Helplessness | Private verbal beratings of self |
| Worthlessness | Spontaneous crying without apparent |
| Guilt | cause |
| Anger (covert or overt) | Dependency |
|  | Passiveness |

Adapted from Keltner NL: Drugs for the treatment of depression and mania. In Shlafer M and Marieb E, editors: The nurse, pharmacology, and drug therapy, Redwood City, Calif., 1989, Addison-Wesley, p 418.

## Box 20-3
## DSM-III-R CLASSIFICATION OF MOOD DISORDERS

| Depressive disorders | | Bipolar disorders | |
|---|---|---|---|
| 296.2x | Major depression, single episode | 296.6x | Bipolar disorder, mixed |
| 296.3x | Major depression, recurrent | 296.4x | Bipolar disorder, manic |
| 300.40 | Dysthymia | 296.5x | Bipolar disorder, depressed |
| 311.00 | Depressive disorder, NOS | 301.13 | Cyclothymia |
|  | (not otherwise specified) | 296.70 | Bipolar disorder NOS |

## Incidence

The DSM-III-R (see Box 20-3) categorizes depressive reactions into major depression (severe) and dysthymia (not as severe). The psychiatric nursing diagnoses (PND-1) for patients with mood disorders are listed in Box 20-4. During any given year about 15% of all adults (18 to 74 years of age) will experience some degree of clinically significant depression. Over the course of a lifetime, it is thought that 5% to 12% of men and 9% to 26% of women will suffer from major depression, and

Box 20-4

PSYCHIATRIC NURSING DIAGNOSES (PND-1) FOR PATIENTS WITH MOOD DISORDERS

*[handwritten: - ineffective individual coping]*
*[handwritten: - Self-care deficit]*
*[handwritten: - potential for self-directed violence]*

| | | | |
|---|---|---|---|
| 01.01.07 | Psychomotor retardation | 01.01.04 | Hyperactivity |
| 01.03.04 | Altered hygiene | 01.04.03 | Insomnia |
| 01.04.02 | Hypersomnia *[handwritten: (major symptom)]* | 02.02 | Altered judgment |
| 01.04.05 | Somnolence | 02.03.02 | Altered intellectual func- |
| 02.01 | Altered decision making | | tioning |
| 04.02.07 | Guilt | 02.07.01 | Delusions |
| 04.02.08 | Sadness | 02.08.02 | Altered concentration |
| 04.02.09 | Shame | 04.02.01 | Anger |
| 05.05.02 | Social isolation/withdrawal | 04.02.03 | Elation |
| 06.01.01 | Distractibility | 05.02.01 | Aggressive/violent |
| 04.02.06 | Grief | | behavior |
| 08.01.02 | Helplessness | 05.02.02.04 | Disorganized behavior |
| 08.01.03 | Loneliness | 05.05.01 | Social intrusiveness |
| | | 06.01.02 | Hyperalertness |
| | | 08.01.04 | Powerlessness |

*[handwritten: - altered self-concept]*
*[handwritten: - dysfunction grieving]*

A. O'Toole, M. Loomis. 1989. "Classifying Human Responses in Psychiatric-Mental Health Nursing," from *Classification Systems for Describing Nursing Practice: Working Papers*, pp. 20-30. Kansas City, MO: American Nurses Association. Reprinted with permission.

*[handwritten left margin: possible 20 hrs of sleep]*

*[handwritten left margin, vertical: Somnolence: condition of becoming sleepy or drowsy; tending to cause sleepiness]*

perhaps as much as 10% of the population will be dysthymic (although only about two thirds will seek professional help). In addition, 35% of all persons hospitalized because of medical illness will suffer depression associated with their illness. Interestingly, major depression is somewhat underrepresented among jail prisoners, comprising only 3.9% of that population (Teplin, 1990).

## Traditional views of depression

Historically, the literature suggests several different ways to categorize depression. These categories are not as discrete as might be expected. In fact, the diagnostic concepts developed for depression over the years have often been unclear and have overlapped. Perhaps depression, among all diagnosable mental disorders, has been the most difficult to trace in the literature because of this redundancy. A brief overview of the major categories is provided to enable the student to understand other professionals who still use "non-DSM-III-R" language and to develop an appreciation for the evolution of our present-day understanding of depression. Each categorization provides a conceptual model and represents efforts to differentiate and understand the major symptoms and etiological factors found in depressed patients (see Table 20-1). These classifications tend to be dichotomous, and each

**TABLE 20-1**   Symptoms and treatments of selected categories of depression discussed in text

| Categories | Symptoms | Treatments |
|---|---|---|
| Endogenous (neuro-chemical) | Lacks specific stressor. Characterized by slowed thinking, speech; poverty of thought and speech; indecision; decreased energy; avolition; anhedonia; decreased productivity; melancholia; diurnal variation of symptoms, usually worse in morning; lack of response to environmental changes (does not find humor in anything); vegetative signs. | Best treated with antidepressants and effective psychotherapeutic management. |
| Reactive | Preoccupation with loss; anxiety, tension, and decreased appetite; able to respond to environmental change (laughs at something funny); symptoms usually self-limiting. This person is often angry. | Antidepressants not usually used because of self-limiting nature of symptoms. Antianxiety drugs, or hypnotics for insomnia, may be very helpful but may cause dependency, hinder understanding, and be countertherapeutic. Psychotherapy and psychotherapeutic management benefits. |
| Neurotic (dysthymia, characterological) | A life-style depression that lacks specific stressors. Poor interpersonal relation skills. Unhappiness with life (job, position, family); dissatisfied with many things (faultfinder, chronic complainer) but refuses to accept blame. Preoccupied with loss or injustices, feels "shortchanged" by life. Emotionally labile, often weeps; is demanding, irritable, angry, dependent, anxious, and hypochondriacal. Able to respond to environmental changes. | Psychotherapy, psychotherapeutic management. Tricyclic antidepressants occasionally given. |

Adapted from Keltner NL: Drugs for the treatment of depression and mania. In Shlafer M and Marieb E, editors: The nurse, pharmacology, and drug therapy, Redwood City, Calif., 1989, Addison-Wesley, p 419.

*Continued.*

**TABLE 20-1**   Symptoms and treatments of selected categories of depression discussed in text—cont'd

| Categories | Symptoms | Treatments |
|---|---|---|
| Melancholia (involutional) | Usually occurs after age 45. Characterized by more somatic symptoms, hypochrondriasis, insomnia, and anorexia than other depressions. Somatic or nihilistic delusions may occur. Anhedonia common. Lifting of depression, even momentarily, is rare. | Tricyclic antidepressants and related drugs. MAOIs often used. Agitated form is helped most by antidepressants. ECT may be very effective. |
| Manic depression | Mood swings encompassing both depressive and manic symptoms are common. High-energy symptoms common during manic phase include flight of ideas, insomnia, hyperactivity, grandiosity, intense irritability, anger, denial of illness, labile affect, manipulativeness, assaultive behavior. | Lithium is the drug of choice. Psychotherapeutic management is very helpful. |
| Drug-induced | Characteristics depend largely on causative agent(s). May be relatively common with some antihypertensives (clonidine, methyldopa, propranolol, reserpine, and pharmacologically similar drugs); benzodiazepines, corticosteroids, general CNS depressants, overtranquilization with antipsychotic drugs. | Identify offending drugs and discontinue if medically permissible. |

focuses on a different aspect of depression. Following are five sets of dichotomous classifications, followed by the critical diagnostic question the nurse must answer (Keltner, 1989). While many of the following terms are still used, only the fifth category is officially endorsed by the DSM-III-R under the heading "Depressive Disorders."

1. Reactive (exogenous) vs endogenous depression: Is the depression a reaction to real-life stressors (exogenous), or is it caused by an internal neurochemical process (endogenous)?
2. Primary vs secondary depression: Is depression the only problem (primary), or is it secondary to another problem such as alcoholism or schizophrenia?
3. Unipolar vs bipolar depression: Is depression the only affective symptom (unipolar), or do depression-dysthymia *and* mania-euphoria occur (bipolar)?
4. Psychotic vs neurotic depression: Is the degree of depression severe enough

to interfere with reality testing, daily life activities, and interpersonal interactions (psychotic), or are the symptoms less disruptive (neurotic)? (The
student should note that the term *neurotic* is purposely deleted from the
DSM-III-R.)

5. Major depression vs dysthymic disorder: How are the symptoms, their severity, and duration classified according to the *Diagnostic and Statistical
   Manual, DSM-III-R,* of the American Psychiatric Association?

This categorization will be discussed later in the chapter.

## Other views of depression

In addition to these more traditional views of depression, some other significant
diagnostic concerns are found in the literature and merit brief mention here. Char-
acterological depression (sometimes referred to as neurotic depression or a depressed personality type) refers to a life-style in which pessimism is the predominant
theme, and the person is easily upset by events, lacks social confidence, and is
introverted. As the descriptor "life-style" suggests, these persons are basically "down"
all the time.

Four other types of depression merit some discussion. First, some drugs cause
depression. Drug-induced depression may be caused by reserpine, propranolol,
methyldopa, guanethidine, diazepam, clonidine, and corticosteroids. Overtranquil-
ization with antipsychotics can also cause depression. For these persons, discontinuance of the offending drug, if medically permissible, should be the first consideration
in alleviating the affective symptoms. Second, a significant number of persons are
depressed either as a reaction to an illness or as part of the illness. For instance,
many persons with schizophrenia are also depressed. Physical illnesses, including
thyroid disease, Addison's disease, and systemic lupus erythematosus, carry a component of depression. Melancholia (sometimes referred to as involutional depression) is another type of depression that is discussed in the literature. There is some
debate as to whether it is a separate subtype of depression or "just" a severe form
of major depression. Its common characteristics include agitation, somatic or nihilistic delusions, loss of pleasure in all or almost all activities, excessive anhedonia,
increased depression in the morning, early morning awakening, and excessive or
inappropriate guilt. Melancholia tends to surface after age 45 and is usually treated
with antidepressants and often with electroconvulsive therapy. Finally, agitated
depression is a type of depression frequently discussed in the clinical setting. Besides
the depressed affect, the nurse is struck by the anger and the pacing, hand wringing,
and agitated behavior manifested by this person.

Although each of the five sets of traditional views capture information about
depression, no single classification scheme seems adequate to fully explain the
complexity of this common mental disorder. Classification of depression as being
reactive or endogenous appears to be the most helpful when discussing the use and
likely success of antidepressant drug therapy, but elements in the other classification
approaches are also important for diagnosis and treatment. For example, life-style
or character traits, age, the presence of another illness, depression-causing drugs,
and other factors must be considered in development of treatment approaches.

As our understanding of depression has evolved, some terms and concepts have been officially dropped from the lexicon in order to fashion diagnostic criteria that are clearly understood, based on universally recognized data, and free of etiological bias or from pseudomedical terms or concepts such as *neurotic depression* (suggesting a Freudian understanding of etiology) has been replaced with the term or concept of *dysthymia.* As a rule of thumb, when the student sees the term *neurotic depression* in older literature, a fair treatment would be to insert the currently accepted term *dysthymia.* Manic-depression is now officially referred to as bipolar illness; however, the term *manic-depression* is still used frequently by psychiatric professionals.

It is important for the student to have a comfort level with the various terms and concepts historically associated with depression, because these terms and concepts are still used in the literature, clinical discussions, and morning report. However, it is also important for the student to recognize the problems associated with these historical terms and concepts. For example, the same severely depressed person might be considered to have psychotic depression, involutional depression, agitated depression, unipolar depression, or major depression, depending on the orientation of the clinician. This book, to be consistent with the latest thinking, to reduce confusion, and to prepare the student for interdisciplinary exchange, emphasizes the use of diagnostic criteria found in the DSM-III-R.

## DSM-III-R terminology and criteria

The DSM-III-R criteria for major depression is found in Box 20-5. The symptoms include a predominant depressed mood during the day, diminished interest in life, weight changes, sleep changes, psychomotor changes, fatigue, feelings of worthlessness or guilt, decreased cognitive ability, and recurrent thoughts of death. When these symptoms begin to dominate and cannot be traced to organic factors, psychosocial stressors (reactive depression), or if reactions to life events are too prolonged, then the diagnosis of major depression is warranted.

Dysthymia is diagnosed when similar criteria are met. The distinction between dysthymia and major depression is subtle and diagnostic confusion is not uncommon. Dysthymia is essentially a diagnosis of chronicity, while severity is the distinguishing factor for major depression. DSM-III-R criteria for dysthymia include poor appetite or overeating, insomnia or hypersomnia, anergia and fatigue, low self-esteem, poor concentration, indecisiveness, and feelings of hopelessness. An elaboration of DSM-III-R criteria is found in Box 20-6. These criteria attempt to rule out competing explanations for depression such as organic and drug-related causes. In addition, since a less severe depression might be expected as a person is recovering from major depression, the revised DSM-III-R reduces the possibility of confusing a gradual recovery from major depression with the less severe dysthymic disorder.

## Behavior

Mrs. B. is a 57-year-old woman who presents with dysphoria, tearfulness, suicidal ideation, loss of energy and sexual interest, and insomnia. Although she feels hopeless about the future and worries that she will never get better. Mrs. B. does accept reassurance that her pessimism is exaggerated and results from her depression. She

Box 20-5

# DSM III R CRITERIA FOR MAJOR DEPRESSIVE EPISODE

Note: A "major depressive syndrome" is defined as criterion A below.

A. At least five of the following symptoms have been present during the same two-week period and represent a change from previous functioning; at least one of the symptoms is either (1) depressed mood, or (2) loss of interest or pleasure. (Do not include symptoms that are clearly due to a physical condition, mood-incongruent delusions or hallucinations, incoherence, or marked loosening of associations.)

1. Depressed mood (or can be irritable mood in children and adolescents) most of the day, nearly every day, as indicated either by subjective account or observation of others.

2. Markedly diminished interest or pleasure in all, or almost all, activities most of the day, nearly every day ( as indicated either by subjective account or observation by others of apathy most of the time).

3. Significant weight loss or weight gain when not dieting ( e.g., more than 5 percent of body weight in a month), or decrease or increase in appetite nearly every day (in children, consider failure to make expected weight gains).

4. Insomnia or hypersomnia nearly every day.

5. Psychomotor agitation or retardation nearly every day (observable by others, not merely subjective feelings of restlessness or being slowed down).

6. Fatigue or loss of energy nearly every day.

7. Feelings of worthlessness or excessive or inappropriate guilt (which may be delusional) nearly every day (not merely self-reproach or guilt about being sick).

8. Diminished ability to think or concentrate, or indecisiveness, nearly every day (either by subjective account or as observed by others).

9. Recurrent thoughts of death (not just fear of dying), recurrent suicidal ideation without specific plan, or a suicide attempt or a specific plan for committing suicide.

B. 1. It cannot be established that an organic factor initiated and maintained the disturbance.

2. The disturbance is not a normal reaction to the death of a loved one (uncomplicated bereavement).

Note: Morbid preoccupation with worthlessness, suicidal ideation, marked functional impairment or psychomotor retardation of prolonged duration suggest bereavement complicated by major depression.

C. At no time during the disturbance have there been delusions or hallucinations for as long as two weeks in the absence of prominent mood symptoms (i.e., before the mood symptoms developed or after they have remitted).

D. Not superimposed on schizophrenia, schizophreniform disorder, delusional disorder, or psychotic disorder NOS.

feels that she is a great burden on her family and blames herself for letting them down and for not bearing her difficulties with dignified stoicism. Her recent inability to achieve orgasm also convinces Mrs. B. that her sexual life and femininity are a thing of the past. (Frances and Hale, 1984.)

Depression results in both objective and subjective behavior. Objective signs, such as agitation, can be observed by the nurse. Subjective symptoms, such as hopelessness, are painful but may be kept hidden by the depressed person. Perhaps more than in schizophrenia, the differentiation between objective signs and subjective symptoms in depression is difficult to develop. Objective signs are typically

**Box 20-6**

**DSM-III-R CRITERIA FOR DYSTHYMIA** – *Chronic depressed mood*

A. Depressed mood . . . for most of the day, more days than not, as indicated either by subjective account or observation of others, for at least two years. *for at least two years*
B. Presence, while depressed, of at least two of the following:
    1. poor appetite or overeating
    2. insomnia or hypersomnia
    3. low energy or fatigue
    4. low self-esteem
    5. poor concentration or difficulty making decisions
    6. feelings of hopelessness
C. During a 2-year period . . . of the disturbance, never without symptoms in A for more than 2 months at a time.
D. No evidence of an unequivocal Major Depression Episode during the first two years . . . of the disturbance.
    Note: There may have been a previous Major Depression Episode, provided there was a full remission (no significant signs or symptoms for 6 months) before development of the Dysthymia. In addition, after these 2 years . . . of Dysthymia, there may be superimposed episodes of Major Depression, in which case both diagnoses are given.
E. Has never had a manic episode or an unequivocal hypomanic episode.
F. Not superimposed on a chronic psychotic disorder, such as schizophrenia or delusional disorder.
G. It cannot be established that an organic factor initiated and maintained the disturbance, e.g., prolonged administration of an antihypertensive medication.

extensions of a subjective state. The nurse is encouraged to observe for visible signs of depression and to be aware of, assess for, and expect subjective anguish and anger.

**Objective signs.** Depressed patients often demonstrate behavior noticeable to others. The depressed patient can be *aggressive,* striking out at family, friends, and staff. The depressed person becomes irritable when disturbed. The patient may seek to be alone, not wanting anyone talking or distracting him from his obsession with his inner world. Two general areas of objective signs are alterations of activity, including activities of daily living (ADL) and altered social interactions.

*Alterations in activity.* The patient may exhibit psychomotor agitation. The patient may be unable to sit still and may pace and engage in handwringing and pulling or rubbing hair, skin, clothing, or other objects. Tying and retying shoes and buttoning and unbuttoning a shirt are typical behaviors. Psychomotor retardation is marked by slowing of speech, increased pauses before answering, soft or monotonous speech, decreased amount of speech (poverty of speech), and muteness. In addition, a general slowing of body movements occurs. The patient may always feel tired, even when he is not physically active. The patient may have a difficult time getting started, for example, rising from a chair to turn off the TV set becomes a major endeavor. The smallest task may seem impossible.

Activities of daily living suffer also. For instance, the same behavior that makes walking to the TV set a struggle also causes the patient to defer basic personal hygiene, such as bathing, shaving, using a napkin, and wiping the nose. However, these latter objective signs are probably caused by more than a lack of energy. Apathy, an inability to be motivated or interested, plays an important role in these undesireable behaviors. An extreme extension of these anergic symptoms is seen in cases in which depressed adults lie in bed and are incontinent or become constipated because of the inability to muster the energy and motivation to walk to the bathroom.

The depressed patient usually has a change in eating behaviors, which results in either a loss or gain of weight. Sleeping behaviors also change. Typically, the patient cannot sleep, but many patients sleep too much (hypersomnia). The insomnia can manifest itself in difficulty going to sleep, difficulty staying asleep, or early morning awakening. The depressed person often denies being depressed but is brought to the attention of the psychiatric community by the complaint of always being tired, of taking too many naps, daytime sleepiness, and so on. The nurse should not confuse the depressed patient's request to "go to my room to lie down" with hypersomnia. Many depressed persons want to lie down but do not sleep. There, in the solitude of an empty room, they descend into uninterrupted, self-defeating ruminations.

*Altered social interactions.* The depressed patient also suffers from poor social skills, which are directly linked to other symptoms of depression. The depressed person underachieves, causing a lack of productivity on the job. This alienating behavior can be quite significant in work situations in which a team approach is used. The patient is easily distracted and is not interested in other people, their ideas, or problems. The self-absorbing nature of depression leaves the depressed person with little to offer others. Conversations are difficult to maintain, and only with great effort can the depressed person sustain a facial indication of interest and concern. The depressed person is also withdrawn. Such a person may withdraw from family and friends and seek social isolation. Hobbies and avocations that once were actively pursued become unimportant and may be abandoned or engaged in half-heartedly. Finally, the body language of depression, saddened expression, and a drooping posture serve as a social barrier.

### Subjective symptoms

*Alterations of affect.* Alterations of affect are the symptoms primarily associated with depression. This is reasonable because these disturbances dominate the internal world of the depressed person. Anger, anxiety, apathy, bitterness, dejection, denial of feelings, despondency, guilt, helplessness, hopelessness, uselessness, loneliness, low self-esteem, sadness, and a sense of worthlessness are all subjective feelings that cause unbearable pain and anguish. Because of this anguish, depressed persons vacillate between sadness and apathy. When the pain becomes too great, they "shut down" and become apathetic.

The overall affective sense is one of low self-esteem. Guilt may include an overreaction to some current failing or may be associated with an indiscretion in the distant past that cannot be forgotten. Guilt can also take the form of accepting responsibility for occurrences in which the person had little impact. For instance, one patient expressed guilt over the death of his son's friend in an automobile accident. The tortured reasoning the man used was as follows: if he had spent more time with the boy, it might have changed the boy's life, and if he had changed the boy's life, the boy might have driven more safely. Guilt can also take the form of obsessional preoccupation with "What if I had only . . . ." The person becomes immobilized with "should have's" and "could have's." An even more morbid extension of guilt is the psychotic delusion of guilt for calamities continents away.

Anxiety is a companion of depression. The depressed person is filled with anxiousness and dread. The ringing phone holds potential for catastrophic news. A siren could mean a loved one injured. A child at school might not return. Although sadly, these terrible things do happen, most of us go on with life somewhat comforted by the knowledge that they probably will not happen if we do not take unusual risks. For many depressed persons, each ringing phone causes the same reaction as all the previous ones.

Worthlessness can range from feeling inadequate to a total devaluation of anything the person has done. The person may even scan the environment for clues of his inadequacy. One patient remarked, "I knew I wasn't any good—it just took awhile to find out."

Finally, although most laymen would consider sadness to be the universal symptom of depression, actually apathy comes closer to being always present in the depressed person.

*Alterations of cognition.* Alterations of cognition include ambivalence and indecision, inability to concentrate, confusion, loss of interest and motivation, pessimism, self-blame, self-depreciation, self-destructive thoughts, thoughts of death and dying, and uncertainty. This inability to make a decision is particularly difficult for others to understand. Faced with even a simple decision, much vacillation is expressed. Once a decision is made, the patient may be obsessed with "what if's." While deliberating, one can be immobilizing.

*Alterations of a physical nature.* Alterations of a physical nature are common in depressed persons. Almost any part of the body can be affected. Common physiological disorders include abdominal pain, anorexia, chest pain, constipation, dizziness, fatigue, headache, indigestion, insomnia, menstrual changes, nausea and vomiting, and sexual dysfunction.

These subjective symptoms come to the attention of nurses because of the numerous somatic complaints of the depressed patient. Some persons become so preoccupied with their bodies that every twinge, every body change, is initially greeted with great alarm and dread. One recovering depressed patient joked, "I have had a hundred heart attacks." Monitoring of body functions is not uncommon in the general population; however, overinvestment in self-assessment by the depressed person is pathological. It is the severity of this thinking that sets the depressed person apart. Panic attacks related to fear of an illness are not uncommon. The chest pain, the unusual spot, the stomach pain can all precipitate a panic attack in some persons.

*Altered perception.* Some depressed persons suffer from altered perceptions. Delusions and hallucinations are typically congruent with the depressed mood, for example, a delusion of persecution because of a moral mistake. Somatic delusions ("my body is full of cancer") and nihilistic delusions ("my brain is dead") are rather common forms of psychotic delusions in the depressed person. Hallucinations tend to be less elaborate than those of the schizophrenic and tend to focus on personal faults (e.g., "You are no good. You don't deserve your family").

## Etiology

The cause of depression can be broadly categorized as either biological or psychological (psychodynamic). Whereas in schizophrenia, mental health professionals tend to defend one view or the other, the discussion of depression does not seem to evoke as much dichotomy. Mental health professionals seem willing to accept a biological explanation for some patients and a psychological explanation for others.

**Biological theories of depression.** The common misconception concerning depression is that it is a reaction to loss or failure. Many depressed persons, however, cannot identify any stressor(s) or conflict in their lives. Sometimes this lack of an objective stressor causes even more feelings of worthlessness and guilt because the patient thinks he has no reason to feel depressed. Many of these persons, suffering from an endogenous depression, experience their symptoms because of neurotransmitter deficiency. Persons with neurotransmitter deficiencies have "vegetative" symptoms, symptoms that affect sleeping and eating. Typically, such a person cannot go to sleep easily, wakes periodically during the night, or more frequently wakes early in the morning and cannot go back to sleep. Appetite is usually decreased, sometimes enough to constitute anorexia with weight loss. Patients with endogenous depression benefit greatly from antidepressant drugs.

The findings of many research studies indicate that a chemical imbalance or deficiency in the brain of certain neurotransmitters cause a mental state of depression. The neurotransmitters (brain amines) are norepinephrine, serotonin, and probably dopamine. The initial interest in neurotransmitter deficiency arose from the use of reserpine, an antihypertensive, in the early 1950s. Patients using reserpine became depressed, and it was found that reserpine lowered norepinephrine, serotonin, and dopamine levels. Conversely, amphetamines elevated mood and increased neurotransmitter levels. From these observations the amine hypothesis of depression was developed. It was postulated that drugs that could increase neurotransmitter availability could be useful in the treatment of depression. Most antidepressants increase the availability of neurotransmitters and are a result of this scientific thinking. A recent National Institute of Mental Health study (Elkin et al., 1989) found that in the treatment of severe depression TCAs were significantly more effective than psychotherapy. Such findings strengthen the argument for a biological base for severe depression. Chapter 13 provides a detailed explanation of antidepressants.

**Psychodynamic theories of depression.** Psychological or psychodynamic explanations of depression can be categorized under three general themes: debilitating early life experiences, intrapsychic conflicts, or reactions to life events.

*Debilitating early life experiences.* According to traditional psychiatric thought, events in one's early life can lay the foundation for adult depression. The developmental theorists previously mentioned (i.e., Freud, Erikson, Sullivan) view the early years of life as foundational to lifelong mental health. Although these theorists use different words to designate life stages, they are similar in their views of the importance of a solid, nurturing early life environment. Early losses, maternal inconsistency, the giving and withholding of love by the caregiver, and various types of abuse are all explained as causative agents for mental illness. Any early life experience that could contribute to or cause lowered self-esteem and that was not dealt with effectively can be a cause for depression later in life. Chapter 2 provides an overview of several developmental theorys.

*Intrapsychic conflict.* Intrapsychic conflict refers to the conflicts people have when they have mixed emotions about some behavior, event, or situation. For instance, the girl or boy who has been brought up to refrain from sexual activity but who also has strong urges to experience sex has a real conflict. To refrain increases sexual frustration and to engage in sexual activity may cause anxiety, guilt, and fear. Since the anxiety, guilt, and fear are uncomfortable, young persons who engage in sexual intercourse may attempt to rationalize their behavior ("my parents are old fashioned," "these are the 90s"), only to find themselves growing more and more depressed. Because the young person has rationalized his behavior, the source of the depression may not be recognized without professional help. People are faced with intrapsychic conflicts all the time. Persistent unsuccessful resolution of these conflicts can lead to depression.

*Reactions to life events.* Most people view depression as a reaction to life stress. Loss is a major theme—loss of a loved one through death or divorce, loss of a job, loss of self-esteem, loss of a sense of control of self and life, loss of familiar surroundings and everything those surroundings represent, and even the loss caused by a psychotic disorder can cause depression (Weiss et al., 1989). It is normal to react to loss with grief and sadness. It is abnormal to overreact. But exactly when normal gives way to abnormal is not clear. Klerman (1980) said; "because clinicians ~~and have arguments for how mixed affect is or the complete range of affective disorders~~ to be diagnosed as psychopathological, the boundary between normal mood and abnormal depression remains undefined." The nurse can assess for degree or severity, for frequency and duration, and for the outcome for the individual, his life-style, and significant others. For example, a grieving person returns to work after a funeral, but the depressed person remains in bed for weeks.

## Special issues related to depression

**Dexamethasone suppression test.** The DST is helpful in the diagnosis of endogenous (neurotransmitter deficiency) depression or depression with vegetative symptoms. A single dose of dexamethasone is given. Blood and urine cortisol levels are drawn before and after. In nonendogenously depressed or normal persons the cortisol levels are suppressed. In persons with endogenous depression these levels are *not* suppressed (nonsuppressors). This test has the potential for establishsing greater accuracy in diagnosis.

**Depression among the elderly.** Depression in the elderly is relatively common, but because of the overlapping symptoms with physical illness and the depressive side effects of many drugs, the diagnosis is complex. The diagnosis is important because treatment flows from such knowledge. To acquaint the nurse with potential confounding variables, a list of depression-causing drugs (Box 20-7) and a list of illnesses that share symptoms with depression (Table 20-2) are presented.

If the depression is related to a physical illness and if the physical illness can be treated, elimination of the physical problem should help the mood return to normal. If the illness is actually depression, appropriate treatment can be instituted. The student should also be aware that some elderly persons who are diagnosed as

### Box 20-7
### DRUGS THAT CAN CAUSE DEPRESSION

| | |
|---|---|
| Digitalis | Corticosteroids |
| Antihypertensives including reserpine and methyldopa | Anticancer drugs |
| Antiparkinson drugs including L-dopa, bromocriptine, carbidopa | Psychotropic drugs including antipsychotic, antianxiety, and antidepressants |

Adapted from Salzman C, and Shader RI: Depression in the elderly. II. Possible drug etiologies: differential diagnostic criteria, J Am Geriatr Soc 26:303, 1978.

**TABLE 20-2**   Physical illnesses of the elderly that share symptoms with depression

| Symptom of depression | Physical illness with same symptom |
|---|---|
| Insomnia | Many medical illnesses; also dyspnea secondary to CHF; also normal if patient naps often |
| Constipation | Normal because of decreased autonomic innervation of GI tract; dehydration; secondary to anticholinergic drugs |
| Anorexia | Chronic infection; malignancy; diabetes |
| Hoplessness, despair | Reaction to severe, chronic, terminal disease |
| Memory loss | Dementia |
| Withdrawal, retardation | Parkinsonism; early CHF |
| Irritability | Reaction to chronic illness |
| Weight loss, pallor | Chronic infection, diabetes, advanced cancer |

Adapted from Salzman C and Shader RI: Depression in the elderly. II. Possible drug etiologies: differential diagnostic criteria, J Am Geriatr Soc 26:303, 1978.

having a dementia are in reality depressed. Since more is known about the treatment of depression, it is important to differentiate depression from dementia. Finally, older men who are depressed are at a high risk of suicide. White men over the age of 50 constitute 10% of the total population but are responsible for 28% of the annual deaths by suicide (Hendin, 1986). It is thought that this group will account for 10,500 suicides annually by the turn of the century.

---

**PSYCHOTHERAPEUTIC MANAGEMENT**

The depressed person is not necessarily the one who is prone to the development of depression but the one who has difficulty recovering from it (Metcalfe, 1974).

The nursing interventions used in the treatment of the depressed patient flow from appropriate development of the nursing care plan. This book is designed around the concept of psychotherapeutic management: the nurse-patient relationship, psychopharmacology, and milieu management. Those concepts are discussed in detail in Units II, III, and IV, respectively. The reader is referred to those units for a full discussion of those intervention strategies.

*PSYCHOTHERAPEUTIC NURSE-PATIENT RELATIONSHIP*   The objective of this chapter is to provide specific principles of therapeutic communication for nurses working with the depressed patient.

1. Depressed persons suffer from low self-esteem. The most effective approach to bolster self-esteem is to accept the patient as he is (negative attitude and all), help him focus on the positive (accomplishments, good points), provide success experiences with positive feedback, keep self-help strategies simple, and help the patient avoid embarrassing social blunders (smelly clothes, unkept appearance). (Also see No. 4.)

2. Development of a meaningful relationship in which the depressed person is valued as a human being is important to his or her sense of personal worth. It is important for the nurse to be nonjudgmental and to work on developing trust. The "trusting relationship" is developed by doing those things that are in the best interest of the patient. For instance, a patient may wish to tell the nurse something of clinical significance but not want the nurse to share the information with other staff members. The nurse builds trust by telling the patient that significant information will be shared with those staff members who have a need to know to be helpful to the patient. The patient learns to trust the nurse as a professional whose dominant concern is the patient's best interest.

3. The nurse working with the depressed patient must have sincere concern for the patient and be empathetic to be effective. For instance, it is not unusual for a nurse to feel a little sad when working with the depressed or suicidal person. The nurse acknowledges the emotional pain and suffering conveyed by the patient and offers to help the patient work through the pain.

4. It is usually not effective to logically outline why the patient is a worthwhile human being. The nurse does point out even small visible accomplishments and strengths, however. ("I'm glad you combed your hair today.") The patient may agree with everything stated and still be just as depressed. Intellectual understanding does not help severely depressed patients. Cognitive therapists, however, have been successful in helping some depressed persons learn to "reprogram" negative thoughts (for example, from "I can't do anything right" to "I can learn from my mistakes.")

5. Depressed persons are typically dependent. After working with the patient, the nurse may notice that he or she (the nurse) is taking on responsibility for the depression. The nurse should recognize but not resent this tendency in the depressed person. The nurse should reward even small decisions or independent actions.

6. The nurse should not attempt to "embarrass" the patient out of being depressed. For instance, pointing out a less fortunate person in the hope that such an action might bring the depressed person to his senses provides, at best, short-lived relief based on the misfortune of others. At worst, it establishes a mind-set that reduces others to object lessons or convinces the person that the whole world is unfair and miserable.

7. Never reinforce hallucinations, delusions, or irrational beliefs. The nurse cannot agree, and arguing seems to reinforce them. Simply state your perception of reality, voice doubt about the patient's perceptions, and move on to discuss "real" people or events.

8. Depressed persons tend to be angry. Sometimes they surprise even themselves with the hateful or hostile things that come out of their mouths. Learn to handle hostility therapeutically by recognizing the anger, not taking it personally, and not retaliating in word, deed, or some passive-aggressive form. Encouraging verbal expressions of anger helps to decrease the "bottled up" tension.

9. The nurse can help the withdrawn patient to emerge from his social isolation by spending time with him (even without speaking), by providing a non-threatening one-to-one relationship, by practicing assertiveness interactions, and by being accepting of the patient.

10. Depressed persons can have difficulty in making decisions, even simple decisions. It is not therapeutic to badger the patient into making a decision, but it is therapeutic to provide decision-making opportunities as the patient is able to comply. Initially the nurse may need to make decisions for the patient, for example, "It is time for your bath." "Here is your apple juice." When possible, the nurse helps guide the patient to appropriate decisions by using problem-solving techniques; that is, what are the options, the pro's and con's of each option, and the potential consequences of each decision.

*PSYCHOPHARMACOLOGY* To understand the range of information required for effective psychopharmacological intervention, the student is encouraged to review Chapter 13, which provides a complete discussion of antidepressant and antimanic drugs. A brief review of critical parameters of antidepressant drug administration is given in Box 20-8 and Table 20-3. (See Tables 13-1 and 13-2 for the usual daily

---

### Box 20-8
## IMPORTANT POINTS FOR ADMINISTERING ANTIDEPRESSANT AND ANTIMANIC DRUGS

■ Most antidepressants have a lag time of 2 to 4 weeks before a full clinical effect occurs. During that time patients gradually begin to feel better and to have more energy. Suicidal tendencies may be greater as antidepressants increase energy and motivation. Lithium has a lag time of 7 to 10 days before it takes effect.

■ Monitor the patient for "cheeking" or hoarding of drugs. At amounts not much greater than the therapeutic amount, antidepressants and lithium can become toxic.

■ Monitor vital signs for patient taking TCAs and MAOIs. TCAs can cause orthostatic hypotension, reflex tachycardia, and arrhythmias. MAOIs have the potential for triggering a hypertensive crisis.

■ Be aware of the drug-drug and food-drug interactions associated with MAOIs.

■ Observe for early signs of toxicity:
  • TCAs: drowsiness, tachycardia, mydriasis, hypotension, agitation, vomiting, confusion, fever, restlessness, sweating
  • MAOIs: dizziness, vertigo, fatigue
  • Lithium: diarrhea, vomiting, drowsiness, muscle weakness, ataxia, giddiness, polyuria

■ Monitor serum lithium levels. Maintenance levels are 0.6 to 1.2 mmol/L.

dosage of antidepressants and MAOIs. The usual daily dosage of lithium ranges from 900 to 1800 mg.)

*MILIEU MANAGEMENT* Milieu management is an important dimension of psychiatric nursing care for the depressed patient. The reader is referred to Unit IV for a complete discussion of milieu management. General principles that specifically address the environment of the depressed patient are considered below.

### The patient with low self-esteem

■ Encourage the patient to participate in activities, including group activities, in which he will be able to experience accomplishment and receive positive

**TABLE 20-3**   Side effects of antidepressant and antimanic drugs and appropriate nursing interventions

| Side effects | Interventions |
|---|---|
| **TRICYCLIC ANTIDEPRESSANTS** *topranil, Prozac* | |
| Dry mouth | Provide sugarless hard candy, sugarless chewing gum, frequent rinses |
| Nasal congestion | Over-the-counter decongestants as approved by PMD (primary medical doctor) or nurse |
| Urinary hesitancy | Running water, privacy, warm water over perineum |
| Urinary retention | Catheterize for residual fluids and encourage frequent voiding |
| Blurred vision | Reassurance; this symptom usually subsides; wear sunglasses outside; caution about driving |
| Constipation | Laxatives as ordered, diet with roughage |
| Sedation, ataxia | Caution to avoid dangerous tasks (i.e., driving); advise that alcohol compounds sedation; daytime sedation is minimized if all TCAs are given at bedtime |
| Confusion | Possibility of tricyclic-induced delirium; withhold drug and notify physician |
| Orthostatic hypotension | Instruct patient to rise slowly; if patient is lying down, should sit on side of bed for 1 full minute before rising to walk; instruct to avoid standing in one place too long and to avoid taking hot baths or showers |
| Arrhythmias, tachycardia, palpitations | Record vital signs; if patient is experiencing tachycardia, withhold drug |
| Decreased sweating | Instruct patient to be cautious about strenuous activity in hot weather |

*Continued.*

**TABLE 20-3**  Side effects of antidepressant and antimanic drugs and
appropriate nursing interventions—cont'd

| Side effects | Interventions |
| --- | --- |
| **MONOAMINE OXIDASE INHIBITORS** | |
| Overstimulation such as agitation, hypo-mania | Withhold MAOIs and notify physician |
| Blurred vision, hypotension, dry mouth, constipation | See TCA interventions |
| Hypertensive crisis related to food-drug or drug-drug interactions | Avoid these food and drug combinations |
| **LITHIUM** | |
| Confusion, restlessness, sleeplessness | Withhold lithium |
| Gastrointestinal symptoms | |
| Nausea | Give lithium with meals |
| Thirst | Instruct patient to drink 10 to 12 8-ounce (240 ml) glasses of water each day |
| Diarrhea | Observe closely for depletion of electrolytes; this can cause higher serum lithium levels |
| Weight gain | Weigh patient weekly; patient may need to be placed on structured diet |
| Sedation, blurred vision, arrhythmias, tachycardia, palpitations, dry mouth, constipation | See TCA interventions |

*[handwritten in left margin: pt teaching is critical ē MAOI]*

feedback. Most people develop a sense of self-worth through mastery or accomplishment. Just telling them that they are "O.K." is not convincing. Provide successful experiences, however small.

■ Provide assertiveness training. Many depressed persons feel like doormats because of their interactional problems. Their communication history is typically a lifetime of being "taken advantage of" punctuated by periodic outbursts of anger when they become "fed up." Assertiveness training helps them learn to take care of their needs and to express their feelings along the way so that the extremes of "doormat" and "flare-up" are avoided.

■ Help the patient avoid embarrassing himself through socially unacceptable appearance or behavior. Many appearance problems are directly related to the depressed person's preoccupation, apathy, and decreased energy level. For instance, food stains on clothes, food in one's beard, an unattended runny nose, uncombed hair, urine on trousers, and an unzipped fly are all commonly seen among depressed persons who "cannot" pay attention to these hygienic concerns. Help patients shower and dress appropriately. Remind the patient to go to the bathroom. In some cases it is better to encourage the patient to walk with the nurse (for example, to the bathroom area or to the shower). Some patients become so apathetic that they "wet their pants."

## The withdrawn patient

- Keep contacts with the patient brief but frequent. Depressed patients often do not want anyone around or, at least, anyone to talk to them. Obviously, their wishes are not a good indicator of what should be done. Spending time with the patient is constructive. Allowing the patient to isolate himself is not. Patients may need to increase physical activity before they are able to verbalize issues.
- Many patients are insistent about going to their room to lie down. They may stay there all day if the nurse does not intervene. Locking the patient's room during the day may be required to keep the withdrawn or isolative patient from disappearing for hours at a time. Sitting in silence during an activity is better than ruminating in isolation.

## The anorexic patient

- Nursing staff must take responsibility for ensuring that the depressed patient eats. It is irresponsible to set a tray down in front of the depressed person, particularly in his room, and then leave. The nurse must encourage the patient to eat and may even spoon-feed him if required.
- Allow patient to participate in selecting preferred foods from menu.
- Promote a proper diet, adequate fluids, and exercise. Provide small, frequent meals. Record intake.
- Constipation is a side effect not only of antidepressants but also of depression itself. A diet with adequate fiber content and sufficient fluids is important.
- If the patient will eat food brought from home, allow him to have such food.

## The patient with sleep disturbances

- Depressed persons want to sleep, but many suffer from insomnia. The tremendous fatigue is real to the patient, since what sleep he does get is usually not restful. The patient often wakes up looking and feeling exhausted. Nursing staff should record the amount and quality of actual sleep. The patient who lies down in the daytime is not necessarily sleeping but may be isolating himself. An accurate understanding of the amount of sleep being obtained helps the nurse formulate an intervention strategy.
- If the patient is taking a sedating TCA, combining the daily dose into a single bedtime dose is known to decrease daytime sedation.
- People suffering from insomnia often engage in self-defeating behaviors, such as daytime napping and drinking stimulants (e.g., coffee, colas). Eliminating these behaviors will increase the likelihood of nighttime sleep.
- Depressed patients who sleep too much (hypersomnia) should have access to their rooms restricted. The goal of working with persons who cannot sleep or who sleep too much is adequate rest (6 to 8 hours per night). Activities can be substituted for the daytime sleeping. Exercise often increases energy levels.

## Case Study

Sylvia Green is a 75-year-old married woman with a long history of depression and hospitalizations. She has been on the unit for 6 weeks. She is experiencing insomnia, anxiety, and anorexia. She does not talk to other patients and tries to stay in her bedroom. Improvements, if any, have been slight. She has multiple physical problems, including hypertension, left-sided weakness due to a cerebral vascular accident, and glaucoma. Her 81-year-old husband of 52 years states that he is at his "wit's end," but wants her to "get well and come home." He reports that she has never been this bad before. Mrs. Green lies in bed when her room is open and on the unit furniture at other times. Her verbal complaints include such statements as: "I'm weak across the back." "My head is driving me crazy." "I can't eat. It goes right through me." "I'm drawn up in a knot." "I can't relax." "My stomach is just quivering and I shake all over." "My head is crawling." "I have terrible thoughts." "I'm so sick I wish I could die."

The nurse finds that Mrs. Green is not suicidal, and the statement "my head is crawling" was not delusional. Mr. Green reports that she has been sick before but always "does real good" after a month in the hospital. He also relates that she has responded to ECT in the past. Mrs. Green is a pathetic figure and feels absolutely hopeless. See the opposite page for Mrs. Green's nursing care plan.

## SUICIDE

> Suicide is a complex phenomenon, influenced by religious, cultural, and psychological factors. Men are far more prone to it than women are, and in the U.S. whites are more likely to kill themselves than are blacks. ("Suicide: the gun factor." *Time,* July 17, 1989, p 61.)

Suicide is a significant cause of death in America. The prototypical victim is an unemployed white man, living alone, who has made a serious suicide attempt in the past. When combined, suicide and homicide are the fourth leading cause of death behind cardiovascular disease, cancer, and accidents (Holinger et al., 1987). About 18,000 suicides a year are related to self-inflicted gunshot wounds (Frierson, 1989). In the last 50 years there has been a 139% increase in suicide by gunshot in the age range of 10 to 24 years (Frierson, 1989). Sixty-four percent of male suicides and 36% of female suicides are committed with guns (Frierson, 1989). The July 17, 1989, issue of *Time* profiled deaths by gunfire during the week of May 1 to 7, 1989. Of the 464 persons killed with guns that week, 216 (47%) killed themselves.

# Nursing Care Plan

NAME: ___Mrs. Sylvia Green___    ADMISSION DATE: _8/12/90_

DSM-III-R DIAGNOSIS: _296.3 Major Depression, recurrent_

### ASSESSMENT:
***Areas of strength***: supportive husband, financial security, history of good adjustment between recurrent episodes of depression. Past treatment with ECT was successful. Patient is not suicidal at this time.

***Problems***: husband (81 y/o) states patient has never been *this* depressed before. Patient making statements about dying. Husband is worn out. States: "I don't know what to do." Patient is isolative, anorexic, cannot sleep, and wants to die.

### DIAGNOSES: Hopelessness related to physical complaints. Exhaustion related to insomnia. Withdrawal related to anxiety.

### PLANNING:                                                        Date met
***Short-term goals:*** Patient will stay out of bed and par-            8/21
ticipate in activities.

Patient will have low-salt diet, low-tyramine food and                  8/21
maintain weight.

Patient will sleep at night.                                            8/18

Husband will attend unit support group.                         _____

***Long-term goals:*** Patient will return to home and hus-     _____
band.

Patient will attend outpatient program.                         _____

Patient will accept psychiatric nursing visits through HHA.             9/12

Husband will attend ongoing support group.                      _____

### IMPLEMENTATION/INTERVENTIONS:
***Nurse-patient relationship:*** Develop a trusting relationship based on honesty and genuine concern for patient. Be empathetic with patient as she verbalizes her negative thoughts. Spend time with patient. Reinforce strengths and accomplishments.

***Psychopharmacology:*** Nardil 15 mg b.i.d.; monitor B/P frequently for both hypotension and hypertensive crisis (from drug-drug and food-drug interactions); Lasix 40 mg qAM; Capoten 25 mg b.i.d.

***Milieu management:*** Minimize patient's tendency to isolate, lock room and assist patient in some activity. Monitor eating and sleeping, eliminate caffeinated drinks and daytime naps. As tolerated, draw patient into small-group situations. Keep environment safe should patient attempt self-injury. Maintain low-tyramine and low-salt diet.

### EVALUATION: Patient still very depressed, isolative, hopeless. Low-salt and low-tyramine diet has been maintained. Some improvement in sleeping behavior. Patient may be candidate for ECT. Consult sent to Dr. Jones to evaluate for ECT.

**TABLE 20-4**   Overall suicide rate for the United States

| Population | Suicides per 100,000 |
|---|---|
| Adult general | 15 - 19 |
| Schizophrenic | 140 |
| Depressed | 230 |
| Alcoholic | 270 |

The overall suicide rate for the general adult population in the United States is high but is still considerably lower than for persons with psychiatric disorders. Table 20-4 compares the suicide rates for the general population with those for mentally disordered persons by diagnostic entity (Clark et al., 1987).

Clark and associates (1987) estimate that over a period of 15 to 20 years 10% to 15% of all patients with schizophrenia, depression, and alcoholism will die by suicide. Becker (1988) finds that 10% of schizophrenics die from suicide. Hendin (1986) states that 90% of older persons who commit suicide have a mental disorder. Persons over 50, although representing only 26% of the population, account for 39% of suicide deaths.

The death by suicide of psychiatric patients is of particular importance to the nurse because of opportunities for assessment and intervention. The psychiatric nurse must continually assess for suicide potential among all patients but especially among schizophrenic, depressed, and alcoholic patients.

Although Table 20-4 provides separate suicide rates for schizophrenics, the depressed, and for alcholics, Hendin points out that when schizophrenics kill themselves they are typically in a depressed phase, and the act is not a product of psychosis (although they do act on command hallucinations at times). Alcoholics usually kill themselves in response to loss (divorce, separation, being fired) and when they have been drinking. Hendin makes the point that suicide most often is the result of depression, diagnosed or not. Drake et al. (1984) depict the most vulnerable psychiatric patients as "young patients with chronic relapsing illness, good educational backgrounds, high-performance expectations, painful awareness of illness, fear of further mental disintegration, and hopelessness about the future."

The major themes in suicidal patients are loss, unbearable psychic pain, helplessness, hopelessness, loneliness, and abandonment ("nobody cares"). These themes complement the common suicidal expressions of a loss of self-esteem, a cry for help, or suicide as a threat (see Box 20-9 for a more complete list of suicidal expressions). Hendin (1986) points out that suicidal patients view and utilize death differently than other people. There is a tendency to use their own death to control others and to maintain control over their own lives. Hence death is viewed as a means of ensuring control.

### Assessment of suicidal patients

It is important for nurses to be able to assess the suicidal potential of mentally disordered patients, because those patients are at higher risk of suicide. Most facilities

**Box 20-9**
## COMMON EXPRESSIONS OF SUICIDAL INDIVIDUALS

| | |
|---|---|
| Cry for help | Admission of inability to handle problem. |
| Escape | "I can't put up with this mess any longer" (especially with embarrassing or traumatic situations). |
| Heroic | To gain respect; some cultures view suicide as a manly alternative to failure; occasionally a patient who is ambivalent about suicide has been taunted into showing he is a real man. |
| Loss of self-esteem | Failure in an area of great personal investment. On 7/18/89 Donnie Moore, a major league baseball pitcher, committed suicide. His former teammates felt it was related to a home run he gave up in a play-off game. |
| Manipulation | This is a coercive measure. "You had better come back to me or I will kill myself." An attempt to control. |
| Martyrdom | "Nobody cares about me. Everyone would be better off without me." |
| Rebirth | Fantasy of getting a new start in life. "Heaven has got to be better than this." |
| Redemption | An attempt to make up for some wrong; for example, a man responsible for the death of a child might kill himself. |
| Relief of pain | "I can't stand the pain (emotional or physical) any longer" (especially with terminal illness). |
| Retaliatory | Suicide is viewed as getting even. "I'll show them." |
| Reunion | Joining a loved one in heaven. "I can't live without her." |

provide the nurse with a format for evaluating suicidal lethality. The crucial variables are the plan, the method, and provision for rescue.

**Plan.** The more developed the plan, the greater the risk of suicide. The person who has carefully developed his suicidal plan is more serious about suicide and presents a greater risk. Although impulsive suicide attempts can result in death, generally they are less lethal because lack of planning sometimes foils the effort.

**Method.** Some methods of suicide are more lethal than others. Accessibility of the means is important also. Having three bottles of pills in hand is more lethal than having to make an appointment with a doctor to ask for a prescription.

A crucial factor in determining the lethality of any particular method is the amount of time between initiation of the suicide method and delivery of the lethal impact of that method. For instance, the person using a gun has no opportunity to avoid the bullet, once the trigger is pulled. On the other hand, sitting in the garage with the motor running affords some time to choose an alternative to self-destruction, as does taking an overdose of some drugs. Very lethal methods include the use of guns, jumping off high places, hanging, drowning, carbon monoxide poisoning, and overdose with certain drugs (e.g., barbiturates, alchohol, and several CNA depressants). Less lethal methods include wrist cutting and overdosing on aspirin or Valium.

**Rescue.** The person who deliberately attempts to deceive would-be rescuers has a high lethality potential. For instance, the person who says he is going to the ocean for the weekend and then drives to the mountains makes it difficult for family and friends to intervene. A person who leaves a note or makes a telephone call before making an attempt is more likely to be rescued.

In summary, the more detailed the *plan,* the more lethal and accessible the *method,* and the more effort to block *rescue,* the greater the likelihood of the suicidal effort being successful. However, impulsive efforts with rescuers in sight have proved fatal, particularly when a lethal method (e.g., gun) has been selected.

## Intervention

**Face to face.** In working face to face with the suicidal patient, several general guidelines are useful for the nurse.

1. Ask the patient if he is planning to hurt himself. It is important for the nurse to understand that
   a. Talking to the patient about his suicidal intentions will not drive him to it. Asking the patient directly provides useful information and often provides a sense of relief. ("Finally someone hears me.")
   b. Many persons die from suicide who did not mean to die but miscalculated. It can be said accurately that many persons who die from suicide die accidentally. The nurse must take all suicidal threats seriously.
2. If the patient is considering suicide, ask him about his plan (when and where), including method and how he thought he would go about doing it (has he planned to frustrate rescue attempts). If he wants to use a gun, ask someone at home to remove the gun or, if by overdose, to throw away the pills. Do not offer a weekend pass. Some clinicians believe if you can block the method of choice, many suicidal patients will not use another method. As an example, a woman who might use a drug overdose would not consider jumping off a building.
3. Ask the patient if he has made previous suicide attempts and then when and how. How did he feel concerning rescue? How did he respond to treatment? Previous attempts put the person at higher risk.
4. Evaluate the patient for depression, recent loss or threat of loss, self-destructive hallucinations, or alchohol or drug use, all which place him at higher risk.
5. Once a patient is hospitalized, most units will protect him by using one of two levels of suicide prevention:
   a. *Level 1:* Used for persons who are not viewed as being at immediate risk of suicide. The nursing staff provides periodic observation (every 15 minutes) and monitors drug taking, eating utensils, shaving gear, and other potentially dangerous devices in the environment. The staff communicates concern and control by this close observation of the patient and his en-

vironment. The patient is asked to sign a contract with the staff that states that he will not harm himself during hospitalization and will seek out a staff member should he begin contemplating self-injurious behavior.

b. *Level 2:* Used for patients who present an immediate and serious threat of suicide behavior. Level 2 may also be instituted for patients who refuse to sign a "no suicide" contract. Occasionally restraints may be used, as can psychotropic medications. Continuous observation is another alternative. This is an expensive use of manpower but provides the needed control coupled with human interaction. The patient at serious risk is usually confined to the unit and has restrictions on visitors, where meals are taken, and so on. Harmful objects are removed from the patient's environment.

**Over the telephone.** Frequently former patients call the unit or outpatient clinic where psychiatric nurses work. Below are helpful guidelines for working with the suicidal person over the telephone (Green and Wilson, 1988).

1. Express genuine concern and a desire to work with the caller. ("Let's see what we can do.") *Give the caller your full attention.*
2. Acknowledge how difficult and painful recent losses must be. ("Its been a tough time for you lately.")
3. Focus on the person's healthy side. ("You called for help. That tells me you want help and that's what we want to do.")
4. Assess lethality, especially if suicidal attempt has begun.
5. Ask about alcohol or drug use. If present, these substances increase the lethality level.
6. Ask caller for his ideas about immediate solutions to his current situation. Assess feasibility, appropriateness, and availability. Suggest alternatives if needed.
7. Obtain the person's name, telephone number, address, and whereabouts during call. Ask how he wants to be addressed. ("Your name is Mr. Robert Smith. What would you like for me to call you?")
8. If other staff members are available, you may need to direct them to call the police or an ambulance. Ask for consent to do so or at least inform the patient of your plans.
9. Ask if anyone else is with the caller. If so, ask to speak to that person to obtain assistance in planning instructions.
10. If family members can be reached, they should be asked to go to the patient and intervene if it is safe to do so (ask for caller consent).
11. Refer caller to walk-in crisis services or regular outpatient counselor.
12. If the caller refuses further help, give the telephone number of a crisis center or a suicide-prevention hotline.

## MANIC EPISODES

Manic episodes are characterized by an elevated or expansive mood. Symptoms are listed in Box 20-10. Manic episodes usually begin suddenly, escalate rapidly, and last from a few days to several months. Judgment is impaired, social blunders occur,

**Box 20-10**
## SYMPTOMS OCCURRING DURING MANIC EPISODES

| Common symptoms | Other symptoms |
|---|---|
| Elevated mood | Lack of awareness of illness |
| Grandiosity | Resistance to treatment |
| Irritability | Labile mood |
| Anger | Depression |
| Insomnia | Delusions |
| Anorexia | Hallucinations |
| Flight of ideas | |
| Distractibility | |
| Hyperactivity | |
| Involvement in pleasurable activities | |
| Loud, rapid speech | |

and involvement with alcohol and drugs is common (an attempt at self-medication). Onset usually occurs in young adulthood. What has been traditionally referred to as manic-depressive illness (mood swings) is now designated as bipolar illness. Manic episodes can also be part of organic mental disorders or another psychotic process. Mania, as a component of bipolar illness, is the focus of this section. Approximately 0.4% to 1.2% of the adult population has had this mental disorder (APA, 1987).

### History

Manic depressive illness can be traced to the earliest recorded history. Thousands of years ago the Greeks recognized the vacillation between extremes of elation and depression. Many people today also have wide mood swings. Often the mood swings are not severe enough to warrant hospitalization (hypomania); however, problems with everyday life still occur. *Hypomania* is the term for an elevated state that is less intense than full mania. Fieve (1975), in his highly respected book, *Moodswings,* points out that many creative people in our society ride the energy from their manic states to success. Fieve also points out that successful playwright Joshua Logan *(South Pacific)* and astronaut Buzz Aldrin (first moon landing) used the tremendous energy from their elevated moods to accomplish great things. Unfortunately for the manic-depressive patient, the trip up the emotional ladder does not stop with elation and excessive energy but moves on into psychotic thinking and behavior. In addition, an equally extreme depression follows these highs. Both Logan and Aldrin required professional help to restore their moods to normal.

### DSM-III-R terminology and criteria

Under the category of bipolar disorders the DSM-III-R defines three different types: manic, mixed, and depressed.

**Box 20-11**
## DIAGNOSTIC CRITERIA FOR BIPOLAR DISORDER, MANIC TYPE

A. An abnormally and persistently elevated mood
B. The presence of
   1. Grandiosity
   2. Decreased need for sleep
   3. Talkativeness
   4. Flight of ideas
   5. Distractibility
   6. Increased goal-directed activity (e.g., social, work/school, sexual) or psychomotor agitation
   7. Excess (e.g., buying sprees, sexual activity, business ventures)
C. Severity of symptoms causes occupational and relational problems or requires hospitalization.

Hypomania includes all of the above criteria except C.

**Bipolar disorder, manic type.** For the diagnosis of manic type to be made, a person must exhibit the symptoms listed in Box 20-11 (APA, 1987).

**Mixed type.** Bipolar disorder, mixed type, is characterized by both manic and depressive symptoms. Secunda et al. (1987) reported that a high percentage of bipolar patients fall into this category. Mixed mania, they believed, suggested a slower response to lithium. The term *rapid cycling* refers to a condition in which there are four or more episodes of mania and depression in 1 year (Kuyler, 1988).

**Depressed type.** Bipolar disorder, depressed type, is characterized by a current state of depression but with a history of at least one manic episode.

**Related disorders**

*Hypomanic episodes.* Hypomania (less than mania) is characterized by a persistent elated mood; however, the extremes found in a manic episode are not present. Hypomania is associated with waves of energy, enthusiasm, and excessive activity. By definition, a hypomanic episode does not require hospitalization.

*Cyclothymia.* Cyclothymia is characterized by numerous hypomanic episodes alternating with periodic depression. These mood swings must be persistent and present for at least 2 years in an adult without a history of major depression or manic episodes. Formerly, this condition, hypomania with depression, was referred to as bipolar II.

**Behavior**

**Objective signs.** The person experiencing a manic episode appears enthusiastic and euphoric. These behaviors are recognized as excessive by others around the person. Objective signs include altered speech patterns; altered social, inter-personal, and occupational relationships; and alteration in activity and appearance.

### Altered speech patterns

> A manic patient stated that a black attendant was a prejudiced Black-Power advocate who hated Jews. She proclaimed that the attendant hated white people and that he was brutalizing patients because of race and religion. She referred to him as a "black bastard" and concentrated on demeaning him and questioning his ability to be helpful to her, based on his low educational level, lack of articulateness, and his presumed prejudice. The nursing attendant, who had presented few overt problems before, became increasingly angry with the patient. He began to avoid talking with her. At times he began to refer to her as a "rich bitch." He became defensive about his lack of education and began to wonder why so few black patients were admitted to the ward and whether blacks were being treated fairly at the hospital (Janowsky et al., 1970, p. 255).

The manic patient may speak loudly in a rapid-fire fashion. He "hogs" the dia-logue, deflecting attempts by others to join in. Conversation is filled with jokes, puns, and clever plays on words. Sarcastic and biting remarks are not uncommon. In fact, even though psychiatric professionals are aware of this tendency, the manic patient's ability to find a "weak spot" often frustrates, embarrasses, and angers the professional person. The tendency to complain often and loudly is also present. The manic patient has the ability to engage staff members in debate and place them on the defensive. Speech is often dramatic, and it is not uncommon for the manic person to burst into song. Speech is often pressured.

The person is also quite easily distracted. While he is in the middle of an apparently meaningful discussion, a bird flying by might distract him onto the topic of flying or some other such irrelevant topic. This phenomenon, in which the person jumps from topic to topic, is called flight of ideas.

### Altered social, interpersonal, and occupational relationships.
It is not surprising that the manic patient irritates others with his faultfinding, anger, and blaming. In a seminal article entitled "Playing the Manic Game," Janowsky et al., (1970) point out five tendencies of the manic patient:

1. *Manipulation of self-esteem of others:* The patient uses techniques to in-crease or decrease another's self-esteem in a coercive fashion. It is easy to fall prey to the manipulation of praise. ("No one here really understands me but you.") It is just as easy to feel the ego-deflating wrath when plans arc thwarted. Some insightful nurses have disclosed the feeling of "having been played like a yo-yo."
2. *Ability to find vulnerability in others:* The manic patient can exploit a weakness in others or create a conflict among staff members.
3. *Ability to shift responsibility:* Through this technique, the patient somehow shifts personal responsibility (e.g., arriving at breakfast on time) to someone else. Nurses are particularly vulnerable in this area since we are trained to take responsibility for many patient concerns.

4. *Limit testing:* The manic patient keeps pushing the limits set on the unit. If one limit is relaxed, the patient will push even more.

5. ⸱⸱⸱⸱⸱⸱⸱⸱⸱⸱⸱⸱⸱ ⸱⸱⸱⸱⸱⸱⸱ The manic patient drives his family away with his behavior.

Because of the tendencies noted by Janowsky et al. (1970), manic-depressive patients have difficulty socially, interpersonally, and occupationally. The same behaviors that drive away family also drive away friends, lovers, bosses, coworkers, ministers, and nonpsychiatric health care providers.

The excess of mood overflows into social, interpersonal, and occupational excesses also. The otherwise faithful husband may become sexually promiscuous; the otherwise thrifty housewife may go on a shopping or spending spree; and the conservative investor may make a dangerously speculative investment.

***Alterations in activity and appearance.*** The manic patient is often hyperactive and agitated. Overt manifestations, such as pacing, flamboyant gestures, colorful dress, singing, and excessive use of make-up, are relatively common. The patient may also dress sloppily and omit personal grooming. The person may not need sleep, or perhaps only a few hours per night. Some have gone for days without sleep, and reports of manic patients dying of exhaustion are not uncommon. Many manic patients suffer from poor nutrition because they quit eating. They simply do not have the patience, the ability to sit still, or the desire to eat.

### Subjective symptoms

***Altered affect.*** The manic patient experiences euphoria and a high regard for self. The inflated self-image can reach levels of grandiosity. Subjectively, the person going through a manic episode experiences an elevated mood, a feeling of joy and greatness. A certain sense of invincibility leads to the social, interpersonal, and occupational problems already discussed.

Another significant symptom is a labile or quickly changing affect. For example, a 64-year-old woman was laughing and talking about her personal acquaintance with the President. ("You know, my husband's name was George." She abruptly began to cry. "He is dead you know.") She quickly returned to the topic of her importance, becoming very excited, with an elevated mood.

***Altered perception.*** Delusions and hallucinations occur, and their content is typically consistent with mood. For instance, if a patient is grandiose about his importance to the government, a mood-congruent delusion could include paranoid thinking related to being pursued by enemy forces.

## Etiology

### Psychodynamic theories

***Family dynamics.*** At one time most psychiatric professionals believed that manic-depressive illness was caused by psychological difficulties. Developmental theorists have hypothesized that faulty family dynamics during early life are responsible for manic behaviors in later life. According to this view the mother (or primary caregiver) enjoys being the "giver of life" and resents autonomy. As the child grows independent, the mother becomes unhappy; to please the mother, the child becomes more dependent. That is, to gain affection, the child at an early age learns to deny his own natural tendencies. The unnatural tension between dependence and independence and the inherent ambivalence in this family environment can be a causative factor in bipolar illness, according to this view.

Others have suggested that the polar events of childhood—for example, receiving praise (elation) and disapproval (depression) or being breast-fed (elation) and being taken from the breast (depression)—are so significant for some people that the result is an adult emotional counterpart to this emotional roller coaster: manic-depressive illness. Still others have suggested that manic-depressive illness is related to an alternating identification with parents—depression with the mother figure and the manic phase with a father figure. Although some of these explanations seem more credible than others, many professionals believe family dynamics play an important role in the genesis of manic-depressive illness.

***Mania as a defense.***  Another psychodynamic hypothesis explains manic episodes as defense against or massive denial of depression. According to this view, these persons go through life appearing independent and excessive in behavior to others—too pushy, too talkative, and too manipulative—only to eventually be blocked by someone who no longer tolerates being pushed, talked to, or manipulated. When this happens, the manic person (who is actually overdependent) may become psychotic.

**Biological theories.**  Although many professionals still hold to the importance of psychological influences, there is a growing awareness of the role of biological considerations. Just as depression seems to be caused by neurotransmitter deficiency, so too, manic episodes seem to be related to excessive levels of norepinephrine, serotonin, and dopamine (Ettigi and Brown, 1977). A related biochemical theory views bipolar illness as an imbalance between cholingeric and noradrenergic systems. According to this view, depression is related to increased cholinergic activity, and mania is related to increased noradrenergic activity.

That genetics has a role in manic-depressive illness seems clear (Gershon et al., 1982; Rosenthal, 1970). Monozygotic (identical) twins have a very high concordancy rate (up to 80% in some studies), whereas dizygotic (fraternal) twins have a higher rate than normal siblings and other close relatives. Siblings and close relatives have a higher incidence of manic-depressive illness than the general population. Cyclothymic personality characteristics are common among family members of bipolar patients.

---

**PSYCHOTHERAPEUTIC MANAGEMENT**

*PSYCHOTHERAPEUTIC NURSE-PATIENT RELATIONSHIP*  The following are specific principles of intervention to be used with the manic patient:

- Safety: It is important for the nurse to prevent the manic patient from hurting himself or others. The manic patient can be very angry when things do not go his way. This pathological irritability leads to arguments, fights, self-injury, (for example, hitting the wall, not paying attention to the environment), and hurting others. By providing emotional support and responding to the patient in a matter-of-fact manner, the nurse conveys both control of the situation and empathy. It is reassuring to the patient to realize that the staff will not let him harm himself or others.

- Clear, concise directions and comments: Working with the hyperactive patient who is very talkative, easily distracted, experiences flights of ideas, and who has poor judgment and a labile affect is difficult. When the nurse is confronted with a very talkative patient, it is not unusual for the nurse to attempt to use familiar skills. For example, most people learn not to interrupt another person until a pause. The pause may never come with a manic patient. To be effective, the nurse may need to raise her hand and say, "Wait just a minute, I do not want to be rude, but I would like to say something." As the patient starts improving, the nurse may be able to work out a nonverbal signal to indicate when the patient needs to stop and let someone else speak. Although the manic patient is talkative, there is a tendency for the talk to be superficial. When talking to the hyperactive patient, the nurse needs to keep remarks brief and simple. The patient literally cannot tolerate a lengthy discussion of anything.
- Limit setting: When the nurse is leading a group, a talkative patient can be disruptive because of the tendencies described by Janowsky et al. (1970):
  - Manipulation of self-esteem of others
  - Ability to find vulnerability of others
  - Ability to shift responsibility to others
  - Limit testing

  This patient has the ability to damage the self-esteem of other patients, ridicule the nurse, blame others, pick fights, create problems between patients, and manipulate others. The nurse needs to protect vulnerable patients and to keep from being drawn into the anger that the manic patient feels. As she is able to remain calm instead of becoming angry, it helps both the manic patient and the other patients in the group. This calmness should be based on an understanding of psychopathology; otherwise, it may simply be an unhealthy defense (that is, "You cannot touch me; you are not important enough"). The nurse absolutely does not want to convey that she is engaged in an adult version of the childish behavior of plugging the ears and saying, "I can't hear you." It is also important to avoid arguing with patients about unit rules and limits. Do not debate these issues with the patient. Simply state the unit policy and move on. Debating and arguing reinforces the tendencies mentioned above.
- Reinforcement of reality: Manic patients also experience disturbances in perception. The intervention strategies outlined for other patients with disturbed perceptions are recommended for the manic patient also.

  *PSYCHOPHARMACOLOGY* Lithium is the drug of choice for manic patients. The starting dose is usually 600 mg three times per day. The typical maintenance dose is 900 to 1200 mg per day. Maintenance blood levels are 0.6 to 1.2 mmol/L. For those persons who are resistant to lithium (10% to 20% [Secunda et al., 1987]) carbamazepine is often prescribed. A full discussion of lithium is found in Chapter 13.

*MILIEU MANAGEMENT* Milieu management is an important dimension of the nursing care of the manic patient because manic patients test the unit perhaps more than any other group of patients.

1. Because of the manic patient's tendency to create conflict, pick on vulnerable persons (patients and staff), blame others, test limits, and shift responsibility to others, the nurse must carefully develop a plan of care. Nursing and other staff members should meet often to defuse conflict and clarify communication. All staff members should be aware of intervention strategies and agree to consistently abide by team decisions. Inexperienced staff members must guard against falling prey to esteem-building statements that tend to split the staff, for example, "You're the only one who understands."

2. Since manic patients are hyperactive, talkative, irritable, and angry, it is important to decrease environmental stimuli. Since the patient is distractible and responds to all sorts of environmental cues, it is important to modify his environment as

   ## Case Study

Mr. Casey Tubbs, a 44-year-old electrician, was admitted to the unit with the diagnosis of bipolar disorder, manic type. He was brought in by police after starting a fight with three Hispanic men in a bar. He had been drinking heavily. He was hyperactive, distractible, irritable, talkative, and demanding upon admission. He demonstrated flight of ideas and was verbally hostile concerning a Hispanic coworker whom he accused of sleeping with his wife and he has vowed to get even. He made several comments about Hispanics in general while looking at Mr. Azteca, a Hispanic nurse. This is Mr. Tubbs' third hospitalization. The first occured 12 years ago after he contracted a *Candida* infection after having sexual intercourse with his wife. The second hospitalization occurred in 1985. No precipitating event was recorded; nor does Mr. Tubbs recollect anything unusual about the second ad-

mission. Mr. Tubbs has responded well to lithium in the past, and during his other hospitalizations also was given chlorpromazine because of his agitation. Between hospitalizations Mr. Tubbs has functioned well and is considered a good worker. His perfectionistic tendencies are appreciated by his boss. Mrs. Tubbs states that Mr. Tubbs has not slept in 3 days and has not stopped to eat for some time (the actual length of time is not clear). She reports a good marriage until Mr. Tubbs stops taking his lithium, which he says he will no longer take. She wants him to "get better and come home." The head nurse decides to streamline the admission process because of Mr. Tubbs' agitated state. He is taken to a quiet area and provided with peanut butter crackers and milk. Mr. Tubbs' nursing care plan is given on the opposite page.

WEEKLY UPDATE: _9/3/90_

NAME: _____Casey Tubbs_____    ADMISSION DATE: _8/27/90_

DSM-III-R DIAGNOSIS: _296.4 Bipolar disorder, manic type_____

### ASSESSMENT:

**Areas of strength:** Patient's marriage is solid between hospitalizations. Patient's boss likes him and is eager for him to return to work. Good adjustment between hospitalizations. He has responded well to lithium in the past.

**Problems:** Patient is threatening and irritating others. Patient has legal problems from bar fight. Patient is threatening to get even with his wife's alledged lover. Patient has not complied with medication regimen recently and states that he will not take lithium.

### DIAGNOSES: Violence related to manic dyscontrol and delusions. Exhaustion related to insomnia. Weight loss related to anorexia and hyperactivity.

### PLANNING:                                                    Date met

**Short-term goals:** Patient will not hurt anyone while in    _____
hospital.
   Patient will comply with medication regimen.              _8/30_
   Patient will become less agitated.                        _9/3_
   Patient will comply with unit norms and limits.           _____

**Long-term goals:** Patient will remain free of manic ep-    _____
isodes.
   Patient will continue to take lithium on outpatient basis.   _____
   Patient will resolve legal problems.                      _____
   Patient will join manic-depressive support group.         _____

### IMPLEMENTATION/INTERVENTIONS:

**Nurse-patient relationship:** Talk to patient in matter-of-fact tone and clearly indicate that aggressive behaviors are not acceptable. Set firm, clear limits. Do not engage in debates over unit policy, limits, etc. Keep comments brief and simple. Do not respond to sarcastic remarks with anger. Reinforce good behavior and confront (carefully) unacceptable behavior.

**Psychopharmacology:** Lithium carbonate, 600 mg t.i.d., p.o. (concentrate); chlorpromazine, 200 mg t.i.d., p.o. (concentrate); chlorpromazine, 50 mg, IM, q.2h. p.r.n for agitation.

**Milieu management:** Provide quiet room and decrease stimuli. Do not include in group activities for a few days. Provide opportunities for rest and monitor sleep. Provide finger foods and weigh daily. Set limits.

### EVALUATION: Mr. Tubbs is less agitated and is taking lithium on schedule. Patient is beginning to talk less about his wife's alleged infidelity. Has not lost weight. Patient continues to test limits.

much as possible. Helpful environmental modifications include a private (if possible), quiet room; limited activities with others; scheduled rest periods; gross motor activities for example, walking, sweeping, or aerobics, to discharge some of his need to be active; and a public room free from a blaring TV or stereo.

3. Manic patients can become hostile and aggressive. It is important for the staff to deal with this aggressiveness in a calm, confident manner. If the patient is escalating, an antipsychotic drug such as haloperidol can be administered to prevent physical aggressiveness and potential weapons (e.g., chairs, pool cues) can be removed. Limits and the consequences of violating those limits should be reviewed. Do not include limits that are not significant. It is countertherapeutic to defend a poor policy, and it is also countertherapeutic to allow this patient to debate a unit issue. It is therapeutic to follow through with appropriate action should the patient violate a unit norm.

4. Since manic patients lose their appetite and are too "busy" to eat, it is the nursing staff's responsibility to ensure that they are adequately nourished. The following are several useful techniques for helping the patient maintain body weight:
   a. Provide the patient with foods that can be eaten on the "run" (sometimes referred to as finger foods). Some patients cannot sit still long enough to eat.
   b. Provide high-protein, high-calorie snacks for the patient. A vitamin supplement may be indicated.
   c. Weigh the patient regularly (sometimes daily weights are needed).

5. Manic patients also experience insomnia. The nurse can help the patient maximize the opportunity for sleep by
   a. Providing a quiet place to sleep
   b. Structuring the patient's day so that there are fewer stimulating activities toward bedtime.
   c. Not allowing caffeinated drinks and providing warm milk before bedtime.
   d. Assessing amount of rest the patient is receiving. Manic patients are not capable of judging their need for rest, and exhaustion and deaths have resulted from lack of rest.

## KEY CONCEPTS

1. Mood disorders are divided into depressive disorders (major depression, dysthymia) and bipolar disorders (bipolar: manic, mixed, or depressed; hypomania; and cyclothymia).

2. The DSM-III-R defines major depression as an episode of depression (apathy, weight changes, sleep changes, psychomotor changes, fatigue, feelings of worthlessness or guilt, decreased cognitive ability, and recurrent thoughts of death) without a history of manic episodes.

3. Reacting to a disappointment or loss with sadness, guilt, or "depression" is normal, however if the sadness, guilt, etc, persists too long, then a diagnosable condition (either dysthymia or major depression) exists.

4. Although there are several approaches to categorizing depression, a particularly appealing approach is to divide depressions between those that are reactions

to loss (reactive) and those for which no identifiable cause can be found (endogenous)

5. Endogenous depression is probably related to deficiencies in certain neurotransmitters such as norepinephrine and serotonin, and probably dopamine.

6. Objective signs of depression include alterations in activity and social interactions.

7. Subjective symptoms of depression include alterations of affect, cognition, physical nature, and perception.

8. Biological explanations for depression include neurotransmitter deficiency; psychodynamic explanations concern debilitating early life experiences, intrapsychic conflicts, and reaction to life events.

9. Psychotherapeutic management includes developing a therapeutic nurse-patient relationship, administering antidepressant drugs when appropriate, and providing a well-managed milieu with particular emphasis on safety because suicide is a prevalent theme among depressed persons.

10. The typical victim of suicide is an unemployed, white man, living alone, who has made a serious attempt in the past.

11. Manic episodes are characterized by an elevated or expansive mood that usually begins suddenly, escalates rapidly, and lasts from a few days up to several months.

12. The DSM-III-R describes three types of bipolar disorder: bipolar manic, bipolar mixed, and bipolar depressed.

13. Objective signs of bipolar illness include altered speech patterns; altered social, interpersonal, and occuptional relationships; and alterations in activity and appearance.

14. Subjective symptoms of bipolar illness include alterations in affect and perception.

15. Psychodynamic theories of bipolar illness include theories about family dynamics (i.e., mother resents the child's growing independence so the child learns to deny his own natural tendencies) and psychoanalytical explanations that view manic behavior as a defense against overwhelming feelings of depression.

16. Biological explanations of bipolar disorder include excessive levels of neurotransmitters (norepinephrine, serotonin, dopamine) and genetics (80% concordancy rates among identical twins in some studies).

17. Lithium is the drug of choice for the treatment of bipolar disorders and, because this drug has a narrow therapeutic index, the nurse must be aware of side effects, toxic effects, and appropriate and inappropriate serum lithium levels.

## REFERENCES

American Psychiatric Association: Diagnostic and Statistical Manual of Mental Disorders, third edition revised, Washington, DC, 1987, The Association.

Becker RE: Depression in schizophrenia, Hosp Community Psychiatry 39:1269, 1988.

Clark DC et al: A field test of Motto's risk estimator for suicide, Am J Psychiatry 144:923, 1987.

Drake RE et al: Suicide among schizophrenics: who is at risk? J Nerv Ment Dis 172:613, 1984.

Elkin I et al: National Institute of Mental Health Treatment of Depression Collaborative Research Program, Arch Gen Psychiatry 46:971, 1989.

Ettigi PG and Brown GM: Psychoneuroendocrinology of affective disorder: an overview, Am J Psychiatry 134:493, 1977.

Fieve RR: Moodswings, New York, 1975, Bantam Books.

Frances A and Hales RE: Determining how a depressed woman's personality affects the choice of treatment (treatment planning), Hosp Community Psychiatry 35:883, 1984.

Frierson RL: Women who shoot themselves, Hosp Community Psychiatry 40:841, 1989.

Gershon ES et al: A family study of schizoaffective, bipolar I, bipolar II, unipolar, and normal control probands. Arch Gen Psychiatry 38:1157, 1982.

Green LW and Wilson CR: Guidelines for nonprofessionals who receive suicidal phone calls, Hosp Community Psychiatry 39:310, 1988.

Hammer M: Psychotherapy with suicidal patients. In Hammer M, editor: The theory and practice of psychotherapy with specific disorders, Springfield, Ill, 1972, Charles C Thomas Publisher, pp 190-218.

Hendin H: Suicide: a review of new directions in research, Hosp Community Psychiatry 37:148, 1986.

Holinger PC, Offer D, and Ostrov E: Suicide and homicide in the United States: an epidemiologic study of violent death, population changes, and the potential for prediction, Am J Psychiatry 144:215, 1987.

Janowsky DS, Melitta L, and Epstein RS: Playing the manic game, Arch Gen Psychiatry 22:252, 1970.

Keltner NL: Drugs for treatment of depression and mania. In Shlafer M and Marieb E, editors: The nurse, pharmacology, and drug therapy, Redwood City, Calif., 1989, Addison-Wesley.

Klerman GI: Overview of affective disorders. In Kaplan HI, Freedmar AM, and Sadock BJ, editors: Comprehensive textbook of psychiatry III, vol 2, Baltimore, 1980, Williams & Wilkins.

Kuyler PL: Rapid cycling bipolar I illness in three closely related individuals, Am J Psychiatry 145:114, 1988.

Loomis M et al: ANA classification of individual human responses, Kansas City, 1986, American Nursing Association.

Metcalfe M: The personality of depressive patients. In Coppen A and Walk A, editors: The psychology of depression: contemporary therapy and research, New York, 1974, John Wiley & Sons.

Meyer J-E and Meyer R: Self-portrayal by a depressed poet: a contribution to the clinical biography of William Cowper, Am J Psychiatry 144:127, 1987.

Rosenthal D: Genetics and abnormal behavior, New York, 1970, McGraw-Hill Book Co., Inc.

Salzman C and Shader RI: Depression in the elderly. II. Possible drug etiologies: differential diagnostic criteria. J Am Geriatr Soc 26:303, 1978.

Secunda SK et al: Diagnosis and treatment of mixed mania, Am J Psychiatry 144:96, 1987.

Teplin LA: The prevalence of severe mental disorder among male urban jail detainees: comparison with epidemiologic catchment area program, Am J Public Health 80:663, 1990.

Weiss KJ, Valdiserri EV, and Dubin WR: Understanding depression in schizophrenia, Hosp Community Psychiatry 40:849, 1989.

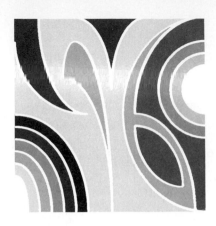

## CHAPTER 21

# Anxiety-related Disorders

LEARNING OBJECTIVES
After reading this chapter you should be able to

- Describe major theories that contribute to the understanding of anxiety, somatoform, and dissociative disorders.
- Recognize special terms related to anxiety, somatoform, and dissociative disorders.
- Describe DSM-III-R criteria for major anxiety, somatoform, and dissociative disorders.
- Describe objective and subjective symptoms of major anxiety, somatoform, and dissociative disorders.
- Develop nursing care plans for persons with major anxiety, somatoform, and dissociative disorders.
- Evaluate the effectiveness of nursing interventions for persons with major anxiety, somatoform, and dissociative disorders.
- Recognize issues related to care of persons with anxiety, somatoform, and dissociative disorders.

The anxiety-related disorders (formerly called neurotic disorders) include disturbances in which felt (subjective) or expressed anxiety (objective) is a major symptom. Currently, the neuroses are viewed as specific illnesses and are classified in the DSM-III-R as anxiety disorders, somatoform disorders, and dissociative disorders (Box 21-1).

To understand the anxiety-related disorders, it is crucial to understand *what* anxiety is, *where* it comes from, *why* it is difficult to deal with, and *how* human beings try to get rid of it (Fig. 21-1).

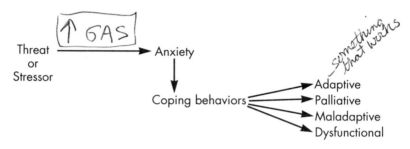

**FIGURE 21-1** Process of anxiety

---

**Box 21-1**

## DSM-III-R CLASSIFICATION OF ANXIETY-RELATED DISORDERS

**Anxiety disorders**

Generalized anxiety disorder
Panic disorder
Obsessive-compulsive disorder
Phobic disorder
Posttraumatic stress disorder

**Somatoform disorders**

Somatization disorder
Somatoform pain disorder

Hypochondriasis
Conversion disorder
Body dysmorphic disorder

**Dissociative disorders**

Psychogenic amnesia
Psychogenic fugue
Depersonalization
Multiple-personality disorder

## RECURRING THEMES OF ANXIETY

Anxiety as a concept and process has been studied, defined, and described by many respected authors: Peplau, 1952; Sullivan, 1954; Lazarus, 1966, Levitt, 1967. The recurring themes are listed below:

- Anxiety is a subjective experience that can be detected only by the objective behaviors that result from it.
- Anxiety is emotional pain.
- Anxiety is apprehension, fearfulness or sense of powerlessness where the threat is less discernible or definable. (Fear, in contrast, has a visible object.)
- Anxiety is a warning sign of a perceived danger or threat.
- Anxiety is an emotional response that triggers behaviors (automatic relief behaviors) aimed at eliminating it.
- Anxiety alerts the person to prepare to defend himself.
- Anxiety occurs in degrees.
- Anxiety is "contagious." It can be communicated from one person to another.
- Anxiety is part of a process, not an isolated phenomenon.

The process of which anxiety is a part is represented in Figure 21-1.

The threat or danger that precipitates anxiety is whatever a person defines as a threat or danger. How people define an event depends on their backgrounds, needs, desires, self-concept, resources, knowledge, skills, personality traits, and maturity. For example, a skilled athlete might define a competitive event as an exciting challenge with a high probability of success. A less skilled athlete might define the same event as an overwhelming test with a high probability of failure. Each athlete, on the basis of his own perception of the situation, will have a different emotional and physical response.

## COMMONLY PERCEIVED THREATS AND DANGERS

There are also commonalities among perceptions of what constitutes a threat or danger. The following is a list of commonly perceived threats or dangers:

1. Loss of health or ability to perform or function
2. Loss of self-esteem or self-respect
3. Loss of control over oneself
4. Loss of control or power over one's life
5. Loss of status or prestige
6. Loss of resources—emotional, physical, financial
7. Loss of loved ones
8. Loss of freedom or independence
9. Unmet needs, goals, desires, expectations

Many of these threats or losses are visible to others (objective). Others are less evident (subjective). The visible losses are more external phenomena; the less evident are more internal. The internal threats may not even be "real or valid"; the perception of threat can be inaccurate, misinterpreted, exaggerated, or unjustified. For example, your best friend turns down your invitation to dinner saying she has to visit her grandmother, who is ill. She has always been honest with you, but you mistakenly begin to doubt if she really cares about you anymore.

## RESPONSES TO ANXIETY

To assess how a person is responding to any given situation, the nurse should ask him to define it and report how he is reacting to it (subjective). Another way of assessing a person's response to a situation is to observe his behaviors (objective) as the situation is occurring or immediately afterward. (See Table 21-1.)

Even a moderate level of anxiety is uncomfortable and cannot be tolerated for very long. As anxiety increases, there is a drive to relieve it as soon as possible. Long-lasting high levels of anxiety are so physically and emotionally draining that a person will do almost anything to escape the pain within a month or two. In some cases, the "almost anything" involves becoming ill (physically or emotionally) or even committing suicide in rare instances. Fortunately, there are many less debilitating ways to cope with anxiety.

## COPING WITH ANXIETY

Methods of coping with anxiety can be divided into four categories according to their degree of effectiveness in decreasing anxiety or eliminating the source of anxiety.

- Adaptive coping: solves the problem causing the anxiety so anxiety is decreased. Example: Anxiety about an upcoming examination is reduced by studying effectively and passing the examination with an A.
- Palliative coping: temporarily decreases the anxiety but does not solve the problem; therefore, the anxiety eventually surfaces. The temporary relief allows a person to come back to the problem with more objectivity, rationality, and energy, making problem solving an easier process. Example: Anxiety about an upcoming examination is temporarily reduced by jogging for half an hour. Effective studying becomes feasible, and a score of A is still possible.
- Maladaptive coping: unsuccessful attempts to decrease the anxiety without attempting to solve the problem. The level of anxiety is usually diminished only enough to allow minimal functioning. Productivity is impaired. Example: Anxiety about an upcoming examination is first ignored by going to a movie and then handled by frantically trying to cram for a few hours. A passing score of C is the likely outcome.
- Dysfunctional coping: is not successful in reducing anxiety or solving the problem. Even minimal functioning becomes difficult, and new problems begin to develop. Example: Anxiety about an upcoming examination is first ignored by going out drinking with friends and then escaped by "passing out" for the night. The result is failing the course and not progressing in school.

Although effectiveness is the primary criterion for evaluating a coping method, outcomes also need to be considered. Sometimes coping reduces the anxiety and solves the problem but at the same time creates other significant problems. Stealing

**TABLE 21-1**  Levels of anxiety

| Severity of anxiety | Physical | Intellectual | Social and emotional |
|---|---|---|---|
| **MINIMAL (near 0)** | Basal levels of: Blood pressure Pulse Respiration rate $O_2$ consumption Pupillary constriction Muscles relaxed | Cognitive activity minimal Disregard for external environmental stimuli; no attempt to actively process information Focus typically on single, nonthreatening mental image States of altered consciousness | No social interaction No attempt to deal with environmental stimuli Minimal emotional activity Feelings of indifference, invulnerability, and contentment prevail |
| **MILD (+1)** | Low-level sympathetic arousal Moderate to low skeletal muscle tension Body relaxed Voice calm, well-modulated | Perceptual field open; able to shift focus of attention readily Passively aware of external environment Self-referent thoughts positive; low concern for unexpected or negative outcomes | Behavior primarily automatic; habitual patterns and well-learned skills Positive feeling of security, confidence, and satisfaction dominate Solitary activities |
| **MODERATE (+2)** | Sympathetic nervous system activation ↑ Blood pressure ↑ Pulse rate ↑ Respiratory rate Pupillary dilation Sweat glands stimulated Peripheral vascular constriction Increased muscular tension Heightened performance of well-learned skills Rate of speech increased, pitch heightened Increased alertness | Narrowing of perception; attentional focus on specific internal or external stimuli Conscious effort in processing of information; optimal level for learning Self-referent thoughts ± mixed; some concern about personal ability or available resources necessary to solve problems; probability of positive outcomes increasingly uncertain | Increased skill in learning and refining of skills; analyzing problematic situations; integrating cognitive and motor domains Feelings of challenge; drive to resolve problems or dilemmas Mixed sense of confidence/optimism with fear, lowered self-esteem, and potential inadequacy |

*[handwritten note in left margin next to MILD row: "learning can happen at this level"]*

Adapted from Longo D, and Williams R: Clinical practice in psychosocial nursing: assessment and intervention, New York, 1986, Appleton-Century-Crofts. From Beck C, Rawlins R, and Williams S: Mental health psychiatric nursing: holistic life-cycle approach, ed 2, St Louis, 1988, The CV Mosby Co.

*Continued.*

**TABLE 21-1**   Levels of anxiety—cont'd

| Severity of anxiety | Physical | Intellectual | Social and emotional |
|---|---|---|---|
| **SEVERE** **(+3)** | Fight-flight response<br>Stimulation of adrenal<br>  medulla<br>  ↑ Catecholamines,<br>    accelerated heart<br>    rate, palpitations<br>  ↑ Blood glucose<br>  ↓ Blood flow to<br>    digestive system<br>  ↑ Blood flow to skel-<br>    etal muscles<br>Muscles extremely<br>  tense<br>Hyperventilation<br>Physical actions in-<br>  creasingly agitated,<br>  pacing, wringing of<br>  hands, fidgeting,<br>  trembling<br>May experience loss<br>  of appetite, nausea,<br>  "cold sweats"<br>Rapid, high-pitched<br>  speech<br>Facial expression:<br>  poor eye contact,<br>  fleeting eye move-<br>  ments | Perceptual capacity<br>  restricted; exclusive<br>  attention to singu-<br>  lar stimuli (internal<br>  or external) or<br>  multifocal, frag-<br>  mented processing<br>  of stimuli<br>Problem soving ineffi-<br>  cient, difficult<br>Some threatening<br>  stimuli disregarded,<br>  minimized, denied<br>Disorientation in<br>  terms of time and<br>  place<br>Expected likelihood<br>  of negative conse-<br>  quences or out-<br>  comes high; esti-<br>  mates of personal<br>  self-efficacy low | Flight behavior may<br>  be manifested by<br>  withdrawal, denial,<br>  depression, somati-<br>  zation<br>Feelings of increasing<br>  threat, need to re-<br>  spond to situation<br>  are heightened<br>Dissociating tendency;<br>  feelings are denied |

*Selective inattention* [handwritten annotation]

class notes from a friend may result in an examination score of A but permanently damages the friendship at the same time. Prolonged late-night studying may also yield an A but also leads to reduced resistance to a virus and an episode of the flu. Excessive studying may also lead to a poorly balanced life of work, love, and play. Thus a coping method must be examined for its primary effectiveness and for its consequences on the person's well-being.

## RELATIONSHIP BETWEEN ANXIETY AND ILLNESS

As anxiety increases to the moderate, severe, and panic levels, the person concomitantly feels more pain and discomfort. To feel better or more comfortable, the person uses behaviors and defense mechanisms to protect himself. The behaviors a person uses are individualized. For instance, a person's biological and genetic

**TABLE 21-1**   Levels of anxiety—cont'd

| Severity of anxiety | Physical | Intellectual | Social and emotional |
|---|---|---|---|
| **PANIC (+4)** | Continued physiological arousal | Perception severely restricted, may be impervious to external stimuli | Emotionally drained, overwhelmed |
|  | Actions disorganized, directionless; unable to execute simple motor tasks; fumbling, gross motor agitation, flailing | Thoughts are random, distorted, disconnected, logical processing impaired | Reliance on earlier, more "primitive" coping behaviors: crying, shouting, curling up, rocking, freezing |
|  | May strike out verbally or physically; may attempt to withdraw from situation | Unable to solve problems; limited tolerance for processing novel stimuli (verbal, auditory, or visual) | Feelings of impotence, helplessness, agony and desperation dominate; may be experienced as horror, dread, defenselessness; may be converted to anger, rage |
|  | Eventual depletion of sympathetic neurotransmitters | Preoccupied with thoughts of highly probable negative outcomes; conclusion may be drawn, negative consequences seen as inevitable |  |
|  | Blood redistributed throughout body |  |  |
|  | Hypotension |  |  |
|  | May feel dizzy, faint, or exhausted |  |  |
|  | Appears pale, drawn, weary |  |  |
|  | Facial expression: aghast, grimacing, eyes fixed |  |  |
|  | Voice louder, higher pitched |  |  |

*[Handwritten margin note: Use of meds (anti-anxiety) part of nursing intervention]*

endowment influences his reaction to stress. An individual is born with his own unique personality traits, predispositions, and physiological and neurological systems. Accordingly, people tend to react to stress in an individualized fashion. If long-term palliative, maladaptive, or dysfunctional coping behaviors are employed, an anxiety-related disorder, a physiological health problem, or even a psychosis may develop.

## ETIOLOGY

**Psychodynamic theory.** Freud viewed the ego as the part of a person that develops defenses to help that person control or deal with anxiety. The need to control anxiety stems from conflicts between the id (our instincts) and the superego (our conscience). Repression of feelings connected with early conflicts occurs. Later in life, as conflicts are once again experienced, repression fails, and these feelings emerge, causing anxiety and discomfort.

**Interpersonal theory.** Sullivan considers interpersonal relations and the socialization process important to how a person feels about himself. Sullivan sees the person striving for security and relief from anxiety to protect his self-system. In childhood a person takes on the values of his parents and family to receive their approval and to feel good about himself. Later in life a threat to the self is based on how the person perceives the danger or threat and how he was taught to handle conflict early in life. Because the child is dependent on others for his feelings of self-worth, he strives to gain approval to feel secure. His sense of self is based on others. Issues of dependency, control, and security and the conflicts related to them form the basis of how anxiety is handled.

**Biological theory.** Selye found that the effects of stress (Fig. 21-1) can be seen by the objective measurement of structural and clinical changes in the body. These changes are called the general adaptation syndrome (see Chapter 2). With activation of the fight-or-flight mechanism, the adrenal cortex and lymph nodes enlarge and hormonal levels increase. Vasoconstriction due to the release of epinephrine and norepinephrine increases blood pressure and the rate and force of cardiac contraction. During adaptation to stress, hormone levels readjust, with the adrenal cortex and lymph nodes returning to normal size. If adaptation does not occur, the adrenal glands enlarge again and hormone production is depleted. The immune response decreases, and lymph nodes increase. Cardiac and renal failure or death can occur if exposure to stress continues (Selye, 1956).

## BEHAVIOR

Persons with an anxiety-related disorder recognize that they are ill and need help. They find their own behavior disturbing. *Subjectively,* they report feeling anxious and easily fatigued. They may complain of dry mouth, nausea, diarrhea, light-headedness, and frequent urination. They may say that they feel keyed up or on edge, have trouble swallowing, or feel as if they have a "lump" in their throat. Sleep difficulties are a common problem and occur as problems in falling asleep or staying asleep. *Objectively,* these persons tremble, twitch, or exhibit restlessness, even pacing. They may experience sweating or clammy hands and chills or flushes. They are often irritable, have difficulty sitting still, are unable to concentrate and startle easily. The discussion of objective and subjective symptoms presented here is not exhaustive but includes only some common manifestations of how anxiety feels to the individual and how it can be observed by others.

## SPECIAL ISSUES

To understand the dynamics of anxiety-related disorders, it is important to understand the concepts of primary gain and secondary gain and how they apply to these persons. Primary gain refers to the person's desire to relieve his anxiety so that he can feel better and feel more secure. Secondary gain refers to the attention or support the person derives from others because he is sick. Family and friends will help him to fulfill his role responsibilities, functions, and duties. For example, "If I am sick I cannot leave the home to go grocery shopping, so I will call my husband at work and tell him to stop at the grocery store on his way home to buy the needed items." This assistance from the husband is called a secondary gain.

Sometimes the attention or the benefit of the secondary gain becomes more important to the person than reducing the anxiety. The continuance of the secondary gains encourages the person to maintain the sick role.

# ■ Anxiety Disorders
## GENERALIZED ANXIETY DISORDERS

In the generalized anxiety disorder (GAD) the anxiety is the predominant characteristic and is directly felt and expressed (see criteria on GAD).

### DSM-III-R criteria, objective and subjective behavior

According to the DSM-III-R (Box 21-2), a person with this disorder spends his days experiencing anxiety or worry beyond what would be a normal reaction to daily stresses. The worry or the anxiety is out of proportion to the original situation. For example, a woman is approaching her fortieth birthday. She spends several hours a day worrying that her husband will start having an affair with his secretary when there is no evidence to support this. Thus this person worries about concrete issues that are not reality based.

In addition the DSM-III-R states that the person experiences symptoms of motor tension, autonomic hyperactivity, and vigilance and scanning. In scanning, the person looks around, pays attention to, and is aware of what is occurring in his immediate environment.

The generalized anxiety disorder rarely occurs by itself. It generally is seen in combination with other anxiety disorders, somatoform disorders, or depression. Persons with GAD are usually admitted to the hospital for relief of their intense symptoms of anxiety which is their immediate concern. Their physiological symptoms have disrupted their interpersonal relationships or social and occupational functioning. The psychiatric nursing diagnoses (PND-I) related to anxiety disorders are listed in Box 21-3.

---

### PSYCHOTHERAPEUTIC MANAGEMENT

*NURSE-PATIENT RELATIONSHIP*  In the nurse-patient relationship, the nurse first of all must assist the patient in reducing his level of anxiety before any problem solving can occur. The nurse's goal ultimately is to assist the patient in developing adaptive coping responses.

Initially, the patient needs support and reassurance from the nurse. Acceptance of the patient's positive and negative feelings, with acknowledgment of his discomfort, promotes trust. Conveying empathy to the patient tells him that the nurse is concerned and understanding and does not minimize the level of distress he is feeling. For example, the nurse might say, "This must be uncomfortable and painful for you."

**Box 21-2**
## DIAGNOSTIC CRITERIA FOR 300.02 GENERALIZED ANXIETY DISORDER

Unrealistic or excessive anxiety and worry (apprehensive expectation) about two or more life circumstances, e.g., worry about possible misfortune to one's child (who is in no danger) and worry about finances (for no good reason), for a period of 6 months or longer, during which the person has been bothered more days than not by these concerns. In children and adolescents, this may take the form of anxiety and worry about academic, athletic, and social performance.

At least 6 of the following 18 symptoms are often present when anxious (do not include symptoms present only during pain attacks):

*Motor tension*

(1) trembling, twitching, or feeling shaky
(2) muscle tension, aches, or soreness
(3) restlessness
(4) easy fatigability

*Autonomic hyperactivity*

(5) shortness of breath or smothering sensations
(6) palpitations or accelerated heart rate (tachycardia)
(7) sweating, or cold clammy hands
(8) dry mouth
(9) dizziness or light headedness
(10) nausea, diarrhea, or other abdominal distress
(11) flushes (hot flashes) or chills
(12) frequent urination
(13) trouble swallowing or "lump in throat"

*Vigilance and scanning*

(14) feeling keyed up or on edge
(15) exaggerated startle response
(16) difficulty concentrating or "mind going blank" because of anxiety
(17) trouble falling or staying asleep
(18) irritability

Reprinted with permission from the *Diagnostic and Statistical Manual of Mental Disorders, Third Edition, Revised.* Copyright 1987 American Psychiatric Association.

**Box 21-3**
PSYCHIATRIC NURSING DIAGNOSES (PND-1):
ANXIETY DISORDERS

| | |
|---|---|
| 04.02.02 | Anxiety |
| 04.02.05 | Fear |
| 04.02.07 | Guilt |
| 02.08.02 | Alteration in concentration |
| 06.01.01 | Distractibility |
| 06.02.02 | Distress |
| 05.05.02 | Social isolation/withdrawal |
| 05.97 | Undeveloped interpersonal processes |
| 05.03 | Altered role performance |

A. O'Toole, M. Loomis. 1989. "Classifying Human Responses in Psychiatric-Mental Health Nursing," from *Classification Systems for Describing Nursing Practice: Working Papers,* pp. 20-30. Kansas City, MO: American Nurses Association. Reprinted with permission.

To help the patient manage and reduce his level of anxiety, the nurse would use the following interventions:

1. Provide a calm and quiet environment by identifying and reducing stimulation, which includes exposure to situations and interactions with patients that could provoke anxiety.
2. Ask the patient to identify what and how he is feeling to help increase his recognition of what is happening to him.
3. Encourage the patient to describe and discuss his feelings with you to help increase his awareness of the connection between feelings and behavior.
4. Help the patient identify possible causes of his feelings to assist him in connecting his feelings with what might have occurred earlier.
5. Listen carefully for the patient's expressions of helplessness and hopelessness. The patient could be suicidal because he wants to escape his pain and does not think that he will ever be better.
6. Ask the patient if he feels suicidal or has a plan to hurt himself. If he does, initiate suicide precautions.
7. Plan and involve the patient in such activities as going for a walk or recreational games to release nervous energy and to discourage preoccupation with self.

After the patient's level of anxiety is reduced to a more manageable and comfortable level, the nurse would begin to assist the patient in examining his coping behaviors. Through the use of problem-solving methods, adaptive coping skills can increase. The nurse would use the following interventions:

1. Discuss with the patient his present and previous coping mechanisms and reinforce effective adaptive behaviors.
2. Discuss with the patient the meaning of problems and conflicts in order to help him appraise the stressor, explore his personal values, and define the scope and seriousness of the problem.
3. Use supportive confrontation and teaching to increase the patient's insight into the negative effects of his maladaptive and dysfunctional coping behaviors.
4. Assist the patient in exploring alternative solutions and behaviors to increase adaptive coping mechanisms.
5. Encourage the patient to test new adaptive coping behaviors through role playing or implementation (in the hospital setting).
6. Teach the patient relaxation exercises to reduce the level of anxiety. These techniques help the patient manage or control anxiety on his own.
7. Promote the use of hobbies and recreational activities to help the patient deal with routine feelings of stress and anxiety.

The process of helping the patient to learn and to use adaptive coping behaviors requires patience and the awareness that each person learns and changes at his own pace. The nurse must also be aware of her own verbal and nonverbal behavior when working with these patients, because anxiety is contagious. The nurse must manage her own stress and anxiety so that the work between the nurse and the patient is not compromised.

*PSYCHOPHARMACOLOGY* The benzodiazepines are most often used for patients with a GAD, primarily alprazolam (Xanax) and lorazepam (Ativan). These medications are usually ordered on a scheduled basis. Additional doses of benzodiazepines are also given on an as-needed basis, depending on the need of the patient and the severity of his anxiety.

Recent studies have shown that patients experiencing pathological anxiety do not usually abuse these medications if they do not have a problem with alcohol or substance abuse (Roy-Byrne and Katon, 1987).

If a patient experiences depression along with a GAD, an antidepressant that has antianxiety properties (e.g., amitriptyline [Elavil]) will be ordered.

The use of benzodiazepines for improving somatic symptoms and buspirone (Buspar) for improving cognitive symptoms of anxiety has been noted to be effective pharmacologic treatment (Roy-Byrne and Katon, 1987; Beeber, 1989).

*MILIEU MANAGEMENT* The patient with a generalized anxiety disorder can benefit from a variety of milieu activities. Recreational activities will help reduce tension and anxiety. The use of relaxation exercises and tapes will help decrease bodily tension and promote relaxation and comfort.

Groups focusing on stress management, problem solving, self-esteem, assertiveness, codependency, and goal setting will assist with stress management. Depending on the issues and concerns of the patient, a variety of groups can be beneficial.

## PANIC DISORDER

### Objective and subjective behavior

In panic disorder, anxiety is the major characteristic. The panic attack is accompanied by intense fear or discomfort that lasts from minutes to, more rarely, hours. The attacks are spontaneous or occur "out of the blue" with no apparent cause or stimulus. These panic attacks may be severe and incapacitating to the person and are more frightening than symptoms experienced with the generalized anxiety disorder. In addition to symptoms of autonomic hypersensitivity (see GAD) experienced by someone with a GAD, the person with a panic disorder can also experience chest pain or discomfort, a choking feeling, the fear of dying or going crazy, depersonalization or derealization, and numbness and tingling (parasthenia). Fear of loss of control over oneself may be another issue experienced by some. The person may become immobilized during an attack and even become suicidal because of helplessness and hopelessness about ever getting better. The fear of having a panic attack in a place where embarrassment could occur, where help might not be available, where escape is impossible can result in agoraphobia. The person who has panic disorder with agoraphobia will restrict activities outside the home or require another person to be with him when outside the home. Thus he becomes agoraphobic because of his fear of having an attack outside the home. Treatment for agoraphobia will be discussed later.

### Etiology

In contrast to the traditional views explained earlier in the chapter, recent studies suggest that panic disorder may be endogenous and, in fact, hereditary. Studies have shown that electroencephalographic changes exist in persons with panic disorders. Lactate, carbon dioxide, and caffeine studies have shown that panic attacks can be induced in patients with panic disorders ("Improving Therapeutic Interventions for the Treatment of Panic Disorders," 1988).

---

#### PSYCHOTHERAPEUTIC MANAGEMENT

*NURSE-PATIENT RELATIONSHIP* The therapeutic relationship is centered around the same issues and interventions discussed for the patient with a generalized anxiety disorder. Interventions specific to a patient experiencing a panic attack are the following:

1. Stay with the patient and acknowledge his discomfort.
2. Maintain a calm style and demeanor.
3. Speak in short, simple sentences and give one direction at a time in a calm tone of voice.
4. If the patient is hyperventilating, give him a brown paper bag and focus on breathing with the patient.
5. If the patient is pacing or crying, allow him to do so to enable him to release tension and energy.

6. Communicate to the patient that you are in control and will not let anything happen to him.
7. Move or direct the patient to a quieter, less stimulating environment.
8. Ask the patient to express his perception or fear about what is happening to him.

*PSYCHOPHARMACOLOGY* An antidepressant such as imipramine (Tofranil) or an MAO inhibitor such as phenelzine (Nardil) and benzodiazepines such as alprazolam (Xanax) and clonazepam (Klonopin) can block or reduce panic attacks ("Improving Therapeutic Interventions for the Treatment of Panic Disorders," 1988; Roy-Byrne and Katon, 1987; Beeber, 1989). These medications will be given as scheduled dosages. However, a p.r.n. benzodiazepine is often ordered to reduce a higher level of anxiety. The nurse must be able to differentiate between anxiety responses and medication side effects.

*MILIEU MANAGEMENT* As the patient's anxiety level decreases from panic to other levels of anxiety, gross motor activities such as walking, jogging, basketball, or volleyball are appropriate to help decrease tension and anxiety. Other milieu interventions are located in the section about the patient with a generalized anxiety disorder.

## OBSESSIVE-COMPULSIVE DISORDER
### DSM-III-R criteria, objective and subjective behavior

According to the DSM-III-R (Box 21-4), obsessions are recurrent and persistent thoughts, ideas, impulses, or images that are experienced as intrusive and senseless. The person recognizes that the thoughts are the product of his own mind. He knows that the thoughts are trivial, ridiculous, or morbid, but he cannot stop, forget, or control them. The thoughts are distressful and anxiety-provoking. An example of a morbid obsession is a mother experiencing an impulse to kill her child. An example of a silly obsession is the rhyme "sticks and stones may break my bones but words will never hurt me."

Compulsions can be defined as repetitive behaviors that are performed in a particular manner in response to an obsession. The person wants to prevent discomfort and bind or neutralize his anxiety. In the obsessive-compulsive disorder the person experiences anxiety if he tries to resist the obsessions or the compulsions. Some examples of compulsions are handwashing, checking doors, counting, and touching. This person knows or recognizes that his actions are absurd, but he is compelled to perform his ritual because if he did not, his tension and anxiety would increase greatly. These persons have a great need to control themselves, others, and their environment. Some find it difficult to express emotions and to be introspective. Depression is a feature associated with this disorder because of its impact on self-esteem and self-worth. The most commonly used defense mechanisms are repression, reaction-formation, isolation, and undoing (Maxmen, 1986). Avoidance of anxiety is also employed in this disorder.

**Box 21-4**
## DIAGNOSTIC CRITERIA FOR 300.30 OBSESSIVE COMPULSIVE DISORDERS

A.  Either obsessions or compulsions:

*Obsessions:* (1), (2), (3), and (4):

(1) recurrent and persistent ideas, thoughts, impulses, or images that are experienced, at least initially, as intrusive and senseless, e.g., a parent's having repeated impulses to kill a loved child, a religious person's having recurrent blasphemous thoughts

(2) the person attempts to ignore or suppress such thoughts or impulses or to neutralize them with some other thought or action

(3) the person recognizes that the obsessions are the product of his or her own mind, not imposed from without (as in thought insertion)

(4) if another Axis I disorder is present, the content of the obsession is unrelated to it, e.g., the ideas, thoughts, impulses, or images are not about food in the presence of an Eating Disorder, about drugs in the presence of a Psychoactive Substance Use Disorder, or guilty thoughts in the presence of a Major Depression

*Compulsions:* (1), (2), and (3):

(1) repetitive, purposeful, and intentional behaviors that are performed in response to an obsession, or according to certain rules or in a stereotyped fashion

(2) the behavior is designed to neutralize or to prevent discomfort or some dreaded event or situation; however, either the activity is not connected in a realistic way with what it is designed to neutralize or prevent, or it is clearly excessive

(3) the person recognizes that his or her behavior is excessive or unreasonable (this may not be true for young children; it may no longer be true for people whose obsessions have evolved into overvalued ideas)

B.  The obsessions or compulsions cause marked distress, are time-consuming (take more than an hour a day), or significantly interfere with the person's normal routine, occupational functioning, or usual social activities or relationships with others.

An important feature to remember about the obsessive-compulsive disorder is that the obsessions or compulsions are so severe that they significantly interfere with a person's normal routine. They are so time consuming that they interfere with occupational and social functioning. The obsessions and compulsions also interfere with the person's interpersonal relationships because he does not have time to relate to others. He is too busy thinking or doing. The person experiencing magical thinking believes that thinking equals doing. For example, "Thinking badly of my father caused him to die" (Maxmen, 1986). Their thinking processes may also be rigid, and they are task-oriented. Relaxation is very difficult. They are very overcontrolled persons and have a strong sense of right and wrong.

In our society, value is placed on performing well in school or at work. Being responsible and perfectionistic is often rewarded by the boss or by family members. Thus, at times, any one of us may be "compulsive." Generally, however, we do not allow our compulsivity to rule our lives. We are able to maintain a balance between work and play, between role expectations and performance. There is a difference between having characteristics or traits and having an illness. Our occasional brooding, rumination, or steadfastness to a task is not considered ridiculous or excessively bothersome to us. They do not rule our lives.

## Etiology

Traditional etiology was described earlier in this chapter. Current views concerning etiology point to genetic transmission for obsessive-compulsive, panic, and phobic disorders. The disorder may run in families (Maxmen, 1986). Obsessive-compulsive disorders are more common among first-degree biologic relatives of persons with this disorder than among the general population (APA, 1987).

---

### PSYCHOTHERAPEUTIC MANAGEMENT

*NURSE-PATIENT RELATIONSHIPS* Therapeutic work between the patient and the nurse focuses on teaching and developing adaptive coping behaviors to deal with anxiety. Therapeutic goals include increasing the patient's expression of feelings and increasing his ability to make decisions concerning conflicts. More specific interventions are listed in Box 21-5.

*PSYCHOPHARMACOLOGY* A new antidepressant, clomipramine (Anafranil), has been shown to be effective for compulsions (Roy-Byrne and Katon, 1987; DeVeaugh-Geiss et al., 1989). Clomipramine has a specific antiobsessional effect and may help alleviate rituals and coexisting depression (Maxmen, 1986; Rapoport, 1989). Other antidepressants have limited efficacy.

*MILIEU MANAGEMENT* A variety of milieu activities and groups are beneficial to this patient after his anxiety decreases and his need for obsessions and compulsions decreases or abates. Of particular importance are stress management groups, recreational or social skills groups, codependency groups, problem-solving groups, and communication or assertive groups. Care is always based on the individual needs of the patient.

**Box 21-5**
## INTERVENTIONS FOR OBSESSIVE-COMPULSIVE DISORDERS

1. Ensure that basic needs of food, rest, and grooming are met since the patient is too busy to attend to these himself. Reminders and specific directions are usually necessary.
2. *Provide the patient with time to perform rituals because he needs to keep anxiety in check.* Later work to decrease the rituals by setting limits, but never take away a ritual or panic may ensue.
3. Explain expectations, routines, and changes to prevent an increase or escalation of anxiety.
4. Be empathetic and aware of the patient's need to perform rituals.
5. Assist the patient with connecting his behaviors to feelings.
6. Structure simple activities, games, or tasks for the patient to help him focus on alternatives to his thoughts and actions.
7. Reinforce and recognize nonritualistic behaviors to increase the patients self-esteem and self-worth.

Exposure treatment and in vivo exposure treatment are effective behavioral treatments used for persons with obsessive-compulsive disorders (Marks, 1988). The patient can perform in vivo exposure treatment on an outpatient basis. The patient not only is encouraged to contact the feared stimuli for a prolonged period of time but also to resist urges to perform rituals (Marks, 1988). Exposure treatment is explained in Chapter 26.

## PHOBIC DISORDERS
### DSM-III-R criteria, objective and subjective behavior

Phobic disorders are intense, irrational fear responses to an external object, activity, or situation. Anxiety is experienced if the person confronts the dreaded object or situation (APA, 1987). Like all anxiety disorders, a phobia is a response to experienced anxiety. It is characterized by a persistent fear of *specific places or things,* whereas in a GAD anxiety is *free-floating.* Thus anxiety is displaced or externalized to a source outside the body.

Phobias persist even though a person recognizes that they are irrational. The person can control the intensity of anxiety by simply avoiding the object or situation he fears.

In the DSM-III-R, phobias are categorized into three types:

1. *Agoraphobia:* fear of being in public or open spaces, places, or situations where escape could be difficult or help might not be available, for example, if the person should faint.

2. *Social phobia:* fear of being humiliated, scrutinized, or embarrassed in public if one should, for example, choke while eating in front of others or stumble while dancing around others.
3. *Simple phobia:* fear of a specific object or situation that is not either of the above. Examples are claustrophobia (a fear of closed places) and a fear of black cats.

## Case Study

Sandra Johnson, a 41-year-old white woman, is being admitted to the psychiatric unit of a general hospital. She is accompanied by her husband and is coming from the emergency room. Her presenting symptoms in the emergency room were shortness of breath, hyperventilation, palpitations, chest pain, and fear of dying. She stated that these symptoms had occurred unexpectedly while she was cooking dinner. She thought that she was having a heart attack.

These attacks had happened three times before. The first attack occurred 2 months ago. After the first attack she went to her family physician, who had given her an electrocardiogram, a stress test, and a complete physical examination. All results were negative for any physiological causation of the symptoms. After the second attack, Mrs. Johnson stated that she took 2 weeks off from work because she was worried about having another attack. She had been employed for 5 years as a secretary for a small insurance agency. Just before she was about to return to work, she experienced another attack. After this third attack, she decided not to return to work and quit her job. She was unable to leave the house to go grocery shopping, to drive the children to activities, and to go out socially with her friends. Her husband, who is 42 years old, stated that he and their three daughters, aged 15, 12, and 9 years, were very concerned about her and had been helping her with daily tasks.

After her husband leaves, Mrs. Johnson begins to cry and states that she is letting her family down. They have tried to help her and she cannot do anything at home, cannot work, and cannot even leave the house because she is so afraid of not being able to control the possibility of another "attack." She does not understand what is happening to her and wants medication to help her feel better.

On the third day of her hospitalization, Mrs. Johnson tells the nurse that she is upset because her husband has not visited her since her admission. As she talks more about her husband, she starts to cry and states that she is afraid of losing him. She reports that 2 or 3 months ago she noticed a change in her husband. He was less affectionate and was spending more time away from home. He suddenly had more business trips. She is afraid he is having an affair. She says: "What am I going to do if he leaves? I can't support myself and my children alone. I don't even have a job. I can't go out of the house. I've lost contact with my friends."

# Nursing Care Plan

NAME: _____Sandra Johnson_____    ADMISSION DATE: _____4/9/90_____

DSM-III-R DIAGNOSIS: _____300.21 Panic Disorder with Agoraphobia_____

### ASSESSMENT:
**Areas of strength:** Managing her role as mother, homemaker, and secretary; was socially active with her friends; in relatively good health.

**Problems:** Fear of dying related to fear of heart attack; unable to leave the house; afraid of losing her husband; feelings of inadequacy.

**DIAGNOSES:** Episodes of severe anxiety related to life stress. Inability to leave home related to anxiety. Fear of losing husband related to feelings of inadequacy.

### PLANNING:                                                      **Date met**
**Short-term goals:**
Patient will discuss fears, her sense of inadequacy and help-   _____
lessness, and anger.
Identify relationship between anxiety and physiological re-   _____
sponses.
Develop strategies for reducing anxiety such as relaxation   _____
techniques.
Use problem solving techniques for life stresses.   _____
**Long-term goals:**
Patient will meet with husband and social worker to discuss   _____
marital issues.
Schedule appointment with outpatient therapist for system-   _____
atic desensitization or self-exposure training.
Identify schedule for attending an agoraphobia support   _____
group.

### IMPLEMENTATION/INTERVENTIONS:
**Nurse-patient relationship:** Empathy and supportive-suppressive techniques to keep anxiety at a minimum; encourage ventilation of feelings and issues; help patient identify relationship between stress, anxiety, and physiological responses; assist with adaptive coping strategies.

**Psychopharmacology:** Xanax, 1 mg q 4h p.r.n.; Tofranil, 25 mg/t.i.d.

**Milieu management:** Decrease stimuli and provide quiet, calm atmosphere; monitor anxiety level to prevent escalation; encourage recreational and diversional activities; use of quiet room if necessary; later encourage problem-solving, assertiveness, communication, problem-centered, self-esteem, and stress management groups.

**EVALUATION:** Patient reports being less anxious last 2 days. Met with husband and social worker, on 4/14.

Exposure to the stimulus results in an anxiety response.

It is common for all of us to have some fears or phobias about certain objects or situations. Some of us are afraid of public speaking, while some of us may be afraid of heights or elevators. However, these fears do not ruin our lives to the extent that we never leave home. We are still able to function and carry on our role expectations, responsibilities, and relationships. Phobic symptoms become phobic disorders when they cause severe distress and impair functioning. It is estimated that 20% of patients with phobic symptoms develop phobic disorders (Maxmen, 1986).

## Etiology

Traditional etiology was discussed earlier in this chapter. Patients are unaware of the unconscious symbolic meaning of their phobia. Repression and displacement are the chief defense mechanisms underlying phobias (Maxmen, 1986). Common repressed conflicts center around sexual and dependency problems. A current view is that agoraphobia runs in families, while most simple and social phobias do not (Maxmen, 1986). In a person with a diagnosis of panic disorder with agoraphobia the phobia usually develops because the person is afraid that he will experience a panic attack outside the home or where help is unavailable. Thus his fear of having an attack leads to another fear that the attack will occur when he is out in public.

---

### PSYCHOTHERAPEUTIC MANAGEMENT

*NURSE-PATIENT RELATIONSHIP*  Patients with phobic disorders are usually treated on an outpatient basis. If the phobia has incapacitated the patient to a severe extent, as in panic disorder with agoraphobia, the patient may be hospitalized. Another example in which hospitalization is indicated is the case of a person who has a phobia about germs and may not eat or drink.

Some interventions useful for persons experiencing phobic disorders are the following:

1. Acceptance of the patient and his fears with a noncritical attitude.
2. Provide and involve the patient in activities that do not increase anxiety but will increase involvement rather than avoidance of others.
3. Help the patient with physical safety and comfort needs.
4. Help the patient recognize that his behavior is a method of coping with anxiety.

*PSYCHOPHARMACOLOGY* Since behavior therapies are the treatments most successful with phobic persons, drugs traditionally have no effect on avoidant behavior. Medication that reduces or blocks panic attacks or reduces depression is used if those features are present. A recent study shows that imipramine in higher doses could enhance the effects of exposure treatment (Roy-Byrne and Katon, 1987). Phenelzine has been effective in the treatment of social phobias (Beeber, 1989). Behavior therapies are the treatment strategies of choice.

*MILIEU MANAGEMENT* Because of these patients' dependency needs, assertiveness-training and goal-setting groups are beneficial. Social skills groups are also necessary to help patients redevelop social skills and to decrease loneliness (Maxmen, 1986).

Behavior therapy, such as systematic desensitization, flooding, exposure, and self-exposure treatments, is most therapeutic for phobic persons (see Chapter 26). Self-exposure treatment is being used more often and is successful for phobics.

## POSTTRAUMATIC STRESS DISORDER
### DSM-III-R criteria, objective and subjective behavior

Post-traumatic stress disorder (PTSD) is somewhat different from the other anxiety disorders. It is a disorder that can develop after experiencing an *out of the ordinary* life-threatening or traumatic event or a series of serious circumstances. Some of the traumatic stressors that may precipitate the development of PTSD are wars, natural and man-made disasters, major fires or accidents, catastrophic illness or injury in self or others, rape, assault, or major personal or business losses (Horowitz, 1986; Karl, 1989). Anyone experiencing such events would be distressed, probably with intense fear, panic, and a sense of powerlessness and helplessness. To an extent, the type and degree of the initial and later reactions to trauma depend on a person's preexisting characteristics, usual coping style and defense mechanisms, personal and social resources, and the definition or meaning of the event to that person. The diagnosis of PTSD is not made because of any initial reactions to the stress or trauma. The diagnosis is based on characteristic symptoms occurring *1 month or more after* the trauma occurred (see Box 21-6).

It is not uncommon for PTSD to be unrecognized for years, sometimes even 10 to 20 years. This is, in part, due to the major characteristic of "numbing of responsiveness" to or reduced involvement with the external world. There is a persistent attempt to avoid situations, activities, and sometimes persons that evoke memories of the trauma. These efforts include trying to avoid thoughts and feelings related to the event. Repression and suppression are common. A constricted or blunted affect or a limitation in the range of feelings may occur, such as not being able to show affection. The patient may feel detached or estranged from family and friends. An inability to trust and love may lead to a withdrawal into isolation from others. There is often a loss of interest in activities, even those unrelated to the traumatic event. There also may be a change in the person's perceptions about the future—a kind of hopelessness, for example, about having a family or a career.

A second major characteristic of PTSD is the reexperiencing of the traumatic event in some way. This may occur as intrusive, unwanted memories, upsetting dreams or nightmares, or even suddenly feeling as if the event were occurring again (flashbacks). There may even be illusions or hallucinations with content related to the traumatic event. It is not known why these unpleasant, even frightening, experiences begin to break through the repression and suppression. The triggers for the reexperiencing episodes may have obvious connections to the trauma, or they may not even resemble the original situation. Therefore the patient may try to avoid even more activities and people in an effort to prevent the reexperiencing episodes.

It is not surprising that other symptoms of PTSD may include irritability, occasional outbursts of anger or rage, disturbances in sleep, and impairment in memory

## Box 21-6
## DIAGNOSTIC CRITERIA FOR 309.89 POST-TRAUMATIC
## STRESS DISORDER

A.  The person has experienced an event that is outside the range of usual human experience and that would be markedly distressing to almost anyone, e.g., serious threat to one's life or physical integrity; serious threat or harm to one's children, spouse, or other close relatives and friends; sudden destruction of one's home or community; or seeing another person who has recently been, or is being, seriously injured or killed as the result of an accident or physical violence.

B.  The traumatic event is persistently reexperienced in at least one of the following ways:

   (1) recurrent and intrusive distressing recollections of the event (in young children, repetitive play in which themes or aspects of the trauma are expressed)

   (2) recurrent distressing dreams of the event

   (3) sudden acting or feeling as if the traumatic event were recurring (includes a sense of reliving the experience, illusions, hallucinations, and dissociative [flashback] episodes, even those that occur on awakening or when intoxicated)

   (4) intense psychological distress at exposure to events that symbolize or resemble an aspect of the traumatic event, including anniversaries of the trauma

C.  Persistent avoidance of stimuli associated with the trauma of numbing of general responsiveness (not present before the trauma), as indicated by at least three of the following:

   (1) efforts to avoid thoughts or feelings associated with the trauma

   (2) efforts to avoid activities or situations that arouse recollections of the trauma

   (3) inability to recall an important aspect of the trauma (psychogenic amnesia)

   (4) markedly diminished interest in significant activities (in young children, loss of recently acquired developmental skills such as toilet training or language skills)

   (5) feeling of detachment or estrangement from others

   (6) restricted range of affect, e.g., unable to have loving feelings

   (7) sense of a foreshortened future, e.g., does not expect to have a career, marriage, or children, or a long life

**Box 21-6**
DIAGNOSTIC CRITERIA FOR 309.89 POST-TRAUMATIC
STRESS DISORDER—cont'd

D. Persistent symptoms of increased arousal (not present before the trauma), as
   indicated by at least two of the following:
   (1) difficulty falling or staying asleep
   (2) irritability or outbursts of anger
   (3) difficulty concentrating
   (4) hypervigilance
   (5) exaggerated startle response
   (6) physiologic reactivity upon exposure to events that symbolize or resemble
       an aspect of the traumatic event (e.g., a woman who was raped in an
       elevator breaks out in a sweat when entering any elevator)
E. Duration of the disturbance (symptoms in B, C, and D) of at least one month.

**Specify delayed onset** if the onset of symptoms was at least six months after the
trauma.

or concentration. There may also be "survivor guilt"—guilt about surviving or the
actions taken in order to survive. For example, a disaster victim or a combat soldier
may feel he survived because of cowardly acts, or a rape victim may feel guilty for
not resisting the attacker. Another consequence in PTSD can be physiological symptoms that develop during exposure to situations resembling the original trauma.
Psychophysiological illnesses may even develop.

If the symptoms of post-traumatic stress develop within 6 months of the traumatic event and last for 1 to 6 months, the disorder is considered to be *acute*. If
the symptoms develop 6 months or more after the trauma, it is considered to be
*delayed* onset. It is sometimes difficult to differentiate PTSD from other disorders.
Persons experiencing PTSD also commonly develop problems with depression, suicidal ideas and attempts, anxiety, and substance abuse. There may also be difficulties,
such as arrests, unemployment, divorce, as well as paranoia toward authority figures
or other persons perceived as directly and indirectly responsible for or not helping
with the original traumatic situation. Initially the patient may appear as if he is more
antisocial, schizoid, schizophrenic, paranoid, or even manic (Allen, 1986).

The family members of persons with post-traumatic stress disorder may develop
problems as well. In some cases the family members experience the same trauma,
as in a major fire or natural disaster, and may develop symptoms themselves. In the
case of rape or war the family, particularly the spouse, may react indirectly to the

trauma itself or to the behaviors of the trauma victim. The family may or may not be able to help in the treatment of their member experiencing PTSD. The whole family or selected members may need treatment themselves.

## PSYCHOTHERAPEUTIC MANAGEMENT

The treatment of the person experiencing post-traumatic stress disorder must be individualized according to the predominant symptoms and the associated problems, such as depression, suicidal ideation, or substance abuse. The overall goal of psychotherapeutic management is progressive recapitulation of each memory, often from the least to the most painful, to integrate the pieces. This involves a move from a victim status to a survivor status, from "I can't go on because of this" to "I have learned from it and can go on with my life." It is often difficult for the person to even seek help or to accept it when offered. Even with help, it may take time for the person to recognize the relationship between current problems and the past traumatic event.

*NURSE-PATIENT RELATIONSHIP* A first priority in the relationship with a patient experiencing PTSD is the development of trust. This may be difficult because of the patient's tendency to be withdrawn, to feel alienated, and even to be suspicious of others. If the patient is aware of the past trauma and its current influence, there is often a tendency for the patient to believe that "No one can understand what I've been through, unless they have been through it too." Therefore the nurse needs to be nonjudgmental, to offer a great deal of empathy and support, and to be honest. A message that can be conveyed by the nurse is "I haven't been through what you have; but the more you tell me, the better I will understand what you have and are experiencing." Depending on the nature of the trauma the patient experienced, the nurse does need to be prepared to hear "horror stories" about hideous injuries, unpredicted behaviors, or gross destruction. If the nurse cannot tolerate the stories of atrocities, the patient is not free to process all the losses and changes that have occurred in his life as a result of and since the trauma.

When the patient is not initially aware of the connection between the original trauma and his current feelings and problems, the nurse gently clarifies those connections as they emerge. The patient needs a significant amount of help in verbally expressing feelings, particularly anger. These feelings have often been ignored or suppressed for a long time, and the patient is afraid to face them. This is especially true if there have been destructive outbursts of anger in the past and the patient is desperately trying to remain in control.

It is important to acknowledge any unfairness or injustices that were part of the original trauma and yet not allow the patient to avoid responsibility for his role and behaviors then and since then. The patient needs to evaluate his past behaviors according to the original context of the situation, not by current values and standards (Huppenbauer, 1982). For example, the rape victim who did not resist the knife-wielding attacker needs to judge her behavior in the context of the life-or-death situation rather than by an acquaintance's comment implying she "must have asked for it." Another example is the Vietnam veteran who must evaluate his killing of a woman holding a grenade within the context of war, not by society's current view of that war as being immoral. It is not easy for the patient to develop a new perspective of the original trauma, and it involves clarification of facts, feelings, and values.

Although the patient struggles through the lengthy process of reintegrating the past experiences, it is also important to take "time outs" to focus on current problems and the potential solutions. These problems, such as divorce or unemployment, and the associated feelings can be just as stressful. The patient needs to be involved in problem solving, decision making, and taking specific actions toward overcoming these stresses. The patient's adaptive coping skills need to be encouraged while the dysfunctional ones, especially the abuse of alcohol and drugs, are discouraged. The patient also needs to try to establish or reestablish relationships that can provide support and assistance. Couple or family counseling may be recommended if appropriate.

*PSYCHOPHARMACOLOGY* The choice of medications for the patient experiencing post-traumatic stress disorder depends on the primary symptoms evidenced. Medications are generally used for short-term therapy during intensive counseling periods or acute crises. *Benzodiazepines* may be prescribed if the major problem is anxiety symptoms. These medications may also help the patient deal with the painful emotions. Sleep disturbances and nightmares are reportedly decreased as well with benzodiazepines. Of course, there is a risk of dependence, especially with patients who are already abusing alcohol or drugs. Benzodiazepines are usually prescribed on a p.r.n. basis rather than on a fixed schedule for PTSD patients. *Propranolol* in low doses, up to 180 mg, may produce responses similar to that of the benzodiazepines. Propranolol can help diminish the peripheral autonomic response associated with fear.

*Lithium carbonate* is sometimes given to patients who are experiencing explosive outbursts and intense feelings of being out of control. It can help decrease hyperarousal, startle response, and nightmares.

*Tricyclic antidepressants* are occasionally used if depression, anhedonia, and sleep disturbances are the primary problems. These, especially amitriptyline, are usually given in one dose at bedtime.

*MAO inhibitors* may be used for the patient with severely constricted affect. These may also help decrease flashbacks and nightmares.

*Hypnotics* are used, but sparingly, if other medications do not work to improve sleep. The risk of dependence must be considered.

*Antipsychotics* are used if the patient also has psychotic thinking. These may be used for hyperarousal in acute crisis periods (Van der Kolk, 1983; Friedman, 1988).

*MILIEU MANAGEMENT* The patient experiencing post-traumatic stress disorder can benefit from many milieu activities. Social activities can help rebuild social skills damaged by the suspiciousness and withdrawal. Recreational and exercise programs can help reduce tension and promote relaxation. Groups that could be useful are ones focusing on self-esteem, decision making, assertiveness, stress management, and relaxation techniques.

*COMMUNITY RESOURCES* A particularly useful therapeutic aid for patients experiencing post-traumatic stress disorders is group therapy with others who have experienced the same or similar trauma. A community may have a veterans outreach center for Vietnam veterans and their spouses and a group for victims of rape or incest, or it may hold meetings for victims after a disaster. There may also be a victim's assistance program for crime victims.

### Adjustment disorders

This separate group of adjustment disorders is not part of the anxiety disorders category but is included here because of its contrasts with post-traumatic stress disorder (PTSD). The diagnosis of adjustment disorder may be made when symptoms develop within 3 months after an identifiable life event that is not severe enough for the criteria of PTSD. The common events or circumstances that may precipitate an adjustment disorder are divorce, moving, marriage, retirement, illness or disability, financial problems, or difficulties in child rearing (Horowitz, 1986).

The symptoms of the maladaptive reactions to the stressful event or circumstances are not as specifically defined as those for PTSD, but they are still considered more severe than a "normal" stress response or grief reaction. The reaction interferes with functioning but lasts no longer than 6 months. The adjustment disorder diagnosis is based on subcategories according to the predominant feature of the person's maladaptive stress reaction. The major feature can be a mood disturbance of anxiety or depression. It can be a disturbance in interpersonal functioning, such as with conduct, physical complaints, work (or academic) inhibition, or withdrawal. There are also subcategories with mixed emotional features and mixed disturbance of emotions and conduct. The psychotherapeutic interventions for patients with adjustment disorders are generally similar to those used with patients experiencing post-traumatic stress disorder. The major goals are to recognize the relationship between the stressful situation and current problems and to review and reintegrate the memories of that original situation.

## ■ Somatoform Disorders

The major characteristic of these disorders is that the patient has physical symptoms for which there is no known organic cause or physiological mechanism. Evidence is present or a presumption exists that the physical symptoms are connected to psychological factors or conflicts. The person is not in control of his symptoms, so they are unconscious and involuntary. The patient expresses conflicts through bodily symptoms and complaints. Somatization is always present.

Patients with these disorders repeatedly seek medical diagnosis and treatment even though they have been told that there is no known physiological or organic evidence to explain their symptoms or disability.

The somatoform disorders that will be discussed here are somatization disorder, somatoform pain disorder, hypochondriasis, and conversion disorder.

## SOMATIZATION DISORDER

According to the DSM-III-R, the main characteristics of this disorder are that the individual verbalizes recurrent, frequent, and multiple somatic complaints for several years with no physiological cause. It usually begins before the age of 30. The person describes his complaints in a vague but dramatic fashion. He has seen many physicians through the years and may even have had exploratory and unnecessary surgical procedures.

This patient may complain about nausea and diarrhea one month and urinary problems the next. Six months later, he may have back problems followed by dizziness or palpitations. The list of symptoms is endless and may have lasted for several years.

These patients may be anxious or depressed. They may feel nervous, have sleep disturbances, and experience suicidal ideation because they experience hopelessness about ever getting better. The psychiatric nursing diagnoses (PND-1) related to somatoform disorders are listed in Box 21-7.

---

### Box 21-7
### PSYCHIATRIC NURSING DIAGNOSES (PND-1):
### SOMATOFORM DISORDERS

| | |
|---|---|
| 01.01 | Altered motor behavior |
| 06.03.01 | Altered body image |
| 01.03 | Altered self-care |
| 05.02.02 | Dysfunctional behaviors |
| 07.05 | Altered neurosensory processes |
| 08.01.04 | Powerlessness |
| 05.01 | Altered communication processess |
| 05.03.06 | Altered work role |
| 05.03.01 | Altered family role |
| 04.02.02 | Anxiety |
| 04.02.05 | Fear |
| 04.02.07 | Guilt |
| 02.08.02 | Alteration in concentration |
| 06.01.01 | Distractibility |
| 06.02.02 | Distress |
| 05.05.02 | Social isolation/withdrawal |
| 05.97 | Undeveloped interpersonal processes |
| 05.03 | Altered role performance |

## SOMATOFORM PAIN DISORDER

In this disorder the chief complaint is severe pain. When the symptom of pain is described, it is inconsistent with anatomical pathways of the nervous system. If the pain mimics a physical disorder, it cannot be accounted for by a physiological reason or cause. The pain must be present for 6 months.

The location or complaint of pain does not change, which is unlike the complaints voiced in the somatization disorder.

In this disorder, there is a known psychological factor related to the development of pain. This information may have been obtained from a family history. In some cases the pain allows the patient to avoid something that he does not want to do. For example, a woman's back pain may be a reason not to vacuum the house. Or a man's chest pain may prevent him from going to work.

Sometimes there is a physiological disorder, but the amount of pain or impairment is greatly exaggerated or out of proportion to it. For example, a person who has experienced a mild myocardial infarction is now convinced that he can no longer engage in such recreational activities as bicycling or swimming.

Patients with somatoform pain disorder are often "doctor shoppers" and may use analgesics excessively without experiencing any relief from their pain. They are often anxious about their symptoms and depressed about ever getting better.

## HYPOCHONDRIASIS

The hypochondriac is preoccupied or worried about getting a serious disease or fears and believes that he has a serious disease. There is no physiological basis for his fear or belief. For example, a person who had one homosexual experience in his life is now seriously worried that he has AIDS. Another example is that a person with a small cut on a finger may produce an exaggerated or unwarranted interpretation that the cut will become infected, lead to gangrene, and result in the finger's needing to be amputated.

A person may also interpret a normal bodily sensation as being a sign of a serious illness. For example, a woman who hears her heart beat at night when her ear is against her pillow, believes that she will have a heart attack.

These patients displace their anxiety into their bodies, and somatic complaints are the result. The hypochondriac fears that he will get a disease, whereas the patient with a somatization disorder focuses on symptoms of disease.

## CONVERSION DISORDER

The major characteristic of the conversion disorder is a loss or alteration of physical functioning that suggests a physical disorder but instead is an expression of a psychological need or conflict (Box 21-8).

The most common conversion symptoms suggest neurological disease such as paralysis, blindness, or seizures.

Primary gain refers to the alleviation of anxiety in that the conflict is kept out of awareness. The secondary gain refers to the gratification received as a result of how people in the patient's environment respond to his illness.

Another characteristic of this disorder is that the symptom is often determined

---

**Box 21-8**
## DIAGNOSTIC CRITERIA FOR 300.11 CONVERSION DISORDER

A. A loss of, or alteration in, physical functioning suggesting a physical disorder.

B. Psychological factors are judged to be etiologically related to the symptom because of a temporal relationship between a psychosocial stressor that is apparently related to psychological conflict or need and initiation or exacerbation of the symptom.

C. The person is not conscious of intentionally producing the symptom.

D. The symptom is not a culturally sanctioned response pattern and cannot, after appropriate investigation, be explained by a known physical disorder.

E. The symptom is not limited to pain or to a disturbance in sexual functioning.

**Specify: single episode or recurrent.**

Reprinted with permission from the *Diagnostic and Statistical Manual of Mental Disorders, Third Edition, Revised.* Copyright 1987 American Psychiatric Association.

---

by the situation that produced it. For example, a soldier suddenly develops paralysis of his hand. As a result, he can no longer engage in combat because he cannot pull the trigger on his gun. The symptom is related to the conflict. This soldier can discuss combat but cannot *connect* his feelings about fighting to the development of his paralysis.

This patient may also have an attitude of *la belle indifference,* meaning that he expresses little concern or anxiety about his distressing disorder. This occurs because his symptom binds his anxiety so it is not behaviorally expressed. Patients with conversion disorders minimize their problems, whereas patients with other somatoform disorders dramatize them (Maxmen, 1986).

Traditional views of this disorder consider repression and conversion as the primary defense mechanism used. At present, patients with conversion disorders are not often seen in an inpatient setting.

Traditional views concerning other somatoform disorders consider repression, denial, and displacement as defense mechanisms used in these disorders. Repression occurs in reference to feelings, conflicts, and unacceptable impulses. Denial of psychological problems is present even though these patients have been told that there is no physiological cause or basis of their symptoms. Displacement occurs when the anxiety is transformed into body symptoms.

Current research suggests that genetic, developmental-learning, personality, and sociocultural factors can predispose, precipitate, and maintain these disorders. Stressful life events can also precipitate bodily concerns and somatization (Lipowski,

1986). Persistent "somatizers" are described as dependent, emotionally needy, frustrated, and chronically resentful persons who seek attention of or want to punish relatives and physicians for not meeting their needs (Lipowski, 1987). If the secondary gains are beneficial and more important than losses and suffering, the sick role will be maintained.

## PSYCHOTHERAPEUTIC MANAGEMENT OF SOMATOFORM DISORDERS

*NURSE-PATIENT RELATIONSHIP* The focus of the nurse-patient relationship is to improve the patient's overall level of functioning by building adaptive coping behaviors. Patients with somatoform disorders often are not able to identify and express their feelings, needs, and conflicts. Teaching them how to appropriately verbalize feelings will help eliminate or diminish the need for physical symptoms. The patient will need time to understand his need for physical symptoms. Awareness and insight will develop slowly as he begins to verbalize his needs. For some patients this awareness and insight will take longer to develop, and they may have only begun to work on this area by the time they are discharged from an inpatient unit.

The physician or psychiatrist will be ordering tests and laboratory work-ups to thoroughly assess the patient physically for the presence of any physiological or organic disease or causation if this has not been done prior to admission. The absence of any relevant medical findings will strongly suggest that somatization is present.

The following nursing interventions are used for patients with somatoform disorders:

1. Use a matter-of-fact caring approach when providing care for physical symptoms to decrease secondary gains and to decrease focusing on physical symptoms.
2. Ask the patient how he is feeling and ask him to describe his feelings to increase his use of verbalization about feelings, especially negative ones, needs, and anxiety rather than somatization.
3. Assist the patient with developing more appropriate ways to verbalize feelings and needs.
4. Use positive reinforcement to increase noncomplaining behavior and set limits by withdrawing attention from the patient when he focuses on physical complaints or makes unreasonable demands.
5. Be consistent with the patient and have all requests directed to the primary nurse providing care to decrease attention-seeking or manipulative behaviors.
6. Use diversion by including the patient in milieu activities and recreational games to decrease rumination about physical complaints.
7. Do not push awareness or insight about conflicts or problems because anxiety will only increase, and the need for symptoms will be maintained.

*PSYCHOPHARMACOLOGY* Because patients with somatoform disorders may be using too much medication and taking a variety of drugs before they are admitted to the hospital, medication will be used temporarily and sparingly.

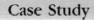 

William Robinson, a 62-year-old white man, was admitted to the psychiatric inpatient unit on June 15 at 10 AM. He walked onto the unit limping and supported by his wife, Harriet. He stated that he was experiencing horrible pain in his left leg and foot. Anger and irritability were evident in his voice.

Mr. Robinson's pain had started suddenly about 7 months ago. Since that time, he had seen numerous physicians to obtain treatment and relief from his pain. He had been told by the last physician that his pain was due to stress and had recommended that he be hospitalized to obtain treatment from a doctor who was trained to manage stress-related disorders. The patient stated that he hoped this doctor would know what to do since none of the others did.

Mrs. Robinson had brought her husband's medications with them. The nurse found that a number of analgesics had been prescribed along with sleeping medication. Mr. Robinson said that he took what he wanted, when he wanted it, and that it was better than not taking anything at all.

The next day, after visiting her husband, Mrs. Robinson told the nurse that Mr. Robinson needed a lot of help with everything. In fact, she had been so physically tired that she had called their only daughter, Sheila, for assistance. Sheila lived 400 miles away and they had not seen her for 3 years. Their daughter was so concerned about her parents that she had come to help for 2 weeks last month.

As the conversation continued, Mrs. Robinson told the nurse that her husband had been in good health, ex-

cept for an occasional cold, up to about 8 months ago. Then suddenly, he started to complain about the awful pain in his leg and foot. He had never in all of his years working for a cabinet manufacturer experienced anything like this before. Mrs. Robinson did not know why all of this pain was happening now, especially since her husband had retired 9 months ago. Actually, he had been forced to retire early because the company he worked for had not been doing well and all employees aged 60 and over were forced to retire. She stated that her husband had never said too much about it and she thought that now they would have time to travel and take fishing trips, which her husband had always enjoyed. They had taken many fishing trips as a family while their daughter was growing up and had enjoyed them immensely. Periodically her husband had also gone fishing with some friends. Since the onset of her husband's pain, they had not done anything socially together or with friends.

Since his admittance to the hospital, Mr. Robinson refused to do anything but sit in a lounge chair in the community room. He needed much assistance from staff to walk to the dining room and to the restroom. At times, his food was brought to him in the community room because he refused to walk to the dining room.

Interactions with the nurse centered on his pain and on requests for pain medication. He described his pain in detail and would talk of little else.

Mr. Robinson was getting Darvon for pain and an antidepressant as ordered by his physician.

# Nursing Care Plan

WEEKLY UPDATE: __6/21/90__

NAME: __William Robinson__          ADMISSION DATE: __6/15/90__

DSM-III-R DIAGNOSIS: _____ 307.80 Somatoform Pain Disorder _____

### ASSESSMENT:
**Areas of strength:** Enjoyed fishing and traveling; had been in good health; wife is very supportive; had worked for many years.

**Problems:** Experiencing pain in his left leg and foot; social functioning has declined; focus with staff is about his pain; secondary gains maintain his sick role.

**DIAGNOSES:** Preoccupation with pain related to inability to express feelings. Decline in social functioning related to not leaving house. Maintenance of sick role related to secondary gains.

### PLANNING:                                                   **Date met**
**Short-term goals:**
Patient will verbalize feelings and needs.                    _____
Patient will verbalize underlying anger due to early retire-  _____
ment.
Patient will verbalize awareness about connecting conflict    _____
with physical symptoms.
Patient will develop adaptive coping behaviors.               _____
**Long-term goals:**
Patient will assume responsibility for self-care and indepen- _____
dent functioning.
Patient will schedule appointments for joint counseling with  _____
his wife.
Patient will identify plans to volunteer in his community.    _____
Patient will plan leisure activities.                         _____

### IMPLEMENTATION/INTERVENTIONS:
**Nurse-patient relationship:** Convey interest and support; focus on assisting the patient to verbalize feelings and needs related to anxiety, self-esteem, and anger; give positive feedback when the patient focuses on issues other than pain; set limits on need for attention and medication.

**Psychopharmacology:** Encourage decrease in use of analgesics.

**Milieu management:** Encourage participation in assertiveness and communication groups as well as problem-solving, discharge-planning, and social skills groups, diversional occupational therapy, and recreational activities.

**EVALUATION:** Patient continues to focus on pain and remains incapacitated. Continue treatment plan.

At times a mild analgesic will initially be prescribed. The TCAs can help decrease somatic complaints if depression is present. Benzodiazepines, such as alprazolam, can help decrease somatic complaints in anxious patients (Lipowski, 1986).

*MILIEU MANAGEMENT* For the patient with a conversion disorder, hypnosis may be used to help in identifying the source of the conflict. Psychological testing and relaxation exercises may also be helpful.

For patients with other somatoform disorders, relaxation exercises and behavioral modification may help.

Assertiveness, decision-making, goal-setting, stress-management, and social skills groups will often benefit these patients.

Outpatient therapy will also be necessary for most patients. Because "somatizers" are most often overusers of medical care, some hospitals and clinics provide psychotherapy groups as part of the medical care for patients identified as somatizers. The groups focus on discussing underlying psychosocial needs and not on physical needs. Some areas of need for these patients are centered on depression, anxiety, loneliness, relationship concerns, and adjustment to chronic disease and disability (Corbin et al., 1988). The success of these types of groups results in decreasing hospital costs while providing more appropriate patient care than a visit to a medical clinic. It is hoped that efficacy of such groups will be recognized and thus used in more hospitals to provide optimal and appropriate patient care.

# ■ Dissociative Disorders

Dissociative states refer to the "splitting off" or removal from conscious awareness of some information, emotion, feeling, or mental function (Maxmen, 1986). According to traditional views, dissociation is an unconscious defense mechanism that protects a person from the emotional pain of experiences or conflicts that have been repressed. Dissociated feelings can be reactivated or reexperienced by a current situation that arouses intense emotional pain, such as the anniversary of someone's death. Dissociation is also linked to extreme stress or trauma, for example, childhood sexual abuse (Ross et al., 1990).

All of us use dissociation at times. We may be so engrossed in a book or a movie that we do not hear anything or anyone around us. This is not pathological. We all forget things or daydream. However, this does not mean that we have an illness.

The DSM-III-R defines dissociative disorders as disturbances or alterations in identity, memory, or consciousness. Most dissociative states are precipitated by a psychosocial trigger, begin suddenly, and end abruptly (Maxmen, 1986). The psychiatric nursing diagnoses (PND-1) related to dissociative disorders are listed in Box 21-9.

## PSYCHOGENIC AMNESIA

Amnesia is a sudden loss of memory or an inability to recall important personal information. It is beyond ordinary forgetfulness. Localized amnesia is the most common type and occurs for the first few hours after an intensely disturbing event (APA,

### Box 21-9
## PSYCHIATRIC NURSING DIAGNOSES (PND-1):
## DISSOCIATIVE DISORDERS

| | |
|---|---|
| 01.04 | Altered sleep/arousal patterns |
| 02.05.03 | Long-term memory loss |
| 02.05.04 | Short-term memory loss |
| 02.06.01 | Confusion |
| 04.02 | Altered feeling patterns |
| 06.03.03 | Altered personal identity |
| 06.03.05 | Altered social identity |
| 07.05.01 | Altered level of consciousness |
| 08.01.01 | Hopelessness |
| 08.01.03 | Loneliness |
| 08.01.04 | Powerlessness |
| 08.02.01 | Spiritual distress |
| 05.05 | Altered social interaction |

A. O'Toole, M. Loomis. 1989. "Classifying Human Responses in Psychiatric-Mental Health Nursing," from *Classification Systems for Describing Nursing Practice: Working Papers,* pp. 20-30. Kansas City, MO: American Nurses Association. Reprinted with permission.

1987). It is important to remember this because sometimes these patients are found wandering aimlessly by the police and are confused and disoriented. They may be taken to a hospital and may be frightened and perplexed. The precipitant is usually something that causes severe psychosocial stress, such as the threat of physical injury or death.

This disorder most often is found in adolescents and young adult women. The military has also provided reports of its occurring in young men during war (APA, 1987).

## PSYCHOGENIC FUGUE

The major feature of psychogenic fugue is sudden, unexpected travel away from home or locale with the assumption of a new identity (partial or complete) and a forgetting of one's previous identity. The travel and behavior appear normal to casual observers, so the person is not wandering in a confused state as someone in psychogenic amnesia (APA, 1987).

Fugue states last from a few hours to a few days. They are usually accompanied by amnesia, so the patient does not remember what happened during the fugue state. Sometimes depression is also present.

Psychogenic fugue usually follows severe psychosocial stress, such as marital quarrels, personal rejections, military conflict, or natural disaster (APA, 1987). The fugue state then allows escape or flight from an intolerable event or situation.

## DEPERSONALIZATION

According to the DSM-III-R, depersonalization is included in this group of disorders because the sense of one's reality is changed but the patient is oriented as to time, place, and person. In depersonalization the person feels detached from parts of his body or mental processes. It involves an altered perception of the self so that the person feels unreal or strange (Coons, 1986). It could also involve feeling like a robot or as if the person were in a dream. Depersonalization is often accompanied by symptoms of derealization in which the person feels that the outside world is changed or unreal. For example, buildings may appear to be leaning or everything seems gray and dull.

A diagnosis of depersonalization is made only when the prevalence or intensity of the disorder causes marked distress and interferes with daily functioning and when it occurs in the absence of any other disorder. This disorder is rare and is often chronic, with remissions and exacerbations. The patient is afraid of going insane and could become suicidal because depersonalization and derealization are so frightening (Coons, 1986).

Symptoms of depersonalization can occur in other disorders, such as schizophrenia, mood disorders, organic mental disorders, personality disorders, and epilepsy (APA, 1987).

## MULTIPLE-PERSONALITY DISORDER

According to the DSM-III-R, the major feature of the multiple-personality disorder (MPD) is the existence within the person of two or more distinct personalities. The transition from one personality to another occurs suddenly and at times of emotional stress. The original personality is unaware of the secondary personalities. However, the secondary personalities are aware of each other in varying degrees and are aware of the original personality (Coons, 1986).

Each personality is quite different from the others and from the original personality. Each personality has its own name, behavior traits, memories, emotional characteristics, and social relations. Secondary personalities are of varying ages, races, and sex (Maxmen, 1986). The most common personality is a fearful, terrified child and the next is a persecutor personality modeled on the abuser(s) (Steele, 1989).

This disorder usually begins in childhood but does not come to clinical attention until later in adolescence or young adulthood and is seen in women more frequently than in men.

A shy, quiet woman may have alternate personalities that are promiscuous or flamboyant, childlike, and aggressive. A woman may awaken one morning and find the living room of her apartment littered with toys or strewn with empty alcohol bottles and leftover food. She does not remember what happened because she has amnesia for that span of time when another personality has taken over or "come out."

Sometimes a switch to another personality is preceded by a headache (Coons, 1986). The patient or original personality may state that she hears voices talking to one another in her head. These could be misdiagnosed as auditory hallucinations and the disorder misdiagnosed as schizophrenia.

These patients are often admitted to inpatient psychiatric units when they are suicidal, meaning that an alternative personality is trying to kill one of them, or when mutilation or uncontrollable impulses to harm the self are present.

Traditional views of this disorder consider dissociation to be a defense against extreme anxiety, which is aroused in highly painful and emotionally traumatic situations such as physical, emotional, and sexual abuse. The "splitting off" of these painful events allows the child to survive the trauma but leaves an impaired personality with disconnected parts or "alters." Studies have asserted that MPD is a result of physical and sexual abuse. The patients are also highly hypnotizable and lack healing or restorative experiences (Anderson, 1988).

Studies have shown that this disorder has a familial pattern (Kluft, 1987). Observations have been made that some male sex offenders in jails had MPD. Assessment of additional male patients may provide a better understanding of this disorder (Kluft, 1987). Ross et al. (1990) found a significant level of MPD among prostitutes and exotic dancers.

## PSYCHOTHERAPEUTIC MANAGEMENT

*NURSE-PATIENT RELATIONSHIP* The nurse's relationship with the person experiencing amnesia and fugue includes interventions to establish trust and support. The patient will be having physiological and neurological workups to rule out organic causations. The nurse will assist with gathering data regarding feelings, conflicts, or situations that the patient experienced prior to his amnesia or fugue state. The patient may also have sessions under hypnosis or Amytal sodium to gather data about forgotten material. The nurse will slowly help the patient to deal with anxiety and conflicts in his life. Patients with a depersonalization disorder usually are not found in an inpatient setting unless they have become suicidal.

With multiple-personality disorder the treatment goal is to ultimately integrate the personalities so that they can live together in the original personality. This takes years of outpatient psychotherapy combined with hypnosis and sodium amobarbital sessions (Coons, 1986).

*PSYCHOPHARMACOLOGY* The symptoms of multiple-personality disorder are not alleviated by medication. If anxiety, somatoform, and depressive symptoms are manifested by these patients, then anxiolytics, sedatives, antidepressants, and mood stabilizers may assist with these features (Kluft, 1987). The individual personalities may respond differently to medications. An antihypertensive medication prescribed for one personality may make another personality hypotensive.

Because of the rarity of the depersonalization disorder, little is known about its treatment. Antidepressants, anxiolytics, and major tranquilizers have not yet proved to be helpful since there is insufficient information about this disorder (Coons, 1986).

*MILIEU MANAGEMENT* If the patient is hospitalized in an inpatient psychiatric unit because of suicidal or uncontrollable attempts to harm himself, the nurse assumes an important role in this patient's care. Provision of a safe environment and a trusting relationship are basic to helping this patient. The patient usually has not had a trusting relationship with anyone else. Assisting with therapy sessions, providing acceptance and support, and helping the patient to deal with daily living concerns are also part of the work of the nurse (Anderson, 1988).

Teaching the patient about his illness and teaching him new ways of coping without dissociation will lead to new behaviors and coping skills for the patient (Anderson, 1988). This work with the patient is very challenging and rewarding to the nurse.

## KEY CONCEPTS

1. Anxiety is an underlying factor in anxiety, somatoform, and dissociative disorders.
2. The effects of anxiety can be assessed by the nurse using the levels of +1 (mild) to +4 (panic). The degrees of dysfunction can range from mild discomfort to total immobilization.
3. In evaluation of coping methods, the effectiveness and outcome of each type of coping are assessed by the nurse and evaluated with the patient.
4. The issues of primary and secondary gains are important to the patient in that primary gain relieves his discomfort while secondary gain may encourage him to maintain his sick role.
5. The patient's anxiety must be reduced to a mild or moderate level before the nurse can work with the patient on problem solving and adaptive coping.
6. In the category of anxiety disorders, symptoms of anxiety are directly felt or expressed.
7. With somatoform disorders, anxiety is expressed through physical symptoms.
8. In dissociative disorders, anxiety is "split off" or removed from conscious awareness, which helps the patient survive extreme emotional pain.
9. Uncovering and linking feelings and conflicts are important aspects of recovery.

## REFERENCES

Allen IM: Posttraumatic stress disorder among black Vietnam veterans, Hosp Community Psychiatry 37:55, 1986.

American Psychiatric Association: Diagnostic and statistical manual of mental disorders, third edition, revised, Washington, DC, 1987, The Association.

Anderson G: Understanding multiple personality disorders, J Psychosoc Nurs 26:26, 1988.

Beeber LS: Treatment of anxiety, J Psychosoc Nurs 27:42, 1989.

Berkseth JK: Legacy of Vietnam, J Psychosoc Nurs 26:24, 1988.

Coons PM: Dissociative disorders: diagnosis and treatment, Indiana Med, p 410, May 1986.

Corbin LJ et al: Somatoform disorders: how to reduce overutilization of health care services, J Psychosoc Nurs 26:31, 1988.

Coughlan K and Parkin C: Women partners of Vietnam veterans, J Psychosoc Nurs 25:25, 1987.

DeVeaugh-Geiss J, Landau P, and Katz R: Treatment of obsessive-compulsive disorder with clomipramine, Psychiatr Ann 19:97, 1989.

Figley C: Stress disorders among Vietnam veterans: theory, research, and treatment, New York, 1978, Brunner/Mazel.

Friedman MJ: Toward rational pharmacotherapy for posttraumatic stress disorder, Am J Psychiatry 145:281, 1988.

Horowitz MJ: Stress-response syndromes: a review of posttraumatic and adjustment disorders, Hosp Community Psychiatry 37:241, 1986.

Huppenbauer SL: PTSD: a portrait of the problem, Am J Nurs 82:1699, November, 1982.

Improving therapeutic interventions for the

treatment of panic disorders, Adv Psychiatr Med Psychiatr Times 5:29, 1988.

Karl GT: Survival skills for psychic trauma, J Psychosoc Nurs 27:15, 1989.

Kluft RP: An update on multiple personality disorder, Hosp Community Psychiatry 38:363, 1987.

Lazarus RS: Psychological stress and the coping process, New York, 1966, McGraw-Hill Book Co.

Levitt E: The psychology of anxiety, Indianapolis, 1967, The Bobbs-Merrill Co.

Lipowski ZJ: Somatization: medicine's unsolved problem, Psychosomatics 28:294, 1987.

Lipowski ZJ: Somatization: a borderland between medicine and psychiatry, Can Med Assoc J 135:609, 1986.

Marks I: Self-exposure treatment in helping patients with anxiety disorders, Psychiatric Times, September, 1988.

Maxmen JS: Essential psychopathology, New York, 1986, WW Norton & Co.

May R: The meaning of anxiety, New York, 1950, The Ronald Press.

Peplau HE: Interpersonal relations in nursing, New York, 1952, GP Putnam's Sons.

Rapoport JL: The biology of obsessions and compulsions, Sci Am, 83, March, 1989.

Reising M: Mental health problems of Vietnam veterans, J Psychiatr Nurs Ment Health Serv 20:40, 1982.

Ross CA, Anderson G, Heber S, and Norton GR: Dissociation and abuse among multiple-personality patients, prostitutes, and exotic dancers, Hosp Community Psychiatry 41:328, 1990.

Roy-Byrne PP and Katon W: An update on treatment of the anxiety disorders, Hosp Community Psychiatry 38:835, 1987.

Selye H: The stress of life, St. Louis, 1956, McGraw-Hill Book Co.

Steele K: Looking for answers: understanding multiple personality disorder, J Psychosoc Nurs 27:5, 1989.

Stuart GW and Sundeen SJ: Pocket guide to psychiatric nursing, St. Louis, 1988, The CV Mosby Co.

Sullivan HS: The psychiatric interview, New York, 1954, WW Norton & Co.

Tyhurst JS: Individual reaction to community disaster, Am J Psychiatry 107:764, 1951.

Uhde TW and Maser JD: Current perspectives on panic disorder and agoraphobia, Hosp Community Psychiatry 36:1153, 1985.

Van der Kolk BA: Psychopharmacological issues in posttraumatic stress disorders, Hosp Community Psychiatry 34:683, 691, 1983.

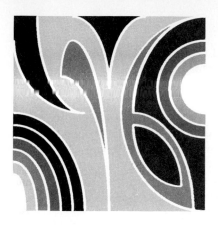

## CHAPTER 22

# Organic Mental Syndromes and Disorders

MIRA KIRK NELSON

LEARNING OBJECTIVES

After reading this chapter you should be able to

- Differentiate the concepts of organic mental syndrome and organic mental disorder.
- Differentiate dementia and delirium.
- Recognize DSM-III-R criteria for delirium and dementia.
- Describe the cardinal symptoms of dementia.
- Understand theories that explain the psychopathology of Alzheimer's disease and other dementias.
- Develop a nursing care plan for a patient with dementia.
- Evaluate the effectiveness of nursing interventions for patients with dementia.

Intellectual functioning is highly valued by all persons because of the importance of the ability to think rationally. The ability to think and to reason is one of the distinguishing features of a human being. Cognitive abilities, including memory, reasoning, orientation, perception, and attention, are processes that allow the person to make sense of experience and to interact productively with the environment. Memory is the foundation of these cognitive processes. Memory is an important cognitive process, as one must remember past experiences to exercise judgment, make decisions, and orient to time and place. Loss of memory is devastating, leaving the affected person in a state of confusion, unable to understand experience, and unable to relate current or past events. This impairment indicates an organic mental disorder.

The terms *organic brain syndrome, organic mental disorder,* and *organic mental syndrome* are often used interchangeably. Technically, it is not correct to do this. A discussion of the differences between and among these terms is presented to facilitate the student's understanding and appreciation of this and other psychiatric literature.

## DSM-III-R TERMINOLOGY AND CRITERIA

*The Diagnostic and Statistical Manual of Mental Disorders,* third edition revised, (DSM-III-R), of the American Psychiatric Association makes the following distinction between organic mental syndromes and organic mental disorders:

- *Organic mental syndrome* refers to a group of psychological or behavioral signs and symptoms without reference to any cause (e.g., delirium or dementia).
- *Organic mental disorder* refers to a particular organic mental syndrome in which the cause is known or presumed, such as alcohol withdrawal delirium, multi-infarct dementia, or Alzheimer's disease.

A psychological or behavioral abnormality associated with transient or permanent dysfunction of the brain is the essential feature of these disorders. The term *organic brain syndrome* is still used by many clinicians, but it has been replaced in the literature by the correct terms just discussed.

### Organic mental syndromes

The most common organic mental syndromes are delirium and dementia, which display variability among persons and in the same person over time. More than one organic mental syndrome may be present in a person simultaneously, such as delirium superimposed on dementia. For example, a person with Alzheimer's disease (a dementia) may also have delirium from systemic infections, metabolic disorders, or psychoactive substance intoxication and withdrawal (American Psychiatric Association, 1986; Cohen and Eisdorfer, 1986a).

### Organic mental disorders

Organic mental disorders are diagnosed

- By recognizing the presence of one of the organic mental syndromes (e.g., symptoms of delirium or dementia)
- By using history, physical examination, or laboratory tests to demonstrate the presence of a specific organic factor (or factors) judged to be etiologically related to the abnormal mental state.

The symptoms of dementia or delirium are usually assumed to be caused by organic factors if a nonorganic mental disorder cannot be identified. That is, the presence of an organic factor can be reasonably assumed to account for the symptoms of dementia if all nonorganic mental disorders that could account for the symptoms, have been ruled out (e.g., depression). Similarly, it can be reasonably assumed that organic factors account for the features of a delirium if nonorganic disorders, such as a manic episode, have been ruled out.

Since organic mental disorders are a heterogeneous group, no single description can characterize them all. The differences in clinical presentation reflect differences in the localization, mode of onset, progression, duration, and nature of the underlying process. For example, the organic factor responsible for an organic mental disorder could be localized primarily in the brain, as in Alzheimer's disease, or it could be a systemic illness, such as a central nervous system infection, that secondarily affects the brain.

According to Cohen and Eisdorfer (1986a), the organic mental disorders are the most prevalent psychiatric disorders of later life. It is estimated that 10% to 20% of the population over the age of 65 have significant cognitive dysfunction or dementia. The estimated prevalence is 1% in persons under the age of 60, 5% in those 65 years of age, 20% in persons 80 years of age, and 50% in those 90 years of age.

This chapter begins with a discussion of the two major classifications of organic mental syndromes, delirium and dementia, and then proceeds to a discussion of significant organic mental disorders, which include the *primary degenerative dementias* of Alzheimer's disease, Parkinson's disease, Huntington's disease, Pick's disease, and Creutzfeldt-Jakob disease. Multi-infarct dementia and transient ischemic attacks (TIAs) will be examined also. Psychotherapeutic management of these organically based disorders will conclude the chapter.

# ■ Organic Mental Syndromes
## DELIRIUM

Delirium is an organic brain syndrome in which there is widespread cerebral dysfunction. Delirium is a common condition; one third to one half of hospitalized patients become delirious at some time during their hospitalization. Although delirium may occur at any age, it more frequently strikes the elderly (Batt, 1989). Delirium has a sudden onset, often starting at night. Its duration is usually brief, about 1 week, and it is rare for it to persist for more than 1 month.

### Objective and subjective behavior

The cerebral dysfunction associated with delirium not only causes subjective problems but also causes visible indications. For instance, the patient with delirium may be incontinent of urine and feces and may have psychomotor agitation, including tremors and choreiform (irregular) movements (Wills, 1986; Gomez and Gomez, 1987).

The essential features of delirium are reduced awareness and attentiveness to the environment, *a reduced state of consciousness,* disorganized thinking, and ram-

**Box 22-1**

## DIAGNOSTIC CRITERIA FOR DELIRIUM

A. Reduced ability to maintain attention to external stimuli (e.g., questions must be repeated because attention wanders) and to appropriately shift attention to new external stimuli (e.g., perseverates answer to a previous question).

B. Disorganized thinking, as indicated by rambling, irrelevant, or incoherent speech.

C. At least two of the following:
   (1) reduced level of consciousness, e.g., difficulty keeping awake during examination
   (2) perceptual disturbances: misinterpretations, illusions, or hallucinations
   (3) disturbance of sleep-wake cycle with insomnia or daytime sleepiness
   (4) increased or decreased psychomotor activity
   (5) disorientation to time, place, or person
   (6) memory impairment, e.g., inability to learn new material, such as the names of several unrelated objects after five minutes, or to remember past events, such as history of current episode of illness

D. Clinical features develop over a short period of time (usually hours to days) and tend to fluctuate over the course of a day.

E. Either (1) or (2):
   (1) evidence from the history, physical examination, or laboratory tests of a specific organic factor (or factors) judged to be etiologically related to the disturbance
   (2) in the absence of such evidence, an etiologic organic factor can be presumed if the disturbance cannot be accounted for by any non-organic mental disorder, e.g., Manic Episode accounting for agitation and sleep disturbance

Reprinted with permission from the *Diagnostic and Statistical Manual of Mental Disorders, Third Edition, Revised.* Copyright 1987 American Psychiatric Association.

bling, irrelevant, or incoherent speech. The syndrome also involves memory impairment, disturbances of the sleep-wake cycle, disturbances in the level of psychomotor activity, and sensory misperceptions, as when a patient listens to a public address system and thinks that God is talking to him. The impaired attentional ability is reflected by disorientation to time, place, and person (Zisook and Braff, 1986). Box 22-1 presents the DSM-III-R diagnostic criteria for patients with delirium, and Box 22-2 presents the psychiatric nursing diagnoses (PND-1) for organic mental syndromes.

## Etiology

Delirium may be caused by chronic or acute physical illnesses and by chemical agents, such as drugs and alcohol. The most common physical illnesses associated with delirium are congestive heart failure, pneumonia, uremia, malnutrition, dehydration, cancer, and cerebrovascular accidents. Other factors include vascular disease, brain damage or disease, impaired vision and hearing, sleep loss, and fatigue. Fever may or may not be associated with these physical illnesses, since the elderly can have a substantial infection with much less change in temperature than younger persons.

Prescription drug intoxication is probably the most frequent single cause of delirium. The central cholinergic system, necessary for memory, learning, attention, and wakefulness, is aggravated by the use of anticholinergic medications. Delirium is most likely when several anticholinergic drugs, such as amitriptyline (antidepressant), thioridazine (antipsychotic), and benztropine mesylate (to correct side effects of tranquilizers) are prescribed at the same time. Therefore, polypharmacy (the prescribing of multiple drugs) should be avoided as much as possible, and the nurse attending the patient should be aware of these dangers (Gomez and Gomez, 1987).

### Box 22-2

## PSYCHIATRIC NURSING DIAGNOSES (PND-I) FOR PATIENTS WITH ORGANIC MENTAL SYNDROME

| | |
|---|---|
| 02.03.02 | Altered intellectual functioning |
| 02.05 | Altered memory |
| 02.06 | Altered orientation |
| 02.06.01 | Confusion |
| 01.03 | Altered self-care |
| 02.06.02 | Delirium |

A. O'Toole, M. Loomis. 1989. "Classifying Human Responses in Psychiatric-Mental Health Nursing," from *Classification Systems for Describing Nursing Practice: Working Papers,* pp. 20-30. Kansas City, MO: American Nurses Association. Reprinted with permission.

## Treatment

If the delirious state is judged to be caused by physical illness, it is important to aggressively and successfully treat the primary problem. For instance, measures for correction of anemia, dehydration, nutritional deficiencies, or electrolyte imbalance should be undertaken. If the delirium is chemically induced, drugs should be withdrawn for a few days, if clinically possible (Wills, 1986). Medications often can be reduced in dosage or discontinued altogether without a significant change in the patient's physiological status. Many times, particularly with older persons, there is a tendency to add new drugs without removing old ones. Most deliriums will improve with removal of the noxious agent or with treatment of the underlying disease. A slow recovery and perhaps, permanent brain damage can result without correct diagnosis and treatment. Batt (1989) recommends manipulating the environment to provide familiarity and decrease the fear of a strange place. Televisions, radios, clocks, newspapers, familiar objects, seasonal decorations, and proper lighting are all helpful in managing delirium.

Delirium is differentiated from dementia by its acute onset and reversibility. Dementia is more often a chronic, irreversible cerebral dysfunction (Foreman, 1986). Distinguishing between delirium and dementia is an extremely important, yet difficult, task. It is difficult to make this distinction because about one third of hospitalized demented patients also experience delirium. In the demented patient, delirium is manifested by apathy and periods of noisy restlessness, as well as by periods of fluctuating cognitive functioning.

## DEMENTIA

Dementia is broadly defined as an altered mental state secondary to cerebral disease. It is usually an irreversible mental state characterized by a decrease in intellectual function, personality change, impaired judgment, and often a change in affect. Dementia is the result of a disease or an abnormal condition, such as a vascular injury. The symptoms are severe enough to interfere with the patient's activities of daily living, work, or social relationships.

### Objective and subjective behavior

The cardinal symptoms of dementia are cognitive symptoms (e.g., orientation, judgment, attention, intellect, memory). These subjective experiences can be objectively observed by the nurse in several ways. The lost patient, the confused patient, the frustrated patient all demonstrate behaviors that are evidence of their neuropathologic state. For instance, impaired judgment commonly manifests itself through the purchase of unneeded or worthless items. Impaired attention span may disrupt the patient's ability to communicate satisfactorily. This disinhibiting effect of dementia may lead to social blunders, such as sexually inappropriate behavior. Many objective manifestations of cognitive degeneration could be listed. The following cognitive disturbances are the fundamental symptoms of dementia. Box 22-3 presents the DSM-III-R criteria for dementia.

**Alterations in memory.** The most prominent symptom of dementia is the impairment of short-term and long-term memory, compounded by significant

TABLE 11-3

# DIAGNOSTIC CRITERIA FOR DEMENTIA

A.  Demonstrable evidence of impairment in short- and long-term memory. Impairment in short-term memory (inability to learn new information) may be indicated by inability to remember three objects after five minutes. Long-term memory impairment (inability to remember information that was known in the past) may be indicated by inability to remember past personal information (e.g., what happened yesterday, birthplace, occupation) or facts of common knowledge (e.g., past Presidents, well-known dates).

B.  At least one of the following:

(1) impairment in abstract thinking, as indicated by inability to find similarities and differences between related words, difficulty in defining words and concepts, and other similar tasks

(2) impaired judgment, as indicated by inability to make reasonable plans to deal with interpersonal, family, and job-related problems and issues

(3) other disturbances of higher cortical function, such as aphasia (disorder of language), apraxia (inability to carry out motor activities despite intact comprehension and motor function), agnosia (failure to recognize or identify objects despite intact sensory function), and "constructional difficulty" (e.g., inability to copy three-dimensional figures, assemble blocks, or arrange sticks in specific designs)

(4) personality change, i.e., alteration or accentuation of premorbid traits

C.  The disturbance in A and B significantly interferes with work or usual social activities or relationships with others.

D.  Not occurring exclusively during the course of Delirium.

E.  Either (1) or (2):

(1) there is evidence from the history, physical examination, or laboratory tests of a specific organic factor (or factors) judged to be etiologically related to the disturbance

(2) in the absence of such evidence, an etiologic organic factor can be presumed if the disturbance cannot be accounted for by any nonorganic mental disorder, e.g., Major Depression accounting for cognitive impairment

## Criteria for severity of Dementia:

**Mild:** Although work or social activities are significantly impaired, the capacity for independent living remains, with adequate personal hygiene and relatively intact judgment.

**Moderate:** Independent living is hazardous, and some degree of supervision is necessary.

**Severe:** Activities of daily living are so impaired that continual supervision is required, e.g., unable to maintain minimal personal hygiene; largely incoherent or mute.

alterations in reasoning, language, and personality. In mild dementia there is moderate memory loss, characterized by forgetting telephone numbers, conversations, or events of the day. In more severe cases, only highly learned material, such as one's own name or previous occupation, is retained, and new information is quickly forgotten. Events that occured many years ago tend to be remembered better than those events that have occurred more recently, although this pattern of loss is variable. In advanced cases of dementia, memory impairment can be so severe that the person forgets his own name, age, occupation, or the names of close relatives (American Psychiatric Association, 1987; Cohen and Eisdorder, 1986a).

**Alterations in abstract thinking.**  Impairment of abstract thinking is noted in reduced capacity for generalization, differentiation, concept formation, and logical reasoning. The patient has difficulty defining words and cannot organize concepts around familiar themes (e.g., if shown a picture in which the task is to identify similar pictures, the patient with dementia could have difficulty). If asked to give the meaning of proverbs such as "don't cry over spilled milk," the patient responds that the milk was dirty. The diminished ability for abstract thinking results in more and more self-preoccupation. A previously caring and responsible person may become extremely self-centered and oblivious to the needs of others (Raskind and Storrie, 1980).

**Alterations in judgment.**  The patient with dementia cannot make the same adequate judgments that he formerly made. For instance, planning may become impossible for him. If a well-intentioned person were to find a stamped envelope near a mailbox, he would most likely put the letter into the mailbox. A well-intentioned person with dementia might not have the good judgment to do so.

**Alterations in perception.** *Hallucinations* are sensory experiences that occur without external stimulus; they may involve all senses but are predominant in the auditory and visual spheres. Patients with dementia experience hallucinations. Abnormal behavior as a result of hallucinations may occur when patients act on these visual and auditory hallucinations (Lucas et al., 1986).

*Delusions* are present at times in relation to a dementia syndrome, although they usually arise out of a reaction to a cognitive deficit. For example, patients are unable to remember where they put a specific item and will accuse others of stealing from them. Hallucinations and delusions must be described and documented accurately, with details concerning frequency, duration, content, and the patient's reaction to these abnormal experiences.

*Illusions* are common in patients with dementia syndromes and are described as misrepresentations of sensory perceptions triggered by environmental stimuli. For example, a tree outside a window may be misperceived as a person standing outside the window. It is important to distinguish an illusion from a hallucination, as the enviromental stimuli can be manipulated to decrease stimulation associated with illusions. Accurate observation and documentation can distinguish between a visual illusion and a visual hallucination and can determine the correct intervention strategy.

## Reversible dementia

Reversible dementia is a term used in the medical literature to describe a dementia that has a specific treatable cause. In the past, dementia has implied a progressive or irreversible course. According to the American Psychiatric Association (1987, p. 104), "Dementia may be progressive, static, or remitting. The reversibility of a dementia is a function of the underlying pathology and of the availability and timely application of effective treatment."

It is estimated that 30% to 40% of persons with memory disturbances have a reversible and, therefore, treatable dementia. Although most of the patients will have physical disorders, psychiatric disturbances such as depression are a significant challenge in the differential diagnosis. Treatment of such conditions as depression, drug-induced dementia, infections, and metabolic disturbances leads to complete restoration of functioning. With prompt diagnosis and appropriate treatment, the dementia can be reversed (Cohen and Eisdorfer, 1986b).

## Nonreversible dementia

When a reversible cause of intellectual impairment cannot be identified, the clinical diagnosis is presumed to be a nonreversible dementia. There are many diseases that can produce a progressive and nonreversible dementia. Most of these are rare and affect adults of all ages; however, when dementia does occur in a younger person, it has been associated with suicide (Margo and Firkel, 1990). The most common nonreversible dementias are Alzheimer's disease, Parkinson's disease, Huntington's disease, Pick's disease, Creutzfeldt-Jakob disease, and multi-infarct dementia (Cohen and Eisdorfer, 1986b). Transient ischemic attacks (TIAs) are included in this category because they can lead to a disabling cerebral infarction.

# ■ Organic Mental Disorders
## ALZHEIMER'S DISEASE
### Description and incidence

Alzheimer's disease is the form of dementia most commonly seen in the elderly. It is the most prevalent of all nonreversible dementias, accounting for between 50% and 70% of all diagnosed cases of dementia. It is defined as an age-related, progressive disorder of the central nervous system, characterized by chronic cognitive dysfunction. The cause of Alzheimer's disease is unknown (Cohen, 1990). It is a nonreversible, insidious, life-threatening disorder that ultimately leads to the premature death of the afflicted person (Kermis, 1986).

The name originated in Tübingen, Germany, in 1907, when Alois Alzheimer, a neuropathologist, detailed the characteristic neurological changes in the brains of affected persons. One of his patients was a 51-year-old woman with symptoms of memory loss, disorientation, hallucinations, and profound dementia. She died 4½ years after the onset of the disease. Postmortem examination revealed brain atrophy and distortions in the cortical neurofibrils. These distortions were later named Alzheimer's tangles and are sometimes referred to as Alzheimer-type changes (Burnside, 1988; Kermis, 1986).

Alzheimer's disease usually begins after the age of 65, and new data suggest a greater prevalence than formally thought. Evans et al (1989) suggest that as many as 10.3% of persons over 65 may have Alzheimer's disease. Prevalence increases with age, and Alzheimer's disease is believed to affect up to 47% of the population over age 85 (Cohen, 1990). Alzheimer's disease is believed to be the fourth or fifth leading cause of death in persons over 65 years of age and accounts for 90,000 to 100,000 deaths per year in this age group. Alzheimer's disease is found more often in women than in men, and a definite diagnosis can be made only on autopsy (Kermis, 1986).

### Progression of the disease

Several stages of Alzheimer's disease have been suggested (Williams, 1986; Cutler and Navang, 1985; Reisberg et al., 1985). Alzheimer's disease is difficult to diagnose, especially in the early stages when it resembles many other disorders. In the last stage the patient eventually becomes emaciated, helpless, and bedridden. The most frequent cause of death is pneumonia and other infections, with malnutrition and dehydration as contributing factors (Kermis, 1986; Williams, 1986). Box 22-4 summarizes the stages of this disease.

### Etiology

The structural changes in the brain of the patient with Alzheimer's disease do not cause the disease. They are the result of something else, and several theories exist as to what this might be. Research has focused on several models or theories proposed as the cause of Alzheimer's disease. A brief discussion of these models follows.

The *genetic model* researches the possibility that there may be one or more faulty genes responsible for Alzheimer's disease. The role of genetics continues to be poorly understood (Cohen, 1990). It is hypothesized that there is some factor in the genetic makeup that renders a person vulnerable to some factor in the environment. In some families several members representing four or five generations have developed a dementia of the Alzheimer's type (Burnside, 1988).

The *toxin model* is based on the belief by some researchers that the salts of aluminum may be contributing to the development of Alzheimer's disease. These salts may be released by aluminum cans, antiperspirants, and utensils or may be added to food and drugs, such as processed cheeses, antacids, and buffered acids. Several researchers have reported higher concentrations of aluminum in the brains of patients with Alzheimer's disease than in those of older persons without dementia (Cohen and Eisdorfer, 1986a; Burnside, 1988). Current research suggests that aluminum in the brains of Alzheimer's patients is an effect of the disease rather than a cause (Cohen, 1990.)

The *acetylcholine model* is based on the hypothesis that some of the cognitive defects that occur in Alzheimer's disease are a result of a reduction in the acetylcholine-mediated transmission of the nerve impulses (Burnside, 1988). Acetylcholine is a neurotransmitter that is important to learning and memory. Intensive research efforts have focused on the study of drugs that might increase the amount of acetylcholine in the brain. Acetylcholine does not enter the brain when taken directly but must be introduced through such substances as lecithin and choline.

## Box 22-4
## STAGES OF ALZHEIMER'S DISEASE

### Stage I

Emotional or mood changes
  Depression
  Anxiety
  Fatigue
  Decreased activity
Memory problems
  Recent
  Delayed
  Concentration
Assistance required in complex tasks
  Finances
  Marketing
  Planning a party

### Stage II

Assistance required with
  Choosing proper clothing
  Putting on clothes
  Bathing properly
  Toileting
Language or motor
  Aphasia: loss of ability to comprehend or express speech
  Apraxia: loss of ability to use objects correctly
  Agnosia: loss of ability to recognize sensory impressions
  Echolalia: automatic repetition by a patient of what is said to him
Wandering, restlessness at night

### Stage III

Urinary or fecal incontinence
Speech limited to a few words
Loss of ability to
  Ambulate
  Sit up
  Smile

When taken orally, these substances are broken down to form acetylcholine, which can enter the brain. However, lecithin and choline compounds have not proved to be beneficial in the treatment of Alzheimer's disease (Cohen and Eisdorder, 1986a).

The *abnormal protein* model is associated with the abnormal protein structures present in the brains of patients with Alzheimer's disease. The brain manufactures the proteins that are used to build internal structures within the nerve cell. Unusual twisted filaments discovered in the neurofibrillary tangles in the brains of patients with Alzheimer's disease prompted research to determine how protein metabolism is disrupted. It still is not known how these abnormal filaments are formed (Burnside, 1988; Cohen and Eisdorfer, 1986a).

The *infectious agent model* was an early hypothesis arising from suggestions that Alzheimer's disease was caused by a slow-growing virus. Research has not isolated a virus and there is no current evidence that Alzheimer's disease can be transmitted from person to person (Cohen and Eisdorfer, 1986).

Through intensified research effort, it is hoped that someday we will be able to learn what causes Alzheimer's disease and what preventive steps, if any, can be taken.

## PARKINSON'S DISEASE
### Description and incidence

Parkinson's disease has become recognized as second only to stroke as the most common neurological disorder in the elderly. The disease was first described by James Parkinson in 1817. As many as 2 million people in the United States are afflicted with Parkinson's disease, and 40,000 to 50,000 new cases are identified annually. Onset is usually between the ages of 55 and 60, and the disease strikes men and women equally (Matteson, 1988; McDowell, 1986).

### Progression of the disease

Parkinson's disease is predominantly a motor disorder, characterized by slowness and weakness of voluntary movement, rigidity, and tremor. Usually there is no clear sign as to when the disease begins. Tremor is usually the initial symptom, beginning on one side of the body in an upper extremity. The tremor often spreads to both sides of the body, and there is a general tendency to move more slowly and to experience difficulty in performing activities of daily living. The slowdown in voluntary movement may be so severe that the person becomes unable to initiate movement. The patient experiences increased difficulty in walking and resorts to short, quick steps or a shuffling of the feet. Older persons have difficulty with balance and may experience frequent falls. They often have trouble bathing and dressing themselves, getting in and out of bed, and turning themselves in bed. Handwriting may become illegible. The patient may have an expressionless face with monotonous speech, excessive salivation, and limited ocular mobility. The patient with Parkinson's disease may become confused, depressed, disoriented, delusional, and hallucinatory (Kermis, 1986; McDowell, 1986; Matteson, 1988).

It is important for patients with Parkinson's disease to remain as physically, socially, and intellectually active as possible. Exercise programs and increased activity are important to maintain optimal performance. The current treatment for

Parkinson's disease includes the administration of antiparkinsonism drugs (see Chapter 11).

## Etiology

The disease is degenerative, affecting the basal ganglia and the extrapyramidal nervous system. The basal ganglia contain short anatomical pathways that connect the basal ganglionic structures to the cerebral cortex. This system has an important role in modifying posture for cortically induced movements. There is a loss of dopamine-generating cells in the substantia nigra, which is a structure in the basal ganglia. These cells are rich in dopamine, and cell loss decreases dopamine levels, leading to the symptoms of Parkinson's disease (Matteson, 1988).

## HUNTINGTON'S DISEASE

Huntington's disease, formerly called Huntington's chorea, involves both motor and cognitive changes. The disease is characterized by uncontrollable quick, jerky, and purposeless writhing movements. Disturbances of gait and slurred speech are noted in the beginning and progress into neurological and intellectual deterioration. These actions can be mistaken for alcoholism, as the victims resemble drunks in their movement and speech. The symptoms include memory loss, paranoia, irritability, impaired impulse control, and lack of tongue and breathing control (Kermis, 1986; Matteson, 1988).

The onset of Huntington's disease usually begins between the ages of 25 and 45, with an average duration of 15 years. It is a hereditary but fairly *rare* disorder, occurring in two to seven of every 100,000 persons in the United States. The only available medical treatment is the administration of drugs to manage the symptoms and decrease choreiform movements. Nursing care and physical, occupational, and speech therapy can help with the problems of dysphagia, malnutrition, impaired communication, functional disabilities, and behavioral abnormalities. Death usually results from heart failure or pulmonary complications caused by asphyxiation or aspiration of food (Wills, 1986; Kermis, 1986; Matteson, 1988).

## PICK'S DISEASE

The onset, course, and clinical presentation of Pick's disease are similar to those of Alzheimer's disease and are usually treated in the same manner. This disease is almost exclusively associated with aging and is found more frequently in women than in men. It usually occurs after the age of 70. Onset is slow, and the disease progresses until death, with an average duration of 4 years (Matteson, 1988).

Symptoms include progressive impairment of cognition, memory, and orientation, which are similar to those of Alzheimer's disease. Language disorders, apathy, and depression are also noted. Treatment is aimed toward management of the symptoms, as there is no known cure. A higher incidence is seen in some families, indicating a genetic predisposition.

Pick's disease is differentiated from Alzheimer's disease in several ways. Whereas Alzheimer's disease is characterized by involvement of higher brain structures, Pick's disease is characterized by shrinkage of localized cortical areas. Neurons decrease in number in Pick's disease, and the preponderance of senile plaques and neurofibrillary tangle found in Alzheimer's disease is not found at postmortem examination.

## CREUTZFELDT-JAKOB DISEASE

Creutzfeldt-Jakob disease is a noninflammatory dementia believed to be caused by a slow-acting virus. The virus has not been isolated, but research is continuing. It is a rapidly progressive disorder of the central nervous system involving severe neurological impairment with marked dysfunction. This disease affects the cerebral cortex through cell destruction. Symptoms include early vision and hearing disturbances, impaired cognition, myoclonus, ataxia, muscle wasting, tremor, hallucinations, and illusions.

Creutzfeldt-Jakob disease is rare, with approximately one case in every 1 million population. It is distinguished clinically by a rapid onset in patients having an average age of 50 to 60 years. There is no known cure, and death occurs within 9 months to 1 year after the onset of symptoms. In the final stage the patient is confined to bed with deterioration of mental and physiological functions (Kermis, 1986; Matteson, 1988).

## MULTI-INFARCT DEMENTIA

Multi-infarct dementia is identified as being a vascular disorder in which there are multiple large and small cerebral infarctions. It is the second greatest cause of dementia, and its features include pseudobulbar palsy with emotional lability, dysarthria, dysphasia, and convulsive seizures. Approximately 25% of all dementia cases are vascular in origin, and arteriosclerosis of the brain and hypertension are closely associated with this disease. Other factors contributing to the disease are smoking, obesity, diabetes, mellitus, arrhythmias, peripheral vascular disease, myocardial infarction, and transient ischemic attacks (Matteson, 1988).

Multi-infarct dementia occurs earlier than the primary degenerative dementias, as the usual age at onset is between 55 and 70 years, with an average of 65 years. It is more common in men than in women, which distinguishes it from the degenerative dementias. The patient will exhibit abrupt ischemic episodes that lead to weakness, slowness, hyperreflexia, and extensor plantar responses (Babinski response). There are also disturbances in memory, abstract thinking, judgment, and impulse control. These behavioral difficulties must be effectively dealt with by the staff; otherwise these disturbances will hamper rehabilitation (Raskind and Storrie, 1980; Kermis, 1986; Matteson, 1988).

## TRANSIENT ISCHEMIC ATTACKS

A transient ischemic attack (TIA), sometimes referred to as a "little stroke," is characterized by transient focal neurological signs and symptoms that occur suddenly and last usually less than an hour but never more than 24 hours.

This syndrome is caused by a microembolism to the brain from atherosclerotic plaques in the aortocranial arteries in about 90% of the persons who experience TIAs. In the remaining 10%, TIAs are caused by mural thrombi, valvular diseases of the heart, vegetations on the heart valve, polycythemia, or some other blood clotting disorder (Harrell, 1988).

Specific symptoms of TIAs vary, depending on the vessel involved, the degree of obstruction of the vessel, and the collateral blood supply. If the posterior (vertebrobasilar) system is involved, symptoms may include tinnitus, vertigo, facial weakness, ataxia, diplopia, and falling without loss of consciousness. If the anterior (carotid) system is involved, the patient may experience ipsilateral blindness, monocular blurring, flashes of light, and headaches.

An elderly person who has a TIA may ignore an attack as the symptoms completely resolve; however, a physician should be consulted to prevent a possible disabling stroke (Harrell, 1988).

---

## PSYCHOTHERAPEUTIC MANAGEMENT

*NURSE-PATIENT RELATIONSHIP* In a nurse-patient relationship the highest priority of nursing care for a patient with delirium is given to interventions that will maintain life. If the patient is unable to attend to basic physiological needs, nursing care must be planned to meet these needs. In a patient with dementia the highest priority should be given to providing nursing care to maintain an optimal level of functioning. This will be different for each individual. Often the attitude of hopelessness evolves in those who work with chronically ill persons. This can result in stereotyping and decreased ability to see and appreciate the individuality of each person. Searching for this individuality can be a challenge for the nurse working with patients who have organic mental disorders.

The nurse should learn as much as possible about the background and life-style of the patient. This information will enable her to individualize a care plan for each patient. The nurse should address the patient on a one-to-one basis by using the title and last name. Use praise, touch, and affection whenever possible. The patient should be dressed in his own clothing during the day with his hair combed. Women should wear makeup, and men should be shaved. These and other actions will promote self-confidence and self-esteem in the patient as well as improved communication between the nurse and the patient.

*PSYCHOPHARMACOLOGY* Antipsychotic medications or neuroleptics are often effective in treating the symptoms associated with organic mental disorders, such as dementia and delirium. These symptoms include agitation, hallucinations, delusions, wandering, and assaultiveness. In general, neuroleptics are recommended for psychotic symptoms, antidepressants for depression, and benzodiazepines for anxiety and insomnia. Neuroleptics are the main drugs for psychotic disorders; however, little is known about the optimal use of these drugs in the elderly.

All antipsychotic medications seem to work equally well, but these drugs differ in the side effects they produce (see Chapter 12). Therefore the selection of an antipsychotic drug must be tailored to the patient on the basis of side effects produced. Also, consideration must be given to patients who are taking other medications and have other physical problems (Cohen and Eisdorfer, 1986b; Nickens et al., 1986).

Antipsychotics, such as haloperidol (Haldol), are as effective in the aged as in young patients, although the dosage levels are lower. Haloperidol is a high-potency antipsychotic, thus producing fewer anticholinergic side effects and more extra-

## Case Study

Mrs. Smith, a 74-year-old retired teacher, lived with her husband of 38 years until his death 2 weeks ago of a massive myocardial infarction. Mrs. Smith has no children or close relatives who are able to care for her.

Irene, a member of Mrs. Smith's church, and Jack, the closest neighbor, have been trying to check on Mrs. Smith daily since her husband's death. Until that time, Irene and Jack were not aware that Mrs. Smith had poor memory. Although she is oriented to person, she does not remember her husband's recent death. She no longer recognizes Irene or any of the neighbors who have lived nearby for several years. She has wandered from home twice in the past 2 weeks. As far as anyone knows, Mrs. Smith is not taking any medication; nor has she seen a physician for several years.

Realizing that Mrs. Smith is unable to care for herself, Irene and Jack decide to contact the Department of Human Services for assistance in caring for her. After evaluation by a social worker, it was recommended that a thorough medical evaluation be done at the local psychiatric hospital.

pyramidal side effects (EPS) than low-potency antipsychotics such as chlorpromazine (Thorazine). Potential side effects that may be intensified in the elderly are sedation, orthostatic hypotension, and EPS, including tardive dyskinesia. If minimum sedation is required, haloperidol has proved to be safe in the elderly and is the drug of choice for this population (see Chapter 12).

Benzodiazepines are the drugs of choice for treating anxiety in elderly patients. In cognitively impaired aged patients, however, benzodiazepines may be contraindicated because they may exacerbate confusion and produce agitation, particularly at night. If tricyclic antidepressants (TCAs) are used, the nurse should monitor TCA serum levels. A TCA-induced delirium due to elevated serum levels is relatively common among elderly patients receiving these drugs.

Age-related physical changes and the presence of chronic illnesses make the use of psychotropic medications in the elderly more difficult than in younger patients (see Chapter 29). Research and accumulated clinical experience will enable those who exhibit mental disorders to be treated more effectively (Nickens et al., 1986).

***MILIEU MANAGEMENT*** Patients with organic mental disorders require a milieu in which they are neither overstimulated nor understimulated. They should be in a safe environment, free from injury, stress, and anxiety. The nurse should maintain an environment free of misleading and frightening stimuli, such as television, a public address system, pictures of animals, and large group activities. Patients should have a warm, caring atmosphere that will facilitate their developing a trusting interpersonal relationship with the caregivers and other patients. The nurse should develop

## Nursing Care Plan

WEEKLY UPDATE: ___8/9/90___

NAME: ___Mrs. Smith___                    ADMISSION DATE: ___7/19/90___

DSM-III-R DIAGNOSIS: _____ 294.10 Dementia _____

*ASSESSMENT:*
*Areas of strength:* Able to feed, dress, and toilet self. Ambulates well. Oriented to person.
*Problems:* Speech is soft and garbled at times. Severe confusion, recent and remote memory loss. Wandering behavior.

*DIAGNOSES:* Fear and anxiety related to confusion and memory loss. Wandering behaviors related to lack of structure. Potential for getting lost related to wandering behaviors.

| | Date met |
|---|---|
| *PLANNING:* | |
| *Short-term goals:* | |
| Patient will remain safe and free of injury. | _____ |
| Patient will express freedom from fear and anxiety. | _____ |
| Patient will establish routine for daily activities. | 8/1/90 |
| *Long-term goals:* | |
| Patient will remain active and independent. | _____ |
| Patient will verbalize acceptance of nursing home place- | 8/7/90 |
| ment. | |

*IMPLEMENTATION/INTERVENTIONS:*
*Nurse-patient relationship:* Address patient as "Mrs. Smith"; use touch, praise, and affection when communicating; express interest in patient's life-style and background; encourage attractive dress and makeup.
*Psychopharmacology:* Haldol 1.0 mg, p.o., q.h.s.
*Milieu management:* Monitor and provide for safety in all ADLs; decrease frightening stimuli; provide relaxing stimuli; encourage participation in quiet activities, including reminiscence therapy.

*EVALUATION:* Patient remains safe and secure; carries out regular ADLs; participates in activities; will transfer to SNF.

a routine the patient can follow daily. Close supervision should be provided during bathing, eating, and other activities. All hot or sharp objects or other hazardous materials should be removed from the patient's surroundings. The doors of the facility should be monitored to prevent elopement. Through these and other management efforts the patient should be able to live in a relatively comfortable and safe environment. To achieve these goals, the nursing staff must be aware of three milieu-related issues: stress, safety, and wandering.

**Stress.** Stress has been shown to be a cause of anxious behavior in demented persons. If the level of stress continues or increases, dysfunctional or catastrophic behavior follows. These dysfunctional behaviors cause excess disability and further limit the patient's ability to function and interact with the environment (Hall and Buckwalter, 1987). Excess disability has been defined as a "reversible deficit that is more disabling than the primary disability, existing when the magnitude of the disturbance in functioning is greater than might be accounted for by basic physical illness or cerebral pathology" (Dawson et al., 1986, p.299).

Hall (1988) lists five groups of stressors that produce disability in the demented person:

1. Fatigue
2. Change of environment, routine, or caregiver
3. Overwhelming or competing stimuli
4. Demands that exceed capacity to function
5. Physical stressors

*Fatigue.* Patients fatigue rapidly from performing basic daily functions and frequently require rest periods both morning and afternoon. These short rest periods should be in a comfortable chair, such as a recliner, so as not to confuse the patient with going to bed. Organized activities, including visits from family members, should be of short duration so as not to interfere with scheduled rest periods. Depending on the progression of the disease, the patient may not be able to tolerate group activities (Hall, 1988).

*Change of environment, routine, or caregiver.* A change of environment, caregiver, or routine can be stressful for patients because of their altered ability to plan, initiate, and carry through voluntary activities. Patients will express frustration at trying to initiate and complete simple tasks and may refuse to attempt any activity they feel they cannot complete. Many patients compensate for this by developing a consistent routine. For some patients it may be helpful for the caregiver to develop a schedule that is posted in the room for the patient to follow. A change in environment, such as holiday decorations, should be limited to specific areas so that the patient's environment remains relatively stable.

*Overwhelming or competing stimuli.* Misleading, overwhelming, or competing stimuli are easily misinterpreted by patients. Elimination of such stimuli as high noise levels, multiple activities, and crowds of people will minimize anxious behavior. Some facilities have smaller self-contained units that minimize competing stimuli and can be used for rest or small-group activities. Meals may be served in a quiet area with one or two other patients present.

*Demands that exceed capacity to function.*  Demands to achieve that exceed their functional capacity can be devastating for patients. Some families and staff members think that frequent testing of the patient to determine the amount of memory loss is important. However, being asked questions they cannot answer and being told they are wrong can be very frustrating (Hall, 1988). Reality orientation is generally helpful to patients with mild cognitive impairments. However, if memory loss is severe, reality orientation probably will not succeed. For these patients, reality orientation seems only to deepen their anxiety. Burnside (1988) states that reminiscence group therapy can be used successfully with severely demented patients because it reinforces identity, acknowledges what was significant and enduring in the person's life, and often compensates for the dullness of the present.

*Physical stressors.*  Physical stressors are identified as anything that causes physical discomfort, such as pain, acute illness, and other psychological alterations. Caffeine is one of the most commonly used physical stressors, and its use should be eliminated. Other common stressors are impacted bowels, full bladder, infections, influenza, and medication reactions and interactions. Patients exhibiting stress-related behavior should be given a physical assessment to determine the presence of any physical stressors (Hall, 1988).

*Safety.*  Safety is an important area that must be addressed in planning care for the patient. As the disease progresses, patients are unable to consider their own safety needs and risks. The disoriented patient with hallucinations may need to be protected from hurting himself or others. These experiences can be frightening, and the patient may try to escape by running away, resulting in injuries to himself or others. Falls are a safety problem, and the nurse should make an evaluation of the environment to eliminate obstacles, slippery floors, throw rugs, and inadequate lighting. Other hazards include such objects as razors and electrical devices, which should be used under supervision. Anything that might harm the patient should not be left at the bedside. Substances that could be ingested, such as toiletries, cleaning solutions, and plants, should be monitored carefully. All caregivers should be aware of and trained to recognize potential hazards to assure a safe environment for the patient (Matteson, 1988; Hall, 1988). Soft restraints should not be used indiscriminately and only when all other nursing interventions have been unsuccessful in protecting the patient.

*Wandering.*  Wandering may be defined as leaving the facility or a designated area without approval of the caregiver. Patients who wander or try to elope present a problem for caregivers, whether at home or in an institution. These patients must be identified and plans made to minimize the risks. The patient's clothing must carry some markings to identify him, and a photograph should be on file to be used in locating the individual. Special alarms should be installed to alert staff if the patient attempts to leave the facility (Burnside, 1988; Hall, 1988).

A patient may wander inadvertently. For example, running an errand or exploring one's surroundings may evolve into aimless wandering. Patients in advanced stages of dementia may simply wander because of disorientation or because of their inability to sustain intentions (Burnside, 1988). A number of risks are involved when a patient "wanders," ranging from simple exposure to being the potential victim of

**Box 22-5**
## CATEGORIES OF WANDERERS AND INTERVENTION STRATEGIES

1. Recreational wanderer—satisfies a need for exercise.
   *Intervention:* Staff takes patient for a walk on a regular basis; develop a routine to enhance orientation.
2. Fantasy or reminiscent wander—desire to elope based on a delusion or fantasy, e.g., going to work.
   *Intervention:* Relieve boredom or tension.
3. Purposeful wander—patient is upset and is preoccupied with leaving the facility. If patient is agitated, he may assault a staff member who attempts to block the exit.
   *Intervention:* Staff should defuse the situation by using diversion or alternate actions.

crime. Consequently the staff must intervene by directing the patient's attention away from doors and hallways, must supervise his walking, and must redirect this attention into safer activities. Several distinct categories of wanderers and intervention strategies are presented in Box 22-5 (Heim, 1986; Burnside, 1988; Hall, 1988).

Other methods of management of wandering include physical or chemical restraints. Use of physical restraints may result in severe physical and emotional problems for the patient. Use of sedatives can compound confusion and add to mental deficits in general. Allowing the patient to wander may be the most feasible alternative; however, patient safety resulting from environmental constraints precludes this alternative in most health care settings (Young et al., 1988).

## KEY CONCEPTS

1. Organic mental syndrome refers to a group of signs and symptoms without reference to a cause, but with organic mental disorder there are known or presumed organic etiological factors.
2. In delirium there is sudden but temporary widespread cerebral dysfunction.
3. The cardinal symptoms of dementia are cognitive symptoms that interfere with daily functioning.
4. Alzheimer's disease is a chronic, nonreversible form of dementia, most commonly seen in the elderly. There are three progressive stages of Alzheimer's disease.
5. Research focuses on five models explaining possible causes of Alzheimer's disease.

6. Parkinson's disease is a degenerative motor disorder related to the loss of dopamine-generating cells in the basal ganglia.
7. Huntington's disease is a rare hereditary disorder involving deterioration of
   both motor and cognitive functions.
8. Approximately 25% of all dementia cases are vascular in origin.
9. Priority nursing interventions with delirium are those that maintain life. Priority
   nursing interventions with dementia are those that maintain an optimal level
   of functioning.
10. Medications prescribed for organic mental syndromes depend on the predom-
    inant type of symptoms, but all are used cautiously with the elderly.
11. Patients with organic mental disorders require a caring, structured milieu that
    minimizes stress, provides for safety, and reduces the possibility of wandering.

## REFERENCES

American Psychiatric Association: Diagnostic and statistical manual of mental disorders, third edition, revised, Washington, DC, 1987, The Association.

Batt LJ: Managing delirium, J Psychosoc Nurs 27:22, 1989.

Burnside IM: Dementia and delirium. In Burnside IM, editor: Nursing and the aged: a self-care approach, ed 3, New York, 1988, McGraw-Hill Book Co, pp 733-767.

Cohen D and Eisdorfer C: The loss of self, New York, 1986, New American Library (a).

Cohen D and Eisdorfer C: Dementing disorders. In Calkins E, Davis PJ and Ford AB, editors: The practice of geriatrics, Philadelphia, 1986, WB Saunders Co, pp 194-205 (b).

Cohen GD: Alzheimer's disease: clinical update, Hosp Community Psychiatry 41:496, 1990.

Cutler NR and Navang PK: Drug therapies, Geriatr Nurs 6:160, 1985.

Dawson P et al: Preventing excess disability in patients with Alzheimer's disease, Geriatr Nurs 7:299, 1986.

Evans DA, Funkenstein HH, Albert MS, et al: Prevalence of Alzheimer's disease in a community population of older persons, JAMA 262:2551, 1989.

Foreman MD: Acute confusional states in hospitalized elderly: a research dilemma, Nurs Res 35:34, 1986.

Gomez GE and Gomez EA: Delirium, Geriatr Nurs 8:330, 1987.

Hall GR: Alterations in thought process, J Gerontol Nurs 14:30, 1988.

Hall GR and Buckwalter KC: Progressively lowered stress threshold: a conceptual model for care of adults with Alzheimer's disease, Arch Psychiatr Nurs 1:399, 1987.

Harrell JS: Age related changes in the cardiovascular system. In Matteson MA and McConnell ES, editors: Gerontological nursing concepts and practice, Philadelphia, 1988, WB Saunders Co, pp 194-217.

Heim KM: Wandering behavior, J Gerontol Nurs 12:4, 1986.

Kermis MD: Mental health in late life: the adaptive process, Boston, 1986, Jones & Bartlett.

Lucas MJ, Steel C, and Bognanni A: Recognition of psychiatric symptoms in dementia, J Gerontol Nurs 12:11, 1986.

Matteson MA: Age-related changes in the neurological system. In Matteson MA and McConnell ES, editors: Gerontological nursing concepts and practice, Philadelphia, 1988, WB Saunders Co, pp 248-263.

McDowell FH: Other neurologic diseases of the elderly. In Calkins E, Davis PJ and Ford AB, editors: The practice of geriatrics, Philadelphia, 1986, WB Saunders Co, pp 225-239.

Margo GM, Finkel JA: Early dementia as a risk factor for suicide, Hosp Community Psychiatry, 41:676, 1990.

National Institute on Aging Task Force: Senility reconsidered: treatment possibilities for mental impairment in the elderly, JAMA 244:259, 1980.

Nickens HW, Crook T, and Cohen GD: Psychotropic drugs. Generations, pp 33-37, Spring, 1986.

Raskind MA, and Storrie MC: The organic mental disorders. In Busse EW and Blazer DG, editors: Handbook of geriatric psychiatry, New York, 1980, Van Nostrand Reinhold, pp 305-328.

Reisberg B, Ferris SH, Franssen E: An ordinal functional assessment tool for Alzheimer's-type dementia, Hosp Community Psychiatry 36:593, 1985.

Williams L: Alzheimer's: the need for caring, J Gerontol Nurs 12:21, 1986.

Wills R: Cognitive changes of normal aging and the dementias. In Carnevali DL and Patrick M, editors: Nursing management for the elderly, ed 2, Philadelphia, 1986, JB Lippincott Co, pp 241-256.

Young SH, Muir-Nash J, and Ninos M: Managing nocturnal wandering behavior, J Gerontol Nurs 14:6-12, 1988.

Zisook S and Braff DL: Delirium: recognition and management in the older patient, Geriatrics 41:67-78, 1986.

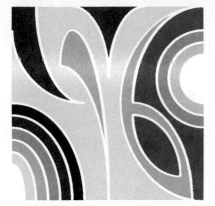

CHAPTER 23

# Personality Disorders

PATRICIA CLUNN AND CAROL E. BOSTROM

LEARNING OBJECTIVES
After reading this chapter you should be able to

- Recognize DSM-III-R criteria for personality disorders.
- Describe behaviors of persons with personality disorders.
- Describe nursing interventions for patients with personality disorders.
- Recognize issues related to the care of patients with personality disorders.
- Describe the two categories of sexual disorders.

$T$his chapter focuses on patients with personality disorders hospitalized in the inpatient psychiatric setting. Except for the patient with a borderline disorder, these patients are not usually hospitalized because of their personality disorders but because of other mental disorders diagnosed on Axis I. The interventions focus primarily on the nurse-patient relationship *unique* to each personality disorder, and this chapter does not repeat the general nurse-patient interventions described in Chapter 6. Neither milieu issues nor medications will be addressed for each disorder because milieu or pharmacological therapy does not exist for each specific disorder. Medication may be given if the patient has an axis I diagnosis or a symptom severe enough to interfere with functioning, such as severe anxiety or depression. The chapter concludes with a review of sexual disorders.

## DSM-III-R CRITERIA AND TERMINOLOGY
### Traits vs disorders

All of us have personality traits and characteristics that make us different, unique, "interesting human beings." "Personality traits are enduring patterns of perceiving, relating to, and thinking about the environment and oneself, and are exhibited in a wide range of important social and personal contexts" (APA, 1987). Personality traits or habits are approaches to the world, expressed in how the person thinks, how he feels, and what he does. Traditionally they have been viewed as unconscious processes. "It is only when personality traits are inflexible and maladaptive and cause either significant functional impairment or subjective distress that they constitute Personality Disorders" (APA, 1987). These traits or behaviors involve lifelong patterns of relating to others and usually cause distress in others. Overall, those with personality disorders do not find their behaviors distressing to themselves. They experience distress because of others' reactions or behaviors toward them. Characteristics displayed by people with personality disorders are inflexible and maladaptive stress responses, inability to relate in work and love, interpersonal conflicts, and the ability to get under others' skin (Kaplan and Sadock, 1985).

### Axis II

Personality disorders are listed on axis II. Axis II can also be used to designate personality traits or habitual use of particular defense mechanisms. For example, compulsive traits are not the same as compulsive personality disorders. Many high-functioning people have compulsive traits, whereas only a few have compulsive personality disorders. Patients benefit from the fact that most nurses have compulsive traits, for example, rechecking labels, dressings, drainage tubes.

## GENERAL ETIOLOGY
### Traditional views

Psychoanalytical theorists, developmentalists, behaviorists, and social learning theorists all believe that personality disorders originate in early childhood experiences. The psychoanalytical theorists and developmentalists agree that unsuccessful mastery of tasks in stages of development leads to anxiety and the resultant use of defense mechanisms. The exclusive use of rigid and maladaptive responses or defenses characterizes personality disorders.

Behavioral and sociocultural factors reinforce and maintain maladaptive social behavior exhibited by people with personality disorders. Responses of others rein-force personality tendencies and traits. Children develop personality characteristics by learning through social experiences. They model their actions after persons around them, particularly their parents. Children repeat actions that bring them rewards and avoid actions that incur punishment. Behavior that has been consistently rewarded from infancy, before the development of understanding, cognition, and language, is the most difficult to unlearn or modify.

### Contemporary views

Genetic factors play a significant role in the genesis of personality disorders. Studies of monozygotic twins indicate that if one twin has a personality disorder, the other twin is more likely to have the same disorder (Kaplan and Sadock, 1985).

Constitutional factors consider that "all forms of neurological insult—especially sedative drug intoxication, postencephalitic states, and temporal lobe epilepsy—increase the incidence and the severity of personality disorders. Children with minimal brain dysfunction may be predisposed to the later development of person-ality disorders" (Kaplan and Sadock, 1985). A careful medical and neurological workup by the physician or psychiatrist would be necessary to rule out an organic basis for personality disorders.

## ■ Personality Disorder Clusters

According to the DSM-III-R, the personality disorders are grouped into three clusters on the basis of descriptive features. Cluster A includes the schizoid, schizotypal, and paranoid disorders characterized by odd or eccentric behaviors. Cluster B includes the narcissistic, histrionic, antisocial, and borderline disorders characterized by dra-matic, emotional, or erratic behaviors. Cluster C includes the dependent, passive-aggressive, avoidant, and obsessive-compulsive disorders characterized by anxious or fearful behaviors (APA, 1987).

When a person exhibits features of more than one specific personality disorder or does not meet the full criteria for any one disorder, the classification of "per-sonality disorder not otherwise specified" is used.

## ■ Cluster A: Odd/Eccentric
### PARANOID PERSONALITY DISORDER

**Characteristics and criteria.** Suspiciousness and mistrust of people charac-terize the patient with a paranoid personality disorder. They interpret the actions of others as deliberately demeaning or threatening (APA, 1987). Therefore tension and the need to scan the environment are evidenced. They are unusually sensitive to other people's motives and feelings but externalize their own emotions; that is, they may project their own desires and traits to others (Millon, 1986). They feel vulnerable because they think others treat them unfairly. Persons with paranoid personality disorders are unable to laugh at themselves and are often humorless and serious. Speech is logical and goal directed, although the bases of arguments are

**Box 23-1**
## DIAGNOSTIC CRITERIA FOR 301.00 PARANOID
## PERSONALITY DISORDER

A.  A pervasive and unwarranted tendency, beginning by early adulthood and present in a variety of contexts, to interpret the actions of people as deliberately demeaning or threatening, as indicated by at least *four* of the following:
(1) expects, without sufficient basis, to be exploited or harmed by others
(2) questions, without justification, the loyalty or trustworthiness of friends or associates
(3) reads hidden demeaning or threatening meanings into benign remarks or events, e.g., suspects that a neighbor put out trash early to annoy him
(4) bears grudges or is unforgiving of insults or slights
(5) is reluctant to confide in others because of unwarranted fear that the information will be used against him or her
(6) is easily slighted and quick to react with anger or to counterattack
(7) questions, without justification, fidelity of spouse or sexual partner
B.  Occurrence not exclusively during the course of schizophrenia or a delusional Disorder.

Reprinted with permission from the *Diagnostic and Statistical Manual of Mental Disorders, Third Edition, Revised.* Copyright 1987 American Psychiatric Association.

false. Thought content includes projection, prejudice, and sometimes ideas of reference. Their affect is restricted, and they may appear to be cold and usually lack sentimental and tender feelings (APA, 1987). Box 23-1 presents the diagnostic criteria for this disorder.

Unlike persons with paranoid schizophrenia, these patients do not have fixed delusions or hallucinations. People with paranoid personality disorders are hospitalized when their behavior is out of control in response to a threat perceived as overwhelming or immediate. Because they are quick to respond with anger or rage if they feel severely threatened, these patients may be brought to the hospital because of their loss of control and potential for violence. Transient psychotic symptoms may be precipitated by extreme stress.

**Unique etiology.** Studies suggest that the paranoid personality disorder tends to occur in families. It appears to have a genetic basis, like schizophrenia (Siever, et al., 1983), and is diagnosed more often in men than in women (APA, 1987).

### PSYCHOTHERAPEUTIC MANAGEMENT

*NURSE-PATIENT RELATIONSHIP* The most important psychotherapeutic task centers on dealing with trust issues. A professional demeanor coupled with honesty and nonintrusiveness will assist with the development of some trust. Since low doses of phenothiazines may be prescribed to manage anxiety and other symptoms, the patient may resist taking medication if basic trust has not been developed (Gunderson, 1988). Clear, simple explanations and requests will reduce the patient's feelings of being threatened or controlled. Patients with paranoid personality disorders do not tolerate group therapies that expect or involve confrontation or much emotional involvement. Behavior therapies threaten their feelings of control (Gunderson, 1988).

## OTHER ODD OR ECCENTRIC DISORDERS
### Schizoid personality disorder

People with schizoid personalities do not want to be involved in interpersonal or social relationships. "Grossly inadequate, cold, or neglectful early parenting" is often seen in their histories (Gunderson, 1988). As a result, the patient learns to withdraw because he does not receive benefits from relationships. "A shy, introverted temperament may be a predisposing factor" (Gunderson, 1988). These persons rarely have close friends and appear uncomfortable about interacting with others. They could be thought of as hermits. They give "short answers to questions and avoid spontaneous conversation" (Kaplan and Sadock, 1985). The defense mechanism of intellectualization is seen in that they describe emotional and interpersonal experiences in a matter-of-fact and impersonal manner (Millon, 1986). Their function at work is successful, especially if little verbal interaction is required. The patients are reality oriented, but fantasy and daydreaming may be more gratifying than realistic persons and situations. For additional characteristics, see DSM-III-R criteria in Box 23-2. These persons are rarely hospitalized because their behaviors do not attract attention.

If such a patient is hospitalized, the nurse-patient relationship will focus on building trust before the nurse assists the patient with identification and appropriate verbal expression of feelings. At first the patient may begin with being on the fringe of the group because of his discomfort and anxiety. Slowly involving the patient in milieu and group activities will help to increase social skills.

### Schizotypal personality disorder

Schizotypal personality disorder is similar to schizophrenia, residual type, except that the psychotic episodes are transient and not as severe (APA, 1987). The patient may need hospitalization during one of these psychotic episodes. Peculiarities of ideation, appearance, and behavior as well as deficits in interpersonal relatedness, are present (APA, 1987). The patients appear to be odd and eccentric in communication and behavior. The diagnostic criteria are listed in Box 23-3. "Magical thinking, ideas of reference, illusions, and derealization are part of his everyday world" (Kaplan and Sadock, 1985). The patient's thinking and communication are disturbed. "Like the schizophrenic, the person with schizotypal personality disorder may not know his own feelings, yet he is exquisitely sensitive to detecting the feelings of others, especially negative affects, like anger" (Kaplan and Sadock, 1985). Schizotypal personality disorders are more common in the biological relatives of chronic schizo-

**Box 23-2**
## DIAGNOSTIC CRITERIA FOR 301.20 SCHIZOID PERSONALITY DISORDER

A.  A pervasive pattern of indifference to social relationships and a restricted range of emotional experience and expression, beginning by early adulthood and present in a variety of contexts, as indicated by at least *four* of the following:
   (1) neither desires nor enjoys close relationships, including being part of a family
   (2) almost always chooses solitary activities
   (3) rarely, if ever, claims or appears to experience strong emotions, such as anger and joy
   (4) indicates little if any desire to have sexual experiences with another person (age being taken into account)
   (5) is indifferent to the praise and criticism of others
   (6) has no close friends or confidants (or only one) other than first-degree relatives
   (7) displays constricted affect, e.g., is aloof, cold, rarely reciprocates gestures or facial expressions, such as smiles or nods
B.  Occurrence not exclusively during the course of schizophrenia or a delusional disorder.

Reprinted with permission from the *Diagnostic and Statistical Manual of Mental Disorders, Third Edition, Revised.* Copyright 1987 American Psychiatric Association.

phrenics than in control groups (Kaplan and Sadock, 1985). Not much has been written about genetic links or the impact of environmental influences on this disorder.

If a person with a schizotypal personality disorder is hospitalized, support, kindness, and gentle suggestions are essential if he is to become involved in activities with others that will improve his interpersonal relationships, social skills, and appropriate behaviors. Social situations are uncomfortable and cause discomfort and anxiety because of the reactions of others to his appearance and behavior. These patients benefit from socializing experiences and may need vocational counseling and assistance with job placement to minimize chances of ridicule and rejection. Low doses of neuroleptic drugs may decrease the severity of symptoms exhibited in the transient psychotic state in relation to thinking, perception, and anxiety. The medications will not affect social and interpersonal adaptation (Gunderson, 1988).

**Box 23-3**
## DIAGNOSTIC CRITERIA FOR 301.22 SCHIZOTYPAL PERSONALITY DISORDER

A. A pervasive pattern of deficits in interpersonal relatedness and peculiarities of ideation, appearance, and behavior, beginning by early adulthood and present in a variety of contexts, as indicated by at least *five* of the following:

   (1) ideas of reference (excluding delusions of reference)

   (2) excessive social anxiety, e.g., extreme discomfort in social situations involving unfamiliar people

   (3) odd beliefs or magical thinking, influencing behavior and inconsistent with subcultural norms, e.g., superstitiousness, belief in clairvoyance, telepathy, or "sixth sense," "others can feel my feelings" (in children and adolescents, bizarre fantasies or preoccupations)

   (4) unusual perceptual experiences, e.g., illusions, sensing the presence of a force or person not actually present (e.g., "I felt as if my dead mother were in the room with me")

   (5) odd or eccentric behavior or appearance, e.g., unkempt, unusual mannerisms, talks to self

   (6) no close friends or confidants (or only one) other than first-degree relatives

   (7) odd speech (without loosening of associations or incoherence), e.g., speech that is impoverished, digressive, vague, or inappropriately abstract

   (8) inappropriate or constricted affect, e.g., silly, aloof, rarely reciprocates gestures or facial expressions, such as smiles or nods

   (9) suspiciousness or paranoid ideation

B. Occurrence not exclusively during the course of schizophrenia or a pervasive developmental disorder.

Reprinted with permission from the *Diagnostic and Statistical Manual of Mental Disorders, Third Edition, Revised.* Copyright 1987 American Psychiatric Association.

## ■ Cluster B: Dramatic/Erratic
### ANTISOCIAL PERSONALITY DISORDER

**Characteristics and criteria.** The main feature of antisocial personality disorder is a pattern of disregard of the rights of others that is usually demonstrated by repeated violation of others' rights in the form of unlawful behaviors. This involves "aggressive or illegal activities, such as repeated thefts, assaults, evasion of financial obligations, and lying" (Gunderson, 1988). The onset of this disorder is before the age of 15, with a history of behaviors diagnosed as conduct disorder (APA, 1987). Affected persons engage in reckless behavior, as evidenced by their driving while intoxicated and engaging in spouse or child beating. They are promiscuous and have no guilt about hurting others. Their criminal behavior places them within the court and prison system more than within the medical system (APA, 1987).

The diagnosis of the antisocial personality disorder is based on history rather than on the mental status examination, in which many areas of disordered life functioning are evident (Kaplan and Sadock, 1985). These persons frequently engage in criminal activity (but not all criminals have antisocial personality disorders). "Despite a normal mental status, there are signs of personal distress including tension, inability to tolerate boredom, depression, and the conviction (often correct) that others are hostile toward them" (APA, 1987).

People with a antisocial personality disorder may appear to be charming and intellectual. They are smooth talkers and deny and rationalize their behavior. Expected anxiety over their predicament is absent. Guilt or loyality is nonexistent. "Psychoactive substance abuse disorders are commonly associated diagnoses" (APA, 1987). This disorder interferes with independent, responsible life functioning, and it is more common in males than in females (APA, 1987). See Box 23-4 for DSM-III-R criteria.

**Unique etiology.** Both genetic and environmental influences are known to influence the development antisocial personality disorder. "Environmental studies have consistently noted the absence of a sustained, stable mother" (Gunderson, 1988). Maternal deprivation in the first 5 years of life is an important element in this disorder (Kaplan and Sadock, 1985). Genetic studies of twin or adoptive siblings and family history data have found significant evidence suggesting a genetic predisposition for the antisocial personality disorder (Siever et al., 1983). "Adoption studies show that both genetic and environmental factors contribute to the risk of this group of disorders, because parents with Antisocial Personality Disorder increase the risk of Antisocial Personality Disorder, Somatization Disorder, and Psychoactive Substance Use Disorders in both their adopted and biologic children" (APA, 1987).

### PSYCHOTHERAPEUTIC MANAGEMENT

*NURSE-PATIENT RELATIONSHIP* Long-term treatment in a therapeutic milieu is necessary for any type of lasting changes to occur. With short-term hospitalization the nurse can initiate the therapeutic process by setting firm limits. These patients try to manipulate staff and bend rules for their wants and needs. The nurse must be steadfast and consistent in confronting behaviors and enforcing rules and policies. Consequences of behavior, both for the unit and for the patient's life, are also focused on. Helping the patient to be aware of consequences is a concrete way to assist the patient in realizing what the results of his behaviors are or will be. Pointing out the effects that his behaviors have on others is also a part of the therapeutic process. He needs to begin to understand how others feel and react to his behaviors and why they react to him the way they do. The nurse must project an attitude of acceptance, avoid moralizing (Frosch, 1983), and assist in identification and verbalization of feelings.

Group membership can help the patient receive parenting that he never received. Because of their deprivation and neglect in childhood, these patients need

**Box 23-4**

## DIAGNOSTIC CRITERIA FOR 301.70 ANTISOCIAL PERSONALITY DISORDER

A. Current age at least 18.

B. Evidence of Conduct Disorder with onset before age 15, as indicated by a history of *three* or more of the following:

   (1) was often truant

   (2) ran away from home overnight at least twice while living in parental or parental surrogate home (or once without returning)

   (3) often initiated physical fights

   (4) used a weapon in more than one fight

   (5) forced someone into sexual activity with him or her

   (6) was physically cruel to animals

   (7) was physically cruel to other people

   (8) deliberately destroyed others' property (other than by fire-setting)

   (9) deliberately engaged in fire-setting

  (10) often lied (other than to avoid physical or sexual abuse)

  (11) has stolen without confrontation of a victim on more than one occasion (including forgery)

  (12) has stolen with confrontation of a victim (e.g., mugging, purse-snatching, extortion, armed robbery)

C. A pattern of irresponsible and antisocial behavior since the age of 15, as indicated by at least *four* of the following:

   (1) is unable to sustain consistent work behavior, as indicated by any of the following (including similar behavior in academic settings if the person is a student):

     *(a)* significant unemployment for six months or more within five years when expected to work and work was available

     *(b)* repeated absences from work unexplained by illness in self or family

     *(c)* abandonment of several jobs without realistic plans for others

   (2) fails to conform to social norms with respect to lawful behavior, as indicated by repeatedly performing antisocial acts that are grounds for arrest (whether arrested or not), e.g., destroying property, harassing others, stealing, pursuing an illegal occupation

   (3) is irritable and aggressive, as indicated by repeated physical fights or assaults (not required by one's job or to defend someone or oneself), including spouse- or child-beating

Reprinted with permission from the *Diagnostic and Statistical Manual of Mental Disorders, Third Edition, Revised.* Copyright 1987 American Psychiatric Association.

*Continued.*

**Box 23-4**
## DIAGNOSTIC CRITERIA FOR 301.70 ANTISOCIAL PERSONALITY DISORDER—cont'd

(4) repeatedly fails to honor financial obligations, as indicated by defaulting on debts or failing to provide child support or support for other dependents on a regular basis

(5) fails to plan ahead, or is impulsive, as indicated by one or both of the following:

    *(a)* traveling from place to place without a prearranged job or clear goal for the period of travel or clear idea about when the travel will terminate

    *(b)* lack of a fixed address for a month or more

(6) has no regard for the truth, as indicated by repeated lying, use of aliases, or "conning" others for personal profit or pleasure

(7) is reckless regarding his or her own or others' personal safety, as indicated by driving while intoxicated, or recurrent speeding

(8) if a parent or guardian, lacks ability to function as a responsible parent, as indicated by one or more of the following:

    *(a)* malnutrition of child

    *(b)* child's illness resulting from lack of minimal hygiene

    *(c)* failure to obtain medical care for a seriously ill child

    *(d)* child's dependence on neighbors or nonresident relatives for food or shelter

    *(e)* failure to arrange for a caretaker for young child when parent is away from home

    *(f)* repeated squandering, on personal items, of money required for household necessities

(9) has never sustained a totally monogamous relationship for more than one year

(10) lacks remorse (feels justified in having hurt, mistreated, or stolen from another)

D. Occurrence of antisocial behavior not exclusively during the course of schizophrenia or manic episodes.

---

to absorb more loving than one person can provide (Kaplan and Sadock, 1985). Groups are also effective in confronting inappropriate and manipulative behaviors. Institutional group programs will help the patient to assume responsibility for his behaviors and to act responsibly toward others (Gunderson, 1988). Inpatient group activities can help this patient to tolerate underlying feelings of emptiness, depression, and anxiety and to develop socially appropriate behavioral responses (Gunderson, 1988).

## BORDERLINE PERSONALITY DISORDER

**Characteristics and criteria.** "Borderline personality disorder is the most common personality disorder found in outpatient and inpatient psychiatric populations where it generally occurs in 15 25 percent of all patients" (Gunderson, 1988). The full range of symptoms and behaviors is not seen in one short-term inpatient hospitalization, which makes persons with this disorder difficult to understand and tolerate. These patients usually require hospitalization when they are in a crisis or exhibit self-mutilating or suicidal behaviors.

The patient with a borderline personality disorder (BPD) exhibits "a pervasive pattern of instability of self-image, interpersonal relationships, and mood" (APA, 1987). According to the DSM-III-R the identity disturbance is seen in the patient who is uncertain about his self-image, sexual orientation, career goals, personal values, and the types of friends to have. Interpersonal relationships alternate between overidealization and devaluation and include manipulation and dependency. This patient experiences great difficulty in being alone. Mood shifts are quick and can include physical fights, displays of temper, and self-mutilating behavior. Complete DSM-III-R criteria for BPD are found in Box 23-5, and psychiatric nursing diagnoses (PND-1) are found in Box 23-6. Impulsive actions, substance abuse, and self-destructiveness are repetitive (Gunderson, 1988). These patients are unstable and changeable. They cannot tolerate stress or delays in gratification and are unable to regulate their affects or moods, which predisposes them to psychic disorganization (Kaplan and Sadock, 1985). At times persons with a BPD experience brief psychotic episodes or symptoms of major depression.

On admission to an inpatient psychiatric unit, the person with a BPD may exhibit his need for attention and affection by contradictory behaviors of manipulation, dependency, or acting-out behaviors. Frustration on the part of the staff may be seen as rejection. This perception by the patient can lead to increased anger and withdrawal. Shifts between depression, anxiety, euphoria, and anger are seen in the patient's labile mood. Under stress the patient regresses to immature behaviors and is unable to cope with conflict (Millon, 1986). The patient vacillates between clinging and disengaged behaviors, as demonstrated by his desiring the hospital and staff to solve all problems or by his viewing the inpatient treatment as unnecessary and meaningless. When progress seems to be occurring, the patient with a BPD may suddenly exhibit opposite behaviors, and it may seem as if the staff will need to start over from the beginning.

**Unique etiology.** Genetic and biological studies are inconclusive. One study indicates that those with a BPD have significantly more relatives with affective illness. There is even less evidence to indicate that a BPD is associated with schizophrenia (Siever et al., 1983). "More important to the etiology of this disorder are enduring patterns of inconsistency and unpredictability in parenting" (Gunderson, 1988). Two types of families are seen in the development of the BPD. One family is neglectful, and the other is characterized by overinvolvement (Gunderson, 1988).

According to Mahler's et al. (1975) concepts of normal development, by the end of the separation-individuation phase (age 2), the child is able to see self and object as separate. The child can retain the images of nurturing figures when they are absent. He can integrate the possibility of good and bad coexisting. The child

**Box 23-5**

## DIAGNOSTIC CRITERIA FOR 301.83 BORDERLINE PERSONALITY DISORDER

A pervasive pattern of instability of mood, interpersonal relationships, and self-image, beginning by early adulthood and present in a variety of contexts, as indicated by at least *five* of the following:

(1)  a pattern of unstable and intense interpersonal relationships characterized by alternating between extremes of overidealization and devaluation

(2)  impulsiveness in at least two areas that are potentially self-damaging, e.g., spending, sex, substance use, shoplifting, reckless driving, binge eating (Do not include suicidal or self-mutilating behavior covered in [5].)

(3)  affective instability: marked shifts from baseline mood to depression, irritability, or anxiety, usually lasting a few hours and only rarely more than a few days

(4)  inappropriate, intense anger or lack of control of anger, e.g., frequent displays of temper, constant anger, recurrent physical fights

(5)  recurrent suicidal threats, gestures, or behavior, or self-mutilating behavior

(6)  marked and persistent identity disturbance manifested by uncertainty about at least two of the following: self-image, sexual orientation, long-term goals or career choice, type of friends desired, preferred values

(7)  chronic feelings of emptiness or boredom

(8)  frantic efforts to avoid real or imagined abandonment (Do not include suicidal or self-mutilating behavior covered in [5].)

Reprinted with permission from the *Diagnostic and Statistical Manual of Mental Disorders, Third Edition, Revised.* Copyright 1987 American Psychiatric Association.

who is developing a BPD fails in this developmental task. The parent may cling to the child and prevent autonomy and individuation. Or the parent may withdraw attention and support, leaving the child with feelings of confusion, rage, and abandonment that continue throughout life. The person with a BPD, in response to his unmet needs for love, dismisses safety and becomes self-destructive in his search for attention and love (Lynch and Lynch, 1977). The conflict between abandonment and domination brings negative feedback from others in response to the person's ambivalent need for attachment and detachment. The person with a BPD vacillates between loving and hating, which is reinforced by the ambivalent reactions of others. The person with a BPD fears abandonment if he grows up and domination if he submits. Attachment is seen in clinging, dependency, and idealization, and detachment is seen in anger, pouting, and devaluation (Melges and Swartz, 1989). The person with a BPD uses the defense mechanism of "splitting": the self and others

## Box 23-6

PSYCHIATRIC NURSING DIAGNOSES (PND I) FOR PATIENTS WITH
PERSONALITY DISORDERS

### Paranoid

| | |
|---|---|
| 06.01.02 | Hyperalertness |
| 06.01.04 | Selective inattention |
| 04.02 | Altered feeling patterns |
| 05.03 | Altered role performance |
| 05.05 | Altered social interaction |
| 02.02 | Altered judgment |
| 02.08.03 | Altered problem solving |
| 02.07.02 | Ideas of reference |
| 05.01 | Altered communication processes |
| 04.98 | Altered emotional processes nos* |

### Schizoid/Schizotypal

| | |
|---|---|
| 05.05.02 | Social isolation/withdrawal |
| 05.03.02 | Altered leisure role |
| 05.01.02 | Altered verbal communication |
| 04.97 | Undeveloped emotional responses |
| 01.03.02 | Altered grooming |
| 03.03 | Altered home maintenance |

### Borderline

| | |
|---|---|
| 05.04 | Altered sexuality processes |
| 06.03.02 | Altered gender identity |
| 06.03.03 | Altered personal identity |
| 06.03.04 | Altered sclf-esteem |
| 06.03.05 | Altered social identity |
| 02.08.01 | Altered abstract thinking |
| 02.08.03 | Altered problem solving |
| 02.02 | Altered judgment |
| 04.98 | Altered emotional processes, self-destructiveness |
| 05.02.01.03 | Aggressiveness/violent behavior toward self nos* |

### Antisocial

| | |
|---|---|
| 05.02 | Altered conduct/impulse processes |
| 02.04 | Altered learning process |
| 05.01.02 | Altered nonverbal communication |
| 05.98 | Altered interpersonal processes nos* |
| 05.02.01.02 | Aggressive/violent behaviors toward others |
| 05.03.01 | Altered family role |
| 05.03.06 | Altered work role |

*Not otherwise specified.

A. O'Toole, M. Loomis. 1989. "Classifying Human Responses in Psychiatric-Mental Health Nursing," from *Classification Systems for Describing Nursing Practice: Working Papers*, pp. 20-30. Kansas City, MO: American Nurses Association. Reprinted with permission.

cannot be viewed as having both good and bad qualities; therefore self and others are either all good or all bad.

This person manifests overwhelming anger and projects the responsibility for his problems onto others. Intense moods of anger and depression are accompanied by chronic feelings of emptiness (Kaplan and Sadock, 1985). Persons with a BPD regress and become suicidal when they feel blocked, frustrated, or stressed. Typically, self-mutilation is a cry for help, an expression of intense anger, or a means to numb psychological pain by inducing physical pain (Kaplan and Sadock, 1985; Favazza, 1989).

## Case Study

Sherry Morgan, a 27-year-old woman, is brought to the psychiatric inpatient unit from the emergency room. Both wrists were bandaged after suturing. She is complaining of nausea and heartburn. She vacillates between being angry and crying. Sherry states, "I know I am bad. I should not have done it. I do not want to die, but I am tired of the hassles." She has brought with her three suitcases filled with her belongings. During the admission interview the nurse finds that Sherry has had three previous admissions to this inpatient unit during the past 8 years. Sherry states that she refuses to return to work because her boss accuses her of bothering the other employees instead of doing her own work. She states her boss is falsely accusing her of using alcohol and drugs and does not accept her reasons for being absent from work. This morning she called her outpatient therapist, whom she had not seen in a year and a half but who agreed to see her at 3 PM. When she called the therapist back at

noon and found he was at lunch, she used her scissors to cut her wrists. "I used to think he understood me, but now I know he doesn't care." Her parents are on vacation out of state, and her only close friend is busy going through a divorce. She had taken some of her mother's Valium, but it did not help calm her down. She has averaged only 3 to 4 hours of sleep each night for the past 5 days and has been unable to eat regular meals. Her attempts to clean her parents' house were never completed. She could not even finish watering her mother's plants. A male acquaintance of 2 weeks was no longer calling her, so she was frequenting several bars and inviting men home. She never heard from these men again, even though she thought that their relationships were sexually satisfying.

Sherry completed 2 years of college and is dressed attractively. She enjoys reading romance novels and has brought five of her favorite books with her.

## PSYCHOTHERAPEUTIC MANAGEMENT

*NURSE-PATIENT RELATIONSHIP* Consistency, limit setting, and supportive confrontation are necessary nursing interventions to provide clear expectations regarding patient behaviors. These patients are adept at avoiding rules and consequences as well as at pitting staff members against each other to get what they want.

## Nursing Care Plan

NAME: _____Sherry Morgan_____

WEEKLY UPDATE: ___12/7/90___
ADMISSION DATE: ___11/25/90___

DSM-III-R DIAGNOSIS: _____Axis I Major Depression_____
_____Axis II Borderline Personality Disorder_____

*ASSESSMENT:*
*Areas of strength:* Well-groomed, neat and clean, intelligent, enjoys reading.
*Problems:* Self-mutilating behavior, absence of support systems, loss of job, decreased sleeping and eating, irresponsible and impulsive sexual behavior.

*DIAGNOSES:* Self-mutilation related to absence of support systems. Labile emotions related to rejection and low self-esteem.

**Date met**

*PLANNING:*
*Short-term goals:* Patient will eliminate self-mutilating
behavior and appropriately verbalize feelings of anger and sadness.      _____

*Long-term goals:* Patient will schedule outpatient appointment and meeting with boss regarding job problems.      _____

*IMPLEMENTATION/INTERVENTIONS:*
*Nurse-patient relationship:* Monitor and set limits on acting-out behaviors. Assist patient with identification and verbalization of feelings. Discuss fears about accepting responsibility for self and decision making. Discuss behaviors interfering with job performance.
*Psychopharmacology:* Phenelzine (Nardil) 15 mg t.i.d.
*Milieu management:* Groups focusing on self-esteem, stress and anger management, assertiveness training, social skills, problem-solving skills, discharge planning.

*EVALUATION:* Patient has not engaged in self-mutilating behavior. Patient beginning to verbalize feelings of anger and sadness. Will meet with Mrs Taylor, R.N. C.S., outpatient coordinator 12/10.

Enforcing unit rules and providing clear structure as well as placing the responsibility for appropriate behaviors on the patient will benefit the person with a BPD. The need to develop realistic short-term goals must be part of the expectations of the nurse and the treatment team if they are to increase the patient's responsibility for self. The nurse will educate the patient on appropriate verbal expression of feelings and assertiveness. The nurse's ability to be empathetic and nonjudgmental is threatened by the BPD patient. It may seem easier to offer superficial solutions to immediate problems, explain rules, and inquire about superficial content of patients' statements than to form a therapeutic, working relationship with the BPD patient (Gallop, et al., 1989).

*PSYCHOPHARMACOLOGY* Since the BPD patient's psychotic states are short term and transient, low-dose neuroleptics for 3 to 12 weeks of treatment are usually sufficient to treat these symptoms. Tricyclic antidepressants are effective for a co-existing axis 1 endogenous major depression. Monoamine oxidase inhibitors (MAOIs) are used for affective symptoms and somatic complaints (Frances and Soloff, 1988). Benzodiazepines may aggravate hostile, impulsive, and self-mutilating behaviors (Gunderson, 1988). Fluoxentine (Prozac) has been reported to help with the BPD symptoms of "anxiety, stress, sensitivity to rejection, mood fluctuations, irritability, obsessional behavior and impulsiveness" (Norden, 1989).

*MILIEU MANAGEMENT* Interventions under the nurse-patient relationship with regard to setting firm limits, consistency, and clear structure are basic to the milieu for the BPD patient. The patient's manipulation of other patients must be dealt with, since the BPD patient can mobilize the other patients against the staff around anger and dependency issues and needs. Consistent communication between staff members is essential to minimize the patient's attempts to divide the staff.

## OTHER DRAMATIC/ERRATIC DISORDERS
### Narcissistic personality disorder

The patient with a narcissistic personality disorder displays grandiosity about his importance and achievements. This grandiosity is unlike the delusions of grandeur seen in schizophrenia or bipolar disorders. The grandiosity of the narcissistic personality disorder is somewhat based in reality but is distorted, embellished, or convoluted to meet the patient's needs of overevaluation of self-importance. For example, the patient may say that he was a star football player in high school and can get a job with the Indianapolis Colts tomorrow. He does not tell the nurse that he barely made the second-string football team in high school.

The narcissistic patient overevaluates himself, is arrogant, and seems indifferent to the criticism of others. Those around him are often seen as superior or inferior. For example, the patient views the nurse who is understanding and supportive as competent or superior, whereas the nurse who questions or confronts him is viewed as incompetent or inferior.

The patient may appear nonchalant or indifferent to criticism while hiding feelings of anger, rage, or emptiness. Relationships with others are shallow but

## Box 23-7
## DIAGNOSTIC CRITERIA FOR 301.81 NARCISSISTIC PERSONALITY DISORDER

A pervasive pattern of grandiosity (in fantasy or behavior), lack of empathy, and hypersensitivity to the evaluation of others, beginning by early adulthood and present in a variety of contexts, as indicated by at least *five* of the following:

(1) reacts to criticism with feelings of rage, shame, or humiliation (even if not expressed)

(2) is interpersonally exploitative: takes advantage of others to achieve his or her own ends

(3) has a grandiose sense of self-importance, e.g., exaggerates achievements and talents, expects to be noticed as "special" without appropriate achievement

(4) believes that his or her problems are unique and can be understood only by other special people

(5) is preoccupied with fantasies of unlimited success, power, brilliance, beauty, or ideal love

(6) has a sense of entitlement: unreasonable expectation of especially favorable treatment, e.g., assumes that he or she does not have to wait in line when others must do so

(7) requires constant attention and admiration, e.g., keeps fishing for compliments

(8) lack of empathy: inability to recognize and experience how others feel, e.g., annoyance and surprise when a friend who is seriously ill cancels a date

(9) is preoccupied with feelings of envy

Reprinted with permission from the *Diagnostic and Statistical Manual of Mental Disorders, Third Edition, Revised.* Copyright 1987 American Psychiatric Association.

meaningful if the patient's self-esteem is positively enhanced. The feelings of others are not understood or considered. These persons use others selfishly to meet their own needs but do not reciprocate. See Box 23-7 for DSM-III-R criteria. This type of patient has a sense of entitlement and expects special treatment. For example, a patient may insist that he must have a private room with a telephone and television because he needs to keep up with the reports on the financial news network. Rationalization is used to blame others, make excuses, and provide alibis for self-centered behaviors (Millon, 1986).

Studies of biological and genetic factors in the narcissistic personality disorder have not been done. Some theorists believe that the self-centered person is arrested at an early developmental stage because "parents do not provide adequate empathetic experiences or adequate exposure to disillusioning realities" (Gunderson, 1988). The parents fail to mirror what is appropriate or inappropriate back to the child (Gunderson, 1988). Consequently the child develops without any feedback about his behaviors.

If this patient is hospitalized, the nurse must deal with decreasing the constant recitation of self-importance and grandiosity. She must mirror what the patient sounds like, especially if contradictions exist, and help him focus on identification and verbal expression of feelings. Supportive confrontation is used to point out discrepancies between what the patient says and what actually exists to increase responsibility for self. Limit setting and consistency in approach are used to decrease manipulation and entitlement behaviors. Realistic short-term goals focused on the here and now are important to decrease the patient's use of fantasy and rationalization and to increase responsibility for self. He needs to be taught that no one is perfect and that he, as well as others, makes mistakes and has imperfections.

### Histrionic personality disorder

The patient with the histrionic personality disorder dramatizes all events and draws attention to himself. He is extroverted and thrives on being the center of attention. His behavior is silly, colorful, frivolous, and seductive. Speech is vague, descriptive, superficial, and overembellished but lacking in detail, insight, and depth. The patient seems to be in a hurry and restless. Temper tantrums and outbursts of anger are seen, as well as overreaction to minor events. "Affective display is common, but when pressed to acknowledge certain feelings, like anger, sadness, and sexual wishes, the patient may respond with surprise, indignation, or denial" (Kaplan and Sadock, 1985). This patient may use somatic complaints to avoid responsibility and support his dependency. Dissociation is seen in putting on a false front or altering self-presentation to avoid unpleasant thoughts and emotions (Millon, 1986). Therefore, this patient cannot deal with his own true feelings. See Box 23-8 for DSM-III-R criteria.

The causes of histrionic personality disorder are unknown but are probably multifactorial (Kaplan and Sadock, 1985). There may be a genetic predisposition (Siever et al., 1983). "Studies show that it occurs in families in which an increased prevalence of antisocial or alcoholic problems is found in relatives" (Gunderson, 1988). In the early mother-child relationship the mother negates the child's inner feelings. The child then turns to his father for nurturance, and the father responds to the child's dramatic emotional behaviors (Gunderson, 1988).

Since the patient is unaware of and does not deal with his feelings, the nurse must help clarify what his true feelings are and help him learn how to express them appropriately. Positive reinforcement in the form of attention, recognition, or praise is given for unselfish or others-centered behaviors. Because the patient needs much reassurance and feels helpless, the nurse works to provide support to facilitate independent problem solving and daily functioning. Working with this type of patient can be frustrating for the nurse, since the patient needs time to internalize the meaning of what the nurse is trying to accomplish.

**Box 23-8**
## DIAGNOSTIC CRITERIA FOR 301.50 HISTRIONIC PERSONALITY DISORDER

A pervasive pattern of excessive emotionality and attention-seeking, beginning by early adulthood and present in a variety of contexts, as indicated by at least *four* of the following:

(1) constantly seeks or demands reassurance, approval, or praise

(2) is inappropriately sexually seductive in appearance or behavior

(3) is overly concerned with physical attractiveness

(4) expresses emotion with inappropriate exaggeration, e.g., embraces casual acquaintances with excessive ardor, uncontrollable sobbing on minor sentimental occasions, has temper tantrums

(5) is uncomfortable in situations in which he or she is not the center of attention

(6) displays rapidly shifting and shallow expression of emotions

(7) is self-centered, actions being directed toward obtaining immediate satisfaction; has no tolerance for the frustration of delayed gratification

(8) has a style of speech that is excessively impressionistic and lacking in detail, e.g., when asked to describe mother, can be no more specific than, "She was a beautiful person."

Reprinted with permission from the *Diagnostic and Statistical Manual of Mental Disorders, Third Edition, Revised.* Copyright 1987 American Psychiatric Association.

## ■ Cluster C: Anxious/Fearful
### DEPENDENT PERSONALITY DISORDER

**Characteristics and criteria.** The DSM-III-R describes the main characteristic of the dependent personality disorder to be a "pervasive pattern of dependent and submissive behavior." Dependent persons will want others to make decisions for them, for example, type of clothes to wear and type of job to look for. They accept direction and need reassurance. "A sense of inferiority, self-doubt, suggestibility, and lack of perseverance are additional characteristics" (Gunderson, 1988). Avoiding responsibility and expressing helplessness, the patient maintains his need to rely on others, for example, "I cannot leave my husband. What would I do?" Or the patient may say, "I could not leave my husband. Look at all that I have done for him throughout our marriage. Where would he be without me?" The dependent person also expects that if he performs good deeds, he will be rewarded by someone doing something for him. An intimate relationship with a spouse who is abusive, unfaithful,

### Box 23-9
### DIAGNOSTIC CRITERIA FOR 301.60 DEPENDENT
### PERSONALITY DISORDER

A pervasive pattern of dependent and submissive behavior, beginning by early adulthood and present in a variety of contexts, as indicated by at least *five* of the following:

(1) is unable to make everyday decisions without an excessive amount of advice or reassurance from others

(2) allows others to make most of his or her important decisions, e.g., where to live, what job to take

(3) agrees with people even when he or she believes they are wrong, because of fear of being rejected

(4) has difficulty initiating projects or doing things on his or her own

(5) volunteers to do things that are unpleasant or demeaning in order to get other people to like him or her

(6) feels uncomfortable or helpless when alone, or goes to great lengths to avoid being alone

(7) feels devastated or helpless when close relationships end

(8) is frequently preoccupied with fears of being abandoned

(9) is easily hurt by criticism or disapproval

Reprinted with permission from the *Diagnostic and Statistical Manual of Mental Disorders, Third Edition, Revised.* Copyright 1987 American Psychiatric Association.

or alcoholic is maintained so as not to disturb his sense of attachment to that individual. Passivity and concealing of sexual feelings and anger are a means of avoiding conflict. Box 23-9 lists the DSM-III-R criteria.

Biochemical and genetic factors have not been correlated with dependent personality disorders. Certain cultures dictate that females should maintain a dependent role. "Overintrusive and oversolicitous early parenting combined with criticism or rejection of the child's signs of assertiveness and independence" is another factor to be considered in persons with this disorder (Kaplan and Sadock, 1985).

### PSYCHOTHERAPEUTIC MANAGEMENT

***NURSE-PATIENT RELATIONSHIP*** The nurse works on decision making with the patient to increase responsibility for self in day-to-day living. The patient needs assistance with managing his anxiety since it will increase as he assumes more responsibility for himself. Assertiveness is an important area of the nurse's teaching so that the patient can clearly state his own feelings, needs, and desires. Verbalization of feelings and how to cope with them is essential.

## OTHER ANXIOUS/FEARFUL DISORDERS
### Passive-aggressive personality disorder

According to the DSM-III-R, this disorder is marked by passive resistance to demands for adequate social and occupational performance, "even when more self-assertive and effective behavior is possible" (APA, 1987). People with this disorder express their passivity through procrastination, dawdling, and inefficiency. For example, after criticizing her secretary for several typing errors, a woman asks the secretary to type two short letters within the next hour. Instead of typing the letters, the secretary spends the hour filing last month's interdepartmental memos. Such a person enjoys the boss's resulting frustration as well as being critical of the boss's minor flaws. The secretary's excuses for not completing tasks and claims of unjust treatment often cause others to do things for her (Kaplan and Sadock, 1985). Box 23-10 lists the DSM-III-R criteria.

**Box 23-10**
### DIAGNOSTIC CRITERIA FOR 301.84 PASSIVE AGGRESSIVE PERSONALITY DISORDER

A pervasive pattern of passive resistance to demands for adequate social and oc-cupational performance, beginning by early adulthood and present in a variety of contexts, as indicated by at least *five* of the following:

(1) procrastinates, i.e., puts off things that need to be done so that deadlines are not met
(2) becomes sulky, irritable, or argumentative when asked to do something he or she does not want to do
(3) seems to work deliberately slowly or to do a bad job on tasks that he or she really does not want to do
(4) protests, without justification, that others make unreasonable demands on him or her
(5) avoids obligations by claiming to have "forgotten"
(6) believes that he or she is doing a much better job than others think he or she is doing
(7) resents useful suggestions from others concerning how he or she could be more productive
(8) obstructs the efforts of others by failing to do his or her share of the work
(9) unreasonably criticizes or scorns people in positions of authority

Reprinted with permission from the *Diagnostic and Statistical Manual of Mental Disorders, Third Edition, Revised.* Copyright 1987 American Psychiatric Association.

Disturbed parent-child interactions thus far are seen as the cause for this disorder. Parental control and inflexibility frustrate the child. In turn, the child uses covert resistance and defiance as a means of expression (Gunderson, 1988). Punishment of normal assertive behaviors by the parents leads to passive inefficiency in the child. Anger is turned against self to protect important relationships (Kaplan and Sadock, 1985).

The nurse teaches assertiveness so that the patient can actively, outwardly, and directly express himself. The patient is accepted, even though passive behaviors are supportively confronted. The nurse encourages autonomy and independent behaviors after clearly stating what behaviors and responsibilities are expected on the unit. When the patient manifests excessive anxiety, relaxation techniques are taught before the patient attempts assertive behavior (McCann, 1988). The nurse teaches the patient about the effects of anger turned inward.

## Avoidant personality disorder

Patients with the avoidant personality disorder are timid, socially uncomfortable, withdrawn, and hypersensitive to criticism. Although they are fearful and shy, they desire relationships and challenges. To keep their anxiety at a minimum level, they avoid risky situations associated with disappointment, rejection, or failure (Gunderson, 1988). When interacting with someone, this patient sounds uncertain and lacks self-confidence. He is afraid to ask questions or speak up in public. He withdraws from others and feels hurt if requests are denied (Kaplan and Sadock, 1985). Vocationally, this patient has rarely received promotions or personal advancement. See the DSM-III-R criteria for this disorder in Box 23-11. "A temperamental predisposition to avoid or to perform inflexibly in new situations may precede the development of this personality type" (Gunderson, 1988). Futher biological or genetic studies have not been conducted.

The nurse helps the patient gradually confront what he fears. Discussing the patient's feelings and fears before and after he does something he is afraid to do is an essential part of the relationship. She supports and directs the patient in the accomplishment of small goals. Helping the patient to be assertive and to develop social skills is necessary. The nurse includes the patient in interactions with others and then progresses to small groups as the patient is able to tolerate them. Because of the patient's anxiety, relaxation techniques are taught to enable him to be successful in interactions. The nurse will give positive feedback to the patient for any real success or attempt to engage in interactions with others to promote self-esteem.

## Obsessive-compulsive personality disorder

The DSM-III-R describes the person with obsessive-compulsive personality disorder as being perfectionistic and inflexible. These patients are overly strict and often set standards for themselves that are too high, so that their work is never good enough. They are preoccupied with rules, trivial details, and procedures. They find it difficult to express warmth or tender emotions. They are afraid of situations that threaten

**Box 23-11**
## DIAGNOSTIC CRITERIA FOR 301.82 AVOIDANT PERSONALITY DISORDER

A pervasive pattern of social discomfort, fear of negative evaluation, and timidity, beginning by early adulthood and present in a variety of contexts, as indicated by at least *four* of the following:

(1)  is easily hurt by criticism or disapproval

(2)  has no close friends or confidants (or only one) other than first-degree relatives

(3)  is unwilling to get involved with people unless certain of being liked

(4)  avoids social or occupational activities that involve significant interpersonal contact, e.g., refuses a promotion that will increase social demands

(5)  is reticent in social situations because of a fear of saying something inappropriate or foolish, or of being unable to answer a question

(6)  fears being embarrassed by blushing, crying, or showing signs of anxiety in front of other people

(7)  exaggerates the potential difficulties, physical dangers, or risks involved in doing something ordinary but outside his or her usual routine, e.g., may cancel social plans because she anticipates being exhausted by the effort of getting there

Reprinted with permission from the *Diagnostic and Statistical Manual of Mental Disorders, Third Edition, Revised.* Copyright 1987 American Psychiatric Association.

their need to be in control (Gunderson, 1988). There is little give and take in their interactions with others, and they are rigid, controlling, and cold. The patient is serious about all of his activities, and it is difficult for him to have fun or to experience pleasure. Because he is afraid of making mistakes, he can be indecisive or will put off decisions until he has accumulated all the facts. His affect is constricted, and he may speak in a monotone. Defense mechanisms used are reaction formation, intellectualization, and displacement (Kaplan and Sadock, 1985). (See Box 23-12 for DSM-III-R criteria.)

Early parent-child relationships around issues of autonomy, control, and authority may predispose a person to this disorder. Some recent studies state that a genetic temperamental predisposition in the form of hypersensitivity to change is possible (Gunderson, 1988). This disorder is more frequently found in men (APA, 1987).

### Box 23-12
## DIAGNOSTIC CRITERIA FOR 301.40 OBSESSIVE COMPULSIVE PERSONALITY DISORDER

A pervasive pattern of perfectionism and inflexibility, beginning by early adulthood and present in a variety of contexts, as indicated by at least *five* of the following:

(1) perfectionism that interferes with task completion, e.g., inability to complete a project because own overly strict standards are not met

(2) preoccupation with details, rules, lists, order, organization, or schedules to the extent that the major point of the activity is lost

(3) unreasonable insistence that others submit to exactly his or her way of doing things, **or** unreasonable reluctance to allow others to do things because of the conviction that they will not do them correctly

(4) excessive devotion to work and productivity to the exclusion of leisure activities and friendships (not accounted for by obvious economic necessity)

(5) indecisiveness: decision making is either avoided, postponed, or protracted, e.g., the person cannot get assignments done on time because of ruminating about priorities (do not include if indecisiveness is due to excessive need for advice or reassurance from others)

(6) overconscientiousness, scrupulousness, and inflexibility about matters of morality, ethics, or values (not accounted for by cultural or religious identification)

(7) restricted expression of affection

(8) lack of generosity in giving time, money, or gifts when no personal gain is likely to result

(9) inability to discard worn-out or worthless objects even when they have no sentimental value

Reprinted with permission from the *Diagnostic and Statistical Manual of Mental Disorders, Third Edition, Revised.* Copyright 1987 American Psychiatric Association.

The nurse needs to support the patient in exploring his feelings and in attempting new experiences and situations. She helps him with decision making and encourages follow-through behavior. At times, there is a need to confront his procrastination and intellectualization. She teaches him the importance of leisure activities and explores his interests in this area. Because he lacks awareness of how he affects others, he needs to look at and understand how others view him. Teaching him that he is human and that it is all right for him to make mistakes helps decrease his irrational beliefs about the necessity to be perfect.

# ■ Sexual Disorders

Every human is a sexual being. Therefore nurses, those professionals who often develop the most intimate relationship with a patient, need to have a basic understanding of sexuality to meet the needs of patients struggling with sexual issues. To be most therapeutic, the nurse must be aware of her own values concerning sexual behavior, must be comfortable in discussing sexuality with patients, and must recognize that not everyone will share her views of appropriate sexual expression. The nurse should not abandon her therapeutic communication skills when she is talking to a person who engages in sexual practices she cannot define as "normal."

Human beings have a wide range of sexual responses that are viewed as *acceptable*. The term "normal" is not often used anymore because what is "normal" to one person is not "normal" to another. Many professionals can agree, however, that sexual behavior is acceptable when it occurs privately between consenting individuals. The point worth emphasizing is that a nurse can intellectually agree that a certain sexual activity is acceptable but emotionally consider it not "normal." *Unacceptable* sexual activities include those in which another person is not the focus of the activity, those in which one of the participants is not consenting or in which one of the consenting individuals is a child, or those in which persons who do not wish to observe the activity are forced to do so.

## DSM-III-R CRITERIA AND TERMINOLOGY

The DSM-III-R (APA, 1987) divides sexual disorders into two groups, the paraphilias and sexual dysfunctions. Paraphilias are characterized by intense sexual urges focused on (1) nonhuman objects, (2) the suffering or humiliation of oneself or one's partner, or (3) children or other nonconsenting persons. Eight paraphilias are described in the DSM-III-R (Box 23-13). Sexual dysfunctions are characterized by inhibition of sexual appetite or psychophysiologic changes that compromise the sexual response cycle (Box 23-14).

### Paraphilias

**Exhibitionism.** The primary characteristic of exhibitionism is sexual pleasure derived from exposing one's genitals to an unsuspecting stranger. The stereotype offender is a young man in a raincoat who flashes a woman while walking down the street. No other sexual activity is attempted. The exhibitionist is stimulated shocking his victim. Exhibitionism only occurs in males.

**Fetishism.** The primary characteristic of fetishism is the sexual pleasure derived from nonliving objects. Common fetish objects are bras, underpants, stockings, and shoes. Less common fetish objects include urine-soaked and feces-smeared items. The person with fetishism often masturbates while holding or rubbing these items.

**Frotteurism.** The primary characteristic of frotteurism is the sexual pleasure derived from touching or rubbing one's genitals against a nonconsenting person's thighs or buttocks. The person with frotteurism may also attempt to fondle the person's breasts or genitals. Frotteurism usually occurs in a crowded place where escape into the crowd is possible.

**Box 23-13**
# DIAGNOSTIC CRITERIA FOR PARAPHILIAS

### 302.40 Exhibitionism

A. Over a period of at least six months, recurrent intense sexual urges and sexually arousing fantasies involving the exposure of one's genitals to an unsuspecting stranger.

B. The person has acted on these urges, or is markedly distressed by them.

### 302.81 Fetishism

A. Over a period of at least six months, recurrent intense sexual urges and sexually arousing fantasies involving the use of nonliving objects by themselves (e.g., female undergarments).
   **Note:** The person may at other times use the nonliving object with a sexual partner.

B. The person has acted on these urges, or is markedly distressed by them.

C. The fetishes are not only articles of female clothing used in cross-dressing (Transvestic Fetishism) or devices designed for the purpose of tactile genital stimulation (e.g., vibrator).

### 302.89 Frotteurism

A. Over a period of at least six months, recurrent intense sexual urges and sexually arousing fantasies involving touching and rubbing against a nonconsenting person. It is the touching, not the coercive nature of the act, that is sexually exciting.

B. The person has acted on these urges, or is markedly distressed by them.

### 302.20 Pedophilia

A. Over a period of at least six months, recurrent intense sexual urges and sexually arousing fantasies involving sexual activity with a prepubescent child or children (generally age 13 or younger).

B. The person has acted on these urges, or is markedly distressed by them.

C. The person is at least 16 years old and at least 5 years older than the child or children in A.
   **Note:** Do not include a late adolescent involved in an ongoing sexual relationship with a 12- or 13-year-old.

**Specify: same sex, opposite sex, or same and opposite sex.**
**Specify if limited to incest.**
**Specify: exclusive type** (attracted only to children), or **nonexclusive type.**

**Box 23-13**
## DIAGNOSTIC CRITERIA FOR PARAPHILIAS—cont'd

### 302.83 Sexual Masochism

A. Over a period of at least six months, recurrent intense sexual urges and sexually arousing fantasies involving the act (real, not simulated) of being humiliated, beaten, bound, or otherwise made to suffer.
B. The person has acted on these urges, or is markedly distressed by them.

### 302.84 Sexual Sadism

A. Over a period of at least six months, recurrent intense sexual urges and sexually arousing fantasies involving acts (real, not simulated) in which the psychological or physical suffering (including humiliation) of the victim is sexually exciting to the person.
B. The person has acted on these urges, or is markedly distressed by them.

### 302.30 Transvestic Fetishism

A. Over a period of at least six months, in a heterosexual male, recurrent intense sexual urges and sexually arousing fantasies involving cross-dressing.
B. The person has acted on these urges, or is markedly distressed by them.
C. Does not meet the criteria for Gender Identity Disorder of Adolescence or Adulthood, Nontranssexual Type, or Transsexualism.

### 302.82 Voyeurism

A. Over a period of at least six months, recurrent intense sexual urges and sexually arousing fantasies involving the act of observing an unsuspecting person who is naked, in the process of disrobing, or engaging in sexual activity.
B. The person has acted on these urges, or is markedly distressed by them.

**Pedophilia.** The primary characteristic of pedophilia is the sexual pleasure derived from sexual activity with children. By definition the child must be younger than 13 years and the person with pedophilia 16 years old or older and at least 5 years older than the victim. The person found guilty of pedophilia often justifies his activity because of its "educational" nature or because he is providing warmth and love a parent refuses to give. Pedophilic behavior can be expressed for opposite sex children or for same sex children. This behavior is a particularly hideous breach of societal norms, yet even this behavior is defended by some in our society. *Time* magazine (1/17/83) reported the activity of the North American Man-Boy Love Society (NAMBLS), which argues for the right to have sex with children. They argue that adult society has no right to limit a child's selection of a sexual partner.

## Box 23-14
# DIAGNOSTIC CRITERIA FOR SEXUAL DYSFUNCTIONS

### 302.71 Hypoactive Sexual Desire Disorder

A. Persistantly or recurrently deficient or absent sexual fantasies and desire for sexual activity. The judgment of deficiency or absence is made by the clinician, taking into account factors that affect sexual functioning, such as age, sex, and the context of the person's life.
B. Occurrence not exclusively during the course of another Axis I disorder (other than a Sexual Dysfunction), such as Major Depression.

### 302.79 Sexual Aversion Disorder

A. Persistent or recurrent extreme aversion to, and avoidance of, all or almost all, genital sexual contact with a sexual partner.
B. Occurrence not exclusively during the course of another Axis I disorder (other than a Sexual Dysfunction), such as Obsessive Compulsive Disorder or Major Depression.

### 302.72 Female Sexual Arousal Disorder

A. Either (1) or (2):
   (1) persistent or recurrent partial or complete failure to attain or maintain the lubrication-swelling response of sexual excitement until completion of the sexual activity
   (2) persistent or recurrent lack of a subjective sense of sexual excitement and pleasure in a female during sexual activity
B. Occurrence not exclusively during the course of another Axis I disorder (other than a Sexual Dysfunction), such as Major Depression.

### 302.72 Male Erectile Disorder

A. Either (1) or (2):
   (1) persistent or recurrent partial or complete failure in a male to attain or maintain erection until completion of the sexual activity
   (2) persistent or recurrent lack of a subjective sense of sexual excitement and pleasure in a male during sexual activity
B. Occurrence not exclusively during the course of another Axis I disorder (other than a Sexual Dysfunction), such as Major Depression.

Reprinted with permission from the *Diagnostic and Statisical Manual of Mental Disorders, Third Edition, Revised.* Copyright 1987 American Psychiatric Association.

**Box 23-14**
DIAGNOSTIC CRITERIA FOR SEXUAL DYSFUNCTIONS—cont'd

### 302.73 Inhibited Female Orgasm

A. Persistent or recurrent delay in, or absence of, orgasm in a female following a normal sexual excitement phase during sexual activity that the clinician judges to be adequate in focus, intensity, and duration. Some females are able to experience orgasm during noncoital clitoral stimulation, but are unable to experience it during coitus in the absence of manual clitoral stimulation. In most of these females, this represents a normal variation of the female sexual response and does not justify the diagnosis of Inhibited Female Orgasm. However, in some of these females, this does represent a psychological inhibition that justifies the diagnosis. This difficult judgment is assisted by a thorough sexual evaluation, which may even require a trial of treatment.

B. Occurrence not exclusively during the course of another Axis I disorder (other than a Sexual Dysfunction), such as Major Depression.

### 302.74 Inhibited Male Orgasm

A. Persistent or recurrent delay in, or absence of, orgasm in a male following a normal sexual excitement phase during sexual activity that the clinician, taking into account the person's age, judges to be adequate in focus, intensity, and duration. This failure to achieve orgasm is usually restricted to an inability to reach orgasm in the vagina, with orgasm possible with other types of stimulation, such as masturbation.

B. Occurrence not exclusively during the course of another Axis I disorder (other than a Sexual Dysfunction), such as Major Depression.

### 302.75 Premature Ejaculation

Persistent or recurrent ejaculation with minimal sexual stimulation or before, upon, or shortly after penetration and before the person wishes it. The clinician must take into account factors that affect duration of the excitement phase, such as age, novelty of the sexual partner or situation, and frequency of sexual activity.

### 302.76 Dyspareunia

A. Recurrent or persistent genital pain in either a male or a female before, during, or after sexual intercourse.

B. The disturbance is not caused exclusively by lack of lubrication or by Vaginismus.

### 306.51 Vaginismus

A. Recurrent or persistent involuntary spasm of the musculature of the outer third of the vagina that interferes with coitus.

B. The disturbance is not caused exclusively by a physical disorder, and is not due to another Axis I disorder.

**Sexual masochism.** The primary characteristic of sexual masochism is the sexual pleasure derived from being humiliated, beaten, or otherwise made to suffer. Bondage, a masochistic variation, is a theme of some pornographic movies and some heavy metal music. Some sexually masochistic persons enjoy being urinated or defecated on and may pay prostitutes to do so. Hypoxyphilia is the act of enhancing sexual arousal by strangulation or other oxygen-depleting activities. Apparently sexual response is heightened by these activities. Unfortunately, a few people have died in their search for the ultimate orgasm.

**Sexual sadism.** The primary characteristic of sexual sadism is the sexual pleasure derived from inflicting psychological or physical suffering on another. Partners can be consenting or nonconsenting. Sadistic behaviors including spanking, whipping, pinching, beating, burning, and restraining. Some sadistic persons derive great pleasure from torturing or even killing their victims. The so-called snuff films, found in the underground of the pornography world, apparently show the actual rape, torture, and murder of women and children for the convenient viewing of sadistic persons in our society.

**Transvestic fetishism.** The primary characteristic of transvestic fetishism is the sexual pleasure derived from cross-dressing. The person with transvestic fetishism may wear only the underwear of a woman or may completely dress as a woman. This apparently occurs only in males.

**Voyeurism.** The primary characteristic of voyeurism is the sexual pleasure derived from observing unsuspecting persons who are naked or undressing or who are engaged in sexual activity. The voyeuristic person is commonly referred to as a "peeping Tom." Voyeurism is differentiated from compulsive pornography viewing because the subjects in a pornographic movie expect to be watched.

## Sexual dysfunctions

The phases of human sexual activity have been called the sexual response cycle. There are four phases: the desire phase, the excitement phase, the orgasm phase, and the resolution phase. Sexual dysfunctions are grouped into disorders that compromise sexual activity at one of these phases. Sexual desire disorders effectively stop the sexual response cycle from getting started. Sexual arousal disorders sidetrack the sexual response cycle at the excitement phase. Orgasm disorders arrest the progression of the cycle in the orgasm phase. Finally, sexual pain disorders can abort the sexual response cycle at any phase.

**Sexual desire disorders.** People with these disorders have little or no sexual desire or have an aversion to sexual contact.

**Sexual arousal disorders.** People with these disorders cannot maintain the physiological requirements for sexual intercourse. Women cannot maintain the lubrication-swelling response of sexual excitement, and men cannot maintain an erection.

**Orgasm disorders.** People with these disorders cannot complete the sexual response cycle because of inability to achieve orgasm. Another orgasm disorder is premature ejaculation, which is found in about 30% of American men. In premature ejaculation a man reaches orgasm with minimal sexual stimulation, frustrating both himself and his partner.

**Sexual pain disorders.** People with these disorders suffer genital pain (dyspareunia) before, during, or after sexual intercourse. Vaginismus, involuntary spasm of the outer third of the vagina, interferes with sexual intercourse.

## KEY CONCEPTS

1. Personality traits are enduring approaches to the world expressed in how the person thinks, how he feels, and what he does. Traditionally they have been viewed as unconscious processes.
2. When traits become rigid, dysfunctional, and cause distress in self and others, they may be diagnosed as a personality disorder. Personal discomfort arises primarily from others' reactions or behaviors toward him.
3. The odd/eccentric cluster of personality disorders includes the
   a. Paranoid, characterized by suspiciousness and mistrust
   b. Schizoid, characterized by hermitlike life-style, aloneness
   c. Schizotypal, characterized by symptoms similar to but less severe than those of schizophrenia.
4. The dramatic/erratic cluster includes the
   a. Antisocial, characterized by disregard of others' rights without guilt
   b. Borderline, characterized by problems with self-identity, interpersonal relationships, mood shifts and self-destructiveness
   c. Narcissistic, characterized by overevaluation of self, arrogance, and indifference to the criticism of others
   d. Histrionic, characterized by dramatic behaviors, attention seeking, and superficiality.
5. The anxious/fearful cluster includes the
   a. Dependent, characterized by submissiveness, helplessness, fear of responsibility, and reliance on others for decision making
   b. Passive-aggressive, characterized by resistance, procrastination, and criticism of authority figures.
   c. Avoidant, characterized by timidity, social withdrawal behavior and hypersensitivity to criticism
   d. Obsessive-compulsive, characterized by indecisiveness, perfectionism, inflexibility and difficulty expressing feelings.
6. Nursing interventions for persons with personality disorders focus on specific behaviors distressing to self or others or both and awareness of dysfunctional and self-defeating patterns.

### REFERENCES

American Psychiatric Association: Diagnostic and statistical manual of mental disorders, ed 3 revised, Washington, DC, 1987, The Association.

Favazza A: Why patients mutilate themselves, Hosp Community Psychiatry 40:137, 1989.

Frances A and Soloff P: Treating the borderline patient with low-dose neuroleptics, Hosp Community Psychiatry 39:246, 1988.

Frosch J: The treatment of antisocial and borderline personality disorders, Hosp Community Psychiatry 34:243, 1983.

Gallop R, Lancee W, and Garfinkel P: How nursing staff respond to the label "borderline personality disorder," Hosp Community Psychiatry 40:815, 1989.

Gunderson JG: Personality disorders. In Nicholi A, editor: The new Harvard guide to psychiatry, Cambridge, Mass, 1988, pp 337-357.

Kaplan H and Sadock B: Modern synopsis of comprehensive textbook of psychiatry, ed 4, Baltimore, Williams & Wilkins, 1985, pp 361-383.

Lynch V and Lynch M: Borderline personality, Perspect Psychiatr Care 15:72, 1977.

Mahler MS, Pine F, and Bergman A: The psychological birth of the human infant: symbiosis and individuation, New York, 1975, Basic Books.

Mark B: Hospital treatment of borderline patients: toward a better understanding of problematic issues, J Psychosoc Nurs Ment Health Serv 17:25, 1980.

McCann J: Passive-aggressive personality disorder: a review, J Pers Disorders 2(2):170, 1988.

Melges T and Swartz M: Oscillations of attachment in borderline personality disorder, Am J Psychiatry 146:1115, 1989.

Millon T: Personality prototypes and their diagnostic criteria. Contemporary directions in psychopathology toward the DSM-IV, New York, 1986, pp 698-710.

Norden M: Is there an effective drug treatment for borderline personality disorder? Harvard Med School Ment Health Letter 6:8, 1989.

Siever L, Insel T, and Uhde T: Biogenetic factors in personalities. In Frosch J, editor: Current perspectives in personality disorders, Washington, DC, American Psychiatric Press, 1983, pp 43-59.

Trull T, Widiger T, and Frances A: Covariation of criteria sets for avoidant, schizoid, and dependent personality disorders, Am J Psychiatry

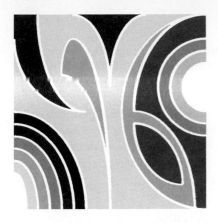

## CHAPTER 24

# Chemical Dependency

MARYLOU SCAVNICKY-MYLANT AND NORMAN L. KELTNER

LEARNING OBJECTIVES
After reading this chapter you should be able to

- Understand the significance of drug abuse in the United States.
- Describe the differences among classes of drugs of abuse.
- Discuss the side effects of drugs of abuse.
- Identify the toxic levels of the drugs of abuse.
- Describe the potential interactions of the drugs of abuse.
- Discuss the implications for patient teaching about the drugs of abuse.
- Identify the recognized medical uses vs. the abuses of drugs.
- Describe the nursing process as it relates to chemical dependency.
- Identify the four levels of recovery for the chemically dependent person.
- Discuss the contributions of other interventions such as Alcoholics Anonymous.

It is estimated that one third to one half of all patients undergoing psychiatric treatment abuse alcohol or drugs (Carey, 1989; Ananth et al., 1989). In addition, the use and abuse of alcohol and drugs among the general population may be the most significant social issue of our time. Statistics are staggering. Newspapers and news magazines carry accounts of national and international problems related to chemicals of abuse in almost every issue. Because of the enormity of the problem, nurses must have a basic understanding of these substances in three major areas to appreciate their addictive qualities and to intervene effectively:

1. The nurse must understand the DSM-III-R criteria used to define chemical dependency.
2. The nurse must understand the nature of the chemicals of abuse.
3. The nurse must understand the nursing process as it relates to chemically dependent persons.

Drugs of abuse fall into four classes: alcohol and other CNS depressants, opioids, stimulants, and hallucinogens (Box 24-1).

## DSM-III-R CRITERIA

The DSM-III-R differentiates between substance abuse and substance dependence (Box 24-2). Dependence is more severe and indicates physiological dependence. Regardless of the substance, behavior patterns that meet these criteria indicate a problem.

Smith et al. (1986) define addiction as a pathological process involving a compulsion to use a psychoactive drug, loss of control over use of the drug, and continued use of the drug despite adverse consequences. The term *dependency* has replaced the term *addiction* for describing compulsive drug use because it more precisely defines the condition. Heroin addiction and alcoholism are correctly referred to as drug dependencies. In 1987 the American Medical Association declared all drug dependencies to be diseases. When chemical dependencies are viewed as diseases, their treatment and understanding are facilitated. Such a view also reduces the guilt and blame traditionally associated with chemical dependency.

Although not all psychiatrists and psychiatric nurses embrace the disease concept of drug dependencies, there are convincing arguments for accepting the disease hypothesis. Using alcoholism as an example, Ohlms (1988) points out that it (1) causes the person to function abnormally, (2) has a characteristic chain of symptoms reflecting specific stages of the disease that are both reliable and predictable, and (3) has the inevitable outcome of death if drinking continues. These three criteria are in concert with a disease model.

Some professionals use a *working definition of chemical dependency* that is less rigid than the criteria outlined in the DSM-III-R. For those professionals, chemicals are a problem for the person when they interfere with and disrupt family, work, or social relationships. If those areas of a person's life are being adversely affected by substance abuse, then the person has a problem and needs treatment.

## Box 24-1
## CATEGORIES OF DRUGS OF ABUSE

**ALCOHOL AND OTHER CNS DEPRESSANTS**

Alcohol (ethanol)
Sedatives-hypnotics, e.g., barbiturates
Minor tranquilizers, e.g., benzodiazepines (diazepam [Valium])
Antipsychotic drugs
Volatile substances (inhalants)

**OPIOIDS**

Morphine
Codeine
Heroin (H, horse, smack, junk)
Methadone

**STIMULANTS**

Cocaine (coke, blow, snow, C, powder, crack, rock)
Amphetamines (bennies, dexies, uppers, black beauties, pep pills, crank, speed)

**HALLUCINOGENS**

LSD (acid)
MDA, STP, DMT, mescaline, psilocybin
Marijuana (pot, grass, hashish, joint, reefer, weed), tetrahydrocannabinols
PCP (angel dust, crystal, super joint, peace pill)

# ■ Alcohol

Alcohol abuse is the No. 1 drug problem in North America and is addressed separately because of the enormity of the problem. The cost to the United States in health problems, lost man hours, family disruption and disintegration, and criminal activity is currently estimated at more than $40 billion annually. An estimated 12.1 million Americans have one or more symptoms of alcoholism (Noble, 1985), and after cardiovascular disease and cancer, alcoholism ranks third among the causes of death and disability in the United States (Whitfield et al., 1986). Alcoholics have a two to four times higher death rate than nonalcoholics have. Approximately 98,000 deaths each year are directly related to alcohol. Cirrhosis and other medical problems, motor accidents, homicides and suicides, and nonvehicular accidents are leading

**Box 24-2**
## DSM-III-R DIAGNOSTIC CRITERIA

### PSYCHOACTIVE SUBSTANCE DEPENDENCE

A. At least three of the following:
  (1) substance often taken in larger amounts or over longer period than the person intended
  (2) persistent desire or one or more unsuccessful efforts to cut down or control substance use
  (3) a great deal of time spent in activities necessary to get the substance (e.g., theft), taking the substance (e.g., chain smoking), or recovering from its effects
  (4) frequent intoxication or withdrawal symptoms when expected to fulfill major role obligations at work, school, or home (e.g., does not go to work because hung over, goes to school or work "high," intoxicated while taking care of his or her children), or when substance use is physically hazardous (e.g., drives when intoxicated)
  (5) important social, occupational, or recreational activities given up or reduced because of substance use
  (6) continued substance use despite knowledge of having a persistent or recurrent social, psychological, or physical problem that is caused or exacerbated by the use of the substance (e.g., keeps using heroin despite family arguments about it, cocaine-induced depression, or having an ulcer made worse by drinking)
  (7) marked tolerance: need for markedly increased amounts of the substance (i.e., at least a 50% increase) in order to achieve intoxication or desired effect, or markedly diminished effect with continued use of the same amount
  **Note:** The following items may not apply to cannabis, hallucinogens, or phencyclidine (PCP):
  (8) characteristic withdrawal symptoms (see specific withdrawal syndromes under Psychoactive Substance-induced Organic Mental Disorders)
  (9) substance often taken to relieve or avoid withdrawal symptoms
B. Some symptoms of the disturbance have persisted for at least one month, or have occurred repeatedly over a longer period of time.

### PSYCHOACTIVE SUBSTANCE ABUSE

A. A maladaptive pattern of psychoactive substance use indicated by at least one of the following:
  (1) continued use despite knowledge of having a persistent or recurrent social, occupational, psychological, or physical problem that is caused or exacerbated by use of the psychoactive substance
  (2) recurrent use in situations in which use is physically hazardous (e.g., driving while intoxicated)
B. Some symptoms of the disturbance have persisted for at least one month, or have occurred repeatedly over a longer period of time.
C. Never met the criteria for Psychoactive Substance Dependence for this substance.

Reprinted with permission from the *Diagnostic and Statistical Manual of Mental Disorders, Third Edition, Revised.* Copyright 1987 American Psychiatric Association.

causes of death associated with alcohol. Low to moderate drinking produces a pleasant, uninhibited feeling. Higher amounts result in significant impairment. The legal blood alcohol level for drunkenness is 0.1% in most states. Five states have lowered the legal blood alcohol level to 0.08% in the hope of reducing highway deaths caused by drunken drivers.

The effects of alcoholism are commonly found among medical and psychiatric patients. It is estimated that among general hospital inpatients 15% to 42% of the men and 4% to 35% of the women are alcoholics (Lewis and Gordon, 1983). Regans (1985) reported that one third of American adults (56 million people) have been adversely affected by alcohol.

## Etiological theories

**Psychodynamic theories.** A number of psychological theories have attempted to explain how people become alcoholics. Traditionally, alcoholics have been viewed as psychologically weak-willed, irresponsible, selfish, self-destructive, and morally bankrupt individuals who easily succumbed to the escape provided by alcohol. Psychoanalytic theory describes alcoholics as having strong oral tendencies related to unresolved issues from the oral stage of development. Drinking alcohol is thought to be an unconscious attempt to satisfy these oral needs. More recent theories have described alcoholics as premorbidly (before they became addicted to alcohol) more phobic, inferior-feeling, dependent, and feminine than nondrinkers. Over time the search for an "alcoholic personality" has given way to a multivariate model that incorporates the biopsychosocial components of the disease (Hough, 1989). Current researchers believe that many of the stereotypical characteristics found among alcoholics such as dependency, low self-esteem, passivity, and introversion are the result of and not the cause of alcoholism.

**Biological theories.** Heredity as an etiological factor has been studied for many years and continues to provide insight into understanding the genesis of alcoholism. Genetic predisposition is considered to be the single most significant piece of information in identifying alcoholism (Ohlms, 1988). Children of alcoholic parents, even if raised in an alcohol-free environment, are more likely to become alcoholics than are the children of nonalcoholic parents (Goodwin et al., 1973). Mueller and Ketcham (1987) found that even when the child of the alcoholic does not drink, an inherited susceptibility to alcoholism is passed on to his children. Hereditary explanations provide a good basis for understanding the vulnerability to alcohol apparent in alcoholics.

## Metabolism

The chemical name for alcohol is ethanol ($CH_3CH_2OH$). It is primarily metabolized in the liver. The oxidation process can be described chemically as follows:

$$CH_3CH_2OH \rightarrow CH_3CHO + H_2 \rightarrow CH_3\text{---}C\text{---}OH\text{---}O \rightarrow CO_2\text{---}H_2O$$

| (ethanol) | (acetaldehyde) | (acetic acid) | (carbon dioxide) | (water) |

At each step of the metabolizing process an enzyme breaks down the chemical. Ethanol is broken down by alcohol dehydrogenase to acetaldehyde and hydrogen. The hydrogen molecule causes the liver to bypass normal energy sources (the hydrogen from fat) and to use the hydrogen from ethanol. Fat accumulates and leads to fatty liver, hyperlipemia, hepatitis, and cirrhosis. Acetaldehyde is toxic to the body. It compromises normal cell function in the liver. If the metabolism of acetaldehyde is impaired, it accumulates in the liver, causing cell death and necrosis. Liver cell loss contributes to cirrhosis. Acetaldehyde interferes with vitamin activation. Aldehyde dehydrogenase breaks down acetaldehyde to acetic acid, which is an innocuous substance. When enzymatic action on acetaldehyde is blocked by the *aldehyde dehydrogenase blocker* disulfiram (Antabuse), acetaldehyde accumulates, causing severe sickness. Recent research confirms an age-old suspicion that women become intoxicated more easily than men, even when studies are controlled for size differences. Frezza et al. (1990) have discovered that the gastrointestinal tissue of women and of alcoholic men contains little alcohol dehydrogenase. The alcohol dehydrogenase in the gastrointestinal tissue of nonalcoholic men oxidizes a significant amount of ethanol in the gut before it enters the bloodstream. The inability of women's bodies to make this "first-pass metabolism" accounts for their enhanced vulnerability to alcohol.

Some researchers believe that some of the excess acetaldehyde travels to the brain and reacts chemically with neurotransmitters to make tetrahydroisoquinolines (TIQs) and β-carbolines (Box 24-3). TIQs are similar to the addictive substance found in heroin and morphine (Mueller and Ketcham, 1987). When TIQs are infused into the brains of monkeys, the monkeys develop an irreversible preference for alcohol over water. β-carbolines have been shown to cause severe anxiety, and it is hypothesized that alcoholics use alcohol in an attempt to reduce the anxiety caused by previous drinks of alcohol (Wallace, 1985).

## Absorption

Alcohol is absorbed partially from the stomach but mostly from the small intestine. Within 20 minutes it is in the bloodstream if it is ingested by a person with an empty stomach. The rate of absorption is affected by the form of alcohol consumed. Alcohol in beer and wine is absorbed more slowly than alcohol in liquor. This may be partially due to dilution. Beer contains 4% ethanol; wine, 12% ethanol; and whiskey, 40% to 50% ethanol. However, slower absorption cannot be totally accounted for by dilution of the alcohol. Food also slows alcohol absorption.

Ethanol is distributed equally in all body tissue according to water content. Larger persons or persons with greater amounts of body water can ingest more alcohol than smaller persons or persons with less body water. Alcohol affects the cerebrum and cerebellum before it affects the spinal cord and the vital centers because the former areas contain more water.

The rate of absorption largely determines how quickly a person will become intoxicated, but the metabolic rate largely determines how long alcohol will affect the body. The metabolic rate is constant. The body can metabolize 10 ml of alcohol (1 ounce of whiskey or 1 glass of beer) every 90 minutes. In persons who drink

Box 24-3

## HOW THE ADDICTIVE PRODUCTS TIQs AND BETA-CARBOLINES ARE FORMED IN THE BODY

Alcohol

Acetaldehyde  ⟶  *Neurotransmitters*  ⟶  *Tetrahydroisoquinolines (TIQs) and beta-carbolines*

       Dopamine + Acetaldehyde  ⟶  Salsolinol

       Dopamine + Dopaldehyde  ⟶  Tetrahydropapaveroline (THP)

       Serotonin + Acetaldehyde  ⟶  Beta-carbolines

Acetate

Excreted from the body

Alcohol is metabolized to acetaldehyde. Acetaldehyde and other aldehydes condense with neurotransmitters to produce tetrahydroisoquinolines (TIQs) and beta-carbolines. These compounds, formed when we drink alcohol, appear to be highly addictive brain substances similar to morphine precursors. Infused into animal brains, they produce what seems to be irreversible addictive thinking.

From Wallace J: Alcoholism: new light on the disease, Newport, RI, 1985, Edgehill Publications.

alcohol frequently over a number of years, hepatic drug-metabolizing levels are increased to hasten alcohol metabolism. Hot coffee, "sweating it out," and other home remedies do not increase alcohol metabolism, nor do they speed the sobering-up process. Attempts by scientists to develop a pill to prevent or decrease intoxication have been unsuccessful. In late-stage alcoholism, tolerance decreases as the abused liver finally can no longer adequately metabolize the alcohol.

*Tolerance* to alcohol occurs and is probably related to elevated hepatic enzyme levels and to cellular adaptation. Where the normal drinker might be noticeably drunk after 10 to 12 drinks, the long-term drinker with tolerance might walk around almost unaffected by drinking the same amount. This is an example of tolerance. "Drinking someone under the table" is a function of "practice" rather than manhood.

## Physiological effects

Initially people drink because alcohol causes a reaction that they desire. Disinhibition, impaired judgment, and fuzzy thinking are initial responses to alcohol ingestion. These signs represent cerebrum intoxication. In many situations this mental relaxation is pleasant. Alcohol depresses psychomotor activity also. Alcohol has been described as a social lubricant because it relaxes self-imposed barriers that tether sociability. Anxiety and tension are relieved, usually for a couple of hours after a drink is taken. Eventually, at least for the alcoholic, drinking becomes defensive; that is, the alcoholic often drinks to avoid the effects of many years of drinking. For instance, once the anxiety-reducing effect wears off, more tension and anxiety are caused, so the drinker must consume more alcohol to regain the "anxiety-free" state again. Many alcoholics, even after drinking all they "can hold," are not able to quell the rebound psychomotor upheaval caused by years of alcohol-related CNS irritation.

The adverse effects of alcohol can be categorized as central (CNS) or peripheral (PNS). CNS effects are related to sedation and toxicity. As the vital centers become affected, a slowed, stuporous to unconscious mental state develops. Large amounts of alcohol can cause sleep, coma, deep anesthesia, and death. Other common symptoms of intoxication include slurred speech, a short retention span, loud talk, and memory deficits. *Blackout* is a period in which an alcoholic functioned socially for which he has no memory.

Historically the brain damage associated with alcoholism was thought to be caused by alcohol-related nutritional deficiencies. Alcoholics do eat poorly, and no doubt such behavior leads to pathological change. However, it is now known that brain damage occurs with drinking even when a nutritious diet is maintained. In fact, all alcoholics will have some brain cell loss.

Increased psychomotor activity as a consequence of alcohol is called the alcohol-withdrawal syndrome. Sedation is the predominant effect of alcohol, but as sedation wears off, psychomotor activity increases. This is referred to as a rebound phenomenon. As the CNS becomes more irritated, the normal drinker feels sick and irritable (a hangover) but lives through it, perhaps vowing "never again." The heavy drinker and the alcoholic have to drink again to "resedate" the psychomotor system. Eventually alcoholics have to drink large amounts just to feel somewhat "normal." Some reach the point where they cannot drink enough, and CNS irritability is not "sedatable." Then alcoholic tremors, sweating, palpitations, and agitation occur. Most often these symptoms occur when alcohol ingestion has stopped, but in some cases they occur while the alcoholic is drinking.

*Alcoholic hallucinosis,* a state of auditory hallucinations, is a phenomenon that alcoholics sometimes experience. The brain begins to "invent" sensory input. Alcoholic hallucinosis usually begins 48 hours or so after drinking has stopped. Usually within the context of a clear sensorium, frightening voices or sounds are heard.

The ultimate level of CNS irritability is delirium tremens (DTs). In DTs the body not only invents sensory input but also has extreme motor agitation. Hallucinations become visual (e.g., the proverbial pink elephants), and the sufferer is tremulous and terrified. Tonic-clonic seizures (grand mal) can occur.

*Wernicke-Korsakoff syndrome* is an organic mental disorder characterized by amnesia, clouding of consciousness, confabulation (falsification of memory) and memory loss, and peripheral neuropathy. This disorder results from the poor nutrition of the alcoholic (specifically, inadequate amounts of thiamine and niacin in the diet) and from the neurotoxic nature of alcohol.

Peripheral nervous system involvement is varied and causes great suffering. For a complete discussion of these various processes the reader is directed to a medical-surgical textbook.

*Cirrhosis* and *peripheral neuritis* are the physical health problems mostly commonly associated with alcohol. Cirrhosis is the fifth leading cause of death in the United States. As the alcoholic's liver function becomes impaired, he is less able to "tolerate" alcohol. The man who once boasted of his drinking exploits is drunk after only a few beers. Physical consequences of cirrhosis include obstructed blood flow (which leads to portal hypertension, ascites, and finally esophageal varices) and decreased liver cell function, low blood protein levels, high ammonia and high bilirubin serum levels, and clotting problems. Peripheral neuritis causes numbness and the subsequent injury in the legs as well as changes in gait.

Alcohol is also an irritant. It burns the mouth and throat and prompts the stomach to secrete more hydrochloric acid. Gastric ulcers are caused and then worsened by alcohol. Alcoholics experience ulcers, gastritis, bleeding, and hemorrhage in the stomach. Ulcers can eventually perforate, creating a life-threatening situation.

The pancreas is affected by alcohol in many direct and indirect ways. Pancreatitis and diabetes are not uncommon consequences of alcoholism. A malabsorption syndrome is caused by irritation of the intestinal lining. This seems to affect B vitamins generally and to lead to a deficiency of vitamin $B_1$ (thiamine) in particular. Thiamine deficiency contributes to peripheral neuritis. Alcohol also has a direct effect on muscle tissue, a condition known as alcoholic myopathy. Other organs affected by alcohol include the eyes (loss of peripheral and night vision), the heart (hypertension, enlarged left ventricle), and reproductive organs (as a depressant, alcohol can cause impotence).

### Nursing issues

**Overdose.** People die from overdoses of alcohol because it depresses the CNS. Vital centers become anesthetized, compromising breathing and heart rate and

## Case Study

C.M., a 30-year-old man, has been brought into treatment from the county jail by his common-law wife. C.M. has a history of alcohol and drug use since the age of 15. He states that his paternal grandfather died of cirrhosis, but C.M. never saw him pick up a drink. C.M. considers his parents to be "teetotalers." They are repulsed by their son's alcohol use.

C.M. has been involved in counseling twice. Both experiences were described as efforts to salvage his marriage or the relationship he was involved in at the time. C.M.'s first marriage ended in divorce at the beginning of this year, after he lost his business. Six years ago he had assaulted his wife, and in June of last year was arrested for child abuse. At both times he was drinking. He also has twice been charged with driving while intoxicated. The first time was 4 years ago, and the charges were dropped. The other was last month, for which he is still being held in custody.

C.M. says he is willing to undergo treatment so that he can get out of this "legal bind" he is presently in, but he feels that alcohol is not a problem in his life right now. He denies suicidal ideation. Blood alcohol level on admission was 0.02. (In most states blood alcohol levels of 0.08 or 0.1 are legal evidence of drunkenness). He enjoys hunting and doing things with his family. Two common-law step-children, ages 4 and 6, live with him at present. C.M. also has a 2-year-old son who lives with his ex-wife.

leading to a comatose state or death. Gastrointestinal bleeding or hemorrhage can occur. Alcohol also causes heat loss, and many people have succumbed to hypothermia in colder climates. People consistently underestimate the potency of alcohol, and deaths have occurred simply because individuals have drunk too much. At least yearly, newspapers report the death of a college student coerced into drinking too much alcohol. Although alcohol alone can kill, most deaths are the result of combining alcohol with other CNS depressants.

**Disulfiram.** Disulfiram (Antabuse) inhibits the breakdown of acetaldehyde by the enzyme aldehyde dehydrogenase. Because acetaldehyde is toxic to the body, the person who drinks alcohol while taking disulfiram will become ill (sweating, flushing of the neck and face, a throbbing headache, nausea and vomiting, palpitations, dyspnea, tremor, and weakness). This combination can also cause arrhythmias, myocardial infarction, cardiac failure, seizures, coma, and death. The unpleasant response to alcohol reinforces the alcoholic's efforts to stop drinking. Disulfiram is usually

## Nursing Care Plan

WEEKLY UPDATE: ___9/6/90___

NAME: _____C.M._____          ADMISSION DATE: __7/31/90__

DSM-III-R DIAGNOSIS: _____Alcohol dependence (or alcoholism)_____

*ASSESSMENT:*
*Areas of strength:* Has no medical problems and denies any suicidal ideation. Has also been in counseling twice and enjoys hunting and doing things with his family.
*Problems:* Has a genetic history of chemical dependency and long-time use of alcohol and drugs. Denies that alcohol is a problem in his life despite family and occupational problems.

*DIAGNOSES:* Alcoholism related to genetic susceptibility and the overtaxing of that susceptibility.

**Date met**

*PLANNING:*
*Short-term goals:* Patient will state that his marital and      ___8/15/90___
occupational problems are due to drinking.
*Long-term goals:* Patient will remain chemical free on      ___8/31/90___
monthly testing, which will be assessed through urine testing
by his probation officer.

*IMPLEMENTATION/INTERVENTIONS:*
*Nurse-patient relationship:* Recognize initial need to use denial; discuss the natural consequences of his drinking and the need for total abstinence; educate regarding the diagnosis concept, offering hope for long-term recovery; encourage attendance at AA meetings.
*Psychopharmacology:* No caffeine or sugar, multivitamin qd.
*Milieu management:* Family treatment; encourage ADL.

*EVALUATION:* C.M. is sober after 1 month according to probation officer started with a single 500 mg dose at bedtime. After 1 or 2 weeks the dose is reduced to a maintenance dose of 250 mg per day.

**Interactions.** Alcohol taken with other CNS depressants causes profound CNS depression, often leading to death. For instance, diazepam, which is seldom lethal when taken alone, even in large doses, can lead to death if it is combined with alcohol. Alcohol should be avoided when a person is taking barbiturates, antipsychotic drugs, antidepressants, benzodiazepines, and other CNS depressants. Chloral hydrate and lorazepam (Ativan) have been associated with intentional sedating of unsuspecting persons in bars. A chloral hydrate and alcohol combination (the legendary "knock out drops") was used years ago to "recruit" men for ship duty or for robbery. The combination of lorazepam and alcohol has been used in recent days by prostitutes to debilitate their clients so they can rob them.

**Use in the elderly.** People with impaired liver function do not metabolize alcohol efficiently and therefore can tolerate little of the drug. Decreased liver function is a product of aging, and consequently many older persons cannot drink much alcohol without becoming inebriated, confused, and sedated. The nurse should be particularly watchful for combinations of alcohol with other CNS depressants in this age group.

**Fetal alcohol syndrome.** Pregnant women who drink alcohol run the risk of seriously harming their unborn child. Fetal alcohol syndrome (FAS) is the result of alcohol's inhibiting fetal development during the first trimester. FAS is the third most commonly recognized cause of mental retardation. Characteristic signs of FAS include microcephaly, cleft palate, altered palmar creases, cardiac defects, anomalous genitalia, severe mental retardation, and a depressed sucking reflex. The risk of FAS is directly related to the amount of alcohol the mother drinks.

**Withdrawal and detoxification.** Withdrawal from alcohol can be painful, scary, and even lethal (Table 24-1). As the person abstains from alcohol, he begins to reap the consequences of the CNS irritation caused by alcohol: tremulousness, nervousness, anxiety, anorexia, nausea and vomiting, insomnia and other sleep disturbances, rapid pulse, high blood pressure, profuse perspiration, diarrhea, fever, unsteady gait, difficulty concentrating, exaggerated startle reflex, and a craving for alcohol or other drugs. As the withdrawal symptoms become more pronounced, hallucinations can occur. The body is experiencing alcohol toxicity and needs detoxification.

Mueller and Ketcham (1987) identify the three crucial elements or the three "Ss" of the detoxification process: secure environment, sedation, and supplements. A calm *secure environment* is important, since the physical experience of withdrawal can be dramatically influenced by emotional and psychological distress. *Sedation* can be used to slow and thus ameliorate the withdrawal process and to calm the anxious, hallucinating, or delirious patient. Chlordiazepoxide (Librium) 50 to 100 mg followed by repeated doses as needed (up to 300 mg per day) is given for acute alcohol withdrawal. Nutritional *supplements* are also recommended during and up to 4 months after detoxification. Supplements include a multivitamin, B-complex, vitamin C, calcium, and magnesium.

# ■ Other CNS Depressants

CNS depressants are relatively new pharmacological agents. Barbiturates were first used medicinally as sedatives in the last half of the nineteenth century. It was not until 1950 that researchers were able to confirm their ability to produce physical dependence. CNS depressants decrease the awareness of and response to sensory stimuli. Two classes of CNS depressants will be discussed in this chapter: barbiturates and inhalants. Antipsychotic drugs and minor tranquilizers (antianxiety agents), which also depress the CNS, are discussed in Chapters 12 and 14.

## BARBITURATES

Barbiturates are used to relieve anxiety or to produce sleep. They have a narrow therapeutic index, the lethal dose being only slightly higher than the therapeutic dose. These drugs produce both physical and psychological dependence.

Barbiturates are classified according to their duration of action: ultrashort (30 minutes to 3 hours), short (3 to 4 hours), intermediate (6 to 8 hours), and long (10 to 12 hours). Uses range from anesthesia (ultra–short acting barbiturates such as thiopental) to long-term use in epilepsy (long-acting barbiturates such as phenobarbital).

### Metabolism

Barbiturates are usually taken orally. They are metabolized by the liver and excreted by the kidneys. When barbiturates are combined with alcohol, dangerous levels of CNS depression can occur.

### Physiological effects

Barbiturates cause CNS depression, thus decreasing awareness of external stimuli, shortening the attention span, and decreasing intellectual ability. Regular sleep patterns are changed, with a loss of rapid eye movement (REM) sleep. Barbiturates are used to treat insomnia, to soften withdrawal from heroin, and as anticonvulsants. Drug abusers take barbiturates to maintain a state of relatively anxiety-free living. These drugs are also taken to counteract the effects of amphetamines, "to come down," or in place of heroin when it is not available. The acutely intoxicated person will have an unsteady gait, slurred speech, and sustained nystagmus. Chronic users have mental symptoms that include confusion, irritability, and insomnia. Persons who regularly use barbiturates develop a tolerance to them.

### Nursing issues

**Overdose.** The toxic dose of barbiturates varies, but in general an oral dose of 1 g results in serious poisoning, and doses of 2 to 10 g can be fatal. Acute overdose is manifested by CNS and respiratory depression. Coma and death are possible. Treatment is supportive.

**Interactions.** Barbiturates interact with many other drugs, but the most significant are those that increase CNS depression. Other CNS depressants such as

TABLE 24-1 Withdrawal courses for addictive drugs

| Drug | Intoxication signs and symptoms | Withdrawal signs and symptoms | Length of acute detoxification | Recurring withdrawal symptoms | Common detoxification agents |
|---|---|---|---|---|---|
| **SEDATIVES** | | | | | |
| Alcohol | Slurred speech, poor coordination, confusion, drowsiness, clumsiness, depressed respirations and blood pressure | Anxiety, sweats, tremors, flushed face, irritability, sleeplessness, confusion, seizures, delirium | 3-5 days | Not usual | Librium, Serax, Vistaril, Valium, alcohol* |
| Valium | | | Slow drug taper up to 2 weeks | Common | Librium, Valium |
| Phenobarbital | | | Slow drug taper for 2-4 weeks | Common | Librium, phenobarbital |
| **NARCOTICS** | | | | | |
| Heroin | Pin-point pupils, euphoria, nodding, sleepiness, anxiety, depressed blood pressure and respiration, elevated pulse | Yawning, dilated pupils, gooseflesh, vomiting, diarrhea, runny nose and eyes, sleeplessness, anxiety, irritability, elevated blood pressure and pulse, craving for narcotics | 3-5 days | Common | Methadone or other tapering opiate or nonopiate withdrawal regimens† |
| Morphine | | | 3-5 days | Common | |
| Demerol | | | 3-5 days | Common | |
| Methadone | | | 2 weeks + | Common | |

| | | | | | Drug intervention |
|---|---|---|---|---|---|
| **STIMULANTS** | | | | | |
| Amphetamines | Rapid pulse, elevated blood pressure, dilated pupils, sweats, tremors, hyperactivity, loss of appetite, irritability, sleeplessness, delirium, seizures | General fatigue, apathy, depression, drowsiness, irritability, paranoia | Common | 3-5 days | usually not required |
| Cocaine | | | Common | 3-5 days | |
| **HALLUCINOGENS** | | | | | |
| Marijuana | Rapid pulse, elevated blood pressure, dilated pupils, flushed face, red conjunctivae, anxiety, hallucinations, time-space disorientation, rambling speech | Few signs of withdrawal; craving for marijuana; general anxiety and restlessness | Possible prolonged craving | 2-3 days | None, usually |

*Low-dose alcohol withdrawal:

Traditionally, alcohol was used by laymen to taper a drunk off a binge. With the advent of sedative medication, this practice was discouraged. The use of general sedatives was thought to be more "clinical" and to achieve better control with less toxicity. In recent years, however, the alcohol withdrawal model has been revived. Leading the way in this detox method is Dr. Walter Gower, M.D., of North Central Alcoholism Research Foundation, Inc., Ford Dodge, Iowa. (*Transition,* "A half-ounce of Prevention for the DT's." September, 1983. "The Relationship of Ethanol to the Occurrence of Delirium Tremens with Prophylactic and Therapeutic Considerations." Presented by Dr. Gower at the National Alcoholism Forum, 1979; abstracted in *Alcoholism Update,* vol. 2, No. 3, Aug-Sept, 1979.)

*Treatment Regimen:* ½ oz. vodka (80-100 proof) with ½ oz. water every 1-6 hours for detox control. Indications for use are the same as for sedative intervention. This can be used alone or in combination with sedatives such as Librium. (Patients with seizure histories are better protected during withdrawal with the combined regimen.)

†Other-opiate-withdrawal protocol:

- Darvon N-100: 1-2 every 4-6 hours to control detox signs and symptoms; taper to discontinue in 3-4 days.
- Catapres: 0.1 mg initially; repeat in 1 hour if needed, then 0.1-0.2 every 6-8 hours as long as blood pressure is no lower than 90/60. This can be used for 7-14 days to control opiate withdrawal symptoms.

From Mueller LA and Ketcham K: Recovering: how to get and stay sober, New York, 1987, Bantam Books.

alcohol, sedatives, tranquilizers, and antihistamines can cause serious CNS depression.

**Use in the elderly.** Barbiturates frequently cause excitement in the elderly. The elderly are also more prone to confusion caused by barbiturates.

**Use during pregnancy.** Barbiturates can cause fetal abnormalities. These drugs cross the placental barrier, and fetal serum levels approach maternal blood levels. Infants born to mothers who take barbiturates during the last trimester of pregnancy experience withdrawal symptoms.

**Withdrawal and detoxification.** Symptoms of withdrawal from barbiturates are severe and can cause death. Symptoms usually begin 8 to 12 hours after the last dose. Minor withdrawal symptoms include anxiety, muscle twitching, tremor, progressive weakness, dizziness, distorted visual perception, nausea and vomiting, insomnia, and orthostatic hypotension. More serious withdrawal symptoms include convulsions and delirium beginning approximately 16 hours after the last dose and lasting up to 5 days. Untreated, withdrawal symptoms may not decline in intensity for some time. Detoxification requires a cautious and gradual reduction of these drugs. One approach is to reduce the patient's regular dose by 10% each day.

## INHALANTS

There are three basic forms of inhalants: hydrocarbon solvents (gasoline), aerosol propellants (the propellants in spray cans), and anesthetics (chloroform, nitrous oxide). Inhalants usually depress the CNS and increase hilarity. They are particularly dangerous because the amount inhaled cannot be controlled. Deaths from asphyxiation have been reported. Inhalants cross the blood-brain barrier quickly. Common side effects include mouth ulcers, gastrointestinal problems, anorexia, confusion, headache, and ataxia.

## ■ Opioids (Narcotics)

Opioids are widely abused. Until the relatively recent "cocaine crisis," the general public viewed heroin as the most significant drug of abuse. Although heroin abuse has been relegated to backpage status for some time, it is again becoming the focus of attention as drug users find it less expensive than cocaine. Illicit drugs can be swallowed, smoked, snorted, injected into soft tissue (skin popping), and "mainlained" (injected intravenously). Parenteral use of heroin, for example, involves (1) "cooking" the substance in a spoon or bottlecap, (2) filtering it with a cotton ball, (3) "sterilizing" a needle with a match, and (4) injecting the drug into a vein. Initially veins in the antecubital space are used, but as vein membranes break down and sclerose ("tracks"), other veins are "used up." The needle is frequently passed from one user to another. Infections, including AIDS, are relatively common. Morphine is the prototype drug of this class and will be discussed in more depth.

### Metabolism

Morphine is metabolized in the liver and is excreted by the kidneys (Table 24-2). It is not absorbed well in the gut but is readily metabolized there and in the liver.

**TABLE 24-2**   Period of time after ingestion that drugs can be detected in the urine

| Drug | Detection period |
|---|---|
| **OPIOIDS** | |
| Heroin | 2-4 d |
| Morphine | " " |
| Meperidine   (Demerol) | " " |
| Methadone | " " |
| Fentanyl | Can be < 1 h |
| **DEPRESSANTS** | |
| Barbiturates | 12 h-3 wk |
| Benzodiazepines | Up to 1 wk |
| **STIMULANTS** | |
| Amphetamines | 2-4 days |
| Cocaine | " " |
| **HALLUCINOGENS** | |
| Marijuana | 3 d to >1 mo |
| PCP | 1 d-1 mo |

Adapted from Sullivan E, Bissell L, and Williams E: Chemical dependency in nursing, Redwood City, Calif., Addison-Wesley, 1988, p. 104.

It can be given orally but is usually given parenterally. Drugs that compete for liver metabolism increase the effect of morphine.

### Physiological effects

Opioids relieve pain by increasing the pain threshold and by reducing anxiety and fear. They do this by stimulating specific neurotransmitter receptor sites in the brain. The naturally occurring neurotransmitters, the endorphins, among other responses, mediate pain and regulate mood. The opioids are endorphin agonists. It is their effect on mood (a feeling of euphoria) that attracts drug abusers. Drug abusers frequently refer to the euphoric mood created by heroin as "better than sex." In addition to the euphoria an overall CNS depression occurs. Drowsiness or "nodding" and sleep are common effects.

Heroin has a higher abuse potential than morphine because it more readily passes the blood-brain barrier. Once heroin enters the brain its chemical structure is changed to that of morphine so it becomes "trapped" in the brain. This property of heroin causes a more sustained high.

*CNS effects* of opioids include respiratory depression related to decreased sensitivity to carbon dioxide stimulation by the medullary center for respiration. Respiratory depression is the primary cause of death among opioid abusers. *PNS effects* include constipation; decreased gastric, biliary, and pancreatic secretions; urinary retention; hypotension; and reduced pupil size. Pinpoint pupils are a sign of opioid overdose. Morphine also causes vomiting.

### Nursing Issues

**Overdose.** At therapeutic doses prescribed and administered by professionals, morphine is a helpful and safe analgesic. Drug abusers are never sure of the amount of the drug they are taking however. Street purchases are not standardized, and occasionally, users obtain "purer" drug than they anticipated. Inadvertent overdose occurs. The primary effect of overdose is respiratory depression. A respiratory rate below 12 per minute is cause for concern. A recognizable symptom pattern for overdose is documented:

- The person become stuporous and then sleeps.
- The skin is wet and warm.
- Next a coma develops accompanied by respiratory depression and hypoxia.
- The skin becomes cold and clammy.
- The pupils dilate.
- Death quickly follows at this point.

Provision of adequate airway and assisted ventilation if needed are treatment priorities. A narcotic antagonist is administered to reverse the effects of opioids.

**Narcotic antagonists.** The opioids are the only class of commonly abused drugs that have a specific antidote. Naloxone (Narcan), a narcotic antagonist, is the drug of choice if opioid overdose is suspected. Naloxone blocks the neuroreceptors affected by opioids, so the patient responds in a few minutes to an intravenous injection of naloxone. Respirations improve, and the patient consciously responds. However, since most opioids have a longer lasting effect than naloxone has, it is often necessary to repeat the antagonist to maintain adequate respirations. The nurse administering naloxone must carefully observe the patient to determine whether additional antagonist will be needed. Nalorphine (Nalline) is also a narcotic antagonist. Narcotic antagonists do not interrupt the effects of nonnarcotics.

**Interactions.** The effects of opioids are increased when they are combined with other CNS depressants. Since the use of multiple drugs is common among drug abusers, the potential for deadly combinations is real. If it is known that heroin was taken and naloxone does not reverse CNS depression, it can be safely assumed that other depressants were taken also. In such cases supportive nursing care is indicated.

**Use in the elderly.** Elderly persons are particularly at risk for decreased pulmonary ventilation associated with these drugs.

**Use during pregnancy.** Women who abuse opioids give birth to babies who suffer withdrawal symptoms. These drugs can cross the placental barrier and produce respiratory depression in neonates.

**Withdrawal and detoxification.** The unassisted withdrawal from alcohol or barbiturates can be fatal, but the unassisted withdrawal from opioids is rarely fatal. Withdrawal symptoms are related to the degree of dependence and the abruptness of the discontinuance. Maximum intensity is reached within 36 to 72 hours and subsides in 5 to 10 days. Withdrawal symptoms can be categorized into early, intermediate, and late appearing. Early symptoms of withdrawal include yawning, tearing, rhinorrhea, and sweating. Intermediate symptoms include flushing, piloerection, tachycardia, tremor, restlessness, and irritability. Late appearing symptoms include muscle spasm, fever, nausea, diarrhea, vomiting, repetitive sneezing, abdominal cramps, and backache. Treatment is primarily symptomatic and supportive.

## Specific drugs

Drugs related to morphine include hydromorphine (Dilaudid), a derivative of morphine and more potent; levorphanol (Levo-Dromoran), a drug whose action is identical to that of morphine but that is used for less severe pain; meperidine (Demerol), a synthetic narcotic analgesic; pentazocine (Talwin), which has weaker analgesic effects than other narcotic drugs, is less addicting, and does not cause euphoria; and several related drugs such as oxymorphone (Numorphan), alphaprodine (Nisentil), anileridine (Leritine), butorphanol (Stadol), and nalbuphine (Nubain). Fentanyl (Sublimaze), an anesthetic, is similar to but 100 times stronger than morphine and 20 to 40 times stronger than heroin. It is said to produce an "unbelievable" high.

**Methadone.** Methadone (Dolophin), although an opioid similar to morphine, is used to prevent withdrawal symptoms. Methadone is given orally and is poorly metabolized in the liver. Accordingly, it has a much longer half-life (15 to 30 hours) than morphine has (1.5 to 2 hours). Because of the long half-life, once-a-day dosing is effective and conducive to outpatient care.

**Heroin.** Heroin is derived from morphine and is referred to as a semisynthetic drug. It was originally thought to be a cure for morphine addiction but proved to be far more addictive than morphine.

**Codeine.** Codeine is used primarily as a cough suppressant. Its abuse preceded the general drug abuse of the mid to late 1960s as it was easily available in over-the-counter cough syrups. Ease of access was eliminated at about the same time that drug abuse became recognized as an emerging national problem. It is not a drug of choice for many substance abusers today.

# ■ Stimulants

Use of stimulants (Box 24-4) by Americans is widespread, for instance, caffeine-containing drinks. Many people feel absolutely sluggish if they cannot start their day with a cup of coffee. Should they remain caffeine free all day, they experience the withdrawal symptoms associated with stimulant withdrawal: headache, nausea, and vomiting. Tobacco is also a stimulant.

## COCAINE

Coca leaves have been used as stimulants for thousands of years. Coca plants grow high in the Andes, and the Inca indians chewed coca leaves long before the Spanish explorers arrived. Cocaine is extracted from the coca plant and is a fine, white, odorless substance with a bitter taste. It was introduced to Western medicine as an anesthetic in 1858. Freud was known to use cocaine and believed it to be a remedy

**Box 24-4**
## STIMULANTS

Cocaine (crack) coca leaves                    Other stimulants
Amphetamines                                        Methylphenidate (Ritalin)
   Amphetamine sulfate (Benzedrine)     Caffeine
   Dextroamphetamine (Dexedrine)
   Methamphetamine (Desoxyn)

for morphine addiction. It was once used in Coca-Cola, and advertisements extolled Coke's ability to "refresh." After the Pure Food and Drug Law was passed in 1906, cocaine was eliminated from Coca-Cola. Cocaine and its offspring *crack* cause perhaps the biggest drug problem today. The list of famous and not so famous persons struck down in their youth by these stimulants is lengthy. The problems associated with these drugs extend to every level of society. The following quote is from a *Bakersfield Californian,* August 1, 1990, article entitled "Murder rampage hits U.S.": "America's murder toll may break a decade-old record this year, the Senate Judiciary Committee said Tuesday in laying the blame on rising stockpiles of assault weapons and shrinking supplies of cocaine."

## Metabolism

Cocaine passes the blood-brain barrier quickly, causing an instantaneous high. When administered intravenously, cocaine is rapidly metabolized by the liver, so the "rush," though exhilarating, does not last long. Cocaine exerts both CNS and PNS effects because of its ability to block norepinephrine and dopamine reuptake into neurons. It depletes these neurotransmitters. Cocaine can also be swallowed (but is poorly absorbed this way) and snorted. Snorting, in which cocaine is absorbed through the nasal mucosa, is the preferred route for drug abusers. Freebasing is another way of using cocaine. Freebasing is a process used to rid "street cocaine" of its adulterants and reduce it to a pure cocaine base. The cocaine base is volatile, and explosions have occurred (e.g., Richard Pryor experienced this and was burned severely). Freebase cocaine is smoked and produces incredibly powerful feelings of euphoria instantaneously. Euphoria is quickly followed by discomfort, so more smoking is required to relieve the discomfort. A vicious cycle ensues.

    Crack or "rock," a form of cocaine, may be the most addictive drug on the streets today. It is produced in a relatively uncomplicated procedure (mixed with baking soda and water, heated, and hardened) and then smoked. It produces an instantaneous high and almost as instantaneous a "crash." An intense desire to smoke again is produced. Crack is cheap (as low as $5 to $10 a purchase) and easy to find.

Tolerance to CNS and PNS effects develops quickly because neuronal norepinephrine stores are depleted, causing a need to increase drug amounts to create
the desired effect. Tolerance develops to otherwise lethal amounts.

## Physiological effects

Cocaine and its derivatives are addicting stimulants. Although physical dependence
is less severe than with opiate abuse, psychological dependence is intense. Abusers
become tongue-tied when attempting to describe the sensations of this drug. Euphoria, increased mental alertness, increased strength, anorexia, and increased sexual
stimulation are major desired effects of these drugs. The number of persons who
have tried cocaine at least once increased from 5.4 million in 1974 to 30 million
in 1989 (DiGregorio, 1990).

Increased motor activity, tachycardia, and high blood pressure are PNS effects.
Sensory and motor nerve endings are numbed, causing blood vessels to contract.
Decreased stimulation occurs. CNS effects include stimulation of the medulla, resulting in deeper respirations, euphoria, increased mental alertness, dilated pupils,
anorexia, and increased strength. The cocaine user also talks a lot and is stimulated
sexually. This latter characteristic no doubt adds to the drug's overall appeal. Less
common reactions are specific hallucinations and delusions. Cocaine users report
"bugs" crawling beneath the skin (formication) and foul smells. Nasal septum per-
foration is associated with snorting cocaine and is due to extreme vasoconstriction,
which impedes blood supply to this area and thus causes nasal necrosis.

## AMPHETAMINES

Amphetamines were developed in 1887. They have medicinal uses, such as short-
term treatment of obesity, attention-deficit disorders in childhood, and narcolepsy.
Although not technically addictive by DSM-III-R criteria, they are highly abused.
The *San Francisco Chronicle,* May 30, 1989, ran a front-page story entitled "Speed
Makes a Comeback on Bay Area Drug Scene." Speed, sometimes known as crank, is
called the poor man's cocaine. Some notable quotations from the article follow.
"Everybody's predicting that it's going to be the next big drug problem .... Only
cocaine and marijuana are used more often.... Speed is gaining on cocaine because
it produces a longer high.... It is also cheaper.... A lot of people arrested for doing
crank say they would never do coke. For some reason they think crank isn't as
addicting.... The greatest percentage of new patients seeking help for speed addiction are teenagers who cannot afford more expensive drugs" (pp A1, A11).

## Metabolism

Amphetamines (speed) are indirect-acting sympathomimetics that cause the release
of norepinephrine from nerve endings. Amphetamines also block norepinephrine
reuptake in presynaptic nerve endings. Amphetamines are well absorbed from the
gastrointestinal tract. They are given orally. Therapeutic parenteral administration
is illegal in the United States, but many speed freaks self-administer amphetamines
intravenously.

## Case Study

John Rice, a 25-year-old, unemployed carpenter, lives with his aunt, who called the sheriff's office when Mr. Rice began tearing the house apart and then locked himself in the bathroom, saying he was going to kill himself. On examination in the emergency room, and with historical information from his aunt, Mr. Rice was noted to have suicidal ideations, auditory hallucinations, delusions of persecution, disorganized thinking, anorexia, insomnia, anxiety, and agitation. He had a difficult time sitting down because of psychomotor agitation and more than once made threatening gestures to the emergency room psychiatric nurse. She finds that his hallucinations are persecutory in nature, for example, he heard coworkers conspire "to get him." When the nurse questions him about his suicide attempt, Mr. Rice states that he does not remember and asks, "Who the hell cares anyway?" The nurse concludes that the suicidal behavior was impulsive and directly related to cocaine intoxication. The nurse obtains a urine sample and sends it to the laboratory.

The aunt states that Mr. Rice has been having difficulties for awhile and that she has suspected drug abuse for about 2 years. On the other hand, she never felt comfortable asking him about drugs so kept her suspicions to herself. She relates that Mr. Rice was fired by the builder he worked for about 3 months ago, but was told that Mr. Rice could return if he ever "cleaned up." She did not ask the builder what "cleaned up" meant.

The emergency room physician decides to keep Mr. Rice in the emergency room until his thinking clears and until concerns about tachycardia, cardiac arrhythmias, and convulsions are alleviated. The physician orders 5 mg diazepam (Valium) to be given intravenously over 2 to 3 minutes and repeated every 10 to 15 minutes as needed if Mr. Rice has seizures and propranolol (Inderal) intravenously (0.1 to 0.15 mg/kg at a rate of 0.5 to 0.75 mg every 1 to 2 minutes) should the patient experience cardiac arrhythmias. After 4 hours no signs of arrhythmias or seizure are noted, and Mr. Rice is transferred to the psychiatric unit.

Upon arrival in the unit Mr. Rice is noticeably irritable, agitated, anxious, and complaining of a headache. His responses to questions indicate continuing difficulty in concentration and some disorganized thinking. The care plan on the opposite page was developed by the psychiatric nurse.

## Nursing Care Plan

NAME: _____John Rice_____      ADMISSION DATE: __5/26/90__

DSM-III-R DIAGNOSIS: _____Psychoactive Substance Dependence Disorder_____

### ASSESSMENT:
*Areas of strength:* Young (25 years old); lives with aunt who wants him to return once he begins to "feel better"; previous employer would hire him if he gets "clean."

*Problems:* Suicidal ideations, hallucinations (auditory), delusions that someone wants to kill him, thinking disorganized (has difficulty completing thought), anorexia, insomnia, anxious (has exaggerated startle reflex), agitated.

**DIAGNOSES:** Potential for self-directed violence related to substance abuse or CNS agitation evidenced by history of suicide attempt. Alterations in perception related to substance abuse or CNS agitation manifested by suicidal ideations, disorganized thinking, and hallucinations and delusions. Alteration in nutrition: less than body requirements related to anorexic effect of cocaine manifested by loss of weight.

| | Date met |
|---|---|
| **PLANNING:** | |
| ***Short-term goals:*** | |
| Patient will not experience physical injury during hospitalization. | 6/2/90 |
| Patient will not experience symptoms of cocaine withdrawal. | 6/2/90 |
| Patient will sleep 6 to 8 hours per night. | 6/2/90 |
| Patient will admit that cocaine is a problem in his life. | 5/28/90 |
| ***Long-term goals:*** | |
| Patient will maintain optimum level of nutrition and maintain at least 90% of normal weight. | |
| Patient will attend outpatient Narcotics Anonymous. | |
| Patient will practice abstinence from psychoactive drugs. | |
| Patient will verbalize and show some evidence of developing non-drug-using friends. | |

*Continued.*

## Nursing Care Plan—cont'd

IMPLEMENTATION/INTERVENTIONS:

*Nurse-patient relationship:* Develop a contract with patient to report to nurse if suicidal thoughts occur. Establish trusting relationship with patient. Provide reality-based conversation. Accept patient. Set limits on behavior; confront the patient with inconsistencies; and do not allow patient to manipulate. All staff must be consistent. Allow patient to verbalize anxiety and fear. Teach patient the effects of drugs on his body. Encourage independence in self-care and reinforce examples of self-denial and delayed gratification.

*Psychopharmacology:* Desipramine 50 mg b.i.d. for cocaine withdrawal for 2 weeks (last dose 0800 6/8). Haldol 5 mg p.o. q4h p.r.n. agitation; Cogentin 2 mg p.o. with first dose of Haldol on the days it is given. Tylenol tabs ii q4h p.r.n. headache.

*Milieu management:* Provide patient with a quiet room to decrease agitation. Provide safe environment including frequent observation by staff, monitoring of smoking, assessing VS p.r.n. Monitor the environment for dangerous objects such as glass, razors, and belts. Provide foods the patient likes to increase interest in food. Provide group setting for patient to explore the issues of substance abuse with other patients and to help the patient get past the notion that no one understands his problem. Orient to surroundings.

*EVALUATION:* Patient has not experienced significant cocaine withdrawal; appetite is returning. Beginning to sleep better (4 to 6 hours). Patient has not attempted self-injury and denies suicidal intent.

## Physiological effects

As with cocaine, people take amphetamines because amphetamines make them feel good. CNS effects include wakefulness, alertness, heightened concentration, energy, improved mood to euphoria, insomnia (sometimes desired, sometimes not), and amnesia.

The most common side effects of amphetamine use are restlessness, dizziness, agitation, and insomnia. PNS effects are palpitations, tachycardia, and hypertension. Respirations also increase because, like cocaine, the amphetamines stimulate the medulla. A psychiatric side effect of amphetamine use is amphetamine-induced psychosis. In the emergency room this psychotic presentation can be almost indistinguishable from paranoid schizophrenia.

### NURSING ISSUES

**Overdose.**  Cocaine overdose has resulted in a number of deaths, primarily due to arrhythmias and respiratory collapse. Freebasing adds to the problem because large amounts reach the system quickly. Toxic levels of amphetamines cause severe hypertension, cerebral hemorrhage, seizures, and coma. Treatment includes induction of vomiting, acidification of the urine, and forced diuresis. In patients with amphetamine psychosis related to toxic levels of these drugs, chlorpromazine or haloperidol given intramuscularly will antagonize the amphetamine effect.

**Interactions.** The effects of cocaine and amphetamines are augmented when they are combined with other CNS stimulants. Many over-the-counter products such as hay fever medications and decongestants contain stimulants. Urinary alkalinizing agents such as sodium bicarbonate decrease the elimination of stimulants while urinary acidifying agents increase the elimination of stimulants.

**Use during pregnancy.** Amphetamines should only be used during pregnancy if clearly needed because harm to the fetus has been demonstrated. Cocaine-addicted mothers give birth to addicted babies with multiple problems. The use of cocaine and crack among pregnant women in New York City is responsible for a dramatic decrease in the birthweight of infants in that city (Joyce, 1990).

**Withdrawal and detoxification.** Although cocaine and amphetamines are highly addictive, physical withdrawal is relatively mild. Psychological withdrawal is severe, however, because the drugs are so pleasurable. For persons withdrawing from amphetamines under medical supervision the withdrawal process is gradual and safe. "Cold turkey" withdrawal without medical supervision causes agitation, irritability, and severe depression. As a rule of thumb, the "low" of withdrawal will be inversely proportional to the "high" experienced. Withdrawal from cocaine causes intense craving for the drug. A number of approaches are used, all aiming to restore depleted neurotransmitters. Amino acid precursors such as tyrosine and phenylaline, tricyclic antidepressants, and the dopamine agonist bromocriptine are three approaches used to increase the availability of neurotransmitters.

# ■ Hallucinogens

Hallucinogens, also referred to as psychotomimetics or psychodelics, alter perception. There are two basic groups of hallucinogens: natural and man made or synthetic. Natural hallucinogenic substances include mescaline (peyote [from cactus]), psilocybin (psilocin [from mushrooms]), and marijuana *(Cannabis sativa).* Synthetic or semisynthetic substances include lysergic acid diethylamide-25 (LSD), 2,5-dimethoxy-4-methyl amphetamine (STP), phencyclidine (PCP), N,N-dimethyltryptamine (DMT), and methylene dioxyamphetamine (MDA).

In general, hallucinogens can heighten awareness of reality or can cause a terrifying psychosis-like reaction. Users report distortions in body image and a sense of depersonalization. Particularly frightful is a loss of the sense of reality. Hallucinations depicting grotesque creatures, such as a "dog with a snake for a tongue," can be extremely frightening. Emotional consequences of such effects are panic, anxiety, confusion, and paranoid reactions. Some persons have experienced frank psychotic reactions after minimal use. In the jargon of the hallucinogens, such an experience is a "bad trip."

## MESCALINE (STP, DMT, MDA)

Mescaline (peyote) is derived from cactus plants found in America. Native Americans harvested peyote "buttons" from cacti and used them in their religious ceremonies. This religious practice is still protected by law and is part of their worship. STP, DMT, and MDA are man-made forms of mescaline.

### Metabolism

Mescaline, whether naturally occurring or synthetically produced, is taken orally and is quickly absorbed. Its site of action is probably the norepinephrine synapses. Mescaline passes the blood-brain barrier within 2 hours and usually takes effect within 30 to 40 minutes. Its effects last up to 12 hours. It is excreted in the urine.

### Physiological effects

With mescaline, colors are vivid, music more beautiful, and sounds more intense. When the user closes his eyes, colors and images can be seen. A distorted sense of space and time occurs. A young man who drove his car after taking peyote stated that it seemed to take an eternity to reach a stop sign no more than 50 feet away. The experience is directly related to preingestion expectations. "Good" experiences include hilarity and joy. The user may feel especially insightful. The answers to such questions as those involving the "meaning of life" may seem very clear. Such insights can easily add to a sense of religious experience.

"Bad" trips are the side effects of concern. Although peyote is less potent than LSD, it still can cause panic, paranoid thinking, and anxiety if the trip is too intense. Dependence does not occur in the strict sense, yet users enjoy the experience and seek to repeat it. Pupil dilation and tremors sometimes occur.

## PSILOCYBIN, PSILOCIN

Psilocybin is derived from mushrooms *(Psilocybe mexicana).*

### Metabolism

Psilocybin is taken orally. Once in the stomach it is converted to psilocin by enzymatic action. Psilocybin decreases the reuptake of serotonin in the brain. Onset of action is experienced in 25 to 40 minutes. Its effects last up to 8 hours.

### Physiological effects

Hallucinations and time, space, and perceptual alterations are experienced and are the sensations that caused Indians to continue its use. Psilocybin dilates the pupils and increases heart rate, blood pressure, and body temperature. Tingling of the skin and involuntary movements can occur. As with other hallucinogens, a sense of unreality can occur. An inability to concentrate may add to feelings of anxiety and lead to panic and paranoia. Hallucinations and illusions may occur. Although no deaths due to psilocybin toxicity have been reported, deaths related to perceptual distortions have occurred.

# MARIJUANA

Marijuana is probably the drug most widely used illegally in the United States; typically it is used by teenagers and young adults. Marijuana (*Cannabis sativa*) and other related drugs (hashish and THC) come from an Indian hemp plant. Marijuana is difficult to categorize. Placement with the hallucinogens seems appropriate, but other categorizations are defensible also.

## Metabolism

The active ingredient in marijuana is $\Delta$-6-3,4-tetrahydrocannabinol (THC). THC is changed to metabolites in the body and is stored in fatty tissues. It remains in the body for up to 6 weeks after it is smoked and can be detected in blood and urine for 2 weeks. The effects of smoked marijuana last between 2 and 4 hours. If marijuana is ingested, effects may last up to 12 hours.

## Physiological effects

Marijuana produces a sense of well-being, is relaxing, and alters perceptions. Euphoria results and is the cause of drug-seeking behaviors. Increased hunger ("munchies") is an effect that makes it useful for anorexic persons (e.g., cancer patients). Marijuana's antiemetic properties make it useful for treating nausea and vomiting associated with chemotherapy.

Balance and stability are impaired for up to 8 hours after marijuana use. Short-term memory, decision making, and concentration are also impaired.

Dry mouth, sore throat, increased heart rate, dilated pupils, conjunctival irritation, and keener sight and hearing are physical responses to marijuana. It has been thought to be amotivational, but not all research supports this thinking.

Other effects associated with the use of marijuana include harmful pulmonary effects (bronchitis), weakening of heart contractions, immunosuppression, and reduction of serum testosterone and sperm count. Anxiety, impaired judgment, paranoia, and panic are not uncommon reactions to marijuana. These terrifying experiences may culminate in some health-compromising behavior.

Flashbacks, more commonly associated with LSD, have also been reported. A flashback is a spontaneous reliving of feelings experienced during a "high."

# LSD (LYSERGIC ACID DIETHYLAMIDE)
## Metabolism

LSD stimulates the sympathetic nervous system by inhibiting the reuptake of serotonin. It is taken orally, and onset of action occurs within 30 to 40 minutes. Effects are experienced for up to 12 hours. Very small amounts of LSD, usually only 50 to 300 µg, produce these effects.

## Physiological effects

LSD causes a phenomenon known as synesthesia. Synesthesia is the blending of senses (for example, smelling a color or tasting a sound). Expectations and environment govern the "quality" of the LSD "trip."

LSD causes an increase in blood pressure, tachycardia, trembling, and dilated pupils. CNS effects include a sense of unreality, perceptual alterations and distortions, and impaired judgment. Another problem with LSD is flashbacks. Flashbacks are scary and can heighten a sense of "going crazy." Bad trips from LSD cause anxiety, paranoia, and acute panic. Some persons have suffered psychotic "breaks" from LSD and have never fully recovered. A number of persons have killed themselves while under the influence of LSD.

## PCP (PHENCYCLIDINE)

PCP, a synthetic drug, traditionally has been used as an animal tranquilizer. Many emergency room nurses are familiar with this drug because PCP-intoxicated persons are often brought to the emergency room. Their unpredictable outbursts of violent behavior are legendary. They literally change from coma to violent behavior and back. Caution must be exercised when one is providing care to these patients because of their unpredictable behavior.

### Metabolism

PCP acts on the brain. It is taken orally and intravenously and is smoked and snorted. Oral PCP takes effect in 5 minutes. Injected or snorted PCP takes effect immediately. Smoking takes longer. PCP is well absorbed by all routes. Effects last for 6 to 8 hours. PCP can be found in the blood and urine for up to 10 days after intake.

### Physiological effects

The user experiences a high. Euphoria and a peaceful, easy feeling can occur and are sought after. Perceptual distortions are common.

Undesired effects of PCP are many and serious. Blood pressure and heart rate are elevated. Other PNS effects include ataxia, salivation, and vomiting. Psychological symptoms include hostile, bizarre behavior, a blank stare, and agitation. A catatonic type of muscular rigidity alternating with violent outbursts is particularly frightening to bystanders.

### NURSING ISSUES

**Overdose.** High doses of mescaline are not generally toxic, but high doses of STP and MDA can cause hyperexcitability. Deaths have occurred because of these drugs. Psilocybin overdose has not been associated with any deaths, and usually a calm environment is all that is needed to assist withdrawal. LSD- and PCP-related deaths are not uncommon. Deaths can be caused by overdose but are more likely to be associated with perceptual disorientation and unresponsiveness to environmental stimuli. Confusion and acute panic can result from an overdose of marijuana. Diazepam (Valium) can be administered for psilocybin, LSD, and mescaline overdoses. PCP presents greater problems. Diazepam may be given for seizures and agitation, and haloperidol (Haldol) for psychotic behavior. Acidifying the urine to a pH of 5.5 accelerates its excretion. Urine screening is the best means of identifying abused substances.

**Interactions.** Mescaline, psilocybin, and LSD can potentiate sympathomimet-ics. Marijuana should not be used with alcohol, because marijuana masks the nausea and vomiting associated with excessive alcohol consumption. Respiratory depres-sion, coma, and death can occur.

**Use during pregnancy.** A number of birth defects have been associated with these drugs.

**Withdrawal and detoxification.** Hallucinogens do not produce physical de-pendence, so there are no withdrawal symptoms. Symptoms of withdrawal from marijuana are insomnia, restlessness, and hyperactivity. One of the biggest concerns for the nurse is development of an approach for dealing with the intoxicated person. Basically, the nurse should provide a calm, reassuring environment.

## ■ Nursing Process for Chemically Dependent Persons

The goal of treatment for the chemically dependent person is abstinence from alcohol *and* drugs. The person who is dependent upon one substance can easily become dependent on another. The term *cross-dependence* describes this condition. Professionals working with chemically dependent persons realize their vulnerability and usually refrain from thinking of anyone as being "cured." Conversely, they tend to view treatment as an ongoing, lifelong process in which the person abstaining from formerly abused substances is "recovering." The term *recovering* indicates a current and dynamic process but also indicates the ever-present possibility of "slip-ping."

### ASSESSMENT

The nurse should assess every patient for chemical dependency. The nurse should always ask if the patient drinks or uses drugs and how he feels about it, if he has had problems associated with alcohol or drugs, and if any relative has had alcohol or drug-related problems.

Whitfield et al. (1986) suggest using open-ended questions to elicit information from the patient. It is also important for the nurse to be positive, receptive, and understanding. Most nurses are not prepared for the extreme defensiveness displayed by the chemically dependent person, but her acceptance of the patient helps to break through this barrier. Furthermore, since many nurses themselves have been personally affected by drugs and alcohol, it is important for the nurse to be in touch with her own feelings regarding these substances and those who use them.

Estes and Heinemann (1986) recommend avoiding the terms *alcoholic* or *addict* early in the assessment process and instead suggest the nurse use phrases such as "problem with drinking" or "difficulties with drug use." It may also be helpful initially to focus on legal or more culturally accepted drugs such as caffeine and nicotine.

The patient's consumption should be evaluated in more detail if the initial assessment data identify him as being at risk, that is, if he has highly suggestive clinical manifestations or has a high-risk complaint such as depression or sexual dysfunction (Box 24-5).

## MEDICAL, PSYCHIATRIC, LEGAL, AND OTHER FINDINGS SUGGESTIVE (0 TO •) TO HIGHLY SUGGESTIVE (•• TO •••) OR DIAGNOSTIC (••••) OF ALCOHOLISM AND OTHER CHEMICAL DEPENDENCE

### PRESENTING COMPLAINT AND HISTORY

•••• Drinking or drug-related problem, recurring

••• Blackouts while drinking

••• Spouse/other complains of patient's drinking

••• Driving-while-intoxicated (DWI) record

••• Prison record

••• Change in alcohol/drug tolerance

••• Frequent requests for mood-changing drugs

•• Gastrointestinal bleeding, especially upper

•• Automobile accident

•• Traumatic injuries, fracture

•• Parent, grandparent or relative alcoholic

•• Friends alcoholic or other chemical dependence

•• Family or other violence

•• Child abuse or neglect

•• First seizure in an adult

•• Job performance problem

• Multiple gastrointestinal complaints

• Untoward responses to a number of medications

• Unexplained syncope

• Frequent infections

• Night sweats

• Depression

• Suicide attempt

• Sexual dysfunction

• Legal problem

• Noncompliance in treatment

• School learning problem

• Hypertension

Heart trouble

Palpitations

Abdominal pain

Amenorrhea

Weight loss

Vagus complaints

Seizure

Insomnia

Anxiety or panic attacks

Marital discord

Financial problem

Behavior problem

### ALCOHOL OR OTHER DRUG USE HISTORY

•••• Alcohol use recurringly interfering with health, job, or social functioning

••• Patient says, "I can stop drinking anytime," or the equivalent; or patient gets evasive or angry, or talks glibly during taking of drinking history

••• Patient states that he has consciously stopped drinking completely for any length of time

••• Word "drinker" said in rounds or report

•• Heavy alcohol use (more than 3 drinks/day or more than 5 drinks at an occasion for a 154-lb person)

•• Other drug misuse or dependence

• Cigarette smoker

From Whitfield C, David J, and Barker L: Alcoholism. In Barker LR, Burton JR, and Zieve PD, editors: Principles of ambulatory medicine, Baltimore, 1986, Williams & Wilkins Co.

## Box 24-5
## MEDICAL, PSYCHIATRIC, LEGAL, AND OTHER FINDINGS SUGGESTIVE (0 TO •) TO HIGHLY SUGGESTIVE (•• TO •••) OR DIAGNOSTIC (••••) OR ALCOHOLISM AND OTHER CHEMICAL DEPENDENCE—cont'd

### PHYSICAL EXAMINATION

- ••• Odor of beverage alcohol on breath
- ••• Parotid gland enlargement, bilateral
- ••• Spider nevi or angioma
- ••• Edematous, "puffy face" (may be subtle); unexplained edema
- ••• Tremulousness, hallucinosis, and/ or 1 or 2 seizures
- •• Cigarette stains on fingers
- •• Breath mints odor
- •• Many scars or tattoos
- •• Hepatomegaly
- •• Gynecomastia
- •• Small testicles
- •• Unexplained bruises, abrasions, or cuts

- • Unexplained arrhythmias, especially chronic borderline tachycardia
- • Thin extremities in proportion to trunk
- • Splenomegaly
- • Hypertension
  Diaphoresis, day or night
  Very neat and clean
  Depression
  Alopecia
  Corneal arcus
  Abdominal tenderness
  Cerebellar signs (*e.g.,* nystagmus)
  Any depressed alteration in consciousness
  Anxiety

### LABORATORY ABNORMALITIES

- •••• Blood alcohol level greater than 300 mg/100 ml
- ••• Blood alcohol level greater than 100 mg/100 ml
- ••• High serum osmolality
- ••• High serum ammonia
- ••• SGOT elevated on admission, and normal by discharge
- ••• GGT elevation
- ••• Negative workups for hyperthyroidism
- •• Creatinine phosphokinase elevation
- •• Blood alcohol level positive, any amount
- •• High amylase

- •• Abnormal liver function tests
- •• Anemia, macrocytic or megaloblastic
- •• Hyperlipoproteinemia-type 4 or 5
- • Positive blood or urine for mood-changing drugs
- • Hyperuricemia (7 to 12 mg/100 ml most often; may be transient)
- • Small intestinal absorption test abnormalities
- • Hypophosphatemia or hypomagnesemia
  Electrolyte imbalance
  Elevated or low blood glucose
  Low white blood cell or platelet count

*Continued.*

Box 24-5

MEDICAL, PSYCHIATRIC, LEGAL, AND OTHER FINDINGS
SUGGESTIVE (0 TO •) TO HIGHLY SUGGESTIVE (•• TO •••) OR
DIAGNOSTIC (••••) OR ALCOHOLISM AND OTHER
CHEMICAL DEPENDENCE—cont'd

**X-RAY FILM FINDINGS**

••• Pancreatic calcification
••• Multiple rib fractures
•• "Aspiration pneumonia"

• Hepatomegaly
• Splenomegaly
• Nonfilling gallbladder

**DIAGNOSIS**

•••• Hepatitis, alcoholic
••• Pancreatitis, acute or chronic (40% to 95%)
••• Cirrhosis (85%)
••• Portal hypertension
••• Wernicke-Korsakoff syndrome
••• Frequent automobile or other accidents
••• Cold injury
••• Nose and throat cancer
•• Hepatitis non-A or B
•• Other chemical dependence
•• Drownings
•• Burns, especially third degree
•• Leaves hospital against medical advice (40% to 80%)

•• Attempted suicide
•• Gastritis
•• Refractory hypertension
•• Cerebellar degeneration
•• Peripheral neuropathy
•• Aspiration pneumonia
• Cerebral
• Cardiomyopathy
•• Anxiety
•• Any symptom or sign, cause not found, or unknown
• Depression
• Marital discord or family problem
• Fatty liver

A comprehensive chemical dependency assessment guide adapted from Estes et al. (1980) has been developed to obtain a nursing history from persons who may be abusing alcohol or drugs. This nursing history is only a guide, and additional appropriate questions may be necessary for clarification purposes. The questions on the guide are organized into specific content areas: demographic data, chief complaint, family history, psychosocial history, general health history, drinking and drug history, and nutritional history (Box 24-6).

**NURSING DIAGNOSIS**

Early diagnosis can mean a better treatment prognosis, as well as the difference between life and death. It is most important that the nurse look for behavioral as

### Box 24-6
## CHEMICAL DEPENDENCY ASSESSMENT GUIDE

**DEMOGRAPHIC DATA**

Name _____ Date _____

Address _____

Age _____ Sex _____ Ethnicity _____

Birthplace _____

Religion _____

Usual source of health care _____

**CHIEF COMPLAINT**

What brought you to the agency today?

What do you most want help with at the present time?

**FAMILY HISTORY**

Describe your ethnic or cultural background (degree of affiliation).

What is your family or marital status? (Describe your relationship with your parents or spouse or significant other.)

Do you have children? (Describe your relationship with your children.)

What is your most important and least important role in the family? (Is this a change from before?)

Was alcohol or drugs used in your family when you were growing up? If so, what was the pattern of use? (For example, did your mother drink or use drugs while she was pregnant?)

Would you describe any of your close relatives—grandparents, parents, siblings—as having an alcohol or **drug** problem?

**PSYCHOSOCIAL HISTORY**

Describe your present living arrangement (e.g., type of residence, persons you live with).

Do any of these people use alcohol or drugs regularly?

Does your present living arrangement differ greatly from the way you have lived in the past?

To whom do you feel close? (Is this a significant change from the past?)

Do they use drugs or alcohol regularly?

Are you presently employed or in school? (What is your usual occupation?)
- If no, what is your source of income?
- If retired, how do you manage your time?
- Is your present place of employment or occupation a significant change from before?

Adapted from Estes N, Smith-DiJulio K, and Heinemann E: Nursing diagnosis of the alcoholic person, St Louis, 1980, The CV Mosby Co.

*Continued.*

**Box 24-6**
## CHEMICAL DEPENDENCY ASSESSMENT GUIDE—cont'd

### PSYCHOSOCIAL HISTORY—cont'd

Describe your relationship with your peers or coworkers.
Are you actively affiliated with a religious group?
What other active affiliations do you have?
How do you spend leisure time?
What hobbies or special interests do you have?
How often and to what degree have you experienced any of the following?
  Depression _____
  Nervousness (anxiety) _____
  Extreme frustration or anger (violence) _____
  Extreme alienation from others _____
  Loneliness _____
  Suicidal thoughts or attempts _____
  Sexual problems _____
  Other emotional problems _____
What do you do when you have these experiences?
Have your ever received treatment for emotional problems (date and place)?
Are you currently taking any medications for emotional problems?
In general, how do you feel about yourself?
To what extent do you live up to expectations you have for yourself?
How successful are you in meeting expectations of others, including your parents
  or spouse, children, teachers or employer, and close friends?

### HEALTH HISTORY

History of present illness:
Describe your usual state of health.
Describe your current state of health.
  • Describe when, where, how long, and how often the problem occurs.
  • Describe the quality of the problem and any associated phenomena.
  • Has anyone in your family had similar problems?

### Past history:

What major illnesses or hospitalizations have you had?
What major accidents or injuries (e.g., head injuries, contusions or broken bones)
  have you experienced?
  • Were they due to fights, falls, auto crashes?

**Box 24-6**
## CHEMICAL DEPENDENCY ASSESSMENT GUIDE—cont'd

### HEALTH HISTORY—*cont'd*

Have you experienced any minor injuries or accidents such as bruises, cigarette burns, cuts?
* Were you using alcohol or drugs at either time?

What prescribed or over-the-counter medications are you currently taking?
* Why and when do you usually take these medications?

Are you allergic to any medications?

What kinds and amounts of beverages (e.g., coffee, soft drinks, tea) do you drink per day?

Do you smoke? Have you ever smoked? (Amount and length of use)

### Family health history:

Record age or age at death and relevant health problems (e.g., cancers of the liver and gastrointestinal tract, unexplained cardiomyopathy, tuberculosis, pneumonia, hypertension, pancreatitis, hepatitis or cirrhosis) of paternal and maternal grand-parents, parents, siblings, spouse, and children.

### Review of systems:

Have you experienced any of the following: sores that heal poorly, dermatitis, hair loss, frequent boils, psoriasis, a change in pigmentation such as large or small bright spots on the skin, presence of blood vessels or reddened palms?

Do you bruise easily?

Have you experienced difficulty in seeing at night, eye infections, or jerking movements of your eyes?

Have you experienced any problems with stomach or abdominal pain, nausea, constipation, vomiting or dry heaves, diarrhea, heartburn or gas, hemorrhoids?

Have you ever vomited blood? If yes, when?

Have you noticed a change in the color (e.g., clay-colored, black, or bright red) in your stools? If yes, when?

Have you ever had stomach ulcers or stomach problems?

Have you ever experienced any tremors, seizures, tingling, pain or numbness, muscle pain or weakness, difficulty in keeping your balance, double vision, mental confusion?
* Was drinking or any drug use involved?

Have you ever been unable to remember later what occurred while you were drinking?

*Continued.*

**Box 24-6**
## CHEMICAL DEPENDENCY ASSESSMENT GUIDE—cont'd

### HEALTH HISTORY—cont'd

Describe any problems you experience with your sleep?
- Do you feel rested?
- What do you do when you are unable to sleep?

Have you experienced any swelling or the hands and feet, chest pain, shortness of breath, rapid or irregular heartbeats, or varicose veins?

Have you ever been told that you have high blood pressure, anemia, or a blood disorder?

Have you experienced frequent colds, tuberculosis, coughing up blood, bronchitis, pneumonia, chronic cough, excessive phlegm?

Have you experienced pain on urination, blood in you rurine, frequent urination, difficulty in passing urine, a change in menses if you are a female, or enlargement in the size of your breasts and/or decrease in the size of your testicles if you are a male?

Are you sexually active? What method of contraception do you use?

Are you pregnant now if you are a female?

Have you given birth to an infant with defects?

Describe any changes in your sex life since your drug and alcohol use?

### DRINKING AND DRUG HISTORY

How old were you when you had your first drink or drug?

Do you recall how you felt?

How much does it take to get the same feeling now? (Is this a lot more or less than a year ago?)

If you were to total up the amount at the end of your day, how much would you say you drink or use drugs?

Have you ever decided to quit drinking or using drugs for a while or to cut down? What reactions did you experience (e.g., tremors, seizures, hear or see things, DT's.)

well as physical clues when she makes her assessment. Denial and the inability to control the use of alcohol or drugs are the two cardinal features of chemical dependency.

## Alcohol

The disease of alcoholism progresses predictably (Fig. 24-1). Early-stage warning signs include an enjoyment of drinking out of proportion to its social benefits and preoccupation with drinking. The amount of alcohol consumed during this stage is not of primary importance.

### Box 24-6
### CHEMICAL DEPENDENCY ASSESSMENT GUIDE—cont'd

Has anyone (parents/spouse, significant other, children, teachers/employers) worried about your drinking or drug use?

Has drinking or drug use interfered with your marriage or your relationship with your parents or significant other?

Do you and your parents, spouse, or significant other socialize often? (Do you go out often?)

Have you had any physical battles with your parents, wife, significant other, or children? Do you get mad more often when you drink or use drugs?

Have you been late to school or work or missed any school or work recently?

Have you ever been suspended from school or laid off or let go from a job? (Was drinking or drugs involved?)

Has anyone at school or your present job complained about your performance?

Have you ever been arrested, including traffic violations, because of drinking or using drugs (e.g., burglary, drunk in public, fights, driving while intoxicated)? Did you know what your blood alcohol level was?

How have you managed any of the above problems?

What previous treatments have you had for alcohol or drug problems?

**NUTRITIONAL HISTORY**

Describe everything you ate in the last 24 hours.

Would you describe it as typical of your usual diet?

During the middle stage the alcoholic begins to experience more and more problems in all areas of his life: interpersonal, occupational, social, and marital. Elaborate alibi systems, broken promises, guilt, self-pity, and loss of self-respect begin to emerge. Most early- and middle-stage alcoholics develop tolerance to alcohol and can drink large amounts without becoming obviously drunk. Nonetheless, drinking begins to take the toll described above.

The alcoholic loses all ability to control his alcohol intake during the late stage of his disease. He is no longer able to restrict his drinking to socially acceptable times and places. Late stage alcoholics lose their tolerance to alcohol and experience severe or life-threatening withdrawal symptoms. As the withdrawal symptoms become more severe, the craving for alcohol becomes more pronounced. The alcoholic is compelled to relieve these withdrawal symptoms and will suffer alcohol-related arrests, accidents, hospitalizations, financial problems, and ethical and moral deterioration to do so (Mueller and Ketcham, 1987).

Symptoms and Stages of Alcoholism

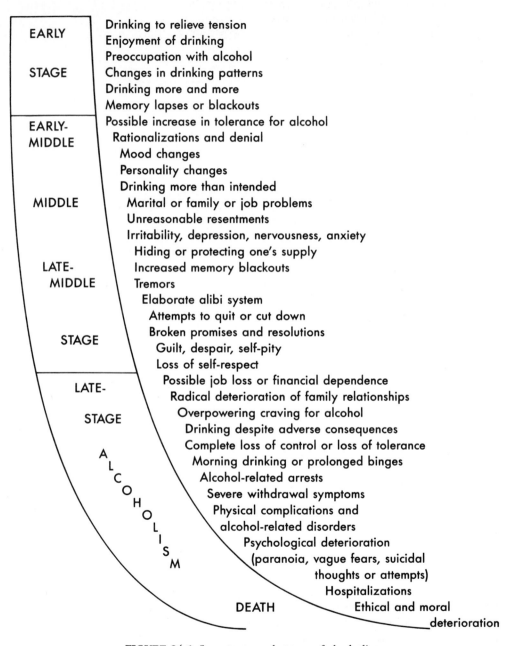

EARLY

STAGE

Drinking to relieve tension
Enjoyment of drinking
Preoccupation with alcohol
Changes in drinking patterns
Drinking more and more
Memory lapses or blackouts

EARLY-
MIDDLE

Possible increase in tolerance for alcohol
Rationalizations and denial
Mood changes
Personality changes
Drinking more than intended

MIDDLE

Marital or family or job problems
Unreasonable resentments
Irritability, depression, nervousness, anxiety
Hiding or protecting one's supply

LATE-
MIDDLE

Increased memory blackouts
Tremors
Elaborate alibi system
Attempts to quit or cut down

STAGE

Broken promises and resolutions
Guilt, despair, self-pity
Loss of self-respect

LATE-

Possible job loss or financial dependence
Radical deterioration of family relationships

STAGE

Overpowering craving for alcohol
Drinking despite adverse consequences
Complete loss of control or loss of tolerance

A
L
C
O
H
O
L
I
S
M

Morning drinking or prolonged binges
Alcohol-related arrests
Severe withdrawal symptoms
Physical complications and
alcohol-related disorders
Psychological deterioration
(paranoia, vague fears, suicidal
thoughts or attempts)
Hospitalizations
Ethical and moral
deterioration

DEATH

FIGURE 24-1 Symptoms and stages of alcoholism.

Potential nursing diagnoses include the following:

- Altered judgment related to unrealistic perceptions
- Ineffective coping related to inadequate coping methods
- Knowledge deficit related to denial of need for information
- Altered self-concept related to perceived failures
- Altered gastrointestinal processes related to abuse of alcohol
- Altered nutrition processes related to drinking alcohol instead of eating

## Drugs

Alcohol abuse and drug abuse have many similarities; however, there are several significant differences: alcohol is legal, whereas many drugs of abuse are illegal; stages of drug abuse tend to advance more rapidly, and drugs can produce their desired effect almost instantly. Potential nursing diagnoses include the following:

- Potential for injury related to drug intoxication
- Altered thought processes related to drug effects
- Knowledge deficit related to lack of interest in learning
- Altered self-concept related to lack of positive feedback
- Potential for self-directed violence related to drug withdrawal

### Screening tests

Several screening questionnaires have been developed to assist the health care professional in diagnosing chemical dependency. The MAST, or Michigan Alcoholism Screening Test (Box 24-7), is a reliable diagnostic screening test that can be given without extensive training (Powers and Spickard, 1984). It can be modified to identify other drug problems.

The CAGE questionnaire is another valid instrument and is easier and less incriminating than the MAST. The following four questions make up this tool:

1. Have you ever felt you should *C*ut down on your drinking?
2. Have people *A*nnoyed you by criticizing your drinking?
3. Have you ever felt bad or *G*uilty about your drinking?
4. Have you ever had a drink first thing in the morning to steady your nerves or get rid of a hangover (*E*ye-opener)?

Two positive responses are suggestive of alcoholism, and three or four positive responses are diagnostic (Whitfield et al., 1986). Schofield (1988) points out that questions 1 and 3 assess introspection and reflection on personal drinking, and question 2 provides reinforcement of this introspection by external cues. Question 4 reflects a change in behavior.

Another tool that distinguishes severity of alcoholism is the Drinking and You self-report instrument (Harrell and Wirtz, 1988). It was specifically developed for use with adolescents and taps four areas: loss of control and social, psychological, and physical symptoms.

The problem with most screening tests has been their susceptibility to faking and denial on the part of the patient (Creager, 1989). The MacAndrew Scale

## Box 24-7
## MICHIGAN ALCOHOLISM SCREENING TEST (MAST)*

|  | YES | NO |
|---|---|---|
| 0. Do you enjoy having a drink now and then? | 0 | |
| 1. Do you feel you are a normal drinker? (By normal we mean you drink less than or as much as most other people and you have not gotten into any recurring trouble while drinking.) | | 2 |
| 2. Have you ever awakened the morning after some drinking the night before and found that you could not remember a part of the evening? | 2 | |
| 3. Does either of your parents, or any other near relative, or your spouse, or any girlfriend or boyfriend ever worry or complain about your drinking? | 1 | |
| 4. Can you stop drinking without a struggle after one or two drinks? | | 2 |
| 5. Do you feel guilty about your drinking? | 1 | |
| 6. Do friends or relatives think you are a normal drinker? | | 2 |
| 7. Are you able to stop drinking when you want to? | | 2 |
| 8. Have you ever attended a meeting of Alcoholics Anonymous (AA)? | 5 | |
| 9. Have you gotten into physical fights when you have been drinking? | 1 | |
| 10. Has your drinking ever created problems between you and either of your parents, or another relative, your spouse, or any girlfriend or boyfriend? | 2 | |
| 11. Has any family member of yours ever gone to anyone for help about your drinking? | 2 | |
| 12. Have your ever lost friends because of your drinking? | 2 | |
| 13. Have you ever gotten into trouble at work or at school because of drinking? | 2 | |
| 14. Have you ever lost a job because of drinking? | 2 | |
| 15. Have you ever neglected your obligations, your school work, your family, or your job for 2 or more days in a row because you were drinking? | 2 | |
| 16. Do you drink before noon fairly often? | 1 | |

*Interpretation: *Standard MAST*—0 to 3 points = probable normal drinker; 4 points = borderline score; 5 to 9 points = 80% associated with alcoholism/chemical dependence; 10 or more = 100% associated with alcoholism.

From Whitfield C, Davis J and Barker L: Alcoholism. In Barker LR, Burton JR, and Zieve PD, editors: Principles of ambulatory medicine. Baltimore, 1986, Williams & Wilkins Co.

### Box 24-7
### MICHIGAN ALCOHOLISM SCREENING TEST (MAST)*—cont'd

|  | YES | NO |
|---|---|---|
| 17. Have you ever been told you have liver trouble? Cirrhosis? | 2 | ___ |
| 18. After heavy drinking have you ever had severe shaking, or heard voices or seen things that really weren't there? | 2(5 DTs) | ___ |
| 19. Have you ever gone to anyone for help about your drinking? | 5 | ___ |
| 20. Have you ever been in a hospital because of drinking? | 5 | ___ |
| 21. Have you ever been a patient in a psychiatric hospital or on a psychiatric ward of a general hospital where drinking was part of the problem that resulted in hospitalization? | 2 | ___ |
| 22. Have you ever been seen at a psychiatric or mental health clinic or gone to any doctor, social worker, or clergy for help with any emotional problem, where drinking was part of the problem? | 2 | ___ |
| 23. Have you ever been arrested for drunk driving, driving while intoxicated, or driving under the influence of alcoholic beverages or any other drug? (IF YES, How many times? ____) | 2 each | ___ |
| 24. Have you ever been arrested, or taken into custody, even for a few hours, because of other drunk behavior, whether due to alcohol or another drug? (IF YES, How many times? ____) | 2 each | ___ |

(MacAndrew, 1965), made up of appropriate items from the Minnesota Multiphasic Personality Inventory (MMPI) scale (Allen et al., 1988), and the Substance Abuse Scale have been developed to overcome denial and lying. The Substance Abuse Scale requires only 10 minutes to complete and claims 90% accuracy of diagnosis (Creager, 1989).

### PLANNING/INTERVENTION

Alcoholism is a highly treatable disease. Success of treatment for abuse of other substances varies, but all chemical dependencies can be helped. The success of treatment, however, depends on the health care professional's skill in interpreting the preceding data and implementing appropriate treatment strategies. The nurse must understand the following general intervention strategies to facilitate her working with *other intervention approaches.*

- Establish a trusting relationship with the patient and limit manipulative behavior.
- Treating the chemically dependent person as if his dependency is secondary to an underlying psychopathology is usually unsuccessful and often countertherapeutic. Accordingly, in-depth psychotherapy is contraindicated early in the treatment process. Chemically dependent persons seem to recover best in a group therapy setting (Whitfield et al., 1986). Groups are especially effective in breaking down the denial process among chemically dependent patients.
- Breaking down denial is the most difficult part of the therapeutic process. All chronic diseases commonly elicit *psychological denial* as a means to handle stress and fear and to suppress the emotional trauma. In *physical denial,* changes in the brain destroy the addict's ability to recognize the disease (Mueller and Ketcham, 1987). During the first weeks of treatment, denial is to be expected, and the nurse should not attempt to introduce reality if the patient is still in a toxic state or in withdrawal. Three effective techniques for breaking down denial are confrontation, offering hope and empathy, and tough love.
- The nurse needs to recognize the symptoms of a still actively addicted mind such as stubbornness, belligerence, mood swings, and violent and aggressive behavior and to confront the patient with them after the withdrawal period. Confrontation involves telling a patient what you observe no matter how strong the denial. For example, "You say that you have not been drinking (or using drugs), but I can smell alcohol on your breath (or found cocaine in your urine sample)."
- Offering the patient hope and empathy is crucial. Explaining to the patient that he has a disease, that it is not his fault, and that it is treatable conveys such a message.
- Tough love primarily involves allowing the patient to take responsibility for his recovery. The patient is often not able to do this initially because of denial.
- Look for potential motivators in the patient's environment. Few people with smooth-running lives suddenly decide to seek help. On the contrary, most patients' lives have begun to crumble before they seek out professional help: The wife is divorcing him, the boss is firing him, the judge is sentencing him. As the nurse understands the patient's motivators, she is better able to support healthy aspects of his motivational system.
- Since marital, occupational, legal, and social problems typically are the reason(s) a person seeks treatment, helping the patient gain stability in these areas is an important intervention strategy. The nurse must guard against taking responsibility for these problems. Many alcoholics and addicts have been enabled to continue in their chemical dependency because well-meaning people have shielded them from their problems.
- It is naive for the nurse to believe that patients in treatment do not use drugs. In some hospitals "pushers" are relatively blatant in their efforts to sell drugs to patients. The only way to know for sure whether a patient is "clean" is to routinely obtain urine samples for laboratory analysis (Table 24-2). Urine

samples must be obtained in such a manner that the nurse positively knows that it is the patient's own urine.

- It is important to create a safe environment for the patient. Fearfulness and anxiety are common themes among patients withdrawing from drugs.
- Teach the patient the effects of chemical abuse on the body.
- Provide for physical and nutritional needs of the patient. Exercise is crucial to increase mental and physical vitality as are relaxation, avoidance of stress, and rest. A balanced diet and vitamin and mineral supplements are essential parts of treatment and recovery.
- Teach patient assertiveness techniques.
- Encourage and arrange for follow-up services such as aftercare, counseling, Alcoholics Anonymous (AA), and Narcotics Anonymous (NA).

## Other interventions

A number of programs exist for the treatment of chemical dependency. That these various programs exist gives testimony to the complexity and seriousness of chemical dependencies in North America.

**Alcoholics Anonymous.** The best known intervention programs are Alcoholics Anonymous (AA) and Narcotics Anonymous (NA). These programs use a self-help, support group model made up of fellow users in various stages of "recovery." Philosophically, AA and NA view psychosocial problems as stemming from substance abuse and reject the idea that an underlying psychopathology is reponsible for drinking or drug use. AA has established the Twelve Step system (Box 24-8), which starts with a man admitting his powerlessness over alcohol and ends with that person's making himself available, night or day, to another alcoholic in need. The popular bumper sticker slogan "Easy does it" reflects a philosophy of taking life one day at a time and avoiding a frenetic life-style. AA and NA subscribe to the belief that only *total abstinence* can free the chemically dependent person from the bondage of alcohol and drugs.

**More traditional programs.** Programs developed by more traditionally oriented mental health professionals may view underlying problems, such as depression or bipolar illness, as the cause of substance abuse. The goal of therapy is to treat the underlying problem. Successful treatment of the underlying problem facilitates resolution of the chemical dependency. Such programs may use a group format or individual therapy format.

**Inpatient specialty hospitals.** Several hospital corporations specialize in treating chemically dependent persons. They advertise on television and market their services to those who can afford them. These facilities have developed programs to help the abuser abstain from taking his "drug of choice." For example, one nationally known facility uses aversive therapy to treat alcoholics. This particular approach to aversive therapy has the patient drink his favorite alcoholic beverage followed by an emetic to make him vomit. The psychological association between the beverage and the vomiting eventually creates an aversion to alcohol.

**Self-help groups.** AA and NA are the best known self-help groups, but there are other, less well known self-help groups that are used by thousands of people. A self-help group by definition is composed of people with something in common. In

**Box 24-8**
## TWELVE STEPS OF ALCOHOLICS ANONYMOUS

1. We admitted we were powerless over alcohol—that our lives had become unmanageable.
2. Came to believe that a Power greater than ourselves could restore us to sanity.
3. Made a decision to turn our will and our lives over to the care of God, as we understood Him.
4. Made a searching and fearless moral inventory of ourselves.
5. Admitted to God, ourselves, and to another human being the exact nature of our wrongs.
6. Were entirely ready to have God remove all these defects of character.
7. Humbly asked Him to remove our shortcomings.
8. Made a list of all persons we had harmed and became willing to make amends to them all.
9. Made direct amends to such people wherever possible except when to do so would injure them or others.
10. Continued to take personal inventory and when we were wrong promptly admitted it.
11. Sought through prayer and meditation to improve our conscious contact with God, as we understood Him, praying only for knowledge of His will for us and the power to carry that out.
12. Having had a spiritual awakening as the result of these steps, we tried to carry this message to alcoholics and to practice these principles in all our affairs.

From *Twelve Steps and Twelve Traditions,* Alcoholic Anonymous World Services, Inc.

the case of substance-abuse self-help groups the commonality is chemical dependency. Self-help groups work because the new member recognizes that others in the group have been where he is and truly understand his situation.

## EVALUATION

Abstinence is the first step in accomplishing the goals of treatment and is the foundation for the four major levels of recovery from chemical dependency: physical, mental, emotional, and spiritual (Mueller and Ketcham, 1987). Knowledge that the addiction is chronic and will always be present is an essential factor in the recovery process.

Appropriate physical and nutritional intervention is essential for *physical recovery* from protracted withdrawal symptoms such as irritability, depression, anxiety, altered nutrition, gastrointestinal problems, insomnia, mood swings, and cravings caused by lingering cell damage, malnutrition, and hypoglycemia. See Box 24-9 for the evaluation criteria for physical recovery.

### Box 24-9
## EVALUATION CRITERIA FOR THE FOUR LEVELS OF RECOVERY FROM CHEMICAL DEPENDENCY

**Physical recovery**

- Decreased levels of stress and anxiety
- Weight gain or stability
- Proper nutritional intake
- Ability and willingness to discuss the relationships between chemical abuse and malnutrition
- Adequate quality and quantity of sleep
- Physiological stability, for example, gastrointestinal system and vital sign stability

**Mental recovery**

- Willingness to meet with the nurse and discuss problems openly
- Taking responsibility for own behavior
- Improvement in problem-solving skills
- Setting and reaching goals
- Attendance at AA or NA meetings
- Repeating information about alcohol or drugs
- Adhering to the treatment program in general, for example, takes Antabuse
- Abstaining from chemicals (no drinking, "clean" urine samples)

**Emotional recovery**

- Ability to discuss feelings, anxieties, and fears
- Ability to make assertive statements
- Working through and subsequent decrease of guilt and grief over past indiscretions
- Improved self-esteem
- Decreased impulsive behavior

**Spiritual recovery**

- Admitting powerlessness over alcohol or drugs
- Working the 12-step program of AA or NA
- Involvement in unit treatment program
- Making amends for past mistakes when possible
- Helping other substance abusers gain and maintain abstinence

*Mental recovery* is based on the patient's ability to identify symptoms of the addicted mind or "stinking thinking": rationalization, denial, minimizing, and projection. The nurse must be aware of these unhealthy defense mechanisms and reinforce the patient as he is able to think in healthier ways. Every alcoholic or addict should be encouraged to attend AA or NA meetings regularly. Regular attendance at AA or NA meetings is strongly correlated with long-term recovery and improved functioning (Vaillant et al., 1983) and is an important evaluation criterion. If a patient is having trouble attending AA or NA for any reason, the nurse should assess and try to solve the problem. See Box 24-9 for the evaluation criteria for mental recovery.

*Emotional recovery* is the third level of recovery. The chemically dependent person has been emotionally anesthetized and developmentally retarded because of his drug use. Self-identity, determination, and love have never had the opportunity to mature appropriately. Thus the patient needs to learn to feel and accept a variety of emotions as well as to communicate them in an assertive manner. The latter may involve the use of support systems, which become available through sobriety such as aftercare, counseling, and AA or NA (Mueller and Ketcham, 1987).

Feelings may also erupt from the way we think about things. The "stinking thinking" identified earlier is an example of thinking that can lead to emotional problems. Applying the theoretical principles of rational emotive therapy (Chapter 2) allows a patient to take responsibility for his emotions and to learn to act upon them and not just react to them. AA or NA also applies this approach by assisting the patient in dealing with his guilt and grief, especially over the past. See Box 24-9 for the evaluation criteria for emotional recovery.

*Spiritual recovery* involves the spirit and spiritual values (Mueller and Ketcham, 1987). Some persons identify this spirit as God, and others think of it as all that is good within us and the world. Whatever this spirit is for the patient, it is stronger and larger than the patient. The building blocks of this spirit are spiritual values such as trust, caring, love, courage, honesty, humility, and forgiveness. Just as one's emotional life needs to be rebuilt during the process of recovery, so does the spiritual life. Spiritual recovery begins with a process called "surrender." Surrender is not defeat but a yielding to a spirit greater than the person and an admission of powerlessness in controlling the disease. Thus the patient is able to reach out and accept help from outside himself. See Box 24-9 for the evaluation criteria for spiritual recovery.

## FOLLOW-UP CARE

Patients and nurses need to be aware that recovery has only begun when an inpatient or outpatient program is completed. The few months immediately following completion of a treatment program are dangerous for the chemically dependent person. Relapse is not uncommon. For this reason follow-up care is essential. The nurse should confirm that arrangements for aftercare, outpatient counseling, and AA or NA are made before discharge.

## KEY CONCEPTS

1. Chemical dependency is a major physical and mental health problem in North America, and most nurses, whether they want to or not, will take care of chemically dependent people.

2. Drugs of abuse can be categorized into four basic groups: *Alcohol and other CNS depressants; opioids* (morphine, heroin), *stimulants* (amphetamines, cocaine, crack, crank), and *hallucinogens,* (mescaline, marijuana, LSD, PCP).

3. The DSM-III-R distinguishes between substance dependence and substance abuse, with substance dependence indicating a more severe, physiological dependence on a drug.

4. Alcohol is the No. 1 drug problem in North America; it exacts a high price economically from our society and is responsible for great suffering and death.

5. Alcohol causes disinhibition and impaired judgment and it is relaxing when first used. The primary concern with respect to alcohol overdose is severe and often fatal CNS depression. Withdrawal causes tremors, nausea, vomiting, tachycardia, diaphoresis, seizures, anxiety, and depression. Withdrawal can be fatal.

6. Other CNS depressants include barbiturates (downers, reds, blues, rainbows), minor tranquilizers such as Librium (green and whites), antipsychotic drugs, methaqualone (ludes), and inhalants (gasoline, cement for model airplanes).

7. Depressants cause relief from anxiety, euphoria, disinhibition, and drowsiness. The primary effect of overdose is respiratory depression. Withdrawal from depressants can be life threatening.

8. Opioids (narcotics) come from the juice of the opium poppy, with opium being the natural product and morphine, codeine, and heroin being easily derived from the poppy juice. Synthetic preparations such as meperidine (Demerol), pentazocine (Talwin), propoxyphene (Darvon), and methadone (Dolophin) have been developed in the vain search for a pain reliever with no addicting qualities.

9. Opioids are taken intravenously, orally, intramuscularly, and subcutaneously ("skin popping"). Overdose can be fatal, with respiratory depression being the most serious side effect. Withdrawal, while miserable (flulike symptoms), is not particularly serious.

10. Nalaxone (Narcan) is a narcotic neuroreceptor blocker and is given in emergency rooms to treat opioid overdose. Nalaxone causes an opioid-abstinence syndrome.

11. Stimulants include amphetamines and cocaine. Stimulants cause elation, grandiose thinking, talkativeness, and other less pleasant effects. The primary concerns in the event of overdose are agitation, tachycardia, cardiac arrhythmias, and convulsions. Withdrawal from stimulants, while miserable, is not particularly serious.

12. Hallucinogens include mescaline, marijuana, LSD, and PCP. Hallucinogens cause illusions, hallucinations, diminished ability to perceive time and distance, anxiety, and paranoid thinking. The primary effects of hallucinogenic overdose are intense "trips," psychotic reactions, and panic. Withdrawal from hallucinogens

can cause anxiety, fear, and panic. However, physical withdrawal has not been found to be particularly serious.

13. While several treatment approaches are effective, the goal for all approaches is abstinence from the substance.
14. Nursing interventions include group work, education, confrontation, tough love, providing for physical and nutritional needs, and helping the patient become involved in AA and NA.
15. Abstinence is the foundation for physical, mental, emotional, and spiritual recovery.

## REFERENCES

Allen JP, Eckardt MJ, and Wallen J: Screening for alcoholism: techniques and issues, Public Health Rep 103:6, 1988.

Ananth J et al: Missed diagnosis of substance abuse in psychiatric patients, Hosp Community Psychiatry 40:297, 1989.

Carey KB: Emerging treatment guidelines for mentally ill chemical abusers, Hosp Community Psychiatry 40:341, 1989.

Creager C: SASSI test breaks through denial, Professional Counselor, p 65, July-August, 1989.

DiGregorio GJ: Cocaine update: abuse and therapy, Am Fam Physician 41:247, 1990.

Estes N and Heinemann ME: Issues in identification of alcoholism. In Alcoholism: development, consequences, and interventions, ed 3, St. Louis, 1986, The CV Mosby Co.

Estes N, Smith-DiJulio K, and Heinemann ME: Nursing diagnosis of the alcoholic person, St. Louis, 1980, The CV Mosby Co.

Frezza M et al: High blood alcohol levels in women, N Engl J Med 322(2):95, 1990.

Goodwin DW et al: Alcohol problems in adoptees raised apart from alcoholic biological parents, Arch Gen Psychiatry 28:238, 1973.

Harrell AV and Wirtz PW: Screening adolescents for drinking problems, Paper presented at 1988 National Alcoholism Forum, Arlington, Va., April 1988.

Hough ESE: Alcoholism: prevention and treatment, J Psychosoc Nurs 27(1):15, 1989.

Joyce T: The dramatic increase in the rate of low birthweight in New York City: an aggregate time-series analysis, Am J Public Health 80:682, 1990.

Lewis DC and Gordon AJ: Alcoholism and the general hospital: the Roger Williams Intervention Program, Bull N Y Acad Med 59:181, 1983.

MacAndrew C: The differentiation of male alcoholic outpatients from non-alcoholic psychiatric outpatients by means of the MMPI, Q J Stud Alcoholism, vol. 26, 1965.

Mueller LA and Ketcham K: Recovering: how to get and stay sober, New York, 1987, Bantam Books.

Noble J: Working paper: projections of alcohol abusers, 1980, 1985, 1990, Washington DC, 1985, NIAAA, Department of Biometry and Epidemiology.

Ohlms D: The disease of alcoholism [videotape], Millstadt, Ill., 1988, Gary Whitaker Corporation.

Peyser HS: Alcohol and drug abuse: underrecognized and untreated, Hosp Community Psychiatry 40:221, 1989.

Powers JS and Spickard A: Michigan alcoholism screening test to diagnose early alcoholism in a general practice. South Med J 77:852, 1984.

Regans P: ABC News/Washington Post Poll, Survey #0190, 1985.

Schofield A: The CAGE questionnaire and psychological health, Br J Addict 83:761, 1988.

Smith AR et al: Trends in psychotropic drug prescribing practice and general medical patients, Postgrad Med J 62:637, 1986.

Vaillant G et al: Prospective study of alcoholism treatment, Am J Med 75:455, 1983.

Wallace J: Alcoholism: New light on the disease, Newport, R.I., 1985, Edgehill Publications.

Whitfield C, Davis J, and Barker L: Alcoholism. In Barker LR, Burton JR, and Zieve PD, editors: Principles of ambulatory medicine, Baltimore, 1986, Williams & Wilkins Co.

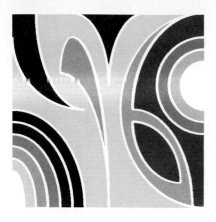

## CHAPTER 25

# Eating Disorders

GALE R. WOOLLEY

LEARNING OBJECTIVES

After reading this chapter you should be able to

- Recognize DSM-III-R criteria and terminology for eating disorders.
- Recognize and describe objective and subjective symptoms of eating disorders.
- Describe biological theoretical explanations for eating disorders.
- Describe psychodynamic theoretical explanations for eating disorders.
- Develop a nursing care plan for a person who has an eating disorder.
- Evaluate the effectiveness of nursing interventions for patients with an eating disorder.

Although eating disorders have been recognized since the late 1600s, they did not receive widespread attention until the 1980s, when the media began to reveal stories of celebrities and young girls suffering from these illnesses. In January 1983 Karen Carpenter, a popular singer, died of complications of anorexia nervosa. Shortly thereafter, Cherry Boone, singer Pat Boone's daughter, revealed her agonizing years with anorexia, and actress Jane Fonda publicly announced her fight with bulimia. Most recently, television personality Oprah Winfrey has disclosed her difficulties with overeating and obesity. Thus the 1980s was a significant decade in the awareness of eating disorders, not only because there was particular attention paid to "thinness" and physical conditioning but also because the public began to realize the life-threatening dangers of these illnesses. What follows in this chapter is a presentation of the psychopathology, a case study, and nursing care plans for patients with anorexia nervosa and bulimia nervosa.

## ANOREXIA NERVOSA
### DSM-III-R criteria

The DSM-III-R diagnostic criteria for anorexia nervosa are found in Box 25-1. The major characteristics include a self-inflicted weight loss aimed at maintaining body weight 15% below minimal normal weight for height and age; an intense fear of becoming fat, even though the person is obviously underweight; a distortion of body image, so that the person perceives herself to be fat when actually she is underweight; and amenorrhea (cessation of the menstrual cycle) for at least 3 consecutive months.

### Box 25-1
### DIAGNOSTIC CRITERIA FOR 307.10 ANOREXIA NERVOSA

A. Refusal to maintain body weight over a minimal normal weight for age and height, e.g., weight loss leading to maintenance of body weight 15% below that expected; or failure to make expected weight gain during period of growth, leading to body weight 15% below that expected.
B. Intense fear of gaining weight or becoming fat, even though underweight.
C. Disturbance in the way in which one's body weight, size, or shape is experienced, e.g., the person claims to "feel fat" even when emaciated, believes that one area of the body is "too fat" even when obviously underweight.
D. In females, absence of at least three consecutive menstrual cycles when otherwise expected to occur (primary or secondary amenorrhea). (A woman is considered to have amenorrhea if her periods occur only following hormone, e.g., estrogen, administration.)

Reprinted with permission from the *Diagnostic and Statistical Manual of Mental Disorders, Third Edition, Revised.* Copyright 1987 American Psychiatric Association.

The DSM-III-R reports that 95% of anorectic patients are female, with the usual age at onset in early to late adolescence. The reported prevalence ranges have varied from 1 in 800 to 1 in 100 girls between the ages of 12 and 18 years.

Although anorexia may be episodic or persist until death, the most common course of illness consists of a single episode with a return to normal weight. Szmukler (1987) states that the illness rarely lasts less than 2 years, with 40% to 60% of those patients who are sick enough to be hospitalized completely recovering, and 20% persisting with a chronic course. The DSM-III-R reports that anywhere from 5% to 18% of those in whom anorexia nervosa is diagnosed die of complications of the illness.

## Behavior

As is true of all psychiatric disorders, the primary symptoms of anorexia nervosa are acutally behaviors. These behaviors are maladaptive in the sense that they are, for the most part, detrimental to the person's well-being.

The onset of anorexia can often be considered insidious (not readily apparent) because the typical adolescent girl who becomes a victim usually portrays an image of being the "perfect little girl," never causing problems for anyone. As dieting and fad foods are such common themes in adolescence, it usually is not until the young woman has lost a significant amount of weight that anyone takes notice.

The term *anorexia* is actually a misnomer, because anorectic patients do not really lose their appetite. On the contrary, they are often quite hungry but suppress their hunger in an effort to remain thin—what they perceive to be attractive. Because the symptoms of anorexia nervosa involve so much of the patient's perceptions (which differ drastically from other people's perceptions of the patient), objective and subjective behaviors will be presented separately.

**Objective signs.** The most obvious observable behavior of anorexia nervosa is the deliberate weight loss. Patients have such a preoccupation with food and such a need to control their weight that their eating behavior changes significantly. Abraham and Llewellyn-Jones (1987) divide patients with anorexia nervosa into two groups: the dieters and the vomiters and purgers. The dieters are those young women who had been in the normal weight range for height and build before the eating disorder began. They view losing weight as more probable if they simply eat less and avoid social situations in which eating is expected. Consequently this group of young women often isolate themselves socially, and others note that they increasingly alienate themselves from their friends and family, often withdrawing into their rooms. It is not uncommon for these young women to be competitive and obsessive about their actitivites. They also are often observed participating in a rigid exercise program to help reduce their weight.

The vomiters and purgers usually were overweight before the eating disorder began. Their weight tends to fluctuate. These young women are more prone to dangerous methods of weight reduction, such as induction of vomiting or excessive use of laxatives. This group of anorectic patients will commonly deny that they are concerned about their weight and will eat normally in a social situation. After the meal they will retreat to the nearest bathroom and purge themselves of the consumed food. Dental problems frequently occur in these patients because the acidic vomitus decays the enamal on their teeth.

Some researchers use the symptom of amenorrhea as a criterion for diagnosing anorexia nervosa, as it is always present in these patients (Mitchell, 1986). It is not uncommon for menstruation to cease early in the illness, before any significant weight loss takes place. The most accepted theory for the cause of the amenorrhea is that the lack of nourishment significantly slows the functioning of the hypothalamus and pituitary glands, which are fundamental to the menstrual cycle. In addition, some studies have shown abnormalities in estrogen metabolism in anorectic patients, which would also affect menstruation (Weiner, 1983).

Since the intake of nutrients, and thus energy, is so low in anorectic patients, the body must try to adjust by using less energy. Consequently, other physiological processes are affected as well. Constipation, hypotension, bradycardia, and hypothermia are commonly reported. In addition, the skin is often dry, and lanugo, or fine, downy hair, appears. Pitting edema occurs in a smaller number of anorectic patients, most often after attempts to gain weight by eating more food. When the young woman notices the swelling, she immediately stops trying to increase her weight and may even be motivated to use diuretics, further complicating the problem.

Many anorectic patients become hyperactive and are unable to relax. It is not uncommon for them to complain of insomnia and to be seen taking early morning walks.

Personality changes in the anorectic patient become obvious. The preoccupation with food seems to involve all aspects of the patient's life. Multiple reading materials on food and dieting appear frequently in the patient's hands, and she often attempts to take control over the family meals since she believes she is the resident authority on nutrition in the household.

Since most anorectic patients are adolescents, they spend much of their time in school. Their performance in school is usually outstanding, most of them often being at the top of their class academically. Their behavior is not overtly a problem. On the contrary, they are usually model students, participating in school activities and achieving honors of some kind.

**Subjective symptoms.**  One of the most outstanding features of anorexia nervosa is the conscious fear the young woman has of losing control over the amount of food she eats and of becoming fat. It is actually this fear that motivates her to begin the diet and weight-losing efforts. The fear may have been triggered by one event that could be considered rather trivial in the minds of many, or one that actually was quite traumatic. Usually the patient at times has felt abandoned or inadequate, which precipitates an overall feeling of helplessness (Casper, 1982). This feeling of helplessness triggers, through the reaction-formation defense mechanism, the need to control. The one aspect of her life that she perceives she has the capability to control is her weight and the amount of food she eats. Consequently, most of her energy becomes invested in this effort.

Control becomes a recurring issue for anorectic patients. Perhaps the most terrifying fear, besides feeling out of control, is of having to be spontaneous at any given time (Flood, 1989). As a result of this fear, the patient will design some rigid structure for almost everything she does. For this reason, anorectic patients are often said to be obsessive-compulsive, as anxiety is experienced if the person cannot perform a task in a specific way.

Anorectic patients will often complain of depression, and their behavior is indicative of this feeling as well. There is usually a loss of interest in social activities, particularly with boyfriends. They prefer more solitary projects, such as writing poems or stories or listening to music. The theme of such endeavors is commonly sad or morbid.

## Etiology

It would be virtually impossible to write a chapter on eating disorders without mentioning the contribution of the psychiatrist Hilde Bruch. Bruch believed that anorexia was caused by a number of specific disturbances (1973). Today most experts agree and have conducted a significant amount of research in recent years to support their beliefs. There now is evidence to suggest that the cause of eating disorders may be both biological and psychodynamic. Many of the modern etiological theories of eating disorders are outgrowths of Bruch's work. The most popular of these theories will be presented.

**Biological theories.** The biological theories of anorexia nervosa stress that there is some type of physical abnormality in the patient. These anatomical or physiological deviations are the main "cause" of the illness, and any psychological disturbances the patient may have stem from the physical problem.

Since the hypothalamus regulates eating and sexual functions, it is believed that perhaps a disturbance in this area is responsible for anorexia nervosa. However, studies on the hypothalamus have been difficult to validate because disturbances in this area might also be a result of starvation. One study has shown that when weight has been restored, the hormonal abnormalities that involve the hypothalamus return to normal (Brown, 1983). Yet numerous studies have shown that disturbances in the hypothalamic-pituitary-ovarian axis, which is responsible for the amenorrhea, do not necessarily resolve soon after weight restoration.

Another biological theory for the development of anorexia nervosa involves disturbances in the neurotransmitters, particularly in the regulation of the dopaminergic systems. Specifically, one study has shown that there is an impaired response of growth hormone to L-dopa (Halmi and Sherman, 1977).

**Psychodynamic theories.** The most widely accepted etiological theories of anorexia nervosa are those that suggest psychological disturbances. One is that the illness is a phobia of normal weight, although in a true phobia the patient is aware that the fear is irrational. The illness involves a regression to a prepubertal state so that the adolescent does not mature physically or emotionally. There is a strong secondary gain of having dependency needs met in this situation, and thus the regression is reinforced. This conscious fear of becoming fat is the symbolic expression of becoming bigger, or growing up, which is the real, unconscious fear of the anorectic patient.

Another theory describes anorexia nervosa as an obsession with weight that stems from a fear of being out of control. In response to this fear the patient, via reaction formation, attempts to organize her life with a whole set of rules and regulations for everything she does. She experiences a tremendous amount of anxiety if one of her rules is broken and attempts to regain control by tightening her rules. Her eating behavior appears to be the most available area of her life through which to achieve her goal.

Bruch (1973) postulated that the three main areas of disturbance in the anorectic patient are body image, interoceptive stimuli, and self-esteem. The disturbed body image means that the patient overestimates the size of her body or body parts. She perceives herself as fat, when in actuality she is grossly underweight. A quick way to assess the severity of the body image disturbance in the anorectic patient is to observe the manner in which she dresses. If the body image disturbance is severe, the patient is likely to be wearing clothes that overweight people wear, such as dresses with no waistlines, baggy pants with elastic waistlines, and large, oversized tops.

The interoceptive disturbance means that the patient has difficulty discriminating between hunger and satiety. In addition, the patient has trouble identifying other stimuli, such as fatigue, cold, and sexual feelings.

The disturbance in self-esteem is reflected in the patient's tremendous sense of inadequacy. Although she is usually quite bright, attractive, and well liked, the anorectic adolescent perceives herself as an ugly and overall ineffective person.

### Special issues related to anorexia nervosa

To understand the complex problems that an anorectic patient presents to the treatment team, two special issues related to this illness must be further discussed: family dynamics and sexuality of anorectic patients.

**Family dynamics of anorectic patients.**  From the time anorexia nervosa was first identified, common familial patterns have been observed. First, most of the families are white, in the upper middle-income level, and able to devote both emotional and financial attention to their daughters. The young women often view their parents as smothering, intrusive, and overprotective. They do not wish to be the center of attention that they frequently are. Their food refusal is thought to be, in part, a form of rebellion against their parents and soon becomes a central issue for the family.

In the early stage of the illness, when the patient begins to refuse food, the family initially tries to coax her to eat. Because the mother is typically the primary provider of the family meals, the conflict seems to intensify between her and the patient. When the coaxing fails, the mother begins to serve the patient's favorite foods and to stress that cooking for her and eating together as a family is one way in which they can express love to each other. Guilt, therefore, becomes a prominent issue because the girl hears the message that, if she really loves her parents, she will eat for them.

As the disease progresses, the family speaks of little but the girl's eating behavior. The girl is confronted with the issue constantly. She attends meals more often and eats minute amounts in an effort to relieve some of the parental pressure to eat.

However, it is not long before her emaciation becomes obvious and the family realizes the need to provide their daughter with medical attention quickly.

**Anorexia and sexuality** Freud believed that the human being has two basic drives: sexual and aggressive. Not surprising, then, is his interpretation of anorexia nervosa. Freud postulated that the appetite is an expression of libido, or sexual drive. Therefore, when one states she does not have an appetite, her sexual drive is also absent. Food and eating are a symbol of nurturing and love. The anorectic patient rejects nurturing. Thus the anorectic patient does not eat because food and sex are repulsive to her.

Today many experts have either modified or rejected many of Freud's theories. However, those working with anorectic patients do admit there are significant sexual issues with their clients. Abraham and Llewellyn-Jones (1987) identify four categories of sexual behavior in patients with eating disorders. The three common in anorexia are:

1. Sexuality denied, in which the young woman suppresses her sexual feelings and has negative attitudes toward puberty, menstruation, masturbation, and sexual intercourse
2. Unsure of sexuality, in which the young woman finds it difficult to form a warm, mature relationship
3. Sexually passive, in which the young woman does not enjoy sexual behavior but accepts and tolerates it to have a socially expected relationship

---

### PSYCHOTHERAPEUTIC MANAGEMENT

As this book is designed around psychotherapeutic management, the nurse-patient relationship, psychopharmacology, and milieu management, these concepts as they relate to anorexia nervosa will be presented. However, there is no specific psychopharmacology that alleviates any eating disorders. Medication is sometimes prescribed to help alleviate some of the symptoms aggravated by the disorder, such as anxiety, depression, or somatic disturbances. Consequently the reader will be referred to Units II to IV for review in these areas.

Psychotherapeutic management is geared toward three major objectives:

1. Increasing self-esteem to the level at which the patient is confident enough of her own self-worth that she does not need the artificial perfection that she believes thinness provides for her
2. Increasing the weight to at least 90% of the average body weight for height and age
3. Helping the patient reestablish appropriate eating behavior

When the patient is in the starvation phase of the illness and malnutrition has become a serious medical problem, treatment usually occurs in a medical environment in which appropriate supplies and equipment, such as intravenous and feeding tube apparatuses are readily available. When the medical crisis is resolved, the patient is transferred to a psychiatric unit or is seen on an outpatient basis where psychotherapeutic intervention can occur effectively.

Working with an anorectic patient usually presents a challenge to the psychotherapeutic team, as the patient continues the struggle to maintain control. When the treatment team requires weight gain, the young woman perceives herself as losing control, which in turn triggers the unconscious feeling of helplessness. Consciously, the patient once again experiences the fear of becoming fat. This fear underlies the need to gain more control, restarting the vicious cycle.

*THE NURSE-PATIENT RELATIONSHIP* As most anorectic patients are in treatment under duress, it is usually a challenge for the nurse to develop a therapeutic alliance (Deering, 1987). The primary belief is that the nurse is there simply to make the patient gain weight, so she is perceived as an enemy rather than an ally. Specific principles of therapeutic communication helpful in facilitating a nurse-patient relationship with an anorectic patient are presented below.

- Convey warmth and sincerity to the patient. The patient needs to believe that the nurse genuinely cares about her and understands her effort to overcome the ambivalence about being in treatment. Increasing the patient's self-esteem is a primary objective in the patient's recovery.
- Listen empathically. Although the patient is likely to deny the weight as a problem, she will admit to feeling extremely lonely and tired of striving to be perfect all the time. A caring, empathic nurse will help foster the patient's ability to express her feelings.
- Be honest. The patient will enter treatment basically distrustful of everyone. For her treatment to be successful, she must establish a trusting relationship with the nurse. Honesty is imperative for this trusting relationship to occur.
- Set limits. Because of her strong need to be in control, the patient will attempt to manipulate the nurse. A clear contract must be established between the nurse and the patient in an effort to establish trust and to minimize power struggles.
- Assist the patient in identifying at least three positive qualities about herself. Because her level of self-esteem is so low, the patient needs to see concrete evidence that she has some redeeming qualities.
- Collaborate with the patient. To elicit cooperation on the part of the patient, it is imperative to engage her in the planning process. This not only will foster the development of trust but also will provide her with a sense of control in her treatment.
- Teach the patient about her illness. The more information the patient receives about anorexia, the harder it is for her to deny her illness. In addition, knowledge of her illness will help the patient understand what is happening with her body, as well as instill confidence that the nurse is capable of helping her.
- Avoid long silences. Although silence is primarily a therapeutic technique that allows the patient time to gather her thoughts, long silences are not necessarily helpful to the anorectic patient, as they may cause the patient to feel abandoned.

- Initiate a behavior-modification program that rewards weight gain with meaningful privileges. Although the idea of gaining weight will be stressful to the patient, it is imperative for her recovery. As soon as a safe weight is attained, allow the patient to regulate her own progression and program.
- Identify non-weight-related interests of the patient. If reactivated, these interests can reduce anxiety, since the patient will be investing energies in areas that do not deal with eating.

*MILIEU MANAGEMENT* The decision to hospitalize an anorectic patient is a controversial one. However, when a young woman has starved herself to the point where she is experiencing serious malnutrition problems or becomes suicidal, hospitalization becomes essential to save her life. As general principles for milieu management were presented in Unit IV, only those that specifically address management of the anorectic patient will be presented here.

- Provide a warm, nurturing atmosphere. It is imperative that the patient feel support from the structure of the hospital to reduce her anxiety and increase her self-esteem.
- Observe the patient closely. The eating behaviors need to be identified so that the staff can plan appropriate interventions. Common eating behaviors include hiding food in a paper napkin to be discarded, leaving bread crusts on the plate and discarding the rest, discarding food into plants or out the window, and holding the food in her mouth and discarding it when she is brushing her teeth (Abraham and Llewellyn-Jones, 1987).
- Encourage the patient to approach a team member when she feels the urge to vomit or purge herself. Expression of feelings reduces anxiety, and the patient might discover another alternative to vomiting.
- Involve the family in treatment. Unless the parents provide emotional consent, treatment efforts are futile. The family needs to understand the illness and how to deal with it if the patient is to recover.
- Maintain consistency. Whatever behavior-modification program or treatment regimen is set up must be adhered to by the entire staff at all times. Otherwise the patient will quickly discover an area that she can manipulate.
- Involve the dietitian in the treatment plan. Proper nutrition needs to be taught to the patient. This can be done while providing the patient with an opportunity to select menus.
- Group therapy. Providing an opportunity for the patient to participate in a group with peers with or without similar problems helps her to see that she is not alone in having difficulty expressing her feelings. Staples and Schwartz (1990) report nurse-led support groups "reinforced and rekindled social alliances and encouraged members to identify and express feelings."

Sarah, a 17-year-old white girl, was brought to the hospital by her parents and her outpatient therapist whom she had been seeing on a weekly basis of 1 month. Sarah and the therapist had a contract that agreed to a 2-pound weight gain every week. However, Sarah had continued to lose weight rather than gain. On admission, she was 5 feet 5 inches tall and weighed 86 pounds. She was strongly opposed to her hospitalization.

Sarah was the youngest of three daughters, ages 27, 24, and 17. She was a late addition to her upper-middle-class family. Her parents admitted she had been steadily losing weight for the past 6 months. At first they believed that Sarah was "just dieting" as teenagers frequently do. However, they soon began to see her ribs and vertebrae through her nightgown and became gravely concerned.

Sarah had recently been named valedictorian of her high school class. She was active in many school activities and was described as a "teacher's dream." Although she appeared to have many friends, Sarah claimed that she only had two real friends.

Sarah said that her obsession with weight began approximately 6 months ago when the family went to visit the oldest daughter, whom Sarah had always idolized. One afternoon the three sisters went berry picking, and the oldest told Sarah, "Don't eat all the berries, or you'll grow into a *real* chub!" Sarah interpreted this to mean that her sister thought she was fat *then.* She became obsessed with food, suddenly deciding to become a vegetarian. She took over the role of planning the menus and educating the family on proper nutrition. When the mother attempted to intervene, Sarah would have a temper tantrum and scream that she knew what she was doing and that she was tired of being treated like a baby. If the mother attempted further control over Sarah's eating behavior, she refused to eat entirely.

The situation in the home deteriorated to the point where there was little communication between any of the family members, particularly with Sarah. The family watched helplessly as she engaged in her irrational rituals and lost weight to a dangerous level. At this point they persuaded Sarah to seek help, as they really loved her and were concerned for her well-being. However, her outpatient experience was not successful.

As Sarah was a charismatic young lady, many of the other adolescents in the hospital were attracted to her and wanted to be her friend. However, they quickly noticed her odd eating habits, such as mixing corn flakes in vanilla pudding and pouring cranberry juice over other cereals. Sarah always dressed in baggy overalls and often wore oversized sweaters. When the other patients asked her if she was cold, she quietly told them that she did not want them to stare at her fat body.

During break times, Sarah was found writing morbid poetry, which often contained subtle suicidal messages. She preferred to be alone and became irritable and rude when asked to participate in group therapy sessions. Sarah tried to be a "good girl," as she was accustomed to doing; however, the lack of control she experienced in the hospital made this difficult. See Sarah's nursing care plan on the opposite page.

## Nursing Care Plan

WEEKLY UPDATE: __1/20/90__

NAME: _____Sarah Hopkins_____          ADMISSION DATE: ___1/6/90___

DSM-III-R DIAGNOSIS: _____307.10 Anorexia nervosa_____

*ASSESSMENT:*

***Areas of strength:*** Intelligence; past achievements; likable; past healthy interpersonal relationships; good personal hygiene; insight into reasons for hospitalization; family support.

***Problems:*** Low weight, disturbed body image, low self-esteem, depressed, lack of accurate knowledge regarding nutrition, manipulative.

***DIAGNOSES:*** Alterations in nutrition: less than body requirements, related to not eating enough nutrients; disturbance in body image, related to feeling fat when actually underweight; disturbance in self-esteem, related to feeling as if she is not a good girl; knowledge deficit in proper nutrition, related to eating imbalanced diet.

*PLANNING:*                                                        Date met

***Short-term goals:*** Patient will gain 2 pounds per week.        _____

Patient will identify three positive qualities about herself.        _____

Patient will discuss feelings of losing control.                    _____

***Long-term goals:*** Patient will gain at least 35 pounds          _____
within 6 months.

Patient will verbalize knowledge of illness and proper              _____
nutrition.

Patient will identify alternative coping mechanisms to              _____
feeling out of control.

Patient will verbalize an increased feeling of self-esteem.          _____

*IMPLEMENTATION/INTERVENTIONS:*

***Nurse-patient relationship:*** Establish a contract to meet at least three times a week to discuss feelings; express concern for the patient; encourage verbalization of feelings about depression and/or lack of control; encourage patient to identify positive qualities about herself.

***Milieu management:*** Encourage patient to attend meals and sit with peers; encourage participation in group therapy to discuss feelings with peers; encourage patient to share positive qualities of herself with peers; maintain consistency of unit rules and make certain patient is adhering to them.

***EVALUATION:*** Patient gained 3 pounds in the first 10 days of hospitalization; attending all unit activities; attending individual therapy with Ms. Mills, RN.

**Box 25-2**
## DIAGNOSTIC CRITERIA FOR 307.51 BULIMIA NERVOSA

A. Recurrent episodes of binge eating (rapid consumption of a large amount of food in discrete period of time).
B. A feeling of lack of control of over eating behavior during the eating binges.
C. The person regularly engages in either self-induced vomiting, use of laxatives or diuretics, strict dieting or fasting, or vigorous exercise to prevent weight gain.
D. A minimum average of two binge eating episodes a week for at least 3 months.
E. Persistent overconcern with body shape and weight.

Reprinted with permission from the *Diagnostic and Statistical Manual of Mental Disorders, Third Edition, Revised.* Copyright 1987 American Psychiatric Association.


## BULIMIA NERVOSA
### DSM-III-R criteria

The DMS-III-R diagnostic criteria for bulimia nervosa is found in Box 25-2. There are three core features of the bulimic patient (Fairburn and Beglin, 1990):

1. Recurrent episodes of overeating (binges)
2. Various behaviors designed to control shape and weight, that is, extreme dieting, excessive exercising, self-induced vomiting, and taking of laxatives or diuretics
3. Persistent overconcern with body shape and weight

The DSM-III-R reports that bulimia nervosa usually begins in adolescence or early adult life, primarily in females. The prevalence of bulimia among adolescent and young adult women is consistently found to be 1%; however, some researchers believe this figure seriously underestimates its incidence (Fairburn and Beglin, 1990). The usual course of the illness is chronic and intermittent over a period of many years. Most commonly the binge periods alternate with periods of normal eating, or with normal eating and fasts. Sometimes, however, there may be no periods of normal eating, merely binges and fasts.

The DMS-III-R states that bulimia nervosa is seldom incapacitating, except in a small number of patients who spend all their time binge eating and vomiting. This group has the potential for experiencing electrolyte imbalances, dehydration, cardiac arrhythmias, and sudden death.

### Behavior

The word *bulimia* actually means to have an insatiable appetite, although it is often used to describe massive overeating and often is used interchangeably with *binge eating* or *binging.* Other names, such as *bulimarexia,* have also been associated with binge and vomiting behaviors.

Until recently, bulimia nervosa was considered to be a part of anorexia nervosa because almost half of those diagnosed with anorexia were observed to have binge-eating episodes. Since the introduction of the third edition of the *Diagnostic and Statistical Manual (DSM-III)* in 1980, bulimia nervosa has been accepted as a separate illness. The true prevalence of bulimia nervosa is unknown, because so many patients hide their behaviors and illness. Only those women who seek medical attention (which usually is for gastrointestinal or menstrual disturbances) are actually identifiable.

The onset of the illness is usually between the ages 15 and 24 years. It often follows a period when the young woman has tried unsuccessfully to diet because she has been concerned about her weight. This concern becomes exaggerated, and a cycle of stringent dieting and binge eating begins.

It is important to distinguish overeating from bulimia. Fairburn et al. (1986) state that there are two conditions that justify a bulimic episode: (1) the person considers the quantity of food eaten to be excessive, and (2) the eating is experienced as involuntary. The subjective behavior (how the binge-eating episode was experienced) is actually the most important consideration in identifying bulimia nervosa.

**Objective signs.** On the whole, patients with bulimia nervosa tend to be much more outgoing and socially assertive than those with anorexia. However, the needs to be perfect and to achieve are similar and are obvious in their behavior.

Most bulimic patients are secretive about their behavior. Some plan for the binge by hiding food beforehand. They usually cook their own simple meals during the binge and then go to various restaurants, where most of their food is eaten. Some bulimics have been observed buying food at multiple food "stands" and eating it immediately. Others have actually been caught shoplifting food.

Observers often consider the eating habits of the bulimic patient during a binge to be repulsive. Bulimic patients are frequently seen eating in a frenzy, gulping their food down while stuffing more into their mouths. Clothing, as well as the area where they have eaten, shows the tell-tale signs of their meal. On the other hand, a small number of bulimic patients are meticulous in their eating, so that their behavior will not be discovered.

Binges usually begin and end suddenly, although most bulimics have specific times when they start, particularly unstructured times such as evenings, weekends, and holidays. The amount of food eaten varies a great deal, and consumption of 5,000 to 10,000 calories per eating episode is not uncommon. A large volume of liquid also may be consumed, particularly if the patient plans to induce vomiting after eating.

Bulimic persons seem to have specific foods that they eat during a binge. In the past it was believed that most binge foods were high in carbohydrates and were classified by many as "junk food." This is not necessarily true. Some bulimic persons eat only foods that are high in protein or fat. What does appear to be true is that each patient prefers certain foods during a binge. Although some eat "everything in sight," this is usually the case in very few patients.

The bulimic episode usually ends when the patient begins to induce vomiting, is physically exhausted, suffers from painful abdominal distension, is interrupted by others, or has simply run out of food (Fairburn et al., 1986). After the binge the patient usually promises herself that she will adhere to a strict diet, vowing never to binge again. Many actually resume their usual schedules as if they had never been interrupted.

Sometimes, when bulimia has been identified in a family, the patient will deliberately binge in front of family members in an attempt to manipulate her significant others. This is an effort to shift the responsibility for her behavior onto those she perceives as having "caused" the problem.

The frequency of binges varies greatly from patient to patient. Some report having several episodes a day, while others report losing control two or three times a week. Still other patients claim that their binge periods occur every few weeks to every few months.

Physical complications in bulimic patients, particularly those who use vomiting or purging as weight-control methods, are common. Almost half the patients examined show some type of fluid-electrolyte imbalance. Several show metabolic alkalosis, hypochloremia, and hypokalemia. Rarely, bulimic patients have renal failure, acute gastric dilatation, and parotid gland swelling. Dental problems are frequent because of the acidic vomitus. Menstrual disturbances are less consistently the problem that they are in anorexia.

Laxative-abuse bulimic patients are significantly more dissatisfied with their bodies and have a greater drive to be thin than do those who vomit (Waller et al., 1990). Laxative abusers also have low serum bicarbonate levels.

**Subjective symptoms.** Although most bulimic patients have a normal body weight, they are gravely concerned about their body shape and weight. The fact that they do not have control over their eating causes them great distress, and they express the same fear of becoming fat as anorexics. Bulimics are torn between two strong conflicting feelings: the fear of being fat and the love of food. To respond to both feelings, the bulimic binges and then vomits and between binges purges, rigidly diets, or does both.

The mood of bulimic patients varies considerably. Patients have reported feeling weak and constrained before a binge, followed by either continued anxiety or relief from tension during the binge (Palmer, 1987). Abraham and Llewellyn-Jones (1987) found that most women report feeling either anxiety, loneliness, boredom, or an uncontrollable craving for food before the binge. The anxiety present before the binge is often replaced with guilt after the binge. If the anxiety is not relieved after the binge, the patient will feel angry and agitated. Many become depressed. Since depression is common in bulimic patients, it will be discussed in the special issues section in this chapter.

More than half the identified bulimic patients induce vomiting to allay the fear of becoming fat. Each patient seems to have her own vomiting ritual. Many stick fingers or eating utensils down their throats, while others contract the diaphragm. Some drink large amounts of water and vomit numerous times to wash out the stomach, and others eat a specific food at the start of the binge and vomit until they recognize that initial food.

Purging is another common behavior that relieves the patient of her fear of becoming fat and removes the contraband food she has eaten. Since many bulimic women are well aware of the fluid-electrolyte imbalances that occur after purging, they are careful to eat foods high in electrolytes such as potassium during the binge to avoid serious complications.

Physically, many bulimic patients complain of feeling bloated or nauseated or of having abdominal pains during a binge. The most common physical complaints after a binge are fatigue and headache.

## Etiology

There has been little research in the etiology of bulimia, and thus the cause remains unknown. The most widely accepted biological and psychodynamic theories are presented below.

**Biological theories.** As is true of anorexia nervosa, one biological theory of bulimia is that there is a dysfunction of the hypothalamus, the hunger center. Studies have shown that when there is either injury or stimulation to the hypothalamus, metabolism of fat, carbohydrates, and water is affected. Other studies have shown that when there is a decrease in glucose utilization in the hypothalamus because of some abnormality such as a lesion, the urge to increase food intake is aroused.

Another biological theory suggests that there is a disturbance in the metabolic feedback mechanism that lets the body know when it has had enough nutrients (Agras and Kirkley, 1986). Specifically, it is believed that bulimics have a disturbance in this feedback mechanism that causes them to crave carbohydrates. When more carbohydrates than proteins are consumed, changes occur in the plasma amino acid levels. This causes an increased amount of tryptophan in the brain, which in turn causes increased release of serotonin. The serotonin enables the body to eat more protein and less carbohydrate at the next meal. The carbohydrate craving occurs again. The person continues to eat in response to these confusing physiological demands. She vomits in an effort to restrict her intake.

**Psychodynamic theories.** The psychodynamic theories of bulimia nervosa are based on the same premise as other psychiatric illnesses: there has been a real or perceived traumatic event in childhood that has been inadequately repressed and transformed by means of defense mechanisms. In bulimia it is believed that the patient has developed ambivalent feelings of self-esteem. The binge-eating–purging behavior expresses the ambivalence that the patient feels toward herself. On the one hand, she believes she is worthy of the nurturing she lacks and, since food is a symbolic form of nurturing, binges. On the other hand, she feels unworthy of the nurturing, so she purges.

Another psychodynamic theory of bulimia suggests that dysfunctional family interaction is the cause of the disorder. This theory postulates that bulimics are rebelling against controlling and powerful parents who persistently demand perfection from them.

A final psychodynamic theory of bulimia must include some sociocultural factors, such as the importance the media and society attach to being thin. The young woman experiences anxiety for a variety of reasons and eats as a means to reduce her anxiety. When she realizes she may become fat as a result of her eating, a tremendous fear is activated, and she attempts to undo her actions by vomiting or purging. However, Reed and Sech (1985) found in one group of bulimic patients that fear had nothing to do with their becoming fat. This group admitted their fear was of intimacy with themselves or others. Their binge-eating–purging behavior encompassed so much of their time that they had no time for intimacy with anyone.

## Special issues related to bulimia nervosa

**Bulimia and depression.** There is a large group of researchers who believe that bulimia nervosa is, in fact, an affective disorder. The depressive symptoms, such as the dysphoric mood, the pathological guilt, hopelessness, and lack of self-esteem, are expressed in similar ways in patients with an affective disorder. In addition, bulimics will often have the same results on a dexamethasone suppression test (DST) that a depressed patient will in that adrenocortical functioning will not be suppressed after a dose of dexamethasone.

The feeling of depression is believed to stem from the feelings of low self-esteem. However, it is compounded by the vicious cycle of the feelings a bulimic appears to experience. First, anxiety is experienced and precipitates the binge-purge behavior. Guilt follows this behavior. Depression and hopelessness surface next, often leading the patient to have suicidal ideation. It should be noted that few bulimics are actually considered to be at risk of suicide.

There is some controversy as to whether the depressive features are secondary to the bulimia nervosa or vice versa. Since many depressive features subside when the patient has regained some control over eating, most professionals do think the bulimia is the primary problem.

Some bulimic patients require and appear to respond to antidepressant medication. Some physicians believe that the monoamine oxidase inhibitors seem to have more of an effect on bulimia than the tricyclics, although more research is needed in this area.

---

### PSYCHOTHERAPEUTIC MANAGEMENT

The psychotherapeutic management of a bulimic patient is often debated among professionals. There are those who believe that the bulimia should not be the center of attention. Rather, the patient needs to work on increasing self-esteem and exploring feelings related to binge-purge behavior. Other therapists practice a behavioral approach that focuses mainly on changing the patient's eating habits, without pursuing the psychodynamics of the behavior. The psychodynamic approach will be presented in this book.

*THE NURSE-PATIENT RELATIONSHIP* The bulimic patient differs from the anorectic patient in the sense that the former is usually desperate for help. She enters therapy of her own volition and is eager to please, behaving so that the therapist will like her. In this effort to please, the bulimic patient has a tendency to become manipulative or possibly not to tell the entire truth in regard to her problem. The desire to be helped is usually the patient's greatest strength. Specific therapeutic communication techniques helpful for these patients follow:

- Create an atmosphere of trust. Bulimic patients have a difficult time with this. The nurse must be honest at all times and follow through with what is said.
- Help the patient identify feelings associated with the binge-purge behavior. Once the feelings are identified, the patient can begin to explore alternative ways of coping with them.
- Accept the patient as a worthwhile human being. The bulimic patient is often ashamed of her behavior and is embarrassed to discuss it. When she realizes that there will be no negative repercussions, she will be more comfortable discussing her problem.
- Encourage the patient to discuss positive qualities about herself. The more she is able to do so, the more her self-esteem will be enhanced.
- Teach the patient about bulimia nervosa. The more she understands, the better control she will be able to exert upon her eating behavior.
- Encourage the patient to explore her interpersonal relationships. Since many bulimics complain of loneliness and problems in the social area, patients need to be encouraged to examine the nature of such problems so that they may be resolved.

*MILIEU MANAGEMENT* Most professionals agree that inpatient treatment of the bulimic is not desirable. First, the patient usually wants treatment and is therefore willing to cooperate with a therapist. Second, the patient needs to learn to find ways to express feelings, other than binging and purging, on a day-to-day basis. A hospital may help with this, but only in a structured setting. A bulimic patient needs to learn to cope in her own unstructured world.

Abraham and Llewellyn-Jones (1987) imply reasons to hospitalize a bulimic:

- To treat a psychiatric or medical crisis, such as suicidal feelings or serious fluid-electrolyte imbalance
- To provide order to an otherwise chaotic life
- To allow the woman to examine her living situation
- To provide treatment to a woman who lives in an area far away from any other services.

Some principles for management of the bulimic patient follow.

- Encourage the patient to adhere to the meal and snack schedule of the hospital. If additional food is not readily available, the patient will have difficulty binging.
- Encourage the patient to approach a staff member when she has the urge to binge and purge. The patient will then have the opportunity to identify and express her feelings that precipitate such episodes and explore alternative ways of coping with them.
- Encourage the patient to attend group therapy sessions. Many professionals believe that this is the most effective modality for the bulimic patient because it not only provides support to the patient but also facilitates her experiencing and resolving the problems she has in relating to others.

- Encourage family therapy. Communication within the family needs to be improved so that these relationships may be strengthened.
- Encourage participation in art, recreation, and occupational therapy. These modalities provide and teach the patient alternative ways to express her feelings.
- Encourage the patient to describe her body image at different ages of her life in the various therapies. When the team has an understanding of how the patient has perceived herself, interventions for helping her change may be devised.

## Case Study

Polly, a 19-year-old white girl, lives at home with her mother, stepfather, and two sisters, 15 and 12 years of age. Her brother, age 22, is away at college. Polly was ready to graduate from a community college and decided to enter treatment because she wanted to go away for her last 2 years of college and she knew her eating behavior would cause massive problems for her.

Polly was 5 feet 6 inches tall and weighed 150 pounds. However, there were times in the last 5 years that she weighed as much as 225 pounds. She admitted to really hating herself when she was fat and was concerned not to become fat again.

Polly always felt that she was not as good as her brother and sisters. She saw herself as less attractive, less intelligent, and less coordinated. She described herself as the "ugly duckling." She has never been on a date and had few girlfriends. She thought that people tolerated her but did not really like her.

Polly began to binge around the age of 15. She would come home from school and eat continuously until time for dinner, which she then ate with her family. When everyone went to bed, Polly would go into the kitchen and eat again. Polly states she would easily eat a loaf of bread, 2 pounds of cheese, a gallon of ice cream, a jar of peanut butter, a box of cookies, and a half-gallon of milk at one sitting. These episodes occurred about two or three times a week. When Polly reached 225 pounds at the age of 17, she entered a diet program and lost 80 pounds. It was soon after this weight loss that Polly felt the urge to binge. Rather than endure a great deal of weight loss again, Polly began to induce vomiting after binging. This behavior has continued for the past year and a half. See Polly's nursing care plan on the opposite page.

# Nursing Care Plan

WEEKLY UPDATE: __11/15/90__

NAME: _____Polly Samuels_____     ADMISSION DATE: __11/8/90__

DSM-III-R DIAGNOSIS: _____307.51 Bulimia nervosa_____

*ASSESSMENT:*
*Areas of strength:* Desire for treatment, sense of humor, past achievement, intelligence, history of self-control long enough to lose 80 pounds, family support.
*Problems:* Low self-esteem, disturbed body image, not able to control binge-vomiting behavior, unable to establish intimate relationships, feels defeated and depressed.

*DIAGNOSES:* Powerlessness, related to feeling not in control over eating habits; disturbance in self-esteem, related to not feeling as worthy as others; disturbance in body image, related to feeling overweight.

*PLANNING:*                                                    **Date met**
*Short-term goals:* Patient will establish and adhere to con-    _____
tract on eating behavior.
  Patient will approach the staff when she feels the urge to     _____
binge or vomit.
  Patient will participate in all unit therapies, including group,   _____
art, recreational, and occupational therapy.
*Long-term goals:* Patient will maintain present weight          _____
without binging or vomiting.
  Patient will participate in physical activity, such as jogging,   _____
when she feels anxious.
  Patient will express several positive qualities about herself.   _____

*IMPLEMENTATION/INTERVENTIONS:*
*Nurse-patient relationship:* Establish a contract that addresses specific eating behavior; be honest and genuine in all contracts with the patient; encourage the patient to identify when she feels the need to binge; help the patient make association between her feelings and her eating behavior.
*Milieu management:* Encourage the patient to attend meals and snacks with peers; encourage the patient to express her feelings in a group setting; encourage the patient to approach the staff when she is feeling out of control; provide diversional activities when patient is feeling anxious.

*EVALUATION:* Patient has maintained her body weight with only one episode of vomiting; attending occupational and recreational therapies consistently, feelings group inconsistently; meeting with individual therapist, Ms. O'Donnell, regularly.

## OBESITY

The issue of whether obesity is actually an eating disorder has been professionally debated for some time. The controversy stems from the concept that eating disorders such as anorexia and bulimia have physiological components; however, these are not as significant as the psychological components. The reverse seems to be true in the case of obesity. Today most experts agree that although obesity has psychological components, it is primarily a genetic or metabolic disorder. The DSM-III-R does not include obesity as a psychiatric disorder. Consequently the reader will be referred to a textbook on pathophysiology for more information.

## KEY CONCEPTS

1. Anorexia nervosa is characterized by self-inflicted weight loss, an intense fear of becoming fat, a distorted body image, and amenorrhea.
2. Anorectic dieters often begin in a normal weight range, tend to isolate themselves socially, alienate themselves from others, are competitive, and exercise excessively.
3. Bulimia is characterized by episodes of binge eating, a feeling of lack of control over eating, self-induced vomiting, use of weight-control methods and laxatives, and overconcern with body shape and weight. Depression commonly coexists with bulimia.
4. Anorectic and bulimic patients suffer a variety of physiological problems that can cause death. Personality and emotional changes are also evident.
5. The anorectic's need to control derives from feeling abandoned or inadequate, a sense of helplessness, and fear of loss of control over food.
6. The cause of eating disorders may be both biological and psychodynamic in nature, including issues of family dynamics and sexuality/intimacy.
7. Nursing interventions with an anorectic patient require a caring, supportive relationship, limit setting, a behavior-modification program, and a consistent milieu. Family involvement and group therapy are also essential.
8. Nursing interventions with a bulimic patient require a caring, supportive relationship, education about the disorder, exploration of feelings and relationships, and group and family therapy. Hospitalization with a structured milieu and antidepressant medications may or may not be needed.

## REFERENCES

Abraham S and Llewellyn-Jones D: Eating disorders: the facts, ed 2, Oxford, 1987, Oxford University Press.

Agras WS and Kirkley BG: Bulimia: theories of etiology. In Brownell KD and Foreyt JP, editors: Handbook of eating disorders, New York, 1986, Basic Books, Inc., pp 367-378.

American Psychiatric Association: Diagnostic and statistical manual of mental disorders, ed 3, revised, Washington DC, 1987, The Association.

Brown GM: Endocrine alterations in anorexia nervosa. In Darby PL et al, editors: Anorexia nervosa: recent developments in research, New York, 1983, Alan R. Liss, pp 231-247.

Bruch H: Eating disorders. New York, 1973, Basic Books, Inc.

Casper RC: Treatment principles in anorexia nervosa. In Feinstein SC et al, editors: Adolescent psychiatry, vol. X, Chicago, 1982, University of Chicago Press, pp 431-454.

Deering CG: Developing a therapeutic alliance with the anorexia nervosa client, J Psychosoc Nurs 25(3):11-13, 1987.

Fairburn CG and Beglin SJ: Studies of the epidemiology of bulimia nervosa, Am J Psychiatry 147:401-408, 1990.

Fairburn CG, Cooper Z, and Cooper PJ: The clinical features and maintenance of bulimia nervosa. In Brownell KD and Foreyt JP, editors: Handbook of eating disorders, New York, 1986, Basic Books, Inc., pp 389-404.

Flood M: Addictive eating disorders. In Zerwekh J and Gordon D, guest editors: The nursing clinics of North America, Vol. 24/No. 1 Philadelphia, 1989, WB Saunders Co, pp 45-53.

Halmi KA and Sherman BM: Dopaminergic and sertoninergic regulations of growth hormone secretion in anorexia nervosa. Psychopharmacol Bull 13:63, 1977.

Mitchell JE: Anorexia nervosa: medical and physiological aspects. In Brownell KD and Foreyt JP, editors: Handbook of eating disorders, New York, 1986, Basic Books, Inc., pp 247-265.

Palmer RL: Bulimia: the nature of the syndrome, its epidemiology and its treatment. In Boakes RA, Popplewell DA, and Burton MJ, editors: Eating habits, Chichester, 1987, John Wiley & Sons, pp 1-23.

Reed G and Sech EP: Bulimia: a conceptual model for group treatment, J Psychosoc Nurs 23:16, 1985.

Staples NR and Schwartz M: Anorexia nervosa support group: providing transitional support, J Psychosoc Nurs 28:6-10, 1990.

Szmukler GI: Anorexia nervosa: a clinical view. In Boakes RA et al, editors: Eating habits, Chichester, 1987, John Wiley & Sons, pp 25-44.

Waller DA, Newton PA, Hardy BW, and Svetlik D: Correlates of laxative abuse in bulimia, Hosp Community Psychiatry 41:797-799, 1990.

Weiner H: The hypothalamic-pituitary-ovarian axis in anorexia and bulimia nervosa. Int J Eating Disorders 2:109, 1983.

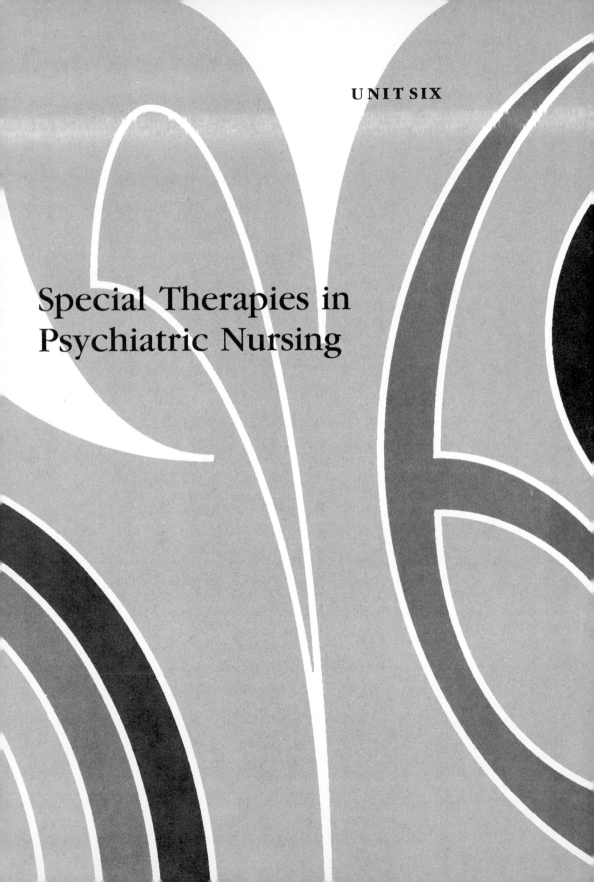

# Special Therapies in Psychiatric Nursing

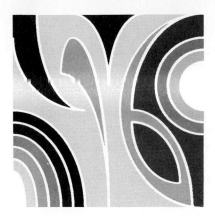

## CHAPTER 26

# Behavior Therapy

SUE MAIN

LEARNING OBJECTIVES

After reading this chapter you should be able to

- Identify three techniques for increasing a behavior.
- Describe two schedules of reinforcement.
- Identify three techniques for decreasing behavior.
- Apply the principles of a token economy.
- Discuss two techniques for helping patients deal with disturbing stimuli.
- Apply the nursing process using behavioral modification principles.

In this chapter a brief overview of classical and operant conditioning will be presented, followed by a discussion of the principles that form the basis of behavioral models and the terms commonly used in behavioral assessment and intervention. Steps for using the behavioral approach will be compared with the nursing process. The use of behavioral intervention in psychiatric nursing will be reviewed, and a guideline for the behavioral nursing process will be presented. Finally, clinical examples illustrating the application of behavioral techniques in nursing will be included.

Behavioral therapy is a distinctive approach to influencing interactions between persons, and between persons and their environment. In a report of the behavior therapy task force of the American Psychiatric Association (1973, p. 2), behavior therapy was defined as the "systematic application of experimentally derived behavior analysis principles to effect observable and, at least in principle, measurable changes in the interaction process." The principles used in behavior therapy were derived from research in conditioned reflex and operant conditioning. As a psychological approach, behavior therapy differs from other psychological theories. In many psychological theories, hypotheses were formulated to explain human behavior; then attempts were made to validate the theories with research. The principles of behavioral therapy came from the repeated research findings, which provided the systematic format for the experimental analysis of human behavior.

## CLASSICAL CONDITIONING

The origin of classical conditioning is credited to Pavlov (1927) and his research on reflexes in laboratory animals. Pavlov was involved in studying reflexes and the various aspects of secretion of gastric juices in dogs when he discovered that the experimental dogs began salivating before they were presented with food. He further studied this process by repeatedly presenting food simultaneously with the sound of a metronome. After several repetitions of this simultaneous presenting, the metronome alone was found to elicit the secretion of saliva in the dogs.

Specific terminology was used in describing these events (Pavlov, 1927). Reflexes are machinelike, inevitable reactions of the organism, called *respondents.* Respondents are involuntary reactions to eliciting stimuli. An *eliciting stimulus* is an environmental event that immediately precedes the reflex behavior or respondent.

$$S \text{ (food)} \longrightarrow R \text{ (salivation)}$$
$$\text{Eliciting stimulus} \qquad\qquad\qquad \text{Respondent}$$

*Respondent conditioning* is the process of pairing a neutral stimulus with an eliciting stimulus so that the neutral stimulus, ultimately alone, elicits the response.

$$S \text{ (food) (metronome)} \longrightarrow R \text{ (salivation)}$$
$$\text{Eliciting plus neutral stimuli} \qquad\qquad\qquad \text{Respondent}$$

$$CS \text{ (metronome)} \longrightarrow R \text{ (salivation)}$$
$$\text{Conditioned stimulus} \qquad\qquad\qquad \text{Respondent}$$

As a result of this type of research, an important principle emerged: When a neutral stimulus is paired repeatedly with an eliciting stimulus, the neutral stimulus (conditioned stimulus) alone elicits the respondent.

The research of Watson and Rayner (1920) demonstrated the application of respondent conditioning with human beings. In an experiment with a young child, Albert, and a white rat (a neutral stimulus), the authors paired the presence of the rat with a loud noise (which had been observed to elicit a fear response in Albert). After noise and the rat were presented simultaneously seven times, the rat alone elicited the fear response in Albert. The fear response was also elicited by stimuli with characteristics similar to those of the rat (rabbit, dog, fur). This process in which the fear response was elicited by stimuli with common characteristics was called *generalization.* The principle here is that neutral stimuli with characteristics similar to those of conditioned stimuli may elicit responses controlled by the conditioned stimuli. Watson's and Rayner's research was one of the classics that have become the foundation for behavioral treatment of phobias.

## OPERANT CONDITIONING

The basis of the operant learning theory was derived from numerous controlled experiments with animals reported originally by B.F. Skinner (1938, 1956). An important distinction of the operant learning theory is the focus on the study of external variables to predict or control behavior (Skinner, 1953). Attention is directed to the events that immediately precede and follow a person's specific behavior, rather than to events that elicit responses. Theoretical inner causes of behavior, such as psychological, neurological, or conceptual states, are not included in this approach. The existence of such inner states is not denied; however, they are not viewed as relevant to the analysis of behavior.

### Terminology

The terminology used in the operant learning theory *(response, stimulus, reinforcement)* sounds familiar and is used in everyday conversation. Each term, however, carries a specific definition that facilitates clearer comprehension of the theory. The following discussion of terms is based on Skinner's (1953) definitions.

A response is any movement or observable behavior. An *operant response,* the unit of analysis in this theory, is behavior emitted by the person. The behavior operates on the environment in relation to consequences. The operant response can be described and measured (frequency, duration, magnitude).

A *stimulus* is an event that immediately precedes or follows a behavior. Three types of stimuli will be defined:

1. A *discriminative stimulus* is an event, immediately preceding a behavior, that predicts or indicates that a response will be followed by reinforcement. A stimulus becomes a discriminative stimulus when a response is repeatedly reinforced in the presence of the stimulus and not reinforced in absence of the stimulus. Discriminative stimuli may be observed, heard, felt (tactile),

or smelled. In interpersonal situations, they may be in the form of subtle verbal or facial expressions, tone of voice, posture, or dress or may be more obvious, as in the presence of a specific person or situation.

2. A *neutral stimulus* is an event that is not associated with reinforcement or that has no effect on changing the probability of behavior.

3. A *reinforcing stimulus* is an event, following a behavior, that strengthens that behavior and increases the probability of the behavior's occurring. Reinforcers can be anything (hugs, smiles, attention, opportunity to play, pay check, chicken dinner) that increases the frequency of a behavior.

*Primary reinforcers* are events of biological importance (food, water, sexual contact, coat on a cold day, bed for sleeping). *Secondary,* or *generalized reinforcers* are events that have been paired repeatedly with a primary reinforcer. Money, tickets, diplomas, and attention of others are examples of secondary reinforcers.

## Major principles

Two important principles have emerged from the research of Skinner and other behavioral psychologists. Operant responses are controlled by the consequences that immediately follow the responses. Specific operant responses are more likely to occur in specific stimulus situations that set the occasion for reinforcement. The basic paradigm for an observation of behavior is

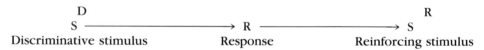

Consider this example: A patient in a hospital room wishes the attention of the nurse. The patient presses a button labeled "nurse" on the paging apparatus. The voice of the nurse, "This is Mrs. White. May I help you?" is heard.

$$S \xrightarrow{D} R \xrightarrow{} S$$

Presence of button          Pressing the button          Voice of the nurse
labeled "nurse"

In this simplified example the presence of a call button labeled "nurse" is the stimulus that signals a patient, who wants the attention of a nurse, to press the button. The signal sets the occasion for attention of a nurse immediately after pressing of the button. Other buttons with the label "Fire," "Emergency," or "TV" do not signal the occasion for the attention of a nurse and therefore are neutral stimuli for the attention of a nurse. The target response also is specific. The patient must press the button for the voice of the nurse to respond. Directing eye contact to the button, talking to the button, or touching the button will not bring the attention of the nurse.

The voice of the nurse serves as the reinforcing stimulus for pressing the button labeled "nurse." When the voice responds immediately and consistently following the pressing of the button, *learning* occurs. The behavior, pressing the button labeled "nurse," will be maintained. If the nurse's voice does not immediately follow pushing of the button, *extinction* occurs. The button-pushing behavior will predictably decrease, and emotional behavior may occur (yelling loudly for the nurse). If the patient receives a painful electrical shock when pushing the button and the response is suppressed, *punishment* has occurred. The patient may exhibit an aggressive response (throwing the paging apparatus against the wall).

## APPLICATION OF BEHAVIORAL THERAPY IN PSYCHIATRIC NURSING PRACTICE

The use of behavior therapy in clinical practice consists of two major steps. First, a detailed functional analysis of behavior and environmental contingencies is carried out (Bellack and Hersen, 1988). Then a treatment program is designed, implemented, and evaluated. The functional analysis requires considerable expertise and, when not carried out appropriately, will result in the failure to achieve expected outcomes from the treatment program.

The application of behavior therapy in general psychiatric practice has been discussed in comprehensive texts by Hersen and Last (1985), Kanfer and Schefft (1987), and Wilson et al. (1987). Behavior therapy is used with children, adolescents, groups, couples, and families. Behavior modification has been used in inpatient settings and in skills-training programs. The use of behavioral therapy with specific problematic behaviors has been reported in the treatment of anxiety, sexual disorders, posttraumatic stress disorders, and addictions. Also, behavioral principles form the basis of self-control treatment programs such as those used for changes in such behaviors as eating, exercise, or assertive communication.

### Behavior modification: Helping patients change behavior

When the patient's problem behavior is reinforced or maintained by consequences of the behavior, operant conditioning, commonly called behavior modification, is the model used. The functional analysis involves a behavioral and reinforcement history. Contingencies that can be controlled by the therapist, patient, or family are altered to create a change in the problematic behavior (Levine & Sandeen, 1985). Several well-known techniques may be applied individually or in combination in the treatment of the patient.

#### Increasing the probability that a behavior will recur

*Conditioning.* Conditioning is the strengthening of a response in the presence of a specific situation. Conditioning results from the repeated reinforcement of that response in the presence of the specific stimulus situation and withholding of reinforcement in neutral stimulus situations. For example, asking for help with assertiveness occurs frequently and is followed by attention and suggestions (reinforcement) in a communication skills group (specific discriminative stimulus). Asking for help with assertiveness rarely occurs and is not followed by reinforcement in a physical exercise group (neutral stimulus).

*Reinforcement.* The process of increasing the probability of a behavior's occurring by immediately following that behavior with a reinforcing stimulus is reinforcement. There are two types of reinforcement: *Positive reinforcement* is the process of presenting a reinforcing stimulus or adding an event to a situation, following a behavior, that increases the probability that the behavior will recur. In the previous example, attention of other group members and suggestions about assertive behavior were positive reinforcement that followed asking for help with assertiveness. *Negative reinforcement* is the process whereby removing a stimulus from a situation immediately after a behavior occurs increases the probability of the behavior's occurring. For example, when a person steps into an uncomfortably hot shower and turns the dial to reduce the water temperature, the behavior (turning the dial) is reinforced. The stimulus (uncomfortably hot water) is removed.

The strength of a reinforcer varies with the situation. *Deprivation* is a condition in which a reinforcing stimulus is withheld. When a person is in a state of deprivation (without water, for example), the effect of the reinforcing stimulus (water) on behavior is increased. *Satiation* is the condition in which a reinforcing stimulus, or a recent effect of it, is present. Water will not function as a reinforcing stimulus for the behavior of a person who has a supply of water or who has just consumed water.

The timing of presentation of a reinforcer is also of importance. *Superstitious behavior* is a term used for behavior that has been reinforced by accident. Athletes provide common examples of superstitious behavior when they display peculiar mannerisms such as tapping a shoe with the bat before stepping up to home plate or tapping the fingers on the strings of a tennis racket before receiving a serve. A reinforcing stimulus will increase the probability that any response will recur. When reinforcers are presented according to a time schedule, for example, rather than being contingent on a particular response, any behavior immediately preceding the reinforcer will be strengthened.

*Premack principle.* When a person is often observed engaging in a particular activity, the opportunity to engage in that activity can be used as a reinforcer for other behaviors that occur less frequently (Premack, 1962). For example, the opportunity to watch television might be used as a reinforcer for cleaning the living area.

*Shaping.* Shaping is a process of reinforcing successive approximations of responses to increase the probability of a behavior that is of low frequency. For example, to increase the probability of a patient's saying "no" in an assertive way, a number of specific responses are identified as prerequisite for the target behavior (successive approximations of voice volume and tone). Each time the patient makes a response that approximates the target response (or gets closer to the target response), reinforcement is presented until that response occurs at a high frequency. Then reinforcement is withheld until the next response more closely approximating the target behavior, and so on until the target behavior is performed. The selective reinforcement of each behavior that more closely approximates the target response is called differential reinforcement and will be described in more detail in the following discussions.

**Schedules of reinforcement.** Schedules are the planned sequences for the presentation of reinforcing stimuli. Each particular schedule of reinforcement results in predictable patterns of behavior frequency (Reynolds, 1968). Each schedule of reinforcement will be described.

*Continuous reinforcement.* Continuous reinforcement is the presentation of the reinforcing stimulus following each occurrence of the selected response. Continuous reinforcement is used primarily during the initial phases of conditioning or shaping of a behavior. This schedule results in a high rate of behavior but is subject to problems of satiation and rapid extinction. Continuous reinforcement is illustrated when a professional provides social reinforcement each time a patient uses appropriate comments during practice and role play of conflict management skills. The patient's use of these skills at home with a spouse may not be reinforced at all and therefore may occur only once.

*Intermittent reinforcement.* Intermittent reinforcement is the presentation of the reinforcer following the target response, according to a selected number of responses (ratio schedule), for example, after every fifth target response, or according to a selected time period (interval schedule), for example, 5 minutes after every target response. Determination of the ratio and interval schedules may be fixed or varied.

Intermittent schedules of reinforcement result in behavior that is more resistant to extinction than behavior that has been reinforced on a continuous schedule. The acts of inserting coins into vending machines and into slot machines will be compared to illustrate the difference. Usually inserting coins into a vending machine is reinforced (with food, e.g.) immediately every time the behavior occurs. When the reinforcer stops (no food is delivered), the act of inserting coins into that particular machine stops rather quickly. Inserting coins into a slot machine, however, is reinforced with tokens or money on an intermittent schedule, not each time. The act of inserting coins into a slot machine continues for a considerable time, even though reinforcers are not presented.

**Decreasing the probability that a behavior will recur**

*Differential reinforcement of other behavior.* Differential reinforcement is a technique used to decrease the frequency of a behavior (Homer and Peterson, 1980; Redman, 1987). When the goal of a treatment program is to decrease a behavior, another behavior incompatible with the target behavior can be reinforced. Target behavior, if emitted, is not reinforced. To decrease the soft speaking of a patient in a group, attention of the group is available only when the patient speaks in a normal audible voice. The soft speaking voice, incompatible with a normal voice, is ignored.

*Extinction.* Extinction is the gradual decrease in the rate of a response when reinforcement is no longer available. The rate of the response may increase for a short time, then begin to decrease gradually. Emotional responses characteristically occur during extinction. A familiar example is the behavior that occurs when one pushes the "up" button to ride an elevator. When the elevator door fails to close, repeated and sometimes rapid button-pushing behavior occurs for a short period, then stops. Banging or pulling on the elevator door (an emotional response) during this time may occur.

*Punishment.* Punishment is the presentation of an event immediately following a response that decreases the probability of that response's recurring. An example would be spanking a child immediately on seeing him playing in the street. Punishment results in the immediate suppression of that response. Punishment may result in emotional behavior or aggressive responses. It is used when other techniques are not applicable in decreasing the frequency of a particular response, or in combination with other procedures.

*Time out.* Time out is a punishment technique in which the person is removed from a setting where ongoing reinforcers are available. When a patient is exhibiting aggressive behavior that is followed by social reinforcement from other patients, the patient may be removed to another room where no social reinforcement is available.

*Response cost.* Response cost, another punishment technique, is the removal of a reinforcer, contingent on a specific behavior (Pazulinec et al., 1983). This technique frequently is used in behavioral programs in inpatient settings where secondary reinforcers, such as points or tokens, are presented for desired behaviors. The reinforcers are removed for inappropriate behavior. In outpatient settings the response cost technique is used in programs in which patients pay a sum of money at the beginning of therapy and are paid back their money contingent on exhibiting specific desired behavior. The money is withheld when inappropriate behavior, such as noncompliance with the treatment contract, is exhibited.

**Skills training.** When behavioral responses are not appropriate for a person's age and life situation, new behaviors are acquired through the use of skills-training procedures. Positive reinforcement and shaping are the basis for these programs. *Modeling* and *imitation* are also used. Modeling is a process in which a patient learns a new behavior by following or imitating the behavior of a model (Baer et al., 1967; Bandura, 1966). The model exhibits the behavior, and the patient receives reinforcement for exhibiting similar behavior. Miller (1989) reports successful nurse modeling of feeling awareness. Her approach integrates more traditional interpersonal techniques with behavioral techniques.

Manderino and Bzdek (1987) provide an example of skills-training techniques in group treatment of hospitalized patients with chronic psychiatric disorders. The nurses made individual assessments of social skills of patients and formed small groups to conduct training of skills that were appropriate for the patients but not used by them in the hospital situation. One group of related skills, carrying on a conversation, was subdivided into specific behaviors: eye contact, posture, voice tone, listening, and beginning, maintaining (clarifying, asking questions, paraphrasing), and ending a conversation. Verbal instructions, modeling of the skill, patient role playing, and homework assignments were used for each skill. Nurses and patients socially reinforced the demonstration of the skills.

**Contingency contracting.** Contingency contracting is the arranging of conditions in therapy so that the patient is able to participate in setting target behaviors and selecting reinforcers. The therapist and the patient jointly specify what, how, when, and where behavioral change will occur. Criteria for the delivery of reinforcement are defined. The type, amount, and schedule of reinforcement are specified. This procedure allows for negotiation between the patient and the therapist (Homme and Tosti, 1971; Steckel, 1980).

**Self-control.** With adult patients in an outpatient treatment setting the direct management of behavioral contingencies by a therapist usually is not practical. A more frequently used approach is the development of a self-control program. Contingency contracting is used, with the patient actually engaging in the process of assessment, behavioral change, delivering the consequences, and evaluating the results in his natural environment (Levine and Sandeen, 1985). Braden (1990) observed that "nurses who can promote enabling skill can make a difference in their patients' life quality."

**Token economy.** Token economy is the term used to describe the use of operant principles in the management of behavior with groups of patients in inpatient or outpatient partial hospital programs. Ayllon and Azrin (1968) conducted early research on the use of a token economy in a hospital setting with patients who had chronic psychiatric disorders. Tokens, tangible conditioned reinforcers, were presented to the patients contingent on specific target behaviors. The tokens could be exchanged for other positive reinforcers, such as privileges and favorite foods.

## Respondent conditioning: Helping patients cope with disturbing stimuli

When the patient's problem behavior is related to a particular stimulus situation, respondent conditioning is the model used. Treatment may involve making changes in the stimulus situation or in control of the problematic behavior (Levine and Sandeen, 1985).

**Reciprocal inhibition.** The process of strengthening alternative responses to fear or anxiety associated with a stimulus is called reciprocal inhibition or counter conditioning (Yates, 1970). Relaxation techniques, for instance, can be taught to highly anxious patients. A person cannot be relaxed and anxious simultaneously.

**Systematic desensitization.** Originally developed by Wolpe (1958) for the treatment of anxiety, systematic desensitization is the planned progressive exposure to stimuli that elicit fear or anxiety while the fear response is suppressed. Hierarchies of the fear-eliciting stimuli are constructed through a detailed assessment. For example, a patient with a fear of being in open and crowded places that limits appropriate shopping behavior may report a hierarchy of fear-eliciting situations as follows: standing outside in the doorway of the house, standing outside several feet from the house, being outdoors two blocks away, then several blocks away from home, being in a small empty store, being in an empty department store, being in an empty shopping center, being in a small crowded store, a crowded department store, then a crowded shopping center. The stimulus least likely to evoke fear or anxiety is introduced initially, followed by gradual exposure to more fearful stimuli.

In the traditional desensitization procedures, presentation or imaging of the fearful stimuli is done while an incompatible response, such as relaxation, assertiveness, or sexual arousal, is used to inhibit the fear or anxiety (Levine and Sandeen, 1985). Simply stated, a person cannot be anxious and relaxed at the same time. Progressive relaxation training (Jacobson, 1938; Bernstein and Borkovec, 1973) or a biofeedback program is used to reach and maintain a state of relaxation during a desensitization procedure. The patient is instructed to tense and then relax specific muscle groups, in a sequence, until general muscular relaxation is achieved. Several sessions of relaxation practice are usually carried out with a therapist, audiotape prompts, or written instructions before the desensitization process begins.

**Other respondent conditioning techniques.** In live or in vivo exposure the patient actually places himself systematically in the least to the most fearful situations. Usually the patient conducts this self-exposure while using incompatible competing responses to fear, such as relaxation. In using these techniques the therapist carefully assists the patient to experience gradual decrease of the fear or anxiety response in the presence of the eliciting stimulus (Ghosh and Marks, 1987). *Flooding* or implosion is a process in which the patient images a magnification of the fearful stimulus or places himself in the fearful situation, that is, he immerses himself in the feared stimulus (Levine and Sandeen, 1985).

## BEHAVIORAL INTERVENTION AND THE NURSING PROCESS

Behavioral nursing process consists of the following:

1. Making an *assessment* of behavior and the related contingencies
2. *Planning* and *implementing* an intervention program to have an impact on this behavior
3. *Evaluating* the results of the intervention.

This series of steps meshes quite naturally with steps of the nursing process. Occasions for conducting this process occur in the day-to-day interaction with patients. These interactions focus on providing a therapeutic milieu, assisting patients with here-and-now living problems, and assisting patients with learning behavior patterns related to emotional health.

### Guidelines for behavioral nursing intervention

The behavioral nursing intervention protocol that follows is derived from the more detailed descriptions of behavioral nursing models by Lebow (1973), Berni and Fordyce (1973), and Loomis and Horsley (1974). This protocol (Box 26-1) illustrates briefly the essence of the important contributions of each of the three books.

The following example illustrates the use of a behavioral approach for skills training in a group of patients with chronic psychiatric disorders who were hospitalized in a facility that used a modified token economy system.

**Baseline observation and assessment.** As part of the treatment program, each patient carried a behavioral rating card that listed specific expected behaviors (self-care activities, management of personal items and living area, attendance at prescribed treatment events). When the patients demonstrated these behaviors, a staff member rated the behavior and initialed the card. At the end of each week the patient's ratings on the behavior cards were tallied, and reinforcement was presented contingent on the score for the week. Examples of the reinforcements were opportunities to engage in the purchase of items at the hospital store, participation in hospital social events, privileges to leave the hospital unit, and home visits.

The skills-training groups consisted of four to six patients and met weekly. The sessions began with a brief orientation period and an introduction of specific skills relevant to that session. Next there was a demonstration and role play using the skills, followed by discussion and homework suggestions.

**Problem specification.** The skills included assertiveness (asking for the treatment or medication that the patient thought was most helpful), communication (starting and continuing a conversation in appropriate and effective ways), moni-

**Box 26-1**

## BEHAVIORAL NURSING INTERVENTION

### Baseline observations

1. Appropriate behavior present
2. Inappropriate behavior present
3. Age-appropriate behavior absent
   Assessment of these behavioral categories includes
   a. Frequency or duration of each response or both
   b. Description of the stimulus conditions that precede responses and follow the behavior
   c. Validation of potential reinforcers

### Problem specification

1. Select the response to be changed
2. Define the response so everyone can recognize it
3. Gather baseline data (frequency, duration of behavior, discriminative and reinforcing stimuli)

### Formulation of treatment plan

1. State the specific response to be changed
2. State how the response is to be changed; include the present status and the target status of the response:
   a. Increase the rate of the response
   b. Decrease the rate of the response
   c. Teach a new response
3. Identify the discriminative and reinforcing stimuli available for use
4. Select and write the intervention plan in detail

### Intervention

1. Implement the treatment plan as written
2. Provide reinforcers for those persons implementing the plan

### Evaluation

1. State the outcome of the intervention
2. Determine whether the response changed as planned
3. Specify what additional changes are required
4. State techniques for maintaining the desirable change

toring of one's condition (reporting changes in self), making a plan for specific methods of self-care, and contracting with staff about treatment events or outcomes.

**Treatment plan.** Specific techniques used by the nurse were positive reinforcement (social reinforcement by the nurse or other patients, initialing the rating card) contingent on appropriate behavior, modeling and imitation, contingency contracting, homework, self-control, and extinction (withholding of reinforcement) following undesired behavior.

**Evaluation.** Each group member's progress was evaluated with use of a recording form that listed the target behaviors. Seven patients showed consistent increases in target behaviors over the period of the group session. These changes would be expected if the group intervention program was effective. One patient demonstrated a relatively high rate of target behaviors during the initial group session and continued this rate. Demonstration of target behaviors by two of the patients was variable and consistently low throughout the sessions. For these two patients the group intervention program was not effective in changing target behaviors during the period of time that they were involved in the group.

## KEY CONCEPTS

1. Classical conditioning is based on the involuntary stimulus—response reaction. After repeated pairing of eliciting and neutral stimuli, the neutral stimulus alone will obtain the expected response.
2. Operant conditioning focuses on the external variables that precede and follow the response to learn which control behaviors. Reinforcers are particularly important.
3. Behavior therapy begins with a functional analysis of behavior and environmental contingencies as the basis for developing a treatment program.
4. Behavior modification programs can be used for a variety of problematic behaviors in a variety of settings.
5. Increasing the probability of a desired behavior can occur with conditioning, reinforcement, or shaping.
6. Decreasing the probability of an undesirable behavior can occur with reinforcement of an incompatible behavior, extinction, and punishment.
7. New behaviors may be acquired in skills training by use of modeling and imitation techniques as well as with reinforcement and shaping.
8. Self-control and token economy programs are varieties of reinforcement approaches.
9. Respondent conditioning is useful in altering an unpleasant response to a specific stimulus. Reciprocal inhibition, systematic desensitization, in vivo exposure, and flooding are varieties of this approach.
10. Behavioral nursing interventions involve baseline observations, analysis of behaviors, problem specification, formulation of treatment plans, intervention, and evaluation.

## REFERENCES

American Psychiatric Association Task Force on Behavior Therapy: Behavior therapy in psychiatry, Washington, DC, 1973, The Association.

Ayllon T and Azrin N: The token economy, New York, 1968, Appleton-Century-Crofts, Inc.

Baer DM, Peterson RF, and Sherman JA: The development of imitation by reinforcing behavioral similarity to a model, J Exp Anal Behav 10:405, 1967.

Bandura A: Behavioral modification through modeling techniques. In Krasner L and Ullman L, editors: Research in behavior modification, New York, 1966, Holt, Rinehart & Winston, Inc.

Bellack AS and Hersen M, editors: Behavioral assessment: a practical handbook, ed 3, New York, 1988, Pergamon Press.

Berni R and Fordyce WE: Behavior modification and the nursing process, St. Louis, 1973, The CV Mosby Co.

Bernstein DA and Borkovec TD: Progressive relaxation training: a manual for the helping professions. Champaign, Ill, 1973, Research Press.

Braden CJ: A test of the self-help model: learned response to chronic illness experience, Nurs Res 39:42-47, 1990.

Ghosh A and Marks IM: Self-treatment of agoraphobia by exposure, Behav Ther 18:3, 1987.

Hersen M and Last CG: Behavior therapy casebook, New York, 1985, Springer Publishing Co.

Homer AL and Peterson L: Differential reinforcement of other behavior: a preferred response elimination procedure, Behav Ther 11:449, 1980.

Homme L and Tosti D: Behavior technology: motivation and contingency management, San Rafael, Calif, 1971, Instruction Learning Systems.

Jacobson E: Progressive relaxation, Chicago, 1938, University of Chicago Press.

Kanfer FH and Schefft BK: Guiding the process of therapeutic change. Champaign, Ill, 1987, Research Press.

Lebow MD: Behavior modification: a significant method in nursing practice, Englewood Cliffs, NJ, 1973, Prentice-Hall Inc.

Levine FM and Sandeen E: Conceptualization in psychotherapy: a models approach, Hillsdale, NJ, 1985, Lawrence Erlbaum Associates, Publishers.

Loomis ME and Horsley JA: Interpersonal change: a behavioral approach to nursing practice, New York, 1974, McGraw-Hill Book Company.

Manderino MA and Bzdek VM: Social skills building, J Psychosoc Nurs 25(9):18-22, 1987.

Miller LE: Modeling awareness of feelings: a needed tool in the therapeutic communication workbook, Perspect Psychiatr Care 25:27-29, 1989.

Pavlov IP: Conditioned reflexes (Anrep GV, translator), London, 1927, Oxford University Press.

Pazulinec R, Meyerrose M, and Sajway T: Punishment via response cost. In Axelrod S and Apsche J, editors: The effects of punishment on human behavior, New York, 1983, Academic Press, pp 71-86.

Premack K: Reversibility of the reinforcement relation, Science 136:255, 1962.

Redman WK: Reduction of physical attacks through reinforcement of other behavior, J Child Adolesc Psychother 4:107-111, 1987.

Reynolds GS: A primer of operant conditioning, Glenview, Ill, 1968, Scott, Foresman & Co.

Skinner BF: The behavior of organisms, New York, 1938, Appleton-Century-Crofts, Inc.

Skinner BF: Science and human behavior, New York, 1953, The Free Press.

Skinner BF: A case history in scientific method, Am Psychol 11:211, 1956.

Steckel SB: Contracting with patient selected reinforcers, Am J Nurs 9:1596, 1980.

Watson JB and Rayner R: Conditioned emotional reactions, J Exp Psychol 3:1, 1920.

Wilson GT et al: Review of behavior therapy, Vol 11, New York, 1987, Guilford Publications, Inc.

Wolpe J: Psychotherapy by reciprocal inhibition, Stanford, 1958, Stanford University Press.

Yates AJ: Behavior therapy, New York, 1970, John Wiley & Sons, Inc.

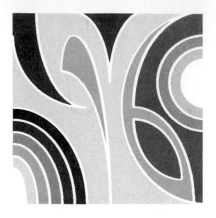

## CHAPTER 27

# Somatic Therapies

NORMAN L. KELTNER AND CLEO METCALF

LEARNING OBJECTIVES
After reading this chapter you should be able to

- Contrast modern electroconvulsive therapy (ECT) with traditional ECT.
- Discuss three indications for ECT.
- Describe the nurse's role in care before and after ECT.
- Describe and discuss the ethical, legal, social, and biological concerns related to psychosurgery.

Somatic therapies are treatment approaches that use physiological or physical interventions to effect behavioral change. The most common forms of somatic therapy, electroconvulsive therapy (ECT) and psychosurgery, are discussed in this chapter. Less common somatic therapy approaches include hydrotherapy, narcotherapy, and Indoklon therapy (for a brief description see Box 27-1).

ECT and psychosurgery emerged as treatment forms in the 1930s. The roots of ECT lie in the misconception of early twentieth century psychiatrists that epilepsy and schizophrenia were incompatible (Coffey and Weiner, 1990). Their advocates envisioned and promised dramatic relief from the curse of mental illness. Over time, inappropriate use and disappointing results coupled with the development of psychotropic drugs and a growing general distrust of psychiatric hospitals created a climate of hostility toward these therapies and their practitioners. Eventually in the 1960s and early 1970s the use of these two therapies came to a virtual standstill. Thompson and Blaine (1987) report that ECT treatments dropped significantly in the years 1975 to 1980. In the past 10 years, however, these two treatments have emerged once again as useful treatment alternatives when more traditional approaches fail. With rigid treatment criteria and careful pretreatment evaluation many psychiatric patients are responding to these somatic therapies.

## ELECTROCONVULSIVE THERAPY (ECT)

ECT's effectiveness in rescuing severely ill patients from the despairing depths of depression or perilous heights of uncontrolled mania is well accepted by psychiatrists. . . . However, ECT, like treatments for every other illness, is not 100% effective; it is not a cure, and it does have some adverse effects (Herbert Pardes, President, American Psychiatric Association, quoted in *Los Angeles Times,* Dec. 22, 1989, p. A-39).

### Box 27-1
### TYPES OF SOMATIC THERAPY

**electroconvulsive therapy** a therapy form based on the therapeutic benefits derived from electrically induced grand mal convulsions.

**hydrotherapy** the use of water (wet sheetpacks, 2- to 10-hour tub baths) for psychotherapeutic purposes.

**indoklon therapy** a convulsive therapy like ECT; however, convulsions are induced by ether rather than by electrical stimulus.

**narcotherapy** the induction of a state of sedation by intravenous administration of sedatives (e.g., amobarbital) or stimulants (e.g., methylphenidate [Ritalin]).

**psychosurgery** surgical interruption of selected neural fibers to reduce psychiatric symptoms.

Electroconvulsive therapy (ECT) was introduced in 1938 by Ugo Cerletti and Luciano Bini, two Italian psychiatrists. ECT is commonly referred to as EST (or electroshock therapy), or just "shock therapy." The latter term is considered unprofessional usage.

During ECT an electric current is passed through the brain, causing an epileptic seizure. Historically this seizure resulted in a full grand mal convulsion accompanied by the various complications of those convulsions, that is, muscle soreness, fractures, dislocations, sprains, tongue lacerations from biting, and so on. These seizures and the grotesque facial grimaces that occur have been dramatically captured on film and graphically detailed in literature. In films and novels ECT has been portrayed as the devious tool used by psychiatrists and psychiatric nurses, themselves demented (see Ken Kesey's *One Flew Over the Cuckoo's Nest* and Sylvia Plath's *The Bell Jar*), to maintain control over sane but highly individualistic patients. This public attack on ECT, when linked with reports of inappropriate use by former patients, virtually stopped the use of ECT in this country. Inappropriate use of ECT included administering ECT for almost all conditions and, from the accounts of former patients, using it as punishment for noncompliant behavior.

In its heyday, ECT was given to almost every patient who did not respond to other treatment forms (i.e., psychopharmacology or psychotherapy). In large state hospitals ECT was given on Mondays, Wednesdays, and Fridays to as many as 20 or more patients on a psychiatric ward. One patient after the other, some under their own power, others literally manhandled and held, would take their place on the bed to be given ECT. Nursing staff would hold the patient in place (to decrease fractures, dislocations, etc.), insert the mouth guard (to prevent tongue bites), put paste on the electrodes and hold the electrodes in place on each side of the head (usually the temple area), and hold the chin and jaw in proper alignment (similar to CPR positioning to prevent dislocation and maintain the airway), and the physician in the background would deliver the shock. As mentioned above, a full grand mal seizure would occur—a tonic seizure followed by a significantly longer clonic seizure. After convulsion activity terminated, the patient was turned on his side and tied in place (to prevent aspiration) while a staff member or "helper patient" stayed at the bedside until consciousness returned. The ECT team moved on to the next patient. This unforgettable scene, the novels and films, and reports from former patients contributed to a growing public fear of ECT. Yet, despite the negative views, ECT remains as a treatment form because many mental health professionals find it to be an effective alternative when other treatment modalities have failed. Simply, ECT has not merited the controversy over its use. It is safe and works where other treatments have failed.

## Modern ECT

During ECT an electric current (70 to 150 volts) is passed through the brain for 0.5 to 2 seconds. The seizure resulting from ECT should last between 30 and 60 seconds to be of therapeutic value. The events leading up to the treatment, including nursing responsibilities, follow.

### Preparation for ECT

- The patient must have a pretreatment evaluation, including physical examination, laboratory work (blood count, blood chemistries, urinalysis), and baseline memory abilities.
- A consent form must be signed. Since ECT is often given as a treatment of last resort, some patients are so profoundly depressed by the time ECT is ordered that "informed consent" is a contradiction in terms. In such cases the nurse should involve family members and request assistance from the facility's legal staff.
- The routine use of benzodiazepines or barbiturates for nighttime sedation should be eliminated because of their ability to raise the seizure threshold (Fink, 1987).
- A trained electrotherapist and an anesthesiologist should be available.
- An electroshock treatment device (e.g., MECTA SR-1, Medcraft B-25) should be available.

### Pretreatment

- The patient should be given nothing by mouth from midnight until after the treatment.
- Atropine as ordered should be given. Atropine can be given 1 hour before treatment or intravenously immediately preceding treatment. Atropine reduces secretions and subsequent risk of aspiration.
- The patient should be asked to urinate before the treatment (seizure-induced incontinence is common).
- The patient's hairpins and dentures should be removed.
- Vital signs should be taken.
- The nurse should be positive about the treatment and attempt to reduce anxiety.

### During treatment

- An intravenous line is inserted.
- Electrodes are attached to the proper place on the head. Electrodes are typically held in place with a rubber strap.
- The bite-block is inserted.
- Methohexital (Brevital) or another short-acting barbiturate is given intravenously for anesthesia. The barbiturate causes immediate anesthesia, preempting the anxiety associated with waiting for the "jolt to hit" and the anxiety caused by succinylcholine (succinylcholine causes paralysis but not sedation, thereby leaving the patient conscious but unable to breathe).
- Succinylcholine (Anectine) is given intravenously. Succinylcholine prevents the external manifestations of a grand mal seizure, thus minimizing fractures, dislocations, etc. while not affecting the "brain seizure."
- The anesthesiologist will mechanically ventilate the patient with 100% oxygen immediately before the treatment.

- The electrical impulse is given—up to 150 volts for 0.5 to 2 seconds.
- The seizure must last between 30 and 60 seconds to be of therapeutic value. If the seizure lasts less than 30 seconds, the physician must decide whether to stimulate another seizure.
- Monitoring devices include those for heart rate and rhythm, blood pressure, and electroencephalography.
- Ventilation and monitoring continue until the patient recovers.

### Posttreatment

- The anesthesiologist will mechanically ventilate the patient with 100% oxygen until the patient can breathe on his own.
- The nurse should monitor for respiratory problems.
- Since ECT causes confusion and disorientation, it is important to help reorient the patient (time, place, person) as he emerges from this groggy state.
- The patient should be observed until he is oriented and is steady on his feet.
- All aspects of the treatment should be carefully documented for the patient's record.

Seizure activity is monitored by an electroencephalographic (EEG) recording. Blood pressure and heart rate are also monitored. Oxygen is administered immediately before the treatment and then after the treatment because of interruption of breathing caused by the succinylcholine and the electrically induced seizure. Typically, patients are given ECT two to three times a week up to a total of 6 to 12 treatments (or until the patient improves or is obviously not going to improve).

### Indications for ECT

At one time ECT was administered to patients with all types of mental illness. Since ECT is not effective for every kind of mental illness, such indiscriminate use contributed to the disrepute into which it fell. ECT is useful in the treatment of delusional depression, and these patients respond better to ECT than to antidepressants (Bowden, 1985). The effects of ECT have a faster onset (Coffey and Weiner, 1990). In addition, depression that has not responded to other treatments, mania, catatonia, and some types of schizophrenia are significantly helped by ECT (Coffey and Weiner, 1990). Patients who are strongly suicidal are also candidates for ECT.

ECT is not useful in the treatment of mild depressions, behavior disorders, phobias, anxiety, or somatoform or personality disturbances.

By far, most ECT patients are severely depressed. Tancer et al. (1989) found that affective disorders accounted for 85% to 89% of all ECT patients. Depressed persons who are candidates for ECT must have vegetative symptoms (insomnia, anorexia, immobility, and muteness) and will often complain of early morning awakening. Anhedonia, the inability to experience pleasure, and delusional experiences are symptoms that also respond to ECT.

### Contraindications for ECT

Coffey and Weiner (1990) state that there are no absolute contraindications for ECT. However most clinicians believe that there is an increased risk when ECT is given to patients with cerebrovascular accidents, space-occupying tumors, and increased intracranial pressure.

## Advantages of ECT

Even with the host of psychotropic agents now available, ECT still represents for some patients the safest, most rapid, and most effective form of treatment." (Frances et al., 1989).

ECT is a safe procedure. Death from it is rare. Runck (1985), after developing a major report for the National Institute of Mental Health, found only 2.9 deaths per 10,000 patients receiving this treatment. Coffey and Weiner (1990) find the mortality rate to be from 0.01% to 0.03% for adults. There is a .01% mortality rate for children, so ECT is comparatively safe. It appears that ECT not only is safe but also more effective than antidepressants. Black et al. (1987) found that 70% of depressed patients and 85% of patients considered schizoaffective showed marked improvement with ECT. Only 48% of those treated with tricyclic antidepressants (TCAs) had similar improvement.

In addition, because it works faster, ECT is more economical. Markowitz et al. (1987) found that patients receiving ECT stayed an average of 13 fewer days in the hospital at a savings of $6,405 per patient. Furthermore, ECT can be given on an outpatient basis in some situations with an additional savings of $9000 (Kramer, 1990). ECT is also safer for patients with heart problems, since it does not produce the cardiovascular side effects associated with TCAs. Suicide by TCA overdose, a persistent concern with depressed patients, is reduced with ECT.

## Disadvantages of ECT

The major disadvantage of ECT is the fact that treatment provides only temporary relief. It does not provide a permanent cure. Certainly many patients are able to remain depression free for long periods of time, and still others may never need treatment again. However, some patients receiving ECT may need another series of treatments within a few months. Some psychiatrists order maintenance or continuation ECT (once per month for 6 to 12 months); however, the benefits of this approach are not clear.

Memory impairment, both retrograde (memory before treatment) and anterograde (ability to learn new things and memory after treatment), has been frequently cited as a side effect of ECT. Events closest in time to ECT are most frequently affected. Although it is true that memory is impaired for events both before and after each treatment and that confusion occurs immediately after each treatment, there does not seem to be any substantial loss of mental function once the treatment series is completed. Furthermore, since depression can cause memory loss too, it is not always clear whether memory impairment is related to ECT or to depression.

Unilateral electrode placement has been shown to reduce anterograde memory loss and posttreatment disorientation. Frances et al. (1989) report that memory actually improved after unilateral nondominant stimulation ECT was begun. When the unilateral approach is used, both electrodes are placed on the nondominant hemisphere (usually the right hemisphere) instead of one on each side of the head. This approach is now a recommended method of delivering ECT.

## How ECT works

It is not clear how this treatment works or why it is so effective. Several hypotheses have been advanced to explain its efficacy, some more reasonable than others:

- Patients recover because they view ECT as punishment or atonement for their guilt.
- Patients recover because they no longer remember why they are depressed.
- ECT causes some of the same biochemical changes that antidepressant drugs cause (i.e., the $5\text{-}HT_2$ serotonin receptor is affected by both ECT and TCAs [Brown and Mann, 1985]).

Although the above explanations may or may not be convincing, the fact remains that ECT is an effective treatment modality for delusional depression, depression resistant to psychopharmacology and psychotherapy, mania, catatonia, and some forms of schizophrenia.

## PSYCHOSURGERY

Earp (1979) defined psychosurgery as, "brain surgery performed on normal or diseased tissues for the relief of intractable personal suffering or for the modification or control of persistent behavior attendant on psychiatric illness." Actually, psychosurgery is not a single procedure but the name given to several different brain operations (Nys, 1988). More than 19 different kinds of psychosurgery have been identified (Buockoms, 1988).

It is difficult to find an area of psychiatry surrounded by more controversy. A review of the literature suggests that medical scientists have strongly-held views on both the efficacy and ethics of this procedure.

## Historical overview

Historically, psychosurgery was first reported in 1891 by Gottlieb Burckhardt, director of the insane asylum in Prefargier, Switzerland. Burckhardt operated on six patients. One died, one developed epilepsy, and one was thought to have improved. He had intended to calm very excitable patients, but the procedure was so vigorously opposed by his medical colleagues that he discontinued this activity (National Commission for the Protection of Human Subjects of Biomedical and Behavioral Sciences, 1977, pp. 1-5). In 1910, Ludwig Puusepp (NCPHSBBS, 1977, pp. 1-5), a Russian neurosurgeon, performed psychosurgery on three manic-depressive patients. The results were unsatisfactory, and he did not perform the procedure again for 25 years (Valenstein, 1980).

The man considered the modern-day pioneer in the field of psychosurgery was Egas Moniz, a Portuguese physician. In 1935, Moniz performed a frontal lobotomy on a depressed, 63-year-old former prostitute (Flor-Henry, 1977). Two months later she was considered cured. In 1949, Moniz received the Nobel Prize in physiology for his research (Davis, 1978).

In 1936, Freeman and Watts performed the first lobotomy in the United States:

In their development of Dr. Moniz' methods, Drs. Freeman and Watts drilled a small hole in the temple on each side of the patient's head where two skull bones meet. Surgeon Watts then inserted a dull knife into the brain, made a fan-shaped incision upward through the prefrontal lobe, then downward a few minutes later. He then repeated the incisions on the other side of the brain. No brain tissues were removed. (In two operations they cut cerebral arteries. Both patients died.) (*Time,* Nov. 30, 1942)

Freeman, a dynamic personality, had manned a booth next to Moniz at the 1935 Neurology Conference in London. Within a decade 6,000 patients had undergone this operation (Flor-Henry, 1977). Before 1960 psychosurgery was used primarily in the treatment of schizophrenia. In the early 1960s some mental health professionals began to believe other forms of mental illness were more responsive to this surgical intervention. Bridges and Williamson (1977), reporting on 10,000 cases of psychosurgery, found two thirds of the patients were schizophrenic and one fourth were depressed; however, depressed patients responded more favorably (50% improved) than did schizophrenic patients (18% improved).

World War II also played a part in the historical development of psychosurgery. Because of the high incidence of mental conditions either hindering admission to the armed forces or precipitating early discharge during the war, the Veterans Administration, in 1943, issued a communication encouraging staff neurosurgeons to obtain special training in prefrontal lobotomy operations. Reduction in soldier attrition rate to increase the number of fighting men was the purpose of this communication.

Psychosurgical intervention was more widely used in the 1940s and 1950s than it is today (see Fig. 27-1). As mentioned above, psychosurgery suffered some of the same public rejection as ECT. The popular novel by Ken Kesey, *One Flew Over the Cuckoo's Nest,* depicted the defiant hero as being the victim of a treacherous state hospital staff. His defiance eventually resulted in the ultimate punishment—a lobotomy. He emerged from the lobotomy room a "vegetable," his defiant character finally conquered. This depiction of psychosurgery may have helped shape public opinion about this procedure.

Flor-Henry (1977), quoting Fulton, states that by 1951, 20,000 persons had

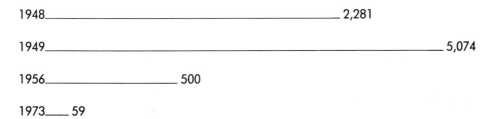

FIGURE 1948_____ 2,281

1949_____ 5,074

1956_____ 500

1973____ 59

**FIGURE 27-1** Psychosurgery performed in the years preceding and following the discovery and introduction of antipsychotic drugs. *(From Valenstein ES: The psychosurgery debate, San Francisco, 1980, WH Freeman and Co.)*

undergone this operation. By his own account, Freeman (1971) estimated his involvement in more than 3500 psychosurgical procedures. Valenstein (1980) estimates that 400 operations were performed each year in the United States for the years 1971, 1972, and 1973. He notes that the rate began to dramatically decline about that time. In the Soviet Union psychosurgery was outlawed in the early 1950s (Nys, 1988). The procedure is rarely performed today; however, some clinicians are beginning to reconsider psychosurgery as a treatment option. Valenstein (1988) laments, "I consider the history of prefrontal lobotomy a cautionary tale from which much can be learned."

### Concerns: Ethical, legal, social, and biological

Many concerns have been voiced regarding the ethical questions related to psychosurgery. The Breggins (1973, 1977, 1984) have been outspoken critics of psychosurgery. Peter Breggin (1973) states, "They mutilate non-diseased tissue, and they blunt the overall emotional and intellectual responsiveness of the mind." He also finds bias among the proponents of psychosurgery; that is, most psychosurgery patients, according to Breggin, are female or black. Freeman (1971) perhaps added to this perception when he stated that lobotomy "proved to be the ideal operation for use in crowded state mental hospitals with a shortage of everything except patients." Thomas Szasz (1977), noted for his critical views of traditional psychiatry, draws an analogy between psychosurgery and abortion, stating that both kill the soul. Bouckoms (1988) lists several ethical concerns that must be addressed, including uncertain efficacy, relative utility of the procedure, the nobility and normality of suffering, and the politics of psychosurgery.

These same concerns have carried over into the courts. Patients have consented to treatment only to find that they had too little information to truly provide informed consent. The procedure is such that the consent of the patient alone is not enough to justify psychosurgical intervention (Nys, 1988). A related concern is the validity of consent when obtained from prisoners (coerced with freedom, for example) or mental patients. The latter, by definition, must be seriously impaired to be considered for this treatment. On the other hand, the court case *Aden vs. Younger* (57 Cal. 3rd 622, 1976) addressed the issue of depriving a person of a potentially helpful treatment because of philosophical bias by the state.

Pakkenberg (1989) found a statistically significant difference between the brain volume (total fixed brain hemispheres, cortex, white matter, and central gray matter) of psychosurgery patients as compared to a control group on postmortem examination. Volume loss was not restricted to the surgical site. Central brain tissue was reduced also, suggesting the risk of morphological changes in the brain besides those intended.

Many mental health professionals find these concerns so complex that they cannot endorse the use of psychosurgery.

### Support for psychosurgery

Supporters of psychosurgery often find themselves defending their position against those who use more traditional treatment approaches. For instance, many detractors are traditional practitioners who question the efficacy of psychosurgery. Supporters of psychosurgery argue that such criticism is inconsistent because the efficacy of psychotherapy itself is difficult to evaluate, and the side effects of neuroleptic agents indicate that psychopharmacology is not without problems also.

A number of writers have spoken out for psychosurgical interventions in pre-scribed situations. Mark (1974) contends that psychosurgery should be used if a recognized pathological process is the primary cause of a patient's unwanted ab-normal behavior. Culliton (1976) points out that the Commission for the Protection of Human Subjects of Biomedical and Behavioral Research approves psychosurgery in carefully defined circumstances. Black (1977) contends that a rationale and an ethical basis for psychosurgery exist if the following criteria are met:

- The illness is disabling and untreatable by nonsurgical means
- The treatment has been demonstrated to be beneficial
- Safeguards such as informed consent, ability to withdraw from treatment, and the availability of a patient advocate are guaranteed

The popular view of a debilitated psychosurgery patient is refuted by several studies. Wehler and Hoffman (1978) compared 28 long-term hospitalized schizo-phrenic patients who had prefrontal lobotomy with 28 counterparts who had not undergone this surgery. IQ tests revealed no differences. Bernstein et al. (1975) studied 43 psychosurgery patients, of whom 35 were virtually symptom free.

## Indications for psychosurgery

Flor-Henry (1975), Tueber (1977), Valenstein (1980), and Reese (1988) state that psychosurgery is helpful for the following mental disorders if or when traditional treatments have failed:

- Depression and anxiety
- Depression-related pain
- Obsessive-compulsive disorders
- Aggression

## Modern psychosurgery

Psychosurgery has changed considerably over the past 50 years. Today radioyttrium rods, thermal probes, electrode implantations, and thermocoagulation have replaced the surgical hammer and leukotome (surgical ice pick) that Freeman used (see Fig. 27-2). Psychosurgical devices are used to destroy small, selected areas of brain tissue as indicated by specific symptoms as opposed to the less specific approach used by Freeman and Watts (1942). Flor-Henry (1977) reports:

> The modern evidence is, on the whole, remarkably convergent: some intractable psychopathological syndromes can be dramatically alleviated by precise, specific lim-bic lesions: orbital-frontal lesions for the affective syndromes; cingulate lesions for certain, but not all, obsessional syndromes; and amygdaloid lesions for some varieties of irresistible explosive violence.

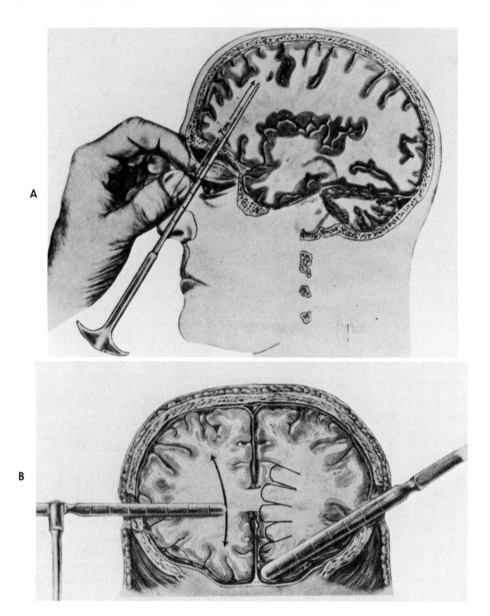

**FIGURE 27-2 A,** Freeman's transorbital lobotomy. **B,** Standard prefrontal lobotomy used by Freeman and Watts. The leukotome (ice pick) was inserted through holes drilled in the side of the frontal region of the skull. *(A from Valenstein ES: The psychosurgery debate, San Francisco, 1980, WH Freeman and Co.; B from Bridges P and Williamson C: Psychosurgery today, Nurs Times 73:1363, 1977.)*

## KEY CONCEPTS

1. Somatic therapies are treatment approaches that use physiological or physical interventions to affect behavioral change.
2. The most common forms of somatic therapy are electroconvulsive therapy (ECT) and psychosurgery.
3. During ECT an electric current is passed through the brain, causing an epileptic seizure.
4. Modern ECT uses anesthesia and muscle relaxants to prevent convulsive jerks that once caused broken bones; oxygen is given to guard against brain damage.
5. An estimated 30,000 to 50,000 Americans are given ECT each year.
6. ECT is indicated for the treatment of delusional depression, depression not responding to other treatments, mania, catatonia, and some types of schizophrenia.
7. Psychosurgery, a controversial brain surgery, is performed to provide relief from mental disorders that have been resistant to other treatment forms.
8. A number of ethical concerns have been raised by critics of psychosurgery, including its efficacy and the possibility of making the person worse.
9. In modern psychosurgery, refinements in the procedure that target very precise and limited brain anatomy have made the procedure safer.

## REFERENCES

Bernstein IC, Callahan WA, and Jaranson JM: Lobotomy in private practice: long term follow-up, Arch Gen Psychiatry 32:1041, 1975.

Black P: The rationale for psychosurgery, Humanist 37:6, 8-9, 1977.

Black DW, Winokur G, and Nasrallah A: The treatment of depression: electroconvulsive therapy v. antidepressants: a naturalistic evaluation of 1,495 patients, Compr Psychiatry 28:169, 1987.

Bowden CL: Current treatment of depression, Hosp Community Psychiatry 36:1192, 1985.

Bouckoms AJ: Ethics of psychosurgery, Acta Neurochir Suppl 44:173, 1988.

Breggin P: Use of psychosurgery as a treatment for hyperactivity in children, Mental Health 58:19, 1984.

Breggin PR: The second wave, Mental Health 57:11, 1973.

Breggin PR: If psychosurgery is wrong in principle...? Psychiatr Opinion 14:23, 1977.

Bridges P and Williamson C: Psychosurgery today, Nurs Times 73:1363, 1977.

Brown RP and Mann JJ: A clinical perspective on the role of neurotransmitters in mental disorders, Hosp Community Psychiatry 36:141, 1985.

Coffey CE and Weiner RD: Electroconvulsive therapy: an update, Hosp Community Psychiatry 41:515-521, 1990.

Culliton BJ: Psychosurgery: National Commission issues surprisingly favorable report, Science 194:299, 1976.

Davis D: Psychosurgery, Operational Psychol 9:70-71, 1978.

Earp JD: Psychosurgery: the position of the Canadian Psychiatric Association, Can J Psychiatry 24:353, 1979.

Fink M: New technology in convulsive therapy: a challenge to training, Am J Psychiatry 144:1195, 1987.

Flor-Henry P: Progress and problems in psychosurgery, Curr Psychiatr Ther 17:282, 1977.

Flor-Henry P: Psychiatric surgery—1936-1973: evolution and current perspectives, Can Psychiatr Assoc J 20:157, 1975.

Frances A, Weiner RD, and Coffey CE: ECT for an elderly man with psychotic depression and concurrent dementia, Hosp Community Psychiatry 40:237, 242, 1989.

Freeman W: Frontal lobotomy in early schizophrenia: long-term follow-up in 415 cases, Br J Psychiatry 119:621-624, 1971.

Freeman W and Watts JW: Time, p 48, Nov. 30, 1942.

Kramer BA: Outpatient electroconvulsive therapy: a cost-saving alternative, Hosp Community Psychiatry 41:361-363, 1990.

Mark VH: A psychosurgeon's case for psychosurgery, Psychol Today 8:28, 30, 33, 84, 86, 1974.

Markowitz J et al: Reduced length and cost of hospital stay for major depression in patients treated with ECT, Am J Psychiatry 144:1025, 1987.

National Commission for the Protection of Human Subjects of Biomedical and Behavioral Sciences: Psychosurgery, Washington, DC, 1977, Department of Health, Education and Welfare.

Nys H: Psychosurgery and personality: some legal considerations, Acta Neurochir Suppl 44:170, 1988.

Pakkenberg B: What happens in the leucotomised brain? A post-mortem morphological study of brain from schizophrenic patients, J Neurol Neurosurg Psychiatry 52:156, 1989.

Reese T: Obsessive-compulsive disorders: a treatment review, J Clin Psychiatry 49:48, 1988.

Runck B: NIMH report: consensus panel backs cautious use of ECT for severe disorders, Hosp Community Psychiatry 36:943, 1985.

Szasz TS: Aborting unwanted behavior: the controversy on psychosurgery, Humanist 37:10, 1977.

Tancer ME et al: Use of electroconvulsive therapy at a university hospital: 1970 and 1980-81, Hosp Community Psychiatry 40:64, 1989.

Thompson JW and Blaine JD: Use of ECT in the United States in 1975 and 1980, Am J Psychiatry 144:557, 1987.

Tueber HC: In National Commission for the Protection of Human Subjects of Biomedical and Behavioral Sciences: Psychosurgery, Sec III, Washington, DC, 1977, DHEW publication No. 77-0001, pp 35-37.

Valenstein ES: Prefrontal lobotomy: author replies, Surg Neurol 30:75, 1988.

Valenstein ES: The psychosurgery debate, San Francisco, 1980, WH Freeman and Co.

Wehler R and Hoffman K: Intellectual functioning in lobotomized long-term chronic schizophrenic patients, J Clin Psychol 34:449-451, 1978.

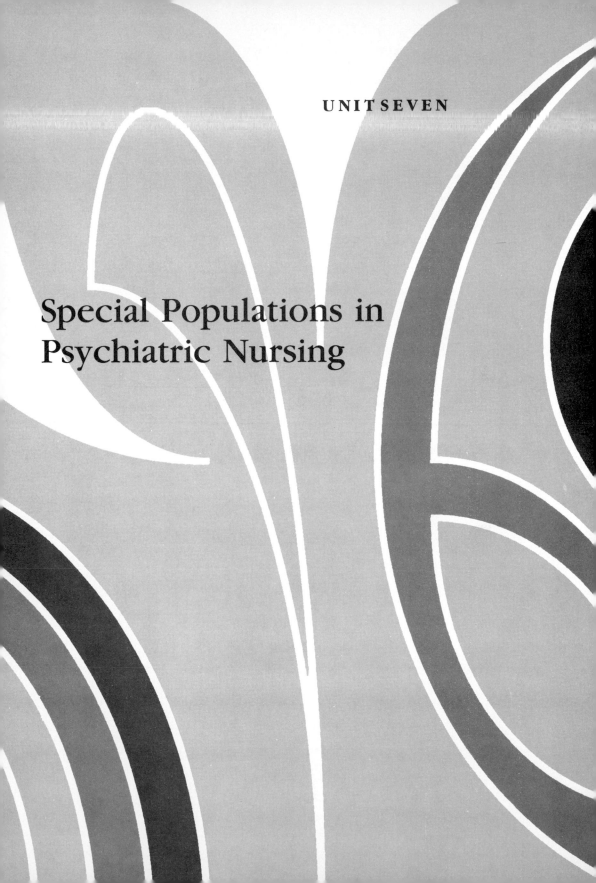

# Special Populations in Psychiatric Nursing

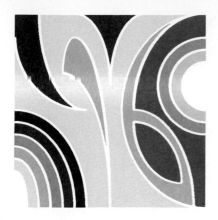

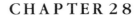

## CHAPTER 28

# Victims of Violent Behavior

LEARNING OBJECTIVES

After reading this chapter you should be able to

- Appreciate the seriousness of violence toward women.
- Describe the emotional reactions of victims of crime, rape, incest, and wife abuse.
- Recognize adult symptoms of victims of childhood incest.
- Understand the cycle of violence and why women stay in abusive relationships.
- Understand the needs of victims of violence.
- Describe strategies for facilitating recovery from violent behavior.
- Develop a nursing care plan for a victim of violent behavior.

The victimization of any person by another is a serious mental health and legal problem. Violence in all forms is increasing in this society (Gest, 1989). Nurses, regardless of area of practice, *will* come in contact with the victims as inpatients, outpatients, home care patients, emergency care patients, parents of patients, friends, and even as relatives. Although the victims are typically seen initially for medical reasons, their psychological needs also require attention if long-term mental health problems are to be prevented.

The major focus of this chapter is the response of adult women to the violent behaviors of others. It begins with general reactions to any crime experienced by any victim, male or female, but then focuses on the victims of rape, adult survivors of childhood incest, and women abused by their partners. It is acknowledged that men may also be raped, sexually abused as children, and abused as adults by their partners; however, statistics indicate that, at most, 5% to 10% of all such victims are male. Although a small number of perpetrators of this kind of violence are female, the most common pattern of victimization is by males against females.

The short- and long-term reactions of victims described in this chapter are *generally* true for both male and female victims, but the more specific differences for males will not be discussed. As a general rule, men have a more difficult time admitting to and dealing with their emotional victimization. The typical male "macho" self-image seems to be the reason men respond so severely to being victimized as adults by women. The great impact on males of sexual violation by other males, both as children and as adults, seems to be the result of their fears about homosexuality (Courtois, 1988).

## VIOLATION BY CRIME
### Emotional reactions

Not all crimes involve physical violence and injury; however, all crimes involve *emotional* violation and injury. As described by Bard and Sangrey (1986), the "violation of self" involves an invisible injury to the very essence of a person. The self is violated even with the loss or destruction of possessions and property because these are an extension of our internal identity. They have more personal significance than their actual monetary value. All crimes also threaten two basic foundations of human development: the sense of trust and the sense of autonomy (Bard and Sangrey, 1986). Crime victims typically experience a loss of trust, not just in the criminal, but to some degree in all other persons. Victims also lose a sense of ability to control their own lives and even themselves (Table 28-1).

The emotional reactions to crime vary greatly according to the person, situational variables, and the meaning of the crime to that person. However, the common reactions are denial, fear, anger, and powerlessness. A sense of failure and guilt are common as the victim thinks of what he did to cause or at least not prevent or stop the crime. Victims commonly feel ashamed and unworthy, as well as contaminated or "dirty," whether they were physically touched by the perpetrator or not. Depression and fantasies of or a wish for revenge are fairly typical (Bard and Sangrey, 1986). The relationships of the victim to family and friends can be disturbed to any degree. This is in part due to the victim's loss of trust but also to the response of the others. Even caring persons can imply that the victim was responsible for the

**TABLE 28-1**    Crimes against people

| Pocket picking, purse snatching | Auto theft | Burglary | Robbery | Robbery with assault | Sexual assault | Homicide |
|---|---|---|---|---|---|---|
| Violation of extension of self: property | Violation of extension of self: home | | Violation of extension of self: personal possessions | Violation of extension of self: personal possessions | Violation of extension of self: clothing | Ultimate violation of self—the destruction of the person |
| Loss of trust | Loss of trust | | Loss of trust | Loss of trust | Loss of trust | |
| Threat to autonomy (control) | Threat to autonomy (control) | | Loss of autonomy (control) | Loss of autonomy (control) | Loss of autonomy (control) | |
| | | | Threat to survival | Threat to survival | Threat to survival | |
| | | | | Physical injury to the external self | Physical injury to the external self | |
| | | | | | Violation of internal self | |

Reprinted with permission from Bard M and Sangrey D: The crime victim's book, New York, 1986, Brunner/Mazel Publishers.

crime, with such questions as: Why were you there alone at night? Why were you carrying so much cash? Why didn't you install the burglar alarm when I suggested it? The victim may then feel alienated and isolated. Hospital personnel, police, and the legal system may also convey a "blaming-the-victim" attitude in their type and manner of questioning and in their focusing on the facts only without any emotional support or empathy.

## Recovery from the trauma

Many theories have been formulated regarding the process of recovery from traumas. Important theorists include Eric Lindeman, Gerald Caplan, Charles Figley, Burgess and Holstrom, Fox and Sherl, and Martha Wolfstein (Bard and Sangrey, 1986). Most theorists agree that the reaction to and recovery from the trauma are influenced by three things: (1) the severity of the trauma, (2) the victim's resources, and (3) the nature of help provided immediately after the event. Typically, three stages of recovery are defined: initially disorganization, then a struggle to adapt, and eventually readjustment (Bard and Sangrey, 1986). The brief summary of these stages is derived from the perspectives of Tynhurst (1951), Fox and Sherl (1972), Burgess and Holstrom (1974), and Stuart and Sundeen (1988). The stages are not clearly separated, and the readjustment process is not smooth. There may be vacillation among the stages, and the length of recovery may take months or years.

**Impact.** The initial reaction to the trauma usually lasts from a few minutes to a few days. The common responses are shock, denial, disbelief, and confusion. There may also be paralyzing fear, or hysteria, a sense of helplessness and vulnerability, and physiological responses that affect sleeping and eating. Some victims react less visibly or in a delayed manner. They will look calm, organized, and rational, and will take all the necessary actions initially needed. It is often later, in private, that the more common delayed reactions described above occur.

**Recoil.** It is in the recoil stage that a victim's struggle to adapt begins. The immediate danger is over, but a great deal of emotional stress remains to be worked through. In the beginning of this phase are periods of time in which the victim looks and acts "normal" and is able to carry out daily routines at home and at work. Activity helps to suppress the fears, anger, and sadness. Later in the phase there is a desire to talk about the trauma and all the feelings. Often a need for support and even a need to be temporarily dependent is felt. Fantasies of revenge are natural during this stage. In the weeks following the crime trauma the victim gradually becomes aware of the full impact the event has had on her life.

**Reorganization.** Reorganization may take months to years to accomplish. Although the trauma is not forgotten, the anxiety, fear, and anger diminish, and the victim reconstructs her life. The beginning of this phase includes reviewing and organizing what happened, attempting to figure out why it happened ("why me"), attributing blame to self, to others, or to both, justifying one's own actions, and regaining a sense of control and self-protection. Grief over the losses resolves slowly as this phase continues. There may be lingering nightmares, frustrations, and disillusionment; however, these also subside as the victim reengages in life and activities. If reorganization is not effective, the victim may experience degrees of symptoms that, in some cases, are clinically diagnosable, as in depression and posttraumatic stress disorder.

### Facilitating recovery from a crime

Although empathy, emotional support, and a willingness to listen are important in all stages of recovery, there are also differences in the kind of help needed at each stage. During the impact stage the focus is on the victim's need for physical safety and emotional security. Reassurance, protection from further harm, and sometimes medical care are needed. The victim often needs clear, simple directions on what to do, where to go, and what to avoid. It is a time for professionals (including nurses) to avoid accusations (blaming) and unnecessary intrusions or invasion of privacy. In most cases this crisis-intervention approach is face-to-face at the scene of the trauma. For those victims who are temporarily calm and in control, the crisis intervention may occur a few hours or days later, when reality hits. A crisis phone or walk-in services can be of help at this time.

During the recoil stage the victim often needs a validation of herself and her rights as a victim. Depending on the type of trauma, referrals can be made to victims assistance or disaster relief programs. Legal or insurance assistance may be needed. If family and friends cannot be fully available during the episodes of emotional turmoil, then short-term counselling or walk-in crisis centers may be beneficial. It is during the struggle to adjust that support groups consisting of other victims can be most useful. Whether the group is short term (6 to 8 weeks) or ongoing and whether the group is professionally or self-led, there is value in receiving information, encouragement, and companionship from others who "have been there too." Many communities have groups for victims of disasters, divorce, death of a loved one, sudden infant death syndrome (SIDS), rape, incest, and physical and emotional abuse, as well as for survivors of suicide, mass murders, and disappearance of children.

In the reorganization stage, most victims are able to recover and grow with minimal assistance. The goal is to move from victim status to survivor status by integrating the memories of the crime or trauma and moving on in life. Sometimes referrals for long-term counseling are needed to overcome anxiety, phobias, depression, suicidal ideation, or other posttraumatic symptoms.

It is uncommon for most victims to need hospitalization beyond any initial medical care. Crisis intervention and short- and long-term counseling on an outpatient basis are usually sufficient. Exceptions include the victim who is unable to function to meet basic needs or who becomes suicidal.

## RAPE AND SEXUAL ASSAULT

U.S. statistics indicate that rape of women is an *under*reported crime, with only 1 in 10 rapes probably reported. Estimates of actual rapes range from one in eight to one in four women being raped after the age of 14. A woman may be raped at any age, but the highest risk occurs between the ages of 15 and 24. One major problem in reporting rape is that laws and attitudes vary in different states and communities. In general, rape is considered forcible penetration of the victim's body by the perpetrator's penis without her consent. Any other form of forced sexual contact (from touch to mutilation) is considered sexual assault. Beyond these definitions, there is little consistency. Some prosecutors will not accept rape as a charge if the two persons know each other, so in those localities "date rape" is considered nonexistent. In other places, by law, husbands cannot be charged with raping their wives. Unfortunately, many members of our society either ignore the issue or, even worse, convey the message that any woman who is raped really asked for it ("blaming the victim"). The laws, applications of these laws, and societal attitudes interfere with both reporting rape and recovering from it. Despite the sexual contact, it is generally acknowledged that rape is not sexually motivated but involves a desire for power and control and a wish to humiliate a woman.

### Surviving rape and sexual assault

As with any crime victim (described earlier), the rape victim experiences a severe violation and all the possible emotions of the impact stage. In addition to internal and external bodily injuries, there may be a threat to life with weapons, a threat to return and rape again if the rape is reported, or actual death at the hands of the perpetrator during or after the rape. The victim may live but wish she had died.

The powerlessness, loss of control, fear, shame, guilt, humiliation, and rage may be overwhelming. A typical reaction of the victim is the wish to regain a sense of control and retreat to a safe place, take a thorough shower, and destroy any damaged belongings. To do so is to destroy most of the evidence that would be required if the woman later decided to report the rape and ask for prosecution.

**Needs of the victim.** Despite an outward appearance of calm composure and denial of need for help, the rape victim needs assistance, information, and support. It may not be until the victim begins the up-and-down struggle of the recoil stage that she recognizes her losses, anger, and needs. An emergency room may or may not be equipped to help a rape victim. Collecting evidence may seem like a priority for staff, but for the victim it is seen only as further intrusion and violation. To staff, the victim may be seen as a resistant, uncooperative patient while the victim is only trying to protect herself and regain a sense of control. Although it is more time and energy consuming, the best approach is to move slowly and supportively at the victim's pace and to always give rationales (as well as descriptions) for any procedures or referrals suggested. Nurses, who are predominantly women, can be particularly helpful to female crime victims. The victims tend to feel safer with a woman and may even refuse to talk to a man, especially alone. Having one nurse stay with the victim through the examinations and interrogations can be particularly reassuring. Many communities have information packets prepared for rape victims and helping personnel (in hospitals, counseling centers, and crisis services) similar to the ones included here (Box 28-1). Victims can be encouraged to keep the

### Box 28-1
### THE NEEDS AND RIGHTS OF RAPE VICTIMS

1. Crisis intervention: information, counseling, and referrals
2. Help with basic needs: housing, transportation, child care, safety
3. Medical information and care: information about pregnancy prevention, follow-up care, and counseling
4. Advocacy for whatever choices are made about reporting or prosecuting
5. Protection of rights: to privacy, confidentiality, gentleness, sensitivity, and explanations of procedures and tests
6. Protection of rights: to refuse collection of evidence, to determine who will and will not be present during examinations, to get copies of all medical and legal reports, and to apply for reimbursement through victim's compensation
7. Fairness, information, and protection of legal rights: during investigations, hearings, and trial, including not being asked about prior sexual experiences with anyone besides the suspect or defendent
8. Reasonable protection against further harm: escorts to court, restraining order, additional patrols, even relocation if necessary

information sheets as well as phone numbers of resources for later use. Especially the "composed, calm" victim who denies the need for help should be encouraged to take materials home. If the services are available, an advocate from a victim's assistance program or a rape crisis counselor can be called to initiate contact in the emergency room and make periodic follow-up days, weeks, and months later.

The ability to make follow-up contact with a rape victim after the impact stage can be beneficial. As stated earlier, it is in the recoil stage that most victims begin to react emotionally to the significant effect rape has on their lives. As with other crime victims, the rape victim may alternately deny and admit to turmoil being experienced. Fear and mistrust are major issues to be addressed. The victim may direct these toward only the perpetrator (or men who resemble him), or she may begin to mistrust everyone around her (especially if others convey any hint of blaming her) and be afraid to leave the one place she designates as safe. More often, the victim is able to go out and be with family and friends but avoids strangers and places similar to the rape scene. If the rape occurred in her own residence, she may move or at least make safety-related changes to prevent recurrence. She may ask for someone to stay with her at night for awhile. Being alone and unprotected is usually frightening for the victim. Although superficial relationships with men friends are usually possible, intimacy, especially sexual relationships, are typically avoided.

In terms of her own view of herself, the rape victim, like other crime victims, experiences shame, loss of a sense of autonomy or control over her life, guilt, and a feeling of being contaminated, "dirty," or like a "damaged, inferior product." These feelings contribute to the avoidance of others and the failure to seek help. The victim needs help to overcome these feelings, especially reaffirming that she is a worthwhile person who did not cause and did not deserve the rape. Her rights and dignity also need reaffirming. She also needs to know that her anger is natural, especially about the violation of person and privacy and the humiliation and sense of powerlessness she has suffered.

**Rape trauma symptoms.** One way to monitor the rape victim's responses to the trauma and recovery process through the recoil and reorganization stages is to use the Rape Trauma Symptom Rating Scale (DiVasto, 1985) (Table 28-2). It is important in using the scale to remember that the victim will vacillate in the recoil stage between repression or suppression and dealing with the trauma. Even progress in the reorganization stage will not be smooth but will have backslides at times, especially if new situations trigger memories of the rape. The victim may need help in overcoming any of the evident symptoms, such as difficulty in sleeping or eating, relationship problems, and lowered self-esteem.

## Facilitating recovery from rape

As with other crime victims, the rape victim needs continual empathy, support, and a willingness to listen from potential helpers. Crisis intervention is still the most appropriate approach during the impact stage. Short-term counseling and a rape support group are beneficial during the recoil stage. These are usually aimed at overcoming guilt and shame, building self-esteem and trust, and assisting in regaining control of one's life and a sense of safety. Support groups are sometimes available for relatives, especially spouses, of the rape victims to help them deal with the

**TABLE 28-2**  Rape trauma symptom rating scale

| | 5 | 4 | 3 | 2 | 1 |
|---|---|---|---|---|---|
| Sleep disorders | No sleep; awake all night most nights; sleep deprived state | Severe: 1-3 hours sleep per night; early morning awaking, stressful nightmares | Moderate: difficulty falling asleep, nightmares | Mild: episodic nightmares; broken sleep | Sleeping well |
| Appetite | Hardly eating at all; prodded by others to eat | Severe: no appetite, eating out of habit | Moderate change; eating less food less frequently | Very little change; not quite as much food intake as before assault | No noticeable change |
| Phobias | Succumbed to fear; will not leave home, answer telephone or talk with nonfamily | Severe: fears dominating life; seeking help; anxiety immobilizing | Moderate suspicion; some fears expressed, change in life-style moderate | Mild suspicion, little change in life-style habits | Calm and relaxed |
| Motor behavior | Uprooting of life (job and home); no activities | Job or home change, reduction in activities, lack of interest, self control | Restlessness and dissatisfaction with indecisiveness, reduction in activities | Mild restlessness; expressed desire to make changes in work or home life | Calm and relaxed |

| | | | | | |
|---|---|---|---|---|---|
| Relations | Denial of or from SOP(s); broken relationship with family, partner, friend | Severe tension, anxiety; relationship(s) disintegrating | Relationship(s) showing stress, nonsupportive, weakened | Relationship(s) intact, strained but supportive | SOP(s) supportive, understanding and patient |
| Self-blame | Overcome with shame; feels cannot forgive self | Severe guilt; blames self, feels dirty, cheap | Moderate guilt; feels responsible | Mild guilt; feels it can be overcome | Free from guilt; accepts event |
| Self-esteem | Feels worthless or hates self; completely unsatisfied with self | Disgusted with self | Disappointed with self; feels badly about self | Occasionally doubts self-worth | Feels good about self |
| Somatic reactions | Compounded symptoms directly related to the assault plus reactivation of symptoms connected to a previous condition; eg, heavy drinking or drug use | Severe symptoms; distressing symptoms described, life-style disrupted | Moderate symptoms, ability to function but some disturbance of life-style | Mild symptoms, minor discomfort reported; ability to talk about discomfort and feeling of control over symptom | No symptoms; none reported and symptoms denied when asked about a specific area |

From DiVasto P: Measuring the aftermath of rape, J Psychosoc Nurs 23(2):33, 1985.

trauma, the stereotyping and myths, and the changes occurring in the victim and themselves. Although uncommon, medications to reduce anxiety and provide for sleep may be used on a *temporary* basis. Long-term counseling should be available if needed and desired during the reorganization stage, especially if the victim decides to prosecute the perpetrator. The lengthy legal process can seriously delay the recovery process. In many trial situations the victim is still treated like a criminal during cross-examinations. On the other hand, conviction and imprisonment of the perpetrator can help the victim feel vindicated, compensated, and more safe in her environment.

If the symptoms on the Rape Trauma Rating Scale are not gradually diminishing and reorganization of life-style does not seem to be occurring, the victim needs to be assessed for newly developed problems, such as anxiety, excessive anger and guilt, depression, acting out, isolation, self-destructive behaviors, substance abuse, phobias, and negative or destructive relationships with others. With any of these behaviors, longer-term counseling is a necessity. As with other crime victims, hospitalization may become essential if lack of functioning or suicidal attempts are apparent.

## ADULT SURVIVORS OF CHILDHOOD INCEST
### Nature of the problem

Recovery from the crime of incest is so difficult for two major reasons: The crime is not a one-time occurrence, and the perpetrator is a known and trusted person. Unfortunately, this is not an uncommon crime. It is estimated that 20% of all females are victims of incest (Russell, 1986). Another estimate is that 2.5 million girls are sexually abused by relatives, friends, and strangers each year (Courtois, 1988). One in ten boys is sexually abused by the age of 18 by relatives or nonrelatives (Burgess, 1984). More recent research indicates that sexual abuse of boys may be much higher than previously thought (Lew, 1988), and among male inpatients as many as one in six have been sexually abused as children (Jacobson and Herald, 1990). Incest includes voyeurism and exhibitionism, which can lead to intercourse and mutilation, but always involves a younger victim who is not capable of giving consent to the older relative. Perpetrators are fathers, uncles, stepfathers, older brothers, and grandfathers. The female victims are all ages, from every social, cultural, ethnic, and economic group. On the average, the incest acts begin as caressing and progress to molestation by 4 years of age and to intercourse by 10 years of age (Courtois, 1988).

Although incest can be violent, it usually is not. Russell's study (1986) found coercion in 68% of the cases but no violence. In 29% of the cases there was mild force, such as pinning the victim down. In only 3% was there some degree of physical violence. Coercion is possible because of the victim's dependent, trusting, and loving relationship with the perpetrator. The victim is urged to maintain the "secret" with various threats such as (1) the victim will be taken away from the family, (2) the perpetrator will be put in a mental hospital or jail, (3) the parents will divorce, (4) the mother will get sick, (5) there will be no abuse of siblings if the victim is compliant, (6) love will be withdrawn, (7) no one would believe the victim anyway, or (8) there will be physical abuse if the victim does not comply.

Even when there is no physical violence, victims usually fear that it will occur if they resist the perpetrator.

Even if the young victims wanted to disclose the incest, it is difficult for them to do so. They often lack the words and concepts to describe what is happening. There is usually an emotional reaction of fear and confusion and some physical pain but not a moral or ethical concept of wrong. Most victims who, as children, tried to tell their mothers were met with disbelief and denial. It is difficult for mothers to believe that the men they love and married are capable of incest. There are also potential benefits from the incestuous relationship: The child is made to feel special, with extra attention and time with the perpetrator that siblings do not enjoy, and a certain power comes from trying to please the adult and from receiving a degree of affection. At times the girl may even have the physical experience of sensual pleasure. However, the emotional pleasure and concept of sexual love are absent. (All girls make bids for attention and affection. Even if they are cute, coy, or flirtatious, these should not be viewed as seduction. The perpetrators choose to misinterpret the behaviors to meet their own needs and still should be held responsible for the crime.)

For the victim the end result is ambivalence about the incestuous experience (both benefits and pain) and denial of what is happening to protect the whole family. The young girl is fulfilling the roles of child and lover to the perpetrator and of child and protector to the rest of the family (protecting them from the "horrible secret"). As a result the child begins a long-term process of parenting others to the exclusion of her own needs (Urbancic, 1987). Basically, the child wishes for love, not sex, but eventually ends up feeling guilty, exploited, betrayed, angry, "dirty," helpless, and responsible. Butler (1978) describes four levels of betrayal: (1) by the abuser, (2) by the lack of response from the other parent or adult relatives, (3) by lack of response from teachers, doctors, nurses, and other professionals who miss the cues, and (4) by herself through denial of the abuse in order to cope. Denial, repression, suppression, rationalization, and even dissociation are mechanisms used by the young victim to cope with this "no-win" situation. Repression is common until victims are in their 20s or 30s and begin having trouble with close relationships. Some victims have repressed even longer, at least one victim for 50 years. She did not "remember" her own incestuous experiences at ages 8 to 10 until her son-in-law revealed that her 40-year-old daughter had also been a victim of the woman's husband during the daughter's childhood.

### Effects of incest

As adolescents, incest victims often show more overt methods of dysfunctional coping, such as impulsive, self-destructive behaviors, including suicide attempts, running away, substance use or abuse, and sexual acting out. The child may have fantasies of revenge and wish for the perpetrator's death. The anger toward the perpetrator and toward the mother or other adults (for not providing protection against the incest) approaches rage but is not directly expressed. The victim may not even be aware of the reason for the rage or realize that the acting-out behaviors are related to the incest.

**Box 28-2**

## MANIFESTATIONS OF CHILDHOOD INCEST OBSERVED IN STUDY GROUP

- Sexual dysfunctioning
  - non-orgasmic to not being able to be touched by a male
- Self-destructive behavior
  - Substance abuse
  - Suicidal behavior
  - Destructive relationships
- Emotional and physical abuse toward children
- Impulsive behavior
  - Eating
  - Spending
- Marital problems
- Difficulty sustaining intimate relationships
- Depression

- Poor self-esteem
- Promiscuity
- Somatic complaints
  - Chronic pain
  - Headaches
  - Nausea
- Feelings of detachment
- Lack of trust
- Feelings of powerlessness
- Needing always to care for others
- Difficulty with authority figures
- Inability to deal with incestuous behavior toward children
- Difficulty in parenting
- Reinvolvement in incestuous assault

From Lowery M: Adult survivors of childhood incest, J Psychosoc Nurs 25(1):27-31, 1987.

Even as adult survivors, women will enter counseling for other reasons, not because of an incestuous relationship. On the surface, the victim may look uninjured because of the denial, dissociation, amnesia, emotional deadening, or repression associated with the incest. They are usually brought to counseling for one or more of the symptoms identified by Lowery (1987) in the study group of adult survivors (Box 28-2). Even if the victim has memories of the incest, she tends to deny or minimize its relationship to any of her current problems. Only later will it become evident that incest has disturbed the victim's whole growth and development process and diminished her self-esteem. The process of surviving as a child and becoming a woman is similar to delayed posttraumatic stress disorder. There is the initial repression of memories (even non-incest-related ones), and then the unwanted intrusive memories begin breaking through. The memories may begin as nightmares, kinesthetic sensations (such as flinching when a boyfriend or husband touches in the same way the perpetrator did), or flashbacks. The memories may return gradually in pieces or in a sudden, overwhelming flood.

Most adult survivors of childhood incest display a variety of clinical symptoms, as can be seen in Box 28-2, but only about 20% reveal serious psychopathology

## REINVOLVEMENT IN INCESTUOUS ASSAULT

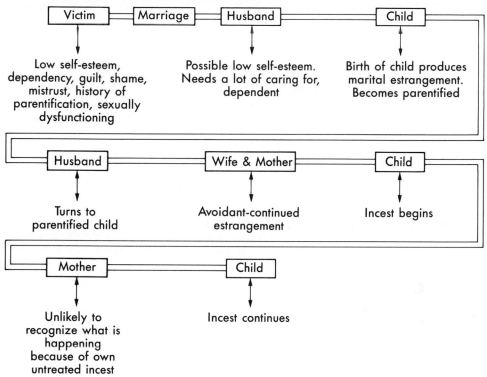

**FIGURE 28-1** Reinvolvement in incestuous assault. *(From Lowrey, M.: Adult survivors of childhood incest. J Psychosoc Nurs 25(1):27-31, 1987.)*

(Courtois, 1988). When there is an axis I diagnosis for outpatients, it is commonly depression (atypical type), a posttraumatic stress disorder, substance-abuse disorder, anxiety disorder, somatoform disorder, dissociative disorder (including multiple personality), or impulse-control disorder. For inpatients, schizophrenia may be diagnosed. Axis II personality disorders may also be diagnosed, such as borderline, narcissistic, histrionic, avoidant, dependent, atypical, or mixed disorder (Courtois, 1988). Receiving a diagnosis is a major problem, not only because of the stigma but also because the diagnosis often becomes the focus of treatment rather than the underlying issue of recovering from the incest. Lack of appropriate treatment carries a major risk, not only for the adult survivor but also for her children, especially if she is still in a stage of repression. There is evidence that an untreated or improperly treated victim may occasionally be a candidate for setting up a dysfunctional, disorganized family that contributes to the incestuous assault of her child or children (Lowery, 1987) (Fig. 28-1). With her own denial, repression, amnesia, or other mechanisms, she has trouble relating to her husband and then is unable to "see" his involvement with her child. There are examples of incest occurring within three and four generations of a family. Breaking this "cycle" is crucial.

## PSYCHOTHERAPEUTIC MANAGEMENT

*NURSE-PATIENT RELATIONSHIP* In some ways, recovery from incest is similar to recovery from any crime or from posttraumatic stress disorder, but it tends to be more difficult and more lengthy. The memories and emotions are painful and confusing. The anger and ambivalence toward the perpetrator are hard for both the survivor and the counselor to handle. The survivor needs to know in the beginning that her symptoms and emotional pain will probably worsen before they improve as the review of experiences occurs. Although therapy often takes 2 years or more, incest survivors tend to engage in treatment sporadically. It is common for the survivor to initially disclose, discuss, vent, and feel "cured." Then, as new crises or relationship problems emerge, she will return to therapy to deal with each issue and maybe its connection to the original incest. It is difficult to get her commitment for continuous long-term treatment, but the counselor can emphasize the desirability and value of at least sporadic counseling.

Much depends on the counselor's ability to quickly develop a trusting relationship with the survivor. Empathy, active support, compassion, warmth, and nonjudgment are crucial. Suggestions for how to respond developed by Courtois (1988) for friends and relatives of survivors is also useful for counselors (Box 28-3).

The survivor needs to be calmly and matter-of-factly asked about the incest, since she is not likely to spontaneously reveal it. As a rule, survivors prefer to be asked about "childhood sexual experiences with adults" or about "an adult's being sexual with her as a child" instead of initially hearing the words *incest, victim,* or *sexual abuse* (Courtois, 1988). The old coercions to keep the "secret" remain strong in the mind of the survivor. She needs to feel quite safe about confidentiality and the counselor's acceptance before disclosure will occur. How much detail is revealed and how soon depends in part on the counselor's ability to be receptive to the experiences *without* being critical of the situation, the perpetrator, and other adults in the family, or of the survivor's loyalty to them. The survivor needs to be reassured that all her experiences and emotions (positive, negative, and ambivalent) are valid and that exploring these is the *beginning* of the process of working through recovery (Courtois, 1988). It is usually helpful for the survivor to be reminded periodically that she was not responsible for and did not deserve incestuous abuse, is not to be blamed, and was not in control of the situation and that the way she coped with it in the past was the best she could do at the time (Courtois, 1988). Education about incest and reassurances about recovery can be useful in correcting faulty perceptions about incest, decreasing self-blame and guilt, and instilling hope for the future despite the inability to change the past. Principles for "retrospective incest therapy" (Courtois, 1988) are summarized below:

1. Establishing a therapeutic trust relationship and educating the patient about the stress recovery process.
2. Breaking the secret, catharsis, and reevaluation of the incest, its circumstances, and its effects.
3. Facilitating the change from victim to survivor and beyond (integrating the positive, negative, and ambivalent trauma experience) and transferring responsibility from herself to perpetrator.

**Box 28-3**

## HOW FRIENDS AND RELATIVES CAN RESPOND TO A DISCLOSURE OF PAST CHILD SEXUAL ABUSE

- Be open to the disclosure. Let the survivor know you are open to discussing what she feels comfortable telling you about her past.
- Appreciate how difficult it is to make a disclosure and to confide long-held secrets.
- Offer her support and understanding. Empathize with her without pitying her. Let her know that you hurt to hear that she had such difficult events to contend with.
- Strive to be sensitive but matter-of-fact in your initial response rather than highly emotional. Know that she needs a calm, accepting, encouraging response.
- Encourage her to tell you details as she chooses to and as she is able. Don't press for details and don't focus on the sexual details. It may suffice for her to tell you only the most minimal of details or she might want you to know more. It is her decision, to do as she is able.
- Don't blame her. Emphasize that, no matter what the circumstance, she was not to blame. Be careful of questions that sound blaming, such as "Didn't you try to stop it?" "Did you tell him that you didn't like it?" "How did you know your mother wouldn't believe you if you didn't try to tell her?" "Maybe you really did enjoy it."
- Don't try to deny that it happened and don't tell her to forget it and get on with her life or otherwise "talk the abuse into going away." It's not "all in her head" and she needs to know that she is believed and supported. Don't tell her she made it up to get attention or "things like that just don't happen in good families," etc. It is especially tempting to deny incest when the perpetrator is a respected and loved member of the family and/or "a pillar of the community."
- Allow her her emotions and expect that she will have positive as well as negative feelings or that her predominant ones might be confusion and ambivalence. Not uncommonly, survivors have feelings of warmth and love towards the perpetrator for the non-exploitive parts of their relationship especially if he was the only family member to offer her nurturance.
- Don't respond with panic. Allow yourself some time to sort out your feelings.
- Don't pressure her and don't try to rush her. She needs to make choices and take action at her discretion. She will also heal at her own pace. Unfortunately, the recovery process is often lengthy—she needs support over its duration.
- Encourage her to seek therapy if she has not yet done so. Let her know that there are professionals who specialize in treating the aftereffects of abuse and who can help her. Offer her hope that she can recover from the effects of the past.

From Courtois CA: Healing the incest wound: adult survivors in therapy, New York, 1988, WW Norton & Co.

*Continued.*

**Box 28-3**

## HOW FRIENDS AND RELATIVES CAN RESPOND TO A DISCLOSURE OF PAST CHILD SEXUAL ABUSE—cont'd

- Encourage her to make choices that are in her best interest. Don't try to stop her from making choices and don't make them for her.
- Don't attempt to be overprotective or rescue her and don't confront the perpetrator or other family members without her knowledge and permission. Be aware that angry and retaliatory behavior can hurt her by making her feel anxious, out of control, and powerless.
- Talk to her about taking action to safeguard children in the family if the perpetrator still poses a risk. Other disclosures and reporting might be necessary. Indicate your support and willingness to explore possible avenues of action.
- Don't treat her like "damaged or spoiled goods" following disclosure. If you are her sexual partner, she needs assurances that she is still lovable and attractive. Try to maintain your normal level of sexual interaction and don't try to "make everything better with sex." Seek out professional assistance or a support group if your feelings are strongly negative or you find yourself obsessing about the details of abuse rather than focusing on the welfare of your partner. It is appropriate to share your feelings of anger, hurt, etc., but be sure they are directed towards the perpetrator and the abuse and are not blaming of the survivor.
- Follow up with her after her initial disclosure to you. Don't let the disclosure "go down a black hole," never to be mentioned again. And don't tell her that you forgot that she had ever made a disclosre to you.
- Maintain your normal expression of affection with the survivor. Touching, holding and hugging can be especially comforting. If you do not have a relationship with the survivor which normally includes physical contact, ask her permission before making any and respect her wishes.
- Support her in future disclosures, confrontations or reporting. Be aware that this may be especially difficult for other family members, who are bound to feel split loyalty and to get caught up in other family roles and interaction patterns.
- Respect her privacy. Do not break her confidence and don't discuss her disclosure without her permission.

4. Helping find meaning in the experience as well as mourning (grieving is a very painful experience).
5. Encouraging ventilation, teaching ways to break the double bind, and fostering separation and individuation from the family and its patterns.
6. Decreasing feelings of isolation and stigma.
7. Facilitating reexperiencing and reworking of the tasks of maturation that were either missed or experienced prematurely.

8. Teaching and encouraging stress management or reduction and expression of feelings and self-acceptance.

9. Teaching about family interactions, family dynamics, and rules and acknowledging the "child within" the survivor.

10. Educating about basic life skills, decision making, conflict resolution, communication, friendships, intimacy, sexuality, parenting, and boundary setting.

Mentally reexperiencing the traumatic experiences is disturbing, to say the least. Only periodic small doses may be tolerable. Both the counselor and the survivor can monitor her tolerance of the process so that she does not become overwhelmed and retreat from treatment. It is also important to consider priorities in each counseling session. Current crises and problems need to be addressed (instead of the incest) as these arise. This is critical for any self-destructive behaviors that are heightened because of counseling, such as suicidal ideation and substance abuse. Hospitalization may be necessary if the crisis is severe.

The overall desired outcomes of treatment are self-esteem and self-acceptance, forgiveness of self, adaptive coping with life and its stresses, the capacity for intimate relationships and genuine sexual pleasure, improvements in mood, and reduced anxiety level and fear.

Confrontation of her family by the survivor is not necessarily an outcome of counseling. This may be done symbolically with the counselor, rather than directly with the perpetrator and other family members. If the survivor chooses to confront directly, much preparation is needed, even rehearsals with the counselor before the event. She needs to consider, plan for, and rehearse her reactions to all the potential responses of family members. The most typical responses are denial, rationalization, and "blaming the victim." The survivor can be helped to debate the benefits and risks of confrontation, as well as the degree and type of contact she wants to have with the family, even if she does not confront them. An important consideration for the counselor and the survivor to discuss is the mandatory reporting of child abuse if currently younger siblings are victims of incest. Such a report is understandably difficult for both counselor and patient but needs to be carefully but directly addressed.

**PSYCHOPHARMACOLOGY** Medications are not always needed or desirable for adult survivors of childhood incest, especially if substance abuse is an additional problem or a potential problem. In the small number of cases with serious psychopathology, medications would be given according to the axis I diagnosis. *Benzodiazapines* may be given on an as-necessary basis to help control the emotional or autonomic arousal that occurs during reexperiencing of traumatic memories. *Antidepressants* may be used if the depressive symptoms are interfering with functioning and sleep.

**MILIEU MANAGEMENT** On an outpatient basis and during any brief hospitalizations, groups can be a useful adjunct to treatment. If available, a short-term or ongoing incest recovery group is beneficial. Self-help groups are beginning to form in some parts of the country: Daughters and Sons United for the survivors and Parents United for the parents.

Other groups recommended depend on symptoms and needs of the survivor, such as Codependency Anonymous, Adult Children of Alcoholics, Alcoholics or Narcotics Anonymous, and Emotions Anonymous. Survivors may also be directed to classes or short-term groups on decision making or problem solving, communication or relationship skills, conflict resolution, parenting skills, and human sexuality.

## VICTIMS OF WIFE ABUSE
### Nature of the problem

An estimated 2 million victims a year suffer from abuse by a male partner: "severe, deliberate and repeated demonstrable physical violence" (Campbell and Humphreys, 1984). The number is even higher when psychological abuse and other violations of rights are considered (see Fig. 28-2 for examples of these). Perhaps 5% of these victims are men. Every 18 seconds a woman is beaten by her male partner (husband, lover, ex-husband, or estranged husband or lover), and most wife abuse goes unreported even when injuries are severe enough to require treatment. Abuse victims, like rape and incest victims, tend to conceal their victimization. Women are acutely aware that disclosure of their plight has previously been met with denial or minimization by friends and relatives and by denial or minimization and increased abuse by their partners. The fact that 29% of all women killed in the United States in 1987 were killed by a husband or a boyfriend supports their fears. When murder by estranged or ex-husbands and lovers was included, the percentage increased to 33%. Women are also known to kill their partners, but 70% of the time it is in self-defense after a history of beatings (Campbell and Humphreys, 1984). Studies show that wife abuse crosses all social, cultural, and economic classes, but more cases are officially reported in the lower socioeconomic class because the women are more often in contact with agencies likely to report it, such as community health nursing, welfare clinics, and inner city emergency rooms (Campbell and Humphreys, 1984).

Rape of a woman by her partner is also a possible concomitant of other forms of abuse. In one study, 36% of the abused women reported spousal rape and exhibited rape trauma symptoms as described earlier in this chapter (Campbell and Humphreys, 1984).

The relationship of alcohol abuse by the male partner to his violent behavior has been the subject of many studies (summarized in Walker, 1979; Campbell and Humphreys, 1984). Some male abusers are abstainers, but more (up to 95%) are abusers of alcohol who batter their partners, whether they are drinking or not. The current view seems to be that men use alcohol as an excuse for their violence and drink when they are about to become violent. There is a correlation between alcohol and the severity of the violence (Walker, 1979). The combination of drinking and violence encourages the women to blame the alcohol rather than to hold the batterers accountable for their violent behaviors. They often describe their men as "Dr. Jekyll and Mr. Hyde" with changing personalities: gentle, loving, and kind at times and rude, uncaring, and violent at other times. (This change is explained in part by the cycle of violence described later.)

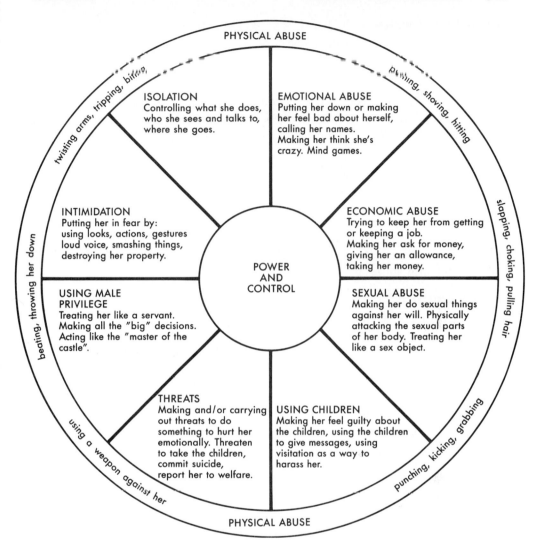

**FIGURE 28-2** Power and control. *(From Domestic Abuse Intervention Project, Duluth, Minnesota.)*

    A factor to be considered in wife abuse is the nature of current society. The portrayal of violence in media (TV, films) is increasing in frequency and severity. Women are still portrayed by the media as second-class citizens. There is also evidence that if a woman becomes more independent (both emotionally and financially), the incidence of violence by spouses increases as well (Campbell and Humphreys, 1984). In addition, it is well documented that the male victims of child abuse tend to become the wife abusers of the next generation (Walker, 1979; Campbell and Humphreys, 1984; Bullock et al., 1989).

## Learned helplessness

The concept of "learned helplessness" is useful in understanding the dynamics of wife abuse (Walker, 1979). Three of the necessary conditions for learned helplessness are certainly present:

1. The victim's behavior is not related to the cause of the beatings.
2. The victim has no control over preventing or stopping the beatings.
3. The victim sees little hope of escaping because of the threats of increased harm if she tries.

Most experts acknowledge the development of learned helplessness, hopelessness, isolation, and resignation in response to ongoing emotional and physical abuse. Few accept a more Freudian-type theory of inherent female masochism (which can be seen as another form of "blaming the victim"). Abused women do *not* report that they enjoy the abuse, but they do have a tendency to believe their partner's view that they deserve the abuse. Box 28-4 presents common reasons why women endure long-term abuse.

## Cycle of violence

Another accepted view of why women endure the abuse is well described by Lenore Walker (1979). The cycle of violence documents several principles:

1. Abuse is not constant, nor is it random.
2. Abuse occurs in a cycle and has three phases, which vary in time and intensity.
3. The last stage ("honeymoon") is the one that convinces the woman that she should stay in the relationship (Table 28-3).

It is during this last stage that the "good side" of the men is evident and the women are reminded of their love and caring and the happy potential of the relationship. Women report that they felt they wanted to and could help their partners overcome their problems and violent behaviors.

It was not until the 1970s that literature about wife abuse began to appear. The earlier lack of attention contributed to the lack of reporting of this crime. The women's movement was in part responsible for making the plight of abused women publicly known. Even so, it was not until 1974 that the first shelter for battered women was opened. Today there is still a shortage of safe places for women to go and of services to help them become independent. Many states still have outdated laws that indirectly perpetuate abuse rather than foster arrest of the man for assault. Arrest is perhaps the major (and maybe the only) way a battering man can get the message that his violence is a crime and not his "right." Other individuals and agencies also need to stop their indirect support of wife abuse as indicated in Box 28-5. It is unlikely that an abused woman will leave her partner until she has realized that the cycle is *not* going to stop, she has the emotional support to do so, and she has a safe place to go. Fearing that the next beating may be fatal, realizing that her partner is also physically or sexually abusing her children, and finding her children are learning to be abusive are also incentives for leaving (Task Force on Families in Crisis). *Text continued on p. 567*

### Box 28-4
## WHY WOMEN STAY AS LONG AS THEY DO

**Situational factors**

- Economic dependence
- Fear of greater physical danger to themselves and their children if they attempt to leave or have partner arrested
- Fear of emotional damage to children because of being without a father
- Fear of losing custody of children
- Lack of alternative housing
- Lack of job skills
- Social isolation resulting in lack of support from family or friends
- Lack of information regarding alternatives
- Fear of involvement in court processes
- Fear of retaliation from partner or partner's family

**Emotional factors:**

- Poor self-image
- Being in a state of denial, and living a "secret"
- Fear of loneliness
- Personal embarrassment and protecting the image of husband and family
- Insecurity over potential independence and lack of emotional support
- Guilt about failures of marriage or relationship
- Fear that partner is not able to survive alone
- Belief that partner is "sick" and needs her help
- Belief that partner will change
- Ambivalence and fear over making formidable life changes and increased responsiblity

**Cultural factors:**

- Knowing batterers are not held accountable for their violent actions
- Believes the abuse is her fault
- Being raised to be passive and submissive
- Developing survival skills instead of escape skills
- Recognition that the legal system is a male-dominated system

### Plus: She still loves him!

Adapted from Sojourner Shelter, Indianapolis, Ind., and Task Force on Families in Crisis, Box 120495, Nashville, Tenn., 37212.

**TABLE 28-3**   Cycle of violence

| Man | Woman |
|---|---|

I
Tension building

II
Serious battering incident

III
Honeymoon

## I. TENSION BUILDING

Minor battering incidents. Verbal abuse. Blaming her for anything that happens.

She's accepting of his behavior; he doesn't try to control; abuse increases.

Aware of inappropriate behavior, doesn't acknowledge it. Afraid that she will be disgusted and leave—increases his jealousy, possessiveness in hope that his brutality will keep her captive.

Excessively high expectations of her. Double-bind situations. Frantic—more control is attempted. Misinterprets her behavior, takes withdrawal as rejection.

Nurturing, compliant, stays out of his way.

She accepts the abuse as being directed against her; she doesn't believe she should be abused but that what she does will prevent his anger from escalating.

Denial: Provides sense of safety. Denies anger, perhaps deserves abuse—it could be worse. Blames external factors—work, alcohol. Escalation will occur. Denies terror and fear of increase of battering; believes she has control.

Frantic—withdraws.

Tension becomes unbearable.

Attempts to alter his behavior as a way of providing safety. Works up to a point; however, crazy part is it appears she has control but doesn't and can't. May call for help at end of this phase.

From THE BATTERED WOMAN by Lenore Walker. Copyright (c) 1979 by Lenore E. Walker. Reprinted by permission of Harper & Row, Publishers, Inc.

**TABLE 28-3**    Cycle of violence—cont'd

| Man | Woman |
|---|---|
| **II. ACTUAL BATTERING INCIDENT** | |
| Almost always occurs privately. | In long-term battering, sometimes she will provoke it. She senses inevitability. |
| Batterer starts out justifying behavior, but not understanding what happens! Double-bind situations. | Anxious, depressed, sleepless, over/under-eating, fatigue, tension headaches. |
| Trigger—external or internal event of man—drinking or other substance use. | Only 1 option—hide. Futility of trying to "resist" further battering. Initial reaction-shock, denial, disbelief. |
| After both rationalize, minimize severity. | Women do not seek help unless severely injured—usually not until a day afterward. |
| Addictive—because stress is relieved. | May call police—calm established. Try to dissuade charges. |
| | Shame—I've allowed someone to do this to me. Feeling of being a victim. Taking responsibility for it. Humiliation (may leave at end of this phase). |
| **III. HONEYMOON** | |
| Loving, contrite behavior. Charming, begs forgiveness, promises. | Victimization complete. Happy, confident, loving. Feels responsible for consequences. |
| Truly believes he will never again abuse. Believes he can control himself. | Believes in permanency of marriage. Easy prey for guilt. |
| Believes he has taught her a lesson—she will never act up. | Believes if she stays he'll get help. Tries to patch things up. |
| Will give up drinking or other behaviors. | Wants to believe she will no longer have to suffer abuse. |
| Pleads, plays on woman's guilty feelings. | Original dream—how wonderful love is. This is what her man is really like. |
| Engages family to do same. | Reduces feeling of victimization. |

**Box 28-5**
## INSTITUTIONAL OR AGENCY SUPPORT OF BATTERING

These are examples of what institutions or agencies have been known to say or do to reinforce the abuser's message that the woman is to blame for his violence.

### Family

Ignores her or does not pick up on cues
Does not ask about injuries or bruises
If told, says "What did you do to cause it?"
Says, "You've made your bed now lie in it" or "Just try harder"
Tell her she's crazy or enjoys it

### Church

Does not ask her about bruises or unusual absences
If told, says "It's a test from God" or "Scripture allows and sanctions it"
"Pray harder"
Tells her to try harder at being a better wife
Attempts marital counseling only

### Medical

Ignores violence and treats injuries only
Does not routinely ask how injury occurred or accepts phony stories
If told, does nothing; does not take photographs or document the incident
Prescribes medicine at three times the rate for nonbattered women

### Mental health counselors

Do not routinely ask about violence
If mentioned, do not treat it first or treat it as a symptom
Ask, "What did you do to make him hit you?"
Agree with man that she is a little "crazy" or is "bitchy" and that she must change first
Ask her what she could have done to deescalate the situation
Do marriage counseling, implying she is equally to blame
Hospitalize her in a mental facility

### Law enforcement

Police choose not to respond to a domestic call
On the scene treat it as a private "family matter"
Only warn the abuser or advise marriage counseling
Fail to take a report or transport her to safety

Adapted from Sojourner Shelter, P.O. Box 88062, Indianapolis, Ind. 46208.

# Facilitating recovery from abuse

## CRISIS INTERVENTION

Just before or during stage II (the serious battering incident) a woman is amenable to crisis intervention. she is most likely to call the police or a crisis service phone line for help. Getting her and her children to a shelter or other safe place (if she will go) is desirable when she is in immediate danger of injury. If she is already injured, she should be encouraged to go to an emergency room. In either case, crisis workers, shelter workers, or nurses can begin the important assessment and information giving that can make a dent in the cycle of abuse. Even if the woman is not yet ready to leave her partner, she can be given an easily concealed wallet-size card (by a crisis or victim's assistance counselor or by the emergency room nurse) with telephone numbers of police, prosecutor, crisis services, victims assistance, shelters, support groups, and perhaps a short message or two about the inevitability of the cycle of violence and the fact that no one deserves to be abused. If contact is only by phone, she can be asked to write down the phone numbers and hide them for future reference.

## PSYCHOTHERAPEUTIC MANAGEMENT

### NURSE-PATIENT RELATIONSHIP

**Assessment.** Since 80% of abused women seek help for their injuries at least once (Campbell and Humphreys, 1984), nurses can be instrumental in offering information and assistance. Nurses in emergency rooms, clinics, doctor's offices, and community health agencies particularly need to know how to recognize an abused woman, make an assessment, and refer her to available services. Some of the common cues to abuse are listed in Box 28-6.

The assessment process is often difficult because of the abused woman's fear of disclosure, embarrassment about the situation, desire to be treated quickly and leave, and sometimes the presence of the abuser. It is important to interview the woman alone, in private, and with sensitivity, empathy, and compassion. Box 28-7 describes other responses that abused women themselves consider to be facilitative and inhibitive.

Each hospital or agency will have its own assessment tool. The most crucial information to document in an initial contact is the following:

1. Length and frequency of abuse
2. Types of abuse (physical, psychological, sexual, financial) and use of weapons
3. Types and locations of injuries (can be written descriptions, but photographs and body maps arc preferred)
4. Duration of episodes of abuse
5. Use and abuse of substances and medications by woman and abuser
6. Current location of abuser
7. Location and safety of any children
8. Types of service she desires (police, legal scrvices, shelter, crisis counseling, social service agencies, transportation)
9. Referrals made

**Box 28-6**
## COMMON CUES TO ABUSE

1. Repeated, vague illnesses that are not confirmed by tests, such as backache, abdominal pain, indigestion, headaches, hyperventilation, anxiety, insomnia.
2. Unexplained injuries or ones with unlikely explanations and embarrassment about them.
3. Hidden injuries such as those in areas hidden by clothes or those visible on physical or x-ray examination only; for example, head injuries, internal injuries, genital injuries, scars, burns, joint pain or dislocations, numbness, hearing problems, fractures, bruises in various stages of healing, or bald spots.
4. Substance abuse and suicidal thoughts or attempts.
5. Attempts to conceal her fear of her partner.
6. Continual efforts to keep partner from getting angry.
7. Denial of any problems in the relationship.
8. Lack of relationships with family and friends.
9. Isolation or confinement to home.
10. Guilt, depression, anxiety, low self-esteem, sense of failure as a wife, concealed anger.
11. Continual justification of her actions and whereabouts to partner.
12. Continual justification of his actions toward her in public—excusing or rationalizing his behaviors.
13. Believes in family unity at all costs and in traditional stereotypes.
14. Believes she can manage by herself, even when help is offered.
15. An oversolicitous partner who doesn't want to leave her alone with hospital or agency staff or even with family and friends.

Adapted from Task Force on Families in Crisis; Campbell, 1984; Loraine, 1981.

Even if the counseling during this initial contact is brief, it is important to convey to the woman that she is not alone in her abuse and that there are those willing to help *whenever she is ready.* She also needs to be told more than once that she does not cause and does not deserve the abuse. The nurse must convey to the woman that she is important and that she has dignity and worth. The woman needs acknowledgment of her mental and physical exhaustion, her fears, her ambivalence about her abuser and about leaving him, and her wish to help him as well as herself. It is difficult for the nurse (and any professionals) to accept that the woman cannot be pushed, rushed, or coerced into leaving the abuser before she is ready. In fact, she may want to try marriage counseling and even personal counseling (if he will not go to counseling) more than once before "giving up hope" of saving the marriage

### Box 28-7
## FACILITATIVE AND INHIBITIVE HELPER RESPONSES

**Facilitative helper responses**

- Helper asking woman if abuse is occuring.
- Helper identifying described behavior as abusive.
- Helper acknowledging seriousness of abuse.
- Helper expressing belief in woman's description of abuse.
- Helper acknowledging that woman does not deserve the abuse.
- Helper being directive in exploring resources.
- Helper telling the man to stop the abuse.
- Helper aiding woman consider full range of available options.
- Helper avoiding telling woman what to do.
- Helper aiding woman to assess her internal strengths.
- Helper suggesting tangible resources (e.g., shelters, financial aid).
- Helper offering support groups with other abused women.
- Helper active in listening and empathizing.

**Inhibitive helper responses**

- Helper demonstrating irritation/anger with woman.
- Helper blaming woman.
- Helper advising woman to accept abuse as better than nothing.
- Helper refusing to help until woman left abuser.
- Helper aligning with abuser.
- Helper disbelieving woman.
- Helper not responding to abuse disclosure.
- Helper advising woman to leave abuser.

From Limandri BJ: The therapeutic relationship with abused women, J Psychosoc Nurs 25(2):9-16, 1987.

and of helping the one she loves. It is important to recognize and to acknowledge that it is common for abused women to leave and go back several times. She need not feel guilty or ashamed of trying to improve the relationship. In fact, the guilt of leaving will be lessened if she has "tried everything" first and finally is able to acknowledge that nothing will change because he is the only one who can control the violence and stop the abuse.

When the abused woman does leave her partner, the problems are not over for her. "If You Have Left an Abusive Man" describes some of the common reactions the abuser may have and ways he may behave (Box 28-8). Abused women frequently

Box 28-8

# IF YOU HAVE LEFT AN ABUSIVE MAN...

Having left the violence of your home does not mean that all your problems are over. The man that has recently and frequently used and abused you may react in several predictible ways. Knowing what he probably will do may have a beneficial effect on your ability to cope with his demands, his attempts to persuade and intimidate, and better enable you to make your decisions without fear.

1. One of his first efforts to locate you will be to go to the friends and family members that he thinks you may go to. Depending on his relationship to them, he will either threaten them or attempt to gain their sympathy. If they do not know where you are, only that you are well, then they cannot be frightened into giving that information. If he uses the sympathy line, his story may be such a distortion of what really happened that they will want to persuade you to return to the poor mistreated fella! Remember, he can be charming and persuasive (that's how he got you in the first place), so be prepared for him to use this on others.

2. If he does make contact with you by whatever means, he will probably first try a great apology line including promises of new ways of behavior, gifts, things for the house and children, anything that he thinks you will believe and will bring you back within his sphere of dominance. Remember, many of these men have indicated that their women are their possessions to do with as they please and they intend to establish and maintain control over you.

3. The next pattern of behavior is generally one of threats and attempts to intimidate. This will often include threats to attack family and friends, threats to kill you or "put out a contract on you," threats that he will take away the children or get custody of them himself, or threats to kill himself. The wisest answer here is to *remind him that he alone is responsible for his actions* and the results of the actions and refuse to listen to further threats.

4. The next step is the counseling/religion step. He will suddenly become a "Christian" and attend church activities in a most obivious manner. Even ministers doubt these sudden conversions! Or he may begin making the rounds of counseling services trying to find a counselor that will call you and tell you that you should go back home and help him sort out his problems.

    Unless a man is willing to go with one counselor and continue his involvement in counseling *whether or not* you come back, he is probably not very sincere in seeking to resolve his personal and marital problems.

5. If the above four steps have not worked there are others he may try, such as: Crying and begging, particularly in a public situation so that you are embarrased and appear to be a "hard-hearted Hannah." Harrassment by phone calls, threats, legal frustrations, showing up at work, hanging around family.

6. One of the main threats that will be used is that he will not let you have the children. Remember, in this case the weight of the law is on your side, that in 99 cases out of 100, the mother will receive custody of the children and has a number of community agencies available to help you deal with the problem of being a single parent. Remember, *you do have rights* and *you do have laws* to help protect your rights. If you allow yourself to be intimidated by his bluffs and false information, then you will continue to lead a life of agony and fear.

From the Salvation Army Domestic Violence Program, Indianapolis, Ind., Dec., 1981.

need longer-term counseling and social services to recover and become independent, even if the abuser is unwilling to participate in marital counseling or an abusers program (often a court-ordered program of group education and counseling lasting 26 weeks or more). Counseling for the woman (individually or in groups) generally focuses on the following:

1. Reiteration of information about abuse, the cycle of violence, and the abuser's accountability
2. Building self-esteem and confidence
3. Sharing of feelings, especially anger, frustration, fear, anxiety
4. Decreasing shame, guilt, embarrassment, manipulation, and isolation
5. Confirmation of personal rights as well as legal rights
6. Stress reduction or management techniques
7. Communication techniques
8. Conflict-resolution techniques
9. Assertiveness training
10. Parenting techniques
11. Decreasing codependency behaviors
12. Building a new, improved support system
13. Goal setting, specific planning for immediate future
14. Resolution of grieving

Referrals may also be needed for job counseling or training, legal assistance, financial aid, and permanent housing. At any stage of working with an abused woman brief hospitalization may be needed because of injuries, suicide attempts, or substance abuse and for treatment of serious problems such as depression, anxiety, or panic attacks.

***PSYCHOPHARMACOLOGY*** Medications normally are not needed but commonly are misprescribed for abused women. The often misprescribed medications are antidepressants, benzodiazepines, and hypnotics.

These same medications may be used appropriately if the abused woman's symptoms of depression, anxiety, sleeplessness, or nightmares are quite severe. Continual assessment is needed to determine when medications are no longer needed and to prevent abuse and addiction.

***MILIEU MANAGEMENT*** Groups in inpatient or outpatient settings that may be relevant for an abused woman would be those focusing on self-esteem, problem solving, assertiveness, relationship issues, stress management, and codependency. Substance-abuse groups could be recommended if this problem exists. In the community a group for abused women would be essential. Two such groups are called Turning Point and Breaking Free.

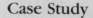

Rachael Grimes, a 26-year-old woman, is married to Richard Grimes. She was previously in a live-in partnership with another man, resulting in one child, Matthew, who is now 8 years old. Richard had one girl and three boys with his former wife. Robert, James, and Daniel, ages 11, 8, and 7, currently live with Rachael and Richard. Angela, age 5, was born to Rachael and Richard, and Andrew was stillborn 2 years ago. Two years ago, Rachael's child, Matthew, was removed from the home because of abuse by Richard's son Robert. Rachael was accused of the abuse and did not deny it.

Rachael initially sought help by attending a group advertised for development of parenting skills and management of difficult child behaviors. The coleaders (both nurses) began the group with five women. After three sessions it became obvious to the leaders and members that the major problem of all five women was wife abuse. By the end of 1 year of weekly meetings, four of the women were able to leave the abusers, support themselves, and begin new lives.

Rachael's situation was more complex and difficult to resolve. Richard was a heavy drinker (as were the male partners of the other four women), and he was beginning to miss days at work and to change jobs more often. He moved downward from car mechanic to junkyard manager to driving a garbage truck. His income declined and was sporadic at times. Expenses did not decline. The hospitalization for the stillbirth was not covered by insurance. Seven-year-old Daniel needed bilateral myringotomy for repeated ear infections, and Rachael had repeated testing and treatment for such problems as menstrual irregularities, back pain, severe headaches, loss of appetite, diarrhea, and bronchitis. She refused treatment for facial bruises, a superficial knife wound to the chest, a sprained wrist, a head wound caused by a beer can, and periodic contusions on the back and abdomen. The abuse of Rachael by Richard began when she was pregnant with Angela 5 years ago. It began with verbal disparagement, yelling, and threats of kicking her out. Within 1 year it escalated to pushing, shoving, and throwing her into walls. By the time she was pregnant with Andrew 2 years ago Richard was punching, slapping, kicking, and hitting her with full beer cans. He slashed her with a knife one time. Rachael is convinced that Andrew died because of Richard's hitting her in her stomach repeatedly during the pregnancy.

At the time Rachael began to attend sessions of the group she was mentally and physically exhausted and never seemed to recover from colds, bronchitis, and episodes of flu. She was still trying to figure out how to be a better wife, how to prevent Richard's anger, and how to help him stop drinking. Richard denied having any problems and blamed his anger and drinking on Rachael's inability to be a good wife and mother. It was not until Richard raped her when she was asleep that Rachael finally believed there was no hope of change and that she needed to leave. This was 9 months after the group began. When Richard realized that she was becoming more assertive and independent, he demanded that she stop going out of the house. He bought a shotgun and threatened to use it if she tried to leave him. He took the starter off the car and got rides to his work with friends.

The group decided to move the meetings to a church close to Rachael's home so that she could still attend. Meeting times were changed periodically so she would not be out of the house the same time and day each week. Members offered her a list of excuses to be away from the house in case Richard called from work. If Richard missed work, Rachael stayed away from the group. Members would call her to check on her safety. Several factors interfered with Rachael's leaving Richard. She had not adopted his children, so she could not take them with her. She was afraid his verbal abuse of the boys would turn to physical violence if she left. There were no shelters for battered women. Any places she thought of going, including her mother's home in a rural area of the state, were known by Richard. It took 4 months to develop, coordinate, and implement the arrangements so that Rachael felt safe in taking Angela and leaving Richard. She told neighbors, friends, and teachers at the boys' school about her abuse and the potential abuse of the boys. She gave all of them the phone number and information about anonymously reporting child abuse. Rachael's mother rented a small trailer in a nearby rural town for Rachael to use when possible. Her mother also obtained forms for Aid to Dependent Children, which Rachael completed and sent to the rural county. Rachael secretly and gradually packed essential clothes and personal items for her and Angela in the trunk of a friend's car.

One night (14 months after the group began) Richard came home drunk, began beating Rachael, and tried to rape her again. She succeeded in fending him off this time because he was so drunk and uncoordinated. She waited until he passed out and then called her friend with the packed car. The friend drove Rachael and Angela to her mother's home. Early the next morning, her mother took them to the trailer.

As expected, when Richard found Rachael and Angela gone, he took his shotgun and, one by one, went to every friend of Rachael's. Legitimately, none of them knew where she was. Fortunately, Richard did not know the friend with the car. The next day he drove to Rachael's mother's home with his shotgun. Her mother called the sheriff the minute his car pulled into her driveway. Richard was escorted out of the county by the sheriff and warned not to return. Within a week after Rachael left, James showed his teacher the bruises his father had given him. The teacher filed a child-abuse report. Within 2 weeks the boys were removed from the home and returned to their natural mother.

Rachael has finally received treatment for the headaches and menstrual irregularities. She is divorced, healthy, going to a job-training program, and maintaining her secret location. Richard has stopped trying to locate her, and she finally feels safe. She is still in counseling once a month to help her complete her emotional recovery from the abuse. She also attends a local support group for battered women once a week.

## Nursing Care Plan

WEEKLY UPDATE: ___1/12/90___

NAME: ___Rachael Grimes___   ADMISSION DATE: ___N/A___

DSM-III-R DIAGNOSIS: _____None_____

*ASSESSMENT:*
*Areas of strength:* Bright, articulate, and capable of problem solving, one friend and mother willing to help; developing trust in group and beginning to process her feelings and rights.
*Problems:* Lack of safe housing and employment; inability to remove his children from the house and fear he will abuse them; fear of increased abuse of her, even death, if she tries to leave.

*DIAGNOSES:* Multiple injuries over time to head, chest, back and abdomen related to physical, emotional and economic abuse. Fear of leaving husband related to potential abuse of sons.

| | Date met |
|---|---|
| *PLANNING:* | |
| *Short-term goals:* | 1/90 |
| Patient will remove bullets from gun; design an escape plan. | 2/90 and 6/90 |
| Patient will verbalize ability to survive on her own; confirm housing in rural county | 6/90 |
| *Long-term goals:* Patient will enroll in job-training program. | 9/90 |
| | 9/90 |
| Patient will obtain legal assistance for divorce. | |
| Patient will seek medical treatment for chronic problems. | |

*IMPLEMENTATION/INTERVENTIONS:*
*Nurse-patient relationship:* Listen nonjudgmentally and empathetically; accept "strange" behaviors related to secrecy and self-protection; avoid disparaging spouse and pressuring to leave; locate resources for training, finances, counseling, and medical care in rural county.
*Psychopharmacology:* Desyrel, 50 mg at bedtime, to alleviate moderate depression and aid to improve sleep. Tylenol #3 p.r.n. for severe headaches.
*Milieu management:* Encourage continuing in local support group; locate support group in rural county; continue assessment of safety of patient and children.

*EVALUATION:* Patient has moved to rural county and joined support group; is receiving counseling and medical care; has appointment with job-training program. Husband's children were removed and placed with natural mother.

## KEY CONCEPTS

1. Not all crimes involve physical violence and injury; however, all crimes involve *emotional* violation and injury. Victims experience a loss of a sense of the ability to control their own lives as well as loss of trust.
2. Progression through the stages of recovery from a crime may take years. Crisis intervention and group meetings with other victims can facilitate recovery.
3. In assisting rape victims, sensitivity to their needs is crucial to build trust and avoid "blaming the victim."
4. Information about counseling resources and support groups can be given to the rape victim for later use, even if there is an initial denial of the need for help.
5. The adult survivor of childhood incest may repress the memories for years as a result of the sense of being betrayed by the abuser and others.
6. Adult survivors of incest typically enter counseling for a variety of overt problems, unaware of how these are related to their childhood trauma.
7. The reexperiencing and working through of the traumatic incest memories is a painful, lengthy, and sometimes sporadic process that requires intense support and empathy.
8. The concepts of "learned helplessness," the cycle of violence, and other situational, emotional, and cultural factors are needed to explain why abused women often remain with their partners.
9. Just before or during a serious battering incident is when abused women are most amenable to crisis intervention and referrals for needed services.
10. Patience, support, and information are critical aspects of nursing interventions with abused women.

## REFERENCES

Bard M and Sangrey D: The crime victim's book, New York, 1986, Brunner/Mazel Publishers.

Barnhill LR: Clinical assessment of intrafamilial violence, Hosp Community Psychiatry 31(8): 543-546, 1980.

Barnhill LR: Basic interventions for violence in families, Hosp Community Psychiatry 3(8): 547-551, 1980.

Borland M, editor: Violence in the family, Atlantic Highlands, NJ, 1986, Humanities Press.

Bullock LF, Sandella FJ, and McFarlane J: Breaking the cycle of abuse: how nurses can intervene, J Psychosoc Nurs 27(8):11, 1989.

Burgess AW: Intra-familial sexual abuse. In Campbell J and Humphreys J, editors: Nursing care of victims of family violence, Reston, Va, 1984, Reston Publishing Co.

Burgess AW et al: Sexual assault of children and adolescents, Lexington, Mass, 1978, DC Heath & Co.

Burgess AW and Holstrom LL: Rape: crisis and recovery, New York, 1979, Prentice-Hall.

Burgess AW and Holstrom LL: Rape trauma syndrome, Am J Psychiatry 131:981-986, 1974.

Butler S: Conspiracy of silence: the trauma of incest, New York, 1978, Bantam Books.

Campbell J and Humphreys J: Nursing care of victims of family violence, Reston, Va, 1984, Reston Publishing Co.

Courtois CA: Healing the incest wound: adult survivors in therapy, New York, 1988, WW Norton & Co.

deYoung M: Incest victims and their offenders: myths and realities, J Psychosoc Nurs 19(10):37, 1985.

DiVasto P: Measuring the aftermath of rape, J Psychosoc Nurs 23(2):33, 1985.

Drake VK: Battered women: a health care problem in disguise, Sigma Theta Tau Image 14(2):40, 1982.

Fleming JB: Stopping wife abuse: a guide to the emotional, psychological and legal implications, Garden City, NY, 1979, Anchor Books.

Fox SS and Scherl DJ: Crisis intervention with rape victims, Soc Work 17:37, January, 1972.

Gest T: Victims of crime, U.S. News & World Report 107:16-19, July 31, 1989.

Green HW: Turning fear into hope, New York, 1984, Thomas Nelson Pub.

Jacobson A and Herald C: The relevance of childhood sexual abuse to adult psychiatric inpatient care, Hosp Community Psychiatry 41:154-158, 1990.

Krach P and Zens D: Incest: nursing interventions for group therapy, J Psychosoc Nurs 26(10):32-34, 1988.

Lew M: Victims no longer, New York, 1988, Nevraumont Publishing Co.

Limandri BJ: The therapeutic relationship with abused women, J Psychosoc Nurs 25(2):9, 1987.

Loraine K: Battered women: the ways you can help, RN, p 23, October 1981.

Lowery M: Adult survivors of childhood incest, J Psychosoc Nurs 25(1):27, 1987.

Martin G: Counseling for family violence and abuse, Waco, Texas, 1987, Word.

Mehta P and Dandrea LA: The battered woman, Fam Pract 37:193, 1988.

Moehling KS: Battered women and abusive partners, J Psychosoc Nurs 26(9):8, 1988.

Power and control, Duluth, Minn., 1987, Domestic Violence Intervention Project.

Rich RF and Burgess AW: Panel recommends program for victims of violent crime, Hosp Community Psychiatry 37:437, 1986.

Roy M: Battered women, New York, 1977, Van Nostrand Reinhold.

Roy M: A psychosocial study of domestic violence, New York, 1977, Van Nostrand Reinhold Co.

Russell DEH: The secret trauma: incest in the lives of girls and women, New York, 1986, Basic Books.

Straus MA, Gelles RJ, and Steinmetz SK: Behind closed doors: violence in the American family, Garden City, NY, 1981, Anchor.

Stuart GW and Sundeen SJ: Pocket nurse guide to psychiatric nursing, St. Louis, 1988, The CV Mosby Co.

Strom K: In the name of submission, Portland, Ore, 1986, Multnomah Publishers.

Task Force on Families in Crisis: Do you know someone who's battered? Nashville, The Task Force.

Tynhurst JS: Individual reactions to community disaster, Am J Psychiatry 107:764, 1951.

Urbancic JC: Incest trauma, J Psychosoc Nurs 25(7):33, 1987.

Walker L: The battered woman, New York, 1979, Harper and Row.

Weingourt R: Never to be alone, J Psychosoc Nurs 23(3):24, 1985.

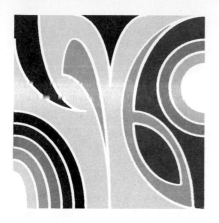

## CHAPTER 29

# Child and Adolescent Psychiatric Nursing

MARYLOU SCAVNICKY-MYLANT AND NORMAN L. KELTNER

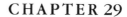

LEARNING OBJECTIVES

After reading this chapter you should be able to

- Discuss the extent of emotional disturbances among children.
- Identify the risk factors associated with childhood psychiatric problems.
- Identify characteristics of resiliency among high-risk children.
- Describe the symptoms and nursing interventions for common child psychiatric disorders.
- Explain the potential emotional effect on children who are raised by mentally ill or alcoholic parents.
- Describe two assumptions underlying preventive efforts directed toward children raised by mentally disordered parents.

**B**ecause of the increasing number of children with emotional disorders all nurses should be sensitive to the emotional needs in this age group. The concept of childhood in this chapter encompasses the developmental spectrum from birth to 17 years of age. An emotional disturbance in a child occurs when the child's personality development is "arrested or interfered with so that the child shows impairment in reasonable and accurate perceptions of the world, impulse control, learning, and social relations with others" (Clunn, 1988). This chapter reviews major emotional disturbances in children and the effect on them of being raised in homes in which one or both parents suffer from mental illness or alcoholism. The nursing care of children, as with adults, includes a sound therapeutic nurse-patient relationship, appropriate psychopharmacology, and milieu management. The reader is referred to these specific units for the older child approaching young adulthood.

## ANA STANDARDS OF CHILD AND ADOLESCENT PSYCHIATRIC AND MENTAL HEALTH NURSING PRACTICE

### Professional practice standards

**Standard I. Theory** The nurse applies appropriate, scientifically sound theory as a basis for nursing practice decisions.

**Standard II. Assessment** The nurse systematically collects, records, and analyzes data that are comprehensive and accurate.

**Standard III. Diagnosis** The nurse, in expressing conclusions supported by recorded assessment and current scientific premises, uses nursing diagnoses and/or standard classifications of mental disorders for childhood and adolescence.

**Standard IV. Planning** The nurse develops a nursing care plan with specific goals and interventions delineating nursing actions unique to the needs of each child or adolescent, as well as those of the family and other relevant interactive social systems.

**Standard V. Intervention** The nurse intervenes as guided by the nursing care plan to implement nursing actions that promote, maintain, or restore physical and mental health, prevent illness, effect rehabilitation in childhood and adolescence, and restore developmental progression.

**Standard V-A. Intervention: Therapeutic Environment** The nurse provides, structures, and maintains a therapeutic environment in collaboration with the child or adolescent, the family, and other health care providers.

From American Nurses' Association: Standards of Child and Adolescent Psychiatric and Mental Health Nursing Practice. 1985. Reprinted with permission of the American Nurses' Association.

**Standard V-B. Intervention: Activities of Daily Living** The nurse uses the activities of daily living in a goal-directed way to foster the physical and mental well-being of the child or adolescent and family.

**Standard V-C. Intervention: Psychotherapeutic Interventions** The nurse uses psychotherapeutic interventions to assist children or adolescents and families to develop, improve, or regain their adaptive functioning, to promote health, prevent illness, and facilitate rehabilitation.

**Standard V-D. Intervention: Psychotherapy\*** The child and adolescent psychiatric and mental health specialist uses advanced clinical expertise to function as a psychotherapist for the child or adolescent and family and accepts professional accountability for nursing practice.

**Standard V-E. Intervention: Health Teaching and Anticipatory Guidance** The nurse assists the child or adolescent and family to achieve more satisfying and productive patterns of living through health teaching and anticipatory guidance.

**Standard V-F. Intervention: Somatic Therapies** The nurse uses knowledge of somatic therapies with the child or adolescent and family to enhance therapeutic interventions.

**Standard VI. Evaluation** The nurse evaluates the response of the child or adolescent and family to nursing actions in order to revise the data base, nursing diagnoses, and nursing care plan.

## Professional performance standards

**Standard VII. Quality Assurance** The nurse participates in peer review and other means of evaluation to assure quality of nursing care provided for children and adolescents and their families.

**Standard VIII. Continuing Education** The nurse assumes responsibility for continuing education and professional development and contributes to the professional growth of others studying children's and adolescent's mental health.

**Standard IX. Interdisciplinary Collaboration** The nurse collaborates with other health care providers in assessing, planning, implementing, and evaluating programs and other activities related to child and adolescent psychiatric and mental health nursing.

**Standard X. Use of Community Health Systems\*** The nurse participates with other members of the community in assessing, planning, implementing, and evaluating mental health services and community systems that attend to primary, secondary, and tertiary prevention of mental disorders in children and adolescents.

**Standard XI. Research** The nurse contributes to nursing and the child and adolescent psychiatric and mental health field through innovations in theory and practice and participation in research, and communicates these contributions.

\*Standards V-D and X apply only to the clinical specialist in child and adolescent psychiatric and mental health nursing.

**Box 29-1**

**AMERICAN ACADEMY OF CHILD AND ADOLESCENT PSYCHIATRY STATEMENT ON CONDITIONS FOR HOSPITALIZATION OF CHILDREN AND ADOLESCENTS**

1. The psychiatric disorder must be of such severity as to significantly impair daily functioning in at least two important areas of the child or adolescent's life such as school performance, social interactions, or family relationships.
2. The treatment must be relevant to the problems diagnosed and judged likely to be beneficial.
3. Least restrictive alternatives must have been considered.
4. The decision to hospitalize a child or adolescent under 16 years of age must be made by a fully trained and qualified child and adolescent psychiatrist unless one is not available, in which case a general psychiatrist must make the decision.
5. Treatment should be conducted in a JCAHO-approved facility.
6. The patient must have an individualized treatment plan based on assessment of biological, psychological, social, and developmental needs.
7. The child or adolescent patient should participate in treatment processes; parents should be kept fully informed of patient progress and treatment goals.

Adapted from the AACAP statement on conditions for hospitalization of children and adolescents, Hosp Community Psychiatry, 40:765, 1989.

Child and adolescent psychiatric nursing is concerned with the mental health needs of all children because of the extent of emotional disturbances found among young people. According to McCellan and Trupin (1989) 5% to 26% of school-aged children have persistent and socially problematic mental health problems; another 30% cannot adjust to school, and adolescent suicides have tripled since 1960. Clunn (1988) estimates that 15% of children in the United States between 3 and 15 years of age can be classified as emotionally disturbed. Wallen and Pincus (1988), in looking at diagnostic characteristics of 7207 children (ages 0 to 17 years) admitted to psychiatric units in general hospitals, found that 40.6% of the children were admitted with depression and that 7.3% were admitted with schizophrenia. Pothier (1984) states that there are 500,000 children with psychotic or borderline psychotic disorders, 1 million children with personality and character disorder, and 1 million children who are institutionalized for emotional disturbances. Some disorders such as psychosis and depression are treated in an inpatient setting, whereas others such as attention-deficit hyperactivity disorder (ADHD) are routinely treated on an outpatient basis. Box 29-1 provides a statement on conditions for hospitalization of children and adolescents.

## RISK FACTORS FOR CHILDHOOD EMOTIONAL DISORDERS

Risk factors include genetic predisposition and biological factors; adverse environmental influences before, during and after birth; social and cultural factors; family system factors; and also as experiences during infancy and childhood.

*Genetic predisposition* involves those influences associated with heredity. Numerous research articles support the claim that mental health problems are passed from parent to child. Children of a parent with bipolar illness are more likely than the general population of children to develop a bipolar illness; children of alcoholics are more likely to develop alcoholism; and children of a parent with schizophrenia are more likely to suffer from schizophrenia. These tendencies hold true even when the child is not raised by his natural parents. *Biological factors* include neurological problems such as ADHD and illness or injuries such as vehicular accidents that impair the child's ability to confront normal developmental issues.

It is believed that any number of environmental factors influence the emotional life of the newborn. *Adverse environmental factors before, during, and after birth* include a variety of noxious elements such as drug ingestion (legal and illegal) or exposure of the mother to toxins; emotional stress of the mother; physical illness of the mother; and lack of a nurturing and loving caregiver.

Examples of *social and cultural influences* are the family's socioeconomic status, the importance of family within a cultural context, and the extent of social support for the child. Children from poorer homes are more likely to suffer from emotional disturbances than children from wealthier homes. Parents in poor families come face to face with primary stressors such as inability to provide their children with adequate food, shelter, and clothing more often than middle-class parents do. These stressors detract from parental energies that could be directed toward the child. Cultural considerations include the importance of the family. Is there a cultural mandate to preserve the integrity of the family? Social support includes a variety of systems that provide an emotional backup for the child. To the extent that the child lives in an adequate socioeconomic environment and has a stable family life and an emotional support system, he is better equipped to deal with the normal stressors of life.

*Family systems* is an important consideration when one is working with children because the family has significant influence on the well-being of the child. Families in turmoil (consistent bickering between parents, threats of divorce) produce children with more emotional problems than families without turmoil do. Families that can tolerate differences among its members are healthier than families that cannot tolerate differences among its members. Families with certain family routines and rituals produce more stable children than families with less predictable behavior do (Keltner et al., 1990). Family systems theory holds that an emotionally disturbed child is but a manifestation of an emotionally disturbed family. It is as if the child has been "chosen" to bear the symptoms for the entire family. Accordingly, family therapy or working with the entire family is the treatment approach of choice.

*Stress experiences* during infancy and childhood take their toll on the child also. Rutter (1979, 1981, 1982, 1984) has demonstrated that stressors in childhood lead to childhood emotional disorders. He found a 6% incidence of emotional disturbance among children who had to deal with two or three stress factors and a 21% incidence of emotional disturbance among children who had to deal with four or more stressors. Mental illness of a parent, an alcoholic parent, drug abuse, venereal disease, economic pressures, early and unwanted sex experiences, school-related stressors, lack of parental involvement, divorce or threat of divorce, single-parent homes, and living in a mobile and competitive society all contribute to a climate that adversely stresses children and makes them vulnerable to emotional disturbances. The effects on children of living with a mentally ill or an alcoholic parent will be discussed separately in this chapter.

## The concept of resiliency

With the many risk factors identified it is a wonder that any child survives childhood. Researchers have sought to find the answer to the question, Why is it that some children who are exposed to many risk factors succumb to those risk factors while others handle those same stressors successfully?

Resiliency is the ability to withstand the problems of an undesireable childhood environment and emerge as a "normal," productive person. Many professionals believe that more attention should be focused on identifying factors associated with resiliency. Early reports focusing on this issue found that competent children of mentally ill mothers had important relationships with others within their family, with other adults, and with peers. These children were appealing to adults and better able to use adults as a substitute parent. The resilient children compensated for their family difficulties with outside activities, a best friend, and school work. Other research has identified family routines as a buffer for the negative effects of poverty. In economically depressed homes where events occur in a predictable fashion, for example, eating the dinner meal together, children are more productive and resilient than in economically equivalent homes where there are no routines (Keltner et al., 1990). As nurses are able to identify factors associated with resiliency in children, they will be able to reinforce those behaviors and develop prevention strategies.

## CHILDHOOD EMOTIONAL DISORDERS
### Attention-deficit hyperactivity disorder

ADHD is the most common pediatric behavioral disorder. ADHD is characterized by inattention, impulsivity, and hyperactivity. Fidgeting and restlessness are more prominent in adolescents, whereas hyperactivity is common in children. ADHD is affected and exacerbated by environmental and social factors. For example, the symptoms of ADHD cause a problem for the child in school, where he is expected to sit still, listen, and learn.

Estimates of incidence range up to 20% of all school-age children (LaGreca and Quay, 1984), but a more accurate estimate is nearer 2% to 3%. Until recently it was thought that ADHD quietly disappeared at puberty because of the developmental changes that take place at that time. Coleman and Levine (1988) found that ADHD symptoms persist into adolescence 50% to 70% of the time, indicating a larger problem during adolescence than previously thought. One third continue to have signs of ADHD into adulthood. Among those children requiring professional intervention, six to nine times more boys are treated than girls (APA, 1987). ADHD is related to other adolescent problems such as antisocial behavior, substance abuse, and poor school performance. Academically the adolescent with ADHD is about 2 years behind his normal counterpart (Manor-Millan and Canteel, 1989).

---

## PSYCHOTHERAPEUTIC MANAGEMENT

*NURSE-PATIENT RELATIONSHIP* The following are strategies the nurse can use to develop a therapeutic relationship with the child with ADHD:

- Differentiate person from behavior (like the person, dislike the behavior). Demonstrate acceptance of individual.
- Be consistent, be honest, follow-through on promises, and confront obnoxious, rude, asocial, manipulative, and destructive behaviors.
- Take time to work with patient to convey worth and to help patient focus on positive accomplishments.
- Reinforce acceptable behaviors immediately. ADHD children change behavior only when rewards are immediate and will not change behavior if rewards are delayed. This type of observation is time consuming, so the nurse must be prepared to expend great energy if a consistent reinforcement program is attempted.
- Refuse to debate unit rules with patient but consistently reinforce acceptable unit behavior.
- Clearly state consequences of violating unit behavior code.
- If patient is going to a formal school, the nurse may work with him on homework assignments.

*PSYCHOPHARMACOLOGY* Central nervous system (CNS) stimulants are the drugs most commonly used to treat young children but are used less often in adolescents, particularly older adolescents. It is a commonly held opinion among many professionals working with ADHD that at about puberty, stimulants lose their effectiveness for treating the hyperactive individual. Others disagree with this position. Methylphenidate is the most commonly used stimulant (about 93% of the time [Safer and Krager, 1988]). Amphetamines (usually dextroamphetamine [Dexedrine]) and pemoline (Cylert) are used also.

### CNS stimulants

- Effect: Paradoxically, CNS stimulants have a calming effect on children with ADHD.
- Metabolism: Methylphenidate is completely metabolized in the liver. Amphetamines are excreted unchanged in the urine.
- Side effects: Nervousness, tachycardia, insomnia, anorexia, stomachache, symptoms of depression, weight loss, and temporary growth retardation are side effects of CNS stimulants in children with ADHD.
- Interactions: CNS stimulants interact with other sympathomimetics and antidepressants. Drugs that alkalinize the urine will delay the excretion of amphetamine.

**TABLE 29-1**   Administration of CNS stimulants for ADHD in children over 6 years of age

|                      | Starting dose (mg) | Maximum dose (mg/d) |
|----------------------|--------------------|---------------------|
| Methylphenidate      | 5 at breakfast     | 60                  |
|                      | 5 at lunch         |                     |
| Dextroamphetamine    | 5 qd or b.i.d.     | 40                  |
| Pemoline             | 37.5 in AM         | 112.5               |

- Dosage (Table 29-1)
  - *Methylphenidate:* In children over 6 years of age 5 mg of methylphenidate before breakfast and lunch is recommended. The optimal daily dose is 0.3 mg/kg/d. Although this dose may not "correct" all social behavior concerns, it is sufficient to increase learning ability.
  - *Dextroamphetamine:* For children 3 to 5 years old 2.5 mg daily taken with or immediately after meals (because loss of appetite is a side effect). The dosage may be raised in 2.5 mg/d increments at weekly intervals as needed. Children 6 years and over may be given 5 mg once or twice a day with an increase of 5 mg/d at weekly intervals as needed.
  - *Pemoline:* In children over 6 years old, 37.5 mg/d in the morning.

*MILIEU MANAGEMENT* The following are strategies the nurse can use to provide a therapeutic milieu for the child with ADHD:

- Provide area for hyperactive child to discharge energy without hurting self or others. The nurse will have to manipulate the environment for safety because the child will not be able to discriminate between safe and unsafe activities.
- Develop group activities to facilitate social development. Group activities should include talking groups in which the patient can learn to work and live with peers. The patient should be reinforced for not talking too much in group and for waiting his turn in group games.
- Help patient stay on task by developing activities that will not strain his limited attention span. Keep explanations short and simple.
- Provide an environment relatively free of extraneous stimuli, which will enable the patient to stay focused and not be distracted.
- If formal educational efforts are made, the classroom should be small with a low-stimulation environment. Frequent communication with the teacher should provide the staff with important information about the effectiveness of treatment.
- Reinforce appropriate appearance.
- Provide a milieu in which all staff consistently reinforce appropriate behavior and block manipulation attempts. Staff should meet regularly to develop a cohesive approach to patient care.

- Teaching concerning appropriate use of behavior modification techniques may be helpful to parents.
- If patient acts inappropriately or acts out, behavioral techniques such as "time out" (patient sitting down out of activity area), seclusion (isolated from others), or "holding" (a staff member controlling the patient by holding the patient's arms) may be used to stop negative behavior.

## Psychotic disorders

Schizophrenia usually emerges in adolescence or early adulthood but can occur in children as young as 5 to 8 years old. Symptoms include hallucinations, delusions, thought disorder, anxiety, inappropriate affect, speech idiosyncracies, morbid thoughts, absence of friends, and concrete thinking. During childhood there is frequently some diagnostic confusion between schizophrenia and autism; however, that confusion is much less prominent during the adolescent years.

Autism is a *pervasive developmental disorder.* Autism is differentiated from schizophrenia by its early onset and lack of hallucinations, delusions, and schizophrenic thought processes. Autism almost always has its onset before the child is 3 years of age, whereas schizophrenia often has its onset during adolescence. Autism, in most cases, continues into adolescence, at which time the cardinal symptoms— social and language skill deficits—may improve or worsen (Dustin Hoffman in the movie *Rain Man* portrayed an autistic person). Adequate history taking precludes misdiagnosis. A reactive depression, that is, a depression caused by the realization that one is "handicapped by autism" is not an uncommon complication of late-adolescent autism.

---

### PSYCHOTHERAPEUTIC MANAGEMENT

*NURSE-PATIENT RELATIONSHIP* The following are strategies the nurse can use to develop a therapeutic relationship with a psychotic or autistic child:

- To improve social interactions and develop a trusting relationship
  - Provide for consistent staff-child interactions so that the child will feel comfortable on unit.
  - Provide an atmosphere of acceptance and warmth when working with child.
  - Reinforce the child's perception that the nursing staff will provide care in the child's best interest and be physically available as the child attempts new social behaviors.
  - Do not allow the child to isolate himself and encourage "protected" socialization.
  - Use eye-to-eye contact to model socialization skills and enhance development of the nurse-patient relationship.
- To enhance reality testing
  - Reinforce reality by focusing on real people and events and do not reinforce delusional thinking.
  - Do not argue with the child about delusional content, but it is appropriate to voice doubt.

- Do not use abstractions, jokes, or puns around the child, as his ability to appropriately interpret these abstractions is limited.
■ To promote orientation and appropriate independence
  - Explain in concrete terms the child's schedule, activities, and routines.
  - Allow child to perform activities of daily living independently but with appropriate supervision. Be prepared to assist as needed.
  - Provide reinforcement for accomplishments.

**PSYCHOPHARMACOLOGY** The goal of drug treatment for the child with psychosis is to decrease thought disorganization so that he can return to a previous "normal" level of functioning. The goal for the autistic child is to decrease behaviors such as biting and head banging or to decrease anxiety. Phenothiazines are often the first drugs used.

### Phenothiazines

- ■ Effect: The neuroleptic effect of phenothiazines is characterized by sedation, emotional quieting, and psychomotor slowing. The antipsychotic effect is manifested by normalization of thought, mood, and behavior. The neuroleptic effect may be more significant for the autistic child, and the antipsychotic effect may be more significant for the child with psychosis.
- ■ Interactions: Phenothiazines interact with other CNS depressants and anticholinergics (for example, cold or hay fever medications).
- ■ Side effects: Extrapyramidal symptoms (EPS), anticholinergic effects (for example, anhidrosis, dry mouth, urinary hesistancy, constipation), sedation, and weight gain are some side effects of phenothiazines.
- ■ Dosage: See Table 29-2.
  - Fluphenazine (Prolixin) is not approved for use in young children, but Joshi et al (1988) found a low maintenance dosage of 0.04 mg/kg/d to be beneficial. Adolescents may respond to low adult doses.
  - Thiothixene (Navane) is not approved for use in young children, but Werry (1978) recommends an average dose of 0.15 to 0.3 mg/kg/d for children with psychosis. Children over 12 years may be given this drug. (See Chapter 12.)

**TABLE 29-2**   Administration of antipsychotics to children*

|  | Inpatients | Outpatients |
|---|---|---|
| Chlorpromazine (Thorazine) (6 months to 12 years old) | 50-100 mg/d | 0.5 mg/kg q 4-6 h as needed |
| Thioridazine (Mellaril) (2 to 12 years old) | 25 mg b.i.d. or t.i.d. | 0.5-3 mg/kg/d |
| Trifluoperazine (Stelazine) (6 to 12 years old) | 1-2 mg qd or b.i.d. | |
| Haloperidol (Haldol) (3 to 12 years old) | 0.05-0.15 mg/kg/d | 0.05-0.075 mg/kg/d |

*See chapter 12 for administration for adolescents.

*MILIEU MANAGEMENT* The following are strategies the nurse can use to create a therapeutic milieu for the psychotic or autistic child:

- Provide a predictable environment.
- Develop an environment that provides physical and emotional safety.
- Orient the child to unit and provide orientation displays to facilitate the child's awareness of his environment (for example, calendar, big clock, list of day's events).
- Remove dangerous items from the environment.
- Protect the autistic child from self-injurious acts such as head banging, biting of arms and hands, and hair pulling. Helmets, arm pads, and mittens may be needed to prevent injury.

## Depression

Until 10 years ago many clinicians debated whether depression actually occurred in children. In a significant study conducted 20 years ago Rutter et al. (1976) carefully observed all 10- to 11-year-old children on the Isle of Wight (2199 children) and found only three who could be described as depressed. Today there is a consensus that childhood depression is a mental health problem; however, it is also recognized that much less is known about the clinical picture of childhood depression than is known about adult depression. Childhood depression can be categorized as primary or secondary depression. Primary or endogenous depression can be defined as a mood disorder in which depression is a presenting problem and the cause cannot be traced to a real life event, situation, or illness. Secondary depression is a reaction to a life event. The reaction often takes the form of grief or anhedonia. Anhedonia, the inability to experience joy, is a major symptom of the depressed child. Most children even when surrounded by a series of unpleasant and "depressing" events, can bounce back and enjoy themselves. The child who is persistently sad and unable to enjoy playing is a tragic figure indeed. Adolescent depression is a growing phenomenon and is related to the alarming rate of suicide in this age group.

---

**PSYCHOTHERAPEUTIC MANAGEMENT**

*NURSE-PATIENT RELATIONSHIP* The following are strategies the nurse can use to develop a psychotherapeutic relationship with a depressed child.

- Assess the patient for suicidal ideations (see the discussion on the self-injurious child, which follows).
- Help patient with low self-esteem to examine self-perceptions. Help patient focus on positive characteristics.
- Accept patient. Willingness to listen to the patient and to accept the patient's feelings communicates your professional commitment to help him.
- Develop a trusting relationship by being honest, consistent, empathetic, and truthful.
- Assist patient to evolve from dependency in decision making to more independence. For example, patient may not be able to decide about what clothes to wear. The nurse should help the patient decide. A frequent example of

early, assisted decision making is the completing of a menu for the next day's meals. The nurse can patiently guide the child through this process.

■ Because of the patient's anergia or apathy he may not talk. The nurse who sits silently with the patient at this time communicates the patient's worth and the nurse's commitment to his recovery.

**PSYCHOPHARMACOLOGY**   The *Physician's Desk Reference (PDR)* does not approve any tricyclic antidepressant (TCA) for use in children under 12 years of age. The prescription of antidepressants not approved for pediatric use must be carefully discussed with the parent and should require that an informed consent form be signed by the parent. TCAs such as imipramine have been used for children by some physicians with beneficial results. Imipramine (Tofranil) is also recommended for the treatment of enuresis in children over the age of 6 years. Lower adult dosages are recommended for adolescents (See Chapter 13.)

### Tricyclic antidepressants

■ Effect: TCAs decrease the level of depression. TCAs do this by increasing the bioavailability of norepinephrine, serotonin, and dopamine. It takes about 2 to 4 weeks for TCAs to have a full clinical effect.

■ Interactions: Sympathomimetics and anticholinergic drugs can intensify the effects of TCAs.

■ Side effects: Anticholinergic side effects (anhidrosis, dry mouth, constipation, urinary hesitancy), a blood pressure higher than 140/90, and a heart rate greater than 130 are cause for alarm (Martin and Agran, 1988). TCAs have a narrow therapeutic index. Children and adolescents are thought to be more sensitive to overdoses than are adults.

■ Dosage
  • *Imipramine (Tofranil):* Puig-Antich et al. (1985) recommend that imipramine be "increased every fourth day from 1.5 to 3, to 4, and to 5 mg/kg/day." Maintaining an appropriate serum level is crucial. The therapeutic serum level for imipramine is 150 to 240 ng/ml (Martin and Agran, 1988).
  • *Desipramine (Norpramin) and amitriptyline (Elavil):* Puig-Antich et al. (1985) recommend a maximum dose of 5 mg/kg/d. The therapeutic serum level for desipramine is 115 ng/ml and for amitriptyline is 100 to 300 ng/ml (Martin and Agran, 1988).

**MILIEU MANAGEMENT**   The following are strategies the nurse can use to provide a therapeutic milieu for the depressed child.

■ Provide a safe environment and observe frequently.

■ If the patient is experiencing insomnia, limit caffeinated drinks, stop daytime naps, and provide for a wind-down period before bedtime (activity before bedtime promotes difficulty going to sleep).

■ If patient is anorexic, monitor food intake accurately, provide foods that are agreeable to patient, and weigh patient regularly.

- Help patient with activities of daily living when needed but promote and move in the direction of self-care.
- Encourage patient participation in groups as tolerated. The nurse should buffer immersion into group activities by supporting the patient directly. Gradually increase social interactions. Do not push the patient too fast.
- Do not allow the patient to isolate himself.

## The self-injurious child

Working with the self-injurious child is of importance to the nurse also. Reported suicides among adolescents have tripled since 1960 (McCellan and Trupin, 1989). Because of underreporting and the reluctance of physicians to identify certain deaths as being caused by suicide, it is thought that the real incidence might be several times higher. Suicides in young people have been linked to depression, psychosis, drug abuse, alcoholism, loss, failure in school, and family turmoil.

---

### PSYCHOTHERAPEUTIC MANAGEMENT

*NURSE-PATIENT RELATIONSHIP* The following are strategies the nurse can use to develop a therapeutic relationship with a self-injurious child:

- Listen to the child and convey an interest in what he is saying. Individuals who are considering suicide need to be assured that someone is listening to them.
- Ask the child if he plans to kill himself. "How are you planning to do it." It is important not to be afraid of this issue. By addressing suicide head-on the nurse reassures the child that the nurse understands and is willing to intimately deal with the child and his problems. Assure the patient that you will not allow him to hurt himself.
- Take the child seriously. A child may be seeking attention, but the nurse cannot afford to disparage the child's motives. Individuals can kill themselves accidentally, so all threats should be taken seriously.
- Maintain a calm attitude and do not spread anxiety to the child. It is important to communicate that you and the rest of the staff are in control. The child needs to believe that the nurse is stronger than the child's impulses.
- Review suicidal thoughts with the child daily. Initially children may feel relief after talking about their self-destructive tendencies, but that relief may pass, so the nurse should be prepared to readdress suicidal issues.

*PSYCHOPHARMACOLOGY* Children and adolescents often receive antidepressants for suicidal thoughts associated with depression (see Pharmacology in Depression discussion). TCAs have a low therapeutic index, so the prescribed dose must be carefully adhered to and monitored.

The potential for suicidal or accidental overdose demands that these drugs be kept away from children, younger adolescents, and potentially suicidal older adolescents.

*MILIEU MANAGEMENT* The following are strategies the nurse can use to develop a therapeutic milieu for the self-injurious child:

- Observe the patient frequently. Most units have at least two levels of suicide observation. Level 1 may provide constant one-to-one supervision, and level 2 may provide periodic (every 15 minute) observation.
- Obtain a written (preferred) or verbal contract from the patient that he will not hurt himself and will contact the staff when he has self-injury impulses.
- Remove dangerous objects from the environment including glass and belts.
- Provide physical outlets for anger, for example, punching bags and physical activity, and encourage child to express anger in acceptable ways, for example, writing down points of anger, discussing anger with nurse, and discussing anger within context of a group.
- Provide restraint and seclusion for the child who has lost control. Communicate to the child that the staff is in control and will not let the child hurt himself.

## Bipolar disorder

Bipolar disorder is not easily recognized in children, and the incidence is not clear. Puig-Antich et al. (1985) have identified the following symptoms in childhood mania: (1) elation, (2) an unrealistic optimism, (3) more activity than usual without fatigue, (4) grandiosity, (5) racing thoughts, (6) flight of ideas, (7) distractibility, and (8) motor hyperactivity. Lithium has been used to treat childhood bipolar illness, although its efficacy has not been clearly demonstrated. As adolescence approaches, mania takes on the characteristics of the adult mania disorder.

## Conduct disorder

The major behavioral theme for conduct-disordered children is violation of age-appropriate social norms and rules. Truancy, stealing, run-away behavior, intentional fire setting, and cruelty to animals are examples of conduct-disordered behavior. Conduct disorders have been treated with antipsychotics.

## Oppositional disorder

Oppositional disorder is characterized by negativistic, hostile, and defiant behavior but without the more serious violations of the basic rights of others demonstrated in conduct disorder.

## Eating disorders

Anorexia nervosa and bulimia nervosa, eating disorders associated with adolescence and young adulthood, are discussed in Chapter 25. Pica or the eating of nonnutritive substances occurs more often in children. Animal droppings, sand, insects, leaves, and pebbles are common items eaten by older children. Complications include lead poisoning and intestinal obstruction. Eating disorders have been treated successfully with TCAs.

## Separation anxiety

The primary symptom of separation anxiety is anxiety associated with separation from significant people in the child's life. Often separation from the child's mother causes the most anguish. The child suffering from separation anxiety finds school intolerable, sleeping overnight at a friend's home frightening, and a week at camp impossible. Children with separation anxiety ruminate about disastrous things happening to their family and themselves. Separation anxiety is treated with TCAs.

## EFFECTS OF LIVING WITH AN IMPAIRED PARENT
### The mentally ill parent

"When a parent dies, the child is able to grieve over the loss and move beyond it. Losing a parent through mental illness, however, continues the hope that the parent will one day recover and the family will be reunited" (Gross, 1989).

Rutter (1966) found that children raised by a mentally ill parent were more likely to develop an emotional disorder than other children were. Research efforts since that time have consistently substantiated his findings (Hammen, 1987; Welner, 1988). Children of mentally ill parents tend to have problems at school, problems relating to other people, and problems emotionally. The effects on children of two types of parental mental illnesses are discussed in this chapter: affective disorders and psychotic disorders.

**Affective disorders.**   Most studies of the children of parents with affective disorders have found some impairment (Beardslee et al., 1985). Beardslee et al. (1988) found that 30% of the children of parents with an affective disorder have an emotional disturbance, and 85% of adolescent children have emotional disturbances when divorce complicates the affective disorder. Depressed mothers are less affectionate and more unresponsive to their infant children (Fleming et al., 1988) and tend to view their children as more difficult to parent (Webster-Stratton and Hammond, 1988). In fact, Grunebaum and Cohler (1983) found that the children of depressed mothers are more vulnerable than are children of schizophrenic mothers.

When a parent has a bipolar illness, families tend to deny feelings, become helpless and dependent in close relationships, have unrealistic standards, displace parental low self-esteem onto the children, and have an absent or passive father (Davenport et al., 1984). Mothers in these families tend to be unhappy, tense, ineffective, disorganized, and overprotective and report more negative feelings toward their children.

**Psychotic disorders.**   The psychotic parent creates an environment of inconsistency, contradictory communication, ambivalent affect, unclear intentions, and irrational acts. Anthony (1974) believes that children are at risk when one or both parents are psychotic because of the aforementioned genetic factor, frequent parental separations, and an environment that provides limited reality testing.

**Research findings.**   More recent studies have shown that children of schizophrenic mothers are less affected by the mental illness if the parent's illness can be clearly labeled as bizarre. For example, the fact that children of depressed mothers are more impaired than children of schizophrenic mothers means that the latter child perceives the schizophrenic behavior as bizarre and inappropriate, whereas the child of the depressed mother may just feel the rejection of his mother's apathy.

Gross (1989, p. 16) summarized the major research findings concerning children raised by mentally ill parents:

- Children of mentally ill parents are at greater risk for psychiatric and developmental disorders than are children of well parents, although it is not clear why this is true.
- The risk to children is greater if the mother rather than the father is the ill parent.
- In studies of depressed versus nondepressed groups, differences in the mother-child interaction are evident as early as 3 months postpartum.
- Many children with emotionally disturbed parents do not become disordered themselves. It appears that a number of factors in the nature of the parent's illness, the child's genetic and constitutional make-up, the family's ability to function despite the illness, and the availability of healthy attachment figures play significant roles in predicting child outcomes.*

## The alcoholic parent

It is estimated that about 7 million youngsters' lives are centered around an alcoholic parent. When these 7 million children are coupled with the 21 million adults who still feel the lingering effects of being raised in an alcoholic household, approximately one out of eight Americans can be said to be negatively affected by alcoholism.

The emotional toll on the child of the alcoholic is significant. The various problems outlined below capture the negative impact that alcohol can have on those dependent on an alcoholic parent for support, love, and nurturance.

**Research Findings.**    Studies of the children of alcoholic parents reveal a number of emotional problems that are more pronounced among these children than among the children of nonalcoholic parents.

- These children are twice as likely to develop alcohol-related problems (Bosma, 1975).
- Adolescent children of alcoholic men are more likely to abuse drugs including speed and cocaine (Johnson et al., 1986).
- Daughters of alcoholics are more likely to marry alcoholic men and continue the cycle of family alcoholism (Nici, 1979).
- The percentage of children of alcoholics who marry alcoholics is 20.7%, versus 12.9% of children of nonalcoholics.
- These children suffer more mental, physical, and emotional problems (Russell et al., 1984).
- Sons of alcoholics from preschool through adolescence have 60% more injuries, are five times more likely to report emotional problems, and are two

*From Gross D: At risk: children of the mentally ill, J Psychosoc Nurs 27(8):16, 1989.

and one-half times more likely to be classified as severely ill or disabled (Putnam, 1985).

■ The daughters of alcoholics are three times more likely to be hospitalized or to attend counseling sessions (Putnam, 1985).

■ Preschool children of alcoholics are 65% more likely to experience illness (Putnam, 1985).

■ Two thirds of children referred for child abuse and neglect have an alcoholic parent(s) (O'Gorman, 1985).

■ Older school-age and adolescent children of alcoholics experience more problems of emotional detachment, dependency, social aggression, decreased attention span, fear, emotional liability, and preoccupation with inner thoughts (Fine et al., 1976).

■ The children of an alcoholic parent:
  • Have difficulty expressing feelings (Black, 1979).
  • Have a higher incidence of psychosomatic complaints (Nylander, 1970).
  • Are excessively dependent (Richards, 1979).
  • Have an impaired self-concept and low self-esteem (Baraga, 1978).
  • Are more delinquent (O'Gorman and Ross, 1984).
  • Are more suicidal (Tishler and McKenry, 1982).
  • Are more antisocial (Chafetz, 1979).
  • Have more interpersonal difficulties (Ellwood, 1980).

Box 29-2 describes the warning signs of parental alcoholism. Perhaps more tragically, the effects of this troubled parenting haunt the child into adulthood. Because of the long-lasting impact of alcoholism on children, a new acronym, ACoAs (adult children of alcoholics), is now part of the nurse's professional vocabulary. ACoAs represent a large aggregate for whom nurses should develop prevention strategies, education, and mental health care (Avery, 1989).

### Intervening with children of impaired parents

The first aim of any treatment program for children at risk is prevention. Primary prevention is the term used to designate a treatment approach that identifies vulnerable children and then develops intervention strategies to minimize the effects of risk factors. Among children of impaired parents a significant subpopulation is at risk, and identifying those children is of primary concern to health professionals.

Prevention and intervention are based on the assumptions that mental health professionals can teach the child and parent new skills and behaviors and that the home environment can be changed. Intervention strategies have included the following:

■ Anthony's (1983, p. 70) risk vulnerability model program, which reduces or neutralizes risk factors and organizes comprehensive support systems.

■ Competency-based programs, such as those that develop problem-solving skills.

■ Significant others–based programs, such as those that use mothers of resilient children to support vulnerable children.

**Box 29-2**

## GENERAL INDICATORS OF PARENTAL ALCOHOLISM

- Frequent absences or truancy, visits to the school nurse, or morning tardiness, especially Mondays.
- History of stress-related illnesses, psychosomatic complaints, accidents, chronic fatigue, sleep disturbances, injuries or bruises, and substance abuse.
- Inappropriate behavior (overly responsible or concerned with pleasing authority figures, passive or controlling, excessive use of humor or acting out).
- Fluctuating or poor nutrition, grooming, hygiene, or clothing.
- Excessive or nonexistent peer contacts.
- Inappropriate school performance (exaggerated concern with achievement, erratic or poor performance without evidence of a learning disability).
- Reports of excessive alcohol consumption (often being negative toward alcohol use), inconsistent or violent discipline, and minimal shared interests among family members. These children also fear any contact between their parents and school personnel.
- Emotional disturbances (absent or extreme emotional response, low self-esteem, feelings of being different or powerless).

- Learning-based programs, such as those that teach people who have learned to be helpless to learn to help themselves.
- Family comprehensive health-based programs, such as psychiatric hospitalization of the entire family to focus on mothering and the mothering role.

## KEY CONCEPTS

1. Estimates of the incidence of emotional disorder among children vary, but all studies indicate this to be a growing concern.
2. Risk factors for childhood emotional disorders include genetic and biological factors; adverse environmental influences before, during, and after birth; social and cultural factors; family system factors; and stress experiences during infancy and childhood.
3. The extent of the negative effects of these risk factors upon children tend to differ according to the degree the risk factors are present as well as according to the characteristics of the child himself.
4. Resiliency is the ability to withstand the problems of an undesirable childhood environment and emerge as a "normal," productive person.
5. Attention-deficit hyperactivity disorder (ADHD) is the most common pediatric behavioral disorder, and CNS stimulants are the drugs most frequently used to treat children with ADHD.

6. Symptoms of childhood psychoses include hallucinations, delusions, thought disorder, anxiety, inappropriate affect, speech idiosyncrasies, morbid thoughts, absence of friends, and concrete thinking.

7. Childhood depression, its existence once debated by clinicians, is considered a significant mental health problem today and pharmacologically is treated with antidepressants.

8. Children with a mentally ill or alcoholic parent are at risk for developing emotional disorders.

9. Prevention efforts assume that positive efforts or adaptive skills can be taught and environments changed.

10. Competence and level of support are important variables to be addressed in a treatment strategy.

## REFERENCES

American Psychiatric Association: Diagnostic and statistical manual of mental disorders, ed. 3 revised, Washington, DC, 1987, The Association.

Anthony EJ: A risk-vulnerability intervention model for children of psychotic parents. In Anthony EJ and Koupernik C, editors: The child in his family: vol. 3, Children at psychiatric risk, New York, 1974, John Wiley and Sons.

Anthony EJ: The preventive approach to children at high risk for psychopathology and psychosis. In Frank M, editor: Children of exceptional parents, New York, 1983, The Haworth Press.

Avery ML: Adult children of alcoholics, J Psychosoc Nurs 27(8):20, 1989.

Baraga DJ: Self-concept in children of alcoholics, Dissertation Abstracts International 39:368B, 1978.

Barlow DJ: Therapeutic holding: effective intervention with the aggressive child, J Psychosoc Nurs 27(1):10, 1989.

Beardslee W, Keller M, and Klerman G: Children of parents with affective disorder, Int J Fam Psychiatry 6:283, 1985.

Beardslee W et al: Psychiatric disorder in adolescent offspring of parents with affective disorder in a non-referred sample, J Affective Disorder 15:313, 1988.

Black C: Children of alcoholics, Alcohol Health Res World, pp 23-27, Fall 1979.

Bosma W: Alcoholism and teenagers, Maryland Med J 24:62, 1975.

Chafetz ME: Children of alcoholics, NYU Educ Quarterly 10:23, 1979.

Clunn PA: The child. In Beck CA, Rawlins RP, and Williams SR, editors: Mental health–psychiatric nursing, St. Louis, 1988, The C.V. Mosby Co.

Coleman WL and Levine MD: Attention deficits in adolescence: description, evaluation, and management, Pediatr Rev 9:287, 1988.

Davenport Y et al: Early child-rearing practices in families with a manic-depressive parent, Am J Psychiatry 141:230, 1984.

Ellwood LC: Effects of alcoholism as a family illness on child behavior and development, Military Med 145:188, 1980.

Fine E et al: Behavior disorders in children with parental alcoholism, Ann NY Acad Sci 273:507, 1976.

Fleming A et al: Postpartum adjustment in first-time mothers: relations between mood, maternal attitudes and mother-infant interactions, Dev Psychol 24:71, 1988.

Gross D: At risk: children of the mentally ill, J Psychosoc Nurs 27(8):14, 1989.

Grunebaum H and Cohler B: Children of parents hospitalized for mental illness: I. Attentional and interactional studies. In Frank M, editor: Children of exceptional parents, New York, 1983, Haworth Press.

Hammen C et al: Maternal affective disorders, illness and stress: risk for children's psychopathology, Am J Psychiatry 144:736, 1987.

Johnson S et al: Children of alcoholics: drinking, driving styles, and drug use. Presented at the

Research Society of America Meeting, San Francisco, April 1986.

Joshi PT, Capozzoli JA, and Coyle JT: Low-dose neuroleptic therapy for children with childhood onset pervasive developmental disorder, Am J Psychiatry 145:335, 1988.

Keltner BR, Keltner NL, and Farren E: Family routines and conduct disorder in adolescent girls, West J Nurs Res 12(2):161, 1990.

LaGreca AM and Quay HC: Behavior disorders in children. In Ender NS and Hunt J McV, editors: Personality and the behavior disorders, ed 2, New York, 1984, John Wiley and Sons.

Martin JE and Agran M: Pharmacotherapy. In Matson JL, editor: Handbook of treatment: approaches in childhood psychopathology, New York, 1988, Plenum Press.

McCellan J and Trupin E: Prevention of psychiatric disorders in children, Hosp Community Psychiatry 40:630, 1989.

Munoz-Millan RJ and Casteel CR: Attention-deficit hyperactivity disorder: recent literature, Hosp Community Psychiatry 40:699, 1989.

Nici J: Wives of alcoholics as "repeaters." J Stud Alcohol 40:677, 1979.

Nylander I: Children of alcoholic fathers, Acta Paediatr Scand 49(suppl. 121):1, 1970.

O'Gorman P: An historical look at children of alcoholics in the juvenile justice system, Alcohol Health Res World 8(4):43, 1985.

O'Gorman P and Ross R: Children of alcoholics in the juvenile justice system, Alcohol Health Res World 8(4):43, 1984.

Pothier PC: Child psychiatric nursing, J Psychosoc Nurs 22:11, 1984.

Puig-Antich J, Ryan ND, and Rabinovich H: Affective disorders in childhood and adolescence. In Wiener JM, editor: Diagnosis and psychopharmacology for childhood and adolescent disorders, New York, 1985, John Wiley and Sons.

Putnam S: Are children of alcoholics sicker than other children: a study of illness experience and utilization behavior in a health maintenance organization. Presented at the annual meeting of the American Public Health Association, Washington, DC, Nov. 1985.

Richards TM: Working with children of an alcoholic mother, Alcohol Health Res World 3:22, 1979.

Russell M, Henderson C, and Blume S: Children of alcoholics: a review of the literature, New York, 1984, Children of Alcoholics Foundation.

Rutter M: The children of sick parents, Maudsley Monograph No. 16, London, 1966, Oxford University Press.

Rutter M: Protective factors in children's response to stress and disadvantage. In Kent M and Rolf J, editors: Primary prevention of psychopathology: vol 3, Social competence in children, Hanover, N.H., 1979, University of New England Press.

Rutter M: Stress, coping, and development: some issues and some questions, Child Psychol Psychiatry 22:323, 1981.

Rutter M: Prevention of children's psychosocial disorders: myth or substance, Pediatrics 70:883, 1982.

Rutter M: Resilient children, Psychol Today, March 1984.

Rutter M et al: Research report: Isle of Wight studies, 1964-1974, Psychol Med 6:313, 1976.

Safer DJ and Krager JM: A survey of medication treatments for hyperactive or inattentive students, JAMA 260:2256, 1988.

Tishler C and McKenry P: Parental negative self-esteem and adolescent suicide attempts, J Am Acad Child Psychiatry 21:404, 1982.

Wallen J and Pincus HA: Care of children with psychiatric disorders in community hospitals, Hosp Community Psychiatry 39:167, 1988.

Webster-Stratton C and Hammond M: Maternal depression and its relationship to life stress, perceptions of child behavior problems, parenting behaviors, and child conduct problems, J Abnorm Child Psychol 16:299, 1988.

Welner Z and Rice J: School-aged children of depressed parents: a blind and controlled study, J Affective Disord 15:291, 1988.

Werry J: Pediatric psychopharmacology, New York, 1978, Brunner/Mazel, Inc.

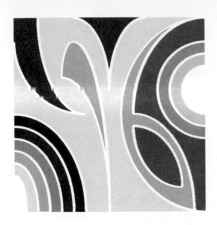

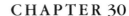
CHAPTER 30

# Working with the Elderly Mentally Ill

MIRA KIRK NELSON

LEARNING OBJECTIVES
After reading this chapter you should be able to

- Identify barriers to mental health care experienced by the elderly.
- Describe unique variations in symptoms of depression evident in the elderly.
- Define the purpose of psychosocial assessment of the elderly.
- Describe the components of assessment of the elderly.
- Identify therapeutic goals for the elderly.
- Identify changes in altered pharmacokinetics as the result of aging.
- Describe strategies of milieu management useful for the elderly.

Aging of the population is one of the most significant trends of this century.

The growth rate of the 65 years and over age group is three times that of the population as a whole and that of the 75 years and over age group is even higher. At the present time, 23 million Americans (one out of nine) are over the age of 65. By the year 2000 there will be approximately 34.9 million people or about 13% of the population over the age of 65 (Tillman-Jones, 1990). Projections indicate that by the year 2040, 68 million Americans (or about 20% of the population) will exceed that age (Sloan, 1986).

The federal government has targeted persons past 75 years of age as having the greatest need for social support, income maintenance, housing, health services, and mental health services. Older persons have a greater incidence of chronic diseases, disabilities, and mental impairments. However, most older persons assess themselves to be in good health. Although many of them may have two or more chronic illnesses, they are not disabled by them. They continue to perform their daily activities, perhaps more slowly but independently (Kermis, 1986).

Psychopathology represents a problem to approximately 15% to 20% of the persons over the age of 65. If one adds persons with dementia (see Chapter 22), up to 25% of the elderly population may, at some time, be in need of neuropsychiatric evaluation and treatment. In addition, psychoactive drugs are prescribed for 25% of the elderly residing in the community and 50% of the institutionalized elderly (Kermis, 1986; Wills, 1986). It is estimated that 65% of elderly persons with psychiatric disorders also have significant medical disease. Depression or other psychiatric disorders should not be considered just a normal response to other disease. If specific therapy is to be initiated, the psychiatric symptoms must be recognized as distinct from those of medical disorders (Wills, 1986).

There has been considerable research documenting the serious and unmet need for mental health care for older adults. The need for mental health services has been underestimated for a variety of reasons:

1. Only 3% to 5% of the elderly seek care in psychiatrists' offices and community mental health clinics.
2. There has been a tendency to overestimate the incidence of dementia while underestimating that of depression.
3. The incidence of alcohol abuse has been minimized.
4. Physician- and patient-induced drug abuse is only now being recognized as a serious problem (Kermis, 1986; Wills, 1986).

This chapter will present an overview of the issues related to working with the mentally ill elderly that are different from issues of working with mentally ill younger adults. Barriers to mental health care, major depression (by far the most common mental disorder among the elderly), schizophrenia, paranoid thinking, and anxiety disorders will be discussed. The process of assessment and the psychotherapeutic management of the elderly mentally ill will also be considered. Finally, a brief discussion of electroconvulsive therapy is provided for the student.

# BARRIERS TO MENTAL HEALTH CARE
## Ageism

Ageism involves the dislike of and discrimination against the elderly by some care-givers and has served as a barrier to effective therapy for the elderly. Behaviors indicative of ageism are the avoidance of older persons on an individual basis and discrimination against the elderly in terms of access to and utilization of social institutions. Historically the elderly have been excluded from psychoanalysis, leading to the relative neglect of the psychodynamic processes of later life (Kermis, 1986).

## Attitudes

The attitudes of the elderly serve as a barrier to mental health services. Older persons tend to define mental health difficulties as unchangeable and are less inclined than younger persons to seek informal or professional outside help for their personal problems. Psychotherapeutic assistance is viewed as financially expensive and time consuming.

## Costs

Costs of mental health services are a major barrier to the elderly seeking mental health services. Most elderly Americans depend on the Medicare program to finance their health care. However, Medicare legislation has established policies that discriminate against mental health care, with limitations on payment for and frequency of care.

# MAJOR DEPRESSION IN THE ELDERLY

Although depression is the most common mental illness in the elderly, it is often overlooked, misdiagnosed, and inadequately treated. Many elderly persons thought to be demented are actually depressed. Tyler and Tyler (1984) estimated that misdiagnosis may occur half the time. The phenomenon of depression appearing to be dementia is referred to as pseudodementia.

Depression is an illness that affects mind and body and causes the elderly person to feel miserable in many ways. Constipation, headaches, dyspnea without a physical basis, and general aches and pains are typical physical complaints. Cognitive symptoms that may mimic dementia include poor memory, disorientation, poor judgment, and agitation (Cohen and Eisdorfer, 1986).

The actual incidence of depression among the elderly is not known. Although the DSM-III-R outlines diagnostic criteria for depression, many clinicians find the criteria difficult to apply to the elderly population. Consequently, prevalence statistics vary greatly. For instance, estimates of depression among all elderly range from 5% to 65% (Hawranik and Kondratuk, 1986; St. Pierre et al., 1986). Whatever the true prevalence of depression among the elderly, epidemiologists agree that the elderly experience more depression than younger age groups. Ronsman (1987) states that fewer than one fourth of all persons with depression receive any type of treatment. Suicide can be the result of untreated depression, and the depressed older person is more likely to commit suicide than is a depressed person in any

### Box 30-1
## COMMON INDICATORS OF DEPRESSION

- Sleep disturbances (one of the earliest symptoms)
- Fatigue, unrelated to hard work or rest
- Loss of sexual interest
- Weight changes (usually loss of weight)
- Gastrointestinal complaints (constipation or stomach distress)
- Multiple vague aches and pains unrelated to a physical cause

other age group (Tillman-Jones, 1990). The prototype older person at risk for suicide is white, male, unmarried, and from a lower socioeconomic class, may have chronic pain or a terminal illness, and uses alcohol or medication to cope (Osgood, 1988).

### Symptoms in the elderly

The detection and diagnosis of true depression in the elderly are difficult because the symptoms may be caused by or imitate those of other common problems, such as dementia, hyperthyroidism, electrolyte disorders, and reactions to terminal illness (Field, 1985). On the other hand, "true" depression is often expressed somatically. Ronsman (1987) states that preoccupation with bodily functions and vague physical complaints may be the only symptoms of which the elderly complain. Alterations in mood or emotional symptoms so characteristic of depression in younger adults may not be present in the elderly and, if present, may not be expressed unless the nurse questions the patient about these feelings.

Chaisson-Stewart (1985) states that somatic symptoms may be the most common indicators of depression among older persons who become depressed. They will often seek help from the family physician with the complaints listed in Box 30-1.

An assessment of the elderly patient is necessary to determine the cause of the depression and to plan for nursing interventions to alleviate or eliminate the problem.

### Life events

Life events, especially loss, are believed to be related to the beginning of depression. Loss is a persistent theme among the elderly. Significant variables of loss include the number of losses, the age of the person, and the meaning of the loss (Wills, 1986). For instance, as the patient ages, there is a general reduction in physical ability. This translates into less energy to fend off the impact of life events. Possible recurrent and serious adverse life events that may result in depression include retirement, inadequate income, loss of friends, loneliness, chronic illness, chronic psychiatric disorders, and alcohol or drug abuse or dependence.

# SCHIZOPHRENIA

Schizophrenia is not a mental disorder that first occurs late in life, but persons with schizophrenia grow old like everyone else and carry that condition into later life. Typically the person has taken antipsychotic drugs for some time. The bizarre delusions and hallucinations associated with Type I schizophrenia are infrequent. Type II symptoms, such as flattened affect, alogia, and autism, are more common among this age group. This probably represents the natural evolution from positive symptoms to negative symptoms that some researchers theorize may happen. Chapter 19 provides a thorough review of schizophrenia.

# PARANOID THINKING

Paranoid thinking is a relatively common problem in the elderly. As coping behaviors are compromised with age, paranoid thinking often emerges as a defense mechanism against a potentially hostile environment. For example, walking to the corner grocery store in some neighborhoods may be perilous for an older person because he is less able to fend off aggressors. The older person finds himself becoming more and more isolated as he retreats to an environment he can control. Although the threat may be based on reality, the resulting isolative and suspicious behavior can lead to unhealthy paranoid thinking. Paranoid thinking may be manifested as exaggerated suspiciousness, ideas of reference, persecutory thoughts, delusions, or a belief that he has a somatic disorder (e.g., cancer of the stomach).

# ANXIETY DISORDERS

Older persons often experience anxiety. Anxiety is characterized by tension, trembling, hyperactivity, anticipation of something terrible happening, vigilance, difficulty in concentrating, impatience, and insomnia. Anxiety among this population is related, in some ways, to the same developmental issues associated with paranoid thinking. As one ages, certain abilities are lost, and the inevitability of physical decline becomes clear. Compounding these issues are the many losses faced by older persons—loss of health, loved ones, status, and so on—that perpetuate anxiety. Anxiety disorders take several forms, including obsessive-compulsive disorder, generalized anxiety disorder, and phobic disorder.

# ASSESSMENT OF THE MENTALLY ILL ELDERLY
## Purpose of psychosocial assessment

According to McConnell and Matteson (1988), the purpose of psychosocial assessment is to characterize the elderly patient's functioning in a particular social environment. The process of assessing the elderly's psychological functioning is necessary for initiating appropriate treatment or management. Assessment of the aged patient provides a basis for setting treatment goals. In the assessment the patient and the caregiver look at the problem, decide what is wrong, and plan what can be done to alleviate or eliminate the problem. Caregivers must understand that old age is a part of the ongoing life process. However, the elderly experience certain tasks, losses, and problems that may require special diagnostic and assessment skills. It is important to remember that chronological age does not tell us much about a person.

A person's ability to function and interact on a day-to-day basis is a far better criterion for assessing performance than is the mere passage of time (Kermis, 1986).

## Assessment strategies

The assessment process begins with the taking of a psychosocial history, which should include both the patient's normal characteristics and those the patient is now exhibiting (Ronsman, 1987). The interview may be highly anxiety producing, as the patient is often reluctant to discuss problems with a stranger, especially a young one. The interview should be held in a comfortable, relaxed, and private setting to reduce any stress or fear the patient may have in talking with the interviewer.

A handshake at the beginning and end of the interview is a valuable tool to reduce anxiety in a confused person. Good eye contact is important, with the interviewer being on the same level as the patient, not standing above and looking down at the bedridden elderly person. Hearing or vision impairments can affect the quality of the communication and should be noted and compensated for as much as possible.

The interviewer must establish a good rapport with the patient. Empathy for the aged patient will reduce the stress that he may feel in the interview situation. This will increase the probability that the required information will be obtained from the patient. For the patient to be open with the interviewer, he must feel that the interviewer accepts him as a person and is not frightened by the physical and mental changes that take place in the elderly. The patient also must feel that the interviewer has the professional skills necessary to work with an older person.

The interviewer should understand that the time of the evaluation may affect its success. As some elderly patients experience fatigue in the early morning or late in the afternoon, it is helpful to schedule the interview at midday. Talking slowly and using simple and concise language will help the patient to understand the meaning of the questions. The interviewer must allow additional time while the older patient gropes for words or expressions to answer the questions.

Interviewers should guard against taking a condescending tone or mannerism in the interview. In our informal society, we are often on a first-name basis with friends and associates. This may be a custom that an older person does not appreciate. Therefore it is always best to call older persons Mr., Mrs., or Miss with the last name until they ask you to call them something else.

Reminiscence, defined as thinking about the past and reflecting on it, can be used by the interviewer as an aid to facilitate communication. There is a tendency for the elderly to reminisce as part of a normal process of life review. The older person, realizing that death is an imminent possibility, attempts to reconstruct his or her past life as a way of accepting its successes and failures. In a mild form of life review the elderly patients tell stories about their past successes and express regrets about their failures. However, others may have extreme forms of life review in which they exhibit anxiety, guilt, depression, and despair. In such cases suicide may result if they cannot resolve or accept the problems (Dreyfus, 1988; Kermis, 1986).

During the interview it is important for the interviewer to be aware of the

**Box 30-2**

### INFORMATION TO OBTAIN DURING THE ASSESSMENT INTERVIEW

- Basic background information, such as age, address, religious activity, family status
- Family history and cultural background
- Economic status and sources of income
- Education and work history
- Life-style and perception of current life situation
- Current living arrangements
- Interests, pleasures, and activities
- Friendship and social interaction patterns
- Medical information or history
- Drugs and dosage
- General psychiatric information, such as mental status, complaints, past history, therapy goals, attitudes, and self-concept
- Goals and plans for the future

persistent themes in the distressed older person, such as somatic concerns, loss reactions, fear of losing control, and fear of death. The interviewer's understanding acceptance of these concerns affirms reality and offers support for the older person, who may have been unable to articulate these anxieties in the past (Kermis, 1986).

### Assessment interview

Each assessment interview attempts to give the caregiver an understanding of the patient's problems. Some of the information that should be obtained in the assessment interview is listed in Box 30-2.

### Physical assessment

After the interview the elderly person suspected of being depressed should be given a thorough physical examination (since depression can often be a "rule-out" diagnosis). Assessment of depression in the elderly is complicated by the many medications that may cause depression as a side effect: analgesics and anti-inflammatory agents, antihistamines, antihypertensive agents, antimicrobials, tranquilizers, and miscellaneous drugs, including alcohol, caffeine, digitalis, propranolol, and amphetamines (Dreyfus, 1988).

Special attention should be given to the possibility of infection, cardiac problems, malignant disease, endocrine disorders, hypothyroidism, hyperthyroidism, and neurological deficits, all of which can produce a secondary depression. Other disorders that may be associated with depression include respiratory, musculoskeletal, gastrointestinal, and renal problems. Laboratory tests are necessary to rule out the possibility of depression secondary to anemia or electrolyte imbalance. Other tests that are helpful in ruling out problems include a complete blood count, urinalysis, thyroid function tests, electroencephalograms, computed tomography (CT scan), positron-emission tomography (PET), and magnetic resonance imaging (MRI) of the brain (Kaszniak et al., 1985; St. Pierre et al., 1986).

## PSYCHOTHERAPEUTIC MANAGEMENT

*NURSE-PATIENT RELATIONSHIP* Depression and other mental disorders have a significant effect on the patient's ability to manage even the simplest of tasks. The nurse should be particularly aware of some of the feelings associated with depression, such as powerlessness, helplessness, hopelessness, guilt, anger, hostility, or low self-esteem. These feelings may cause the patient to regress to a point of such self-neglect that he refuses to wash, bathe, or shave. Eating may become a monumental task. Sleep and wake cycles are interrupted. Meeting these basic needs is a nursing priority, whether in the acute-care hospital or the psychiatric setting.

The success or failure of a plan of care depends on the quality of the relationship established between the nurse and the elderly mentally ill patient. The nurse must focus on providing care for the patient and help the patient and his family manage the activities and demands of daily living (Hawranik and Kondratuk, 1986).

**Realistic goals.** Nursing interventions to assist elderly mentally ill patients include the setting of realistic small goals that can be achieved. A discussion should be held with the patient to stress the importance of setting goals to accomplish each of the daily living activities. Developing a schedule of activities for each day can assist the patient in making decisions and coping with these demands. The caregiver must be gentle and supportive, as additional time may be needed to achieve these goals. Some examples of daily living activities include bathing, dressing, eating, taking medications, keeping appointments, going shopping, and paying bills. The caregiver should encourage participation in these activities, knowing how far to push the patient and when to back off if the activity proves to be too strenuous or agitating for the patient (Hawranik and Kondratuk, 1986; Patrick, 1986).

**Levels of psychological intervention.** Therapeutic intervention with the elderly has two main goals: the alleviation of anxiety and the maintenance or restoration of psychological functioning. Three levels of psychological intervention can be used, depending on the problem of the elderly patient:

1. Total prevention of the occurrence of mental impairment through prestress counseling, improvement of living conditions, and ensuring adequate nutrition and socialization
2. Restoration to the previous functional level through early intervention to remedy nutritional deficiencies, inadequate oxygenation, biochemical aberrations, and psychosocial stresses
3. Therapeutic programs to slow the rate of social, intellectual, and emotional deterioration in the elderly person (Kermis, 1986).

The choice of intervention is determined by the presenting symptoms, the patient's level of functioning, and the resources available to assist in ongoing treatment.

PSYCHOPHARMACOLOGY Although Unit III covers psychopharmacology, it is important to understand the use of these drugs by the mentally ill elderly. Sloan (1986) reports that a national health care expenditure study found that patients who are 65 years of age or over averaged 10.8 prescriptions annually. On discharge from the hospital, 25% of the patients in this age group receive prescriptions for six or more drugs. Of all elderly patients in nursing homes or other institutions, 95% are receiving one or more drugs, with some patients receiving as many as 12 to 15 drugs concurrently. Therefore it is easy to understand why an elderly person living alone with poor vision and hearing would have difficulty complying with a medical regimen involving several drugs. In addition, the patient could be taking several nonprescription drugs without the knowledge of the physician. Polypharmacy is common, and the caregiver should be aware of these potential problems. Patient compliance is a significant problem in approximately 60% of the elderly patients, especially those who have disabilities and live alone. Box 30-3 provides guidelines for use of psychotropic drugs in the elderly.

**Box 30-3**
## GUIDELINES FOR USE OF PSYCHOTROPIC DRUGS IN THE ELDERLY

**Initial dose**

• Start with small dose and gradually increase until therapeutic effect or adverse side effects occur.
• Usually one third to one half younger-adult dose.

**Daily dose**

• Use smallest dose that will produce relief.

**Individualization**

• Elderly persons are the most heterogeneous age group in American society.
• Each individual will need thoughtful attention.
• Partial symptom relief may well the the most judicious and realistic goal.

**Discontinuance**

• The elderly should be gradually tapered off psychotropic drugs.
• If the elderly patient can manage without drug therapy, he should be allowed to do so.

**TABLE 30-1**  Physiological changes in the elderly resulting in pharmacokinetic alteration

| Physiological change | Pharmacokinetic alteration |
| --- | --- |
| Increased gastric pH | Decreased absorption |
| Increased body fat | Decreased fat-soluble drug concentration |
| Decreased body water | Increased water-soluble drug concentration |
| Decreased serum albumin | Increased unbound drug leading to increased drug activity |
| Decreased cardiac output | Decreased metabolism of drugs |
| Decreased renal function | Decreased metabolism of drugs |
| Decreased liver mass, blood flow | Decreased metabolism of drugs |

**Altered pharmacokinetics.**  According to Sloan (1986), the elderly demonstrate altered responses to drug therapy and increased adverse effects. The aging process produces numerous bodily changes that bring about changes in the absorption, distribution, metabolism, and excretion of drugs (see Table 30-1). Because the elderly have diminished gastric acidity, fewer active cells and enzymes, and slowed arterial blood flow, drug absorption is considered to be slower and less complete.

Distribution is determined by the alterations in blood flow, plasma albumin concentration, and body composition that can occur in the course of aging. Blood flow to the renal and hepatic systems is decreased to maintain adequate flow to the cerebral and coronary systems, resulting in altered patterns of drug metabolism and excretion. Total systemic diffusion is decreased because of decreases in plasma volume, total body water, and extracellular fluid in the elderly. The proportion of lean body mass to total body weight decreases with age. Lipid-soluble drugs such as barbiturates, phenothiazines, benzodiazepines, and phenytoin will be absorbed into the increased amount of fatty tissue and retained by the body.

Serum albumin concentration is another major factor that affects the distribution of drugs in the elderly. Although healthy older adults may have only mild reductions in serum albumin, substantial reductions are noted in those who are malnourished and chronically ill. Phenytoin, diazepam, warfarin, digitoxin, and naproxen are examples of drugs that are highly bound to plasma proteins. A large proportion of these drugs is confined to the intravascular space, and only a small fraction is distributed to the pharmacological site of action. A reduction in the amount of total plasma albumin will decrease the number of binding sites and increase the amount of free or active drug. When hypoalbuminemia is present, drug serum level is not an accurate predictor of free drug. Therefore a normally therapeutic serum drug level could be a toxic amount of free drug.

A delay in transporting drugs to the liver caused by problems in distribution can diminish metabolism of drugs in the elderly. As there is a significant decrease in the size of the liver with normal aging, a person's drug-metabolizing capacity may be affected. Although a decrease in the number of enzymes available to metabolize drugs has been demonstrated, it has not been shown to be of any clinical significance in the absence of specific organ disease.

The kidney, also affected by the aging process, is responsible for drug excretion. Drugs are excreted by active tubular secretion, glomerular filtration, or both. Renal function is more accurately measured by creatinine clearance than by serum creatinine. Creatinine clearance decreases significantly with age, along with a decrease in renal size, blood flow, glomerular filtration rate, and the number of functioning glomeruli. Creatinine-clearance studies show that renal function drops significantly in persons over 30 years of age, declining at a rate of 6% to 10% per decade, with an increased rate of decline after the age of 65. Because of a decrease in lean body weight and creatinine production, the creatinine clearance can be greatly reduced in the presence of a normal serum creatinine. For example, 60% to 90% of digoxin is excreted unchanged. In an elderly person whose renal excretion of the drug is prolonged, the daily dose of digoxin may have to be reduced to prevent an adverse reaction due to an accumulation of the drug (Martilla and Anderson, 1979; Sloan, 1986).

The nurse must be aware of the therapeutic goals of the patient's drug regimen and should observe the patient for the effects of the therapy. The nurse contributes to the ongoing care plan by reporting both the therapeutic and adverse effects of drug therapy and ensures that unneeded medications are discontinued. Common side effects of psychotropic drugs in the elderly are listed in Table 30-2.

**Antidepressants.** The most common drugs chosen for treatment of depression are the tricyclic antidepressants and the monamine oxidase inhibitors. Methylphenidate may also be prescribed for apathetic or withdrawn patients. The adverse effects of these drugs often complicate their use in the aged, and the dosage requirements are generally much lower. Antidepressants may cause sedation, anticholinergic effects, and signs of tremulousness, sweating, and cardiovascular effects. The latter effects are of primary concern in the elderly, particularly abnormally low blood pressure on change to an upright position that leads to possible falls and fractures. Peripheral anticholinergic effects, such as urinary retention, bowel immobility, acute glaucoma, tremors, and blurred vision, are additional side effects of concern in the elderly. Antidepressant medications can cause a central anticholinergic syndrome of delirium, confusion, and acute psychosis that may be indistinguishable from dementia (Nickens et al., 1986).

**Antipsychotics.** Antipsychotic drugs are used in the treatment of schizophrenia, acute psychosis, aggressive behavior, and agitation. A complete explanation of antipsychotic drugs is found in Chapter 12. In that chapter antipsychotic drugs are categorized as high potency or low potency. The high-potency drugs such as haloperidol (Haldol), fluphenazine (Prolixin), and thiothixene (Navane) are associated with extrapyramidal side effects. The low-potency antipsychotics such as chlorpromazine (Thorazine) and thioridazine (Mellaril), are associated with sedation and anticholinergic and cardiovascular side effects (i.e., orthostatic hypotension). Since sedation and anticholinergic and cardiovascular side effects are particularly bothersome to older persons, the *high-potency* antipsychotic drugs are prescribed more

**TABLE 30-2**   Common side effects of psychotropic drugs in older adults and appropriate nursing interventions

| Side effects | Nursing interventions |
| --- | --- |
| Dry mouth | • Provide frequent sips of water; hard, sugarless candy or sugarless gum. Petroleum jelly may help dentures fit better. |
| Nasal congestion | • Over-the-counter nasal decongestants may be suggested; however, over-the-counter drugs can interact with many prescribed drugs. Physician should be consulted. |
| Urinary hesistancy | • Running water, privacy, warm water run over perineum; evaluate for enlarged prostate. |
| Urinary retention, bladder distension | • Catheterize for residual; give fluids; encourage frequent voiding, evaluate for enlarged prostate. |
| Blurred vision | • Reassurance; blurred vision is a temporary side effect of many drugs. |
| Constipation | • Give laxatives as ordered and provide appropriate diet with roughage. |
| Eye pain | • Instruct the older adult to report eye pain immediately, as this may indicate exacerbation of undiagnosed glaucoma. |
| Orthostatic hypotension | • Instruct the older adult to get out of bed slowly, to then sit on the edge of the bed for a short while, and to rise slowly.<br>• Observe closely to ascertain whether a change of drug might be appropriate. |

often for them. Dosages for older persons tend to be half or less than half those given to younger patients. Box 30-4 provides an overview of side effects and appropriate nursing responses.

**Antianxiety agents.** Anxiety is a common theme among the elderly, and consequently antianxiety agents (Chapter 14) are frequently used. The benzodiazepines are the antianxiety drugs most often prescribed. The benzodiazepines are categorized as long-acting and short-acting drugs. The long-acting benzodiazepines are not given to older persons because they take longer to clear the system. Long-acting benzodiazepines include chlordiazepoxide (Librium), clorazepate (Tranxene), diazepam (Valium), and prazepam (Centrax). The short-acting benzodiazepines, which are ordered for older persons, include lorazepam (Ativan), oxazepam (Serax), clonazepam (Klonopin), and alprazolam (Xanax). Since a withdrawal syndrome (including a withdrawal seizure) can occur in persons taken off of an antianxiety agent after 30 days or more of use, benzodiazepines should be withdrawn slowly for a period of several weeks. Benzodiazepines are relatively safe drugs when taken alone but can cause severe sedation and respiratory suppression when combined with alcohol or other sedatives (see Table 30-3). A new antianxiety drug, buspirone (Buspar), is not a benzodiazepine and seems to have some advantages over the benzodiazepines. Its chief advantage is that it *does not* react with alcohol and other

Box 30-4

# SPECIAL CONSIDERATIONS FOR ELDERLY PATIENTS TAKING PSYCHOTROPIC DRUGS

### Antidepressant drugs: TCAs

- Orthostatic hypotension is a major concern; nortriptyline, as opposed to other TCAs, does not seem to cause as severe a hypotensive episode.
- Amitriptyline produces the *most* anticholinergic side effects.
- Desipramine, trazodone, and fluoxetine produce the *fewest* anticholinergic side effects.
- CNS symptoms of toxicity include disorientation, confusion, and memory loss.
- Caution should be observed when TCAs are given to elderly persons with cardiovascular disease.

### Antipsychotic drugs

- Haloperidol, fluphenazine, and thiothixene cause more extrapyramidal symptoms (EPS) than most other antipsychotics.
- The elderly are more prone to EPS because of age-related CNS changes.
- Thioridazine and the new antipsychotic drug clozapine (Green and Salzman, 1990) have a low incidence of EPS.
- The elderly are particularly susceptible to tardive dyskinesia.
- Agranulocytosis is most common in elderly women and is a particular risk with clozapine.
- Anticholinergic side effects are particularly troublesome for the elderly.
- Long-acting or depot antipsychotics are not usually prescribed for elderly patients because of the long half-lives of these drugs.

### Antianxiety agents: benzodiazepines

- Up to one third of all elderly persons take these drugs.
- The half-lives of several benzodiazepines are lengthened by age-related changes that prolong sedation, cause poor coordination and disorientation, and may lead to misdiagnosis.
- Benzodiazepines with a long half-life include chlordiazepoxide (Librium), chlorazepate (Tranxene), diazepam (Valium), and prazepam (Centrax). *These benzodiazepines are not usually ordered for elderly patients.*
- Benzodiazepines with shorter half-lives that *typically are prescribed* for elderly patients include lorazepam (Ativan), oxazepam (Serax), clonazepam (Klonopin), and alprazolam (Xanax).

### Antimanic agent: lithium

- Because of age-related changes in the kidneys, excretion of lithium is slowed, creating the opportunity for prolonged side effects.
- Sodium depletion from diet or diuretics will increase serum lithium levels.
- A lower blood level of lithium may be appropriate for elderly patients.
- Caution should be exercised if lithium is combined with an antipsychotic drug because of the risk of neuroleptic malignant syndrome.

**TABLE 30-3**  Alcohol and psychotropic drug interactions in the elderly

| Class of psychotropic drug | Additive effect |
| --- | --- |
| Antidepressant drugs | |
| Tricyclic antidepressants (TCAs) | Lowered seizure threshold, hypotension |
| Monoamine oxidase inhibitors (MAOIs) | Hypertensive crisis, especially with Chianti wine, beer, ale, or sherry |
| Antipsychotic drugs | |
| Phenothiazines | Respiratory depression, lowered seizure threshold, impaired hepatic function, hypotension |
| Antianxiety drugs | |
| Benzodiazepines | CNS depression, respiratory depression, sedation |
| Barbiturates | |
| Secobarbital, pentobarbital | Vomiting, severe motor impairment, unconsciousness, coma, and death. (The lethal dose is reduced by 50% when barbiturates are taken with alcohol.) |

sedatives to cause sedation and respiratory problems. A major disadvantage is a slow onset of action: it takes up to 2 weeks before a clinical response is experienced.

**Antimanic agent.**  Lithium is the drug of choice for bipolar illness. Because of the decreased rate of excretion in the elderly there is a higher incidence of toxicity in this age group. Chapter 13 provides a thorough review of this drug.

*MILIEU MANAGEMENT* Approximately 5% of the elderly in America reside in long-term institutions such as nursing homes, state hospitals, and adult homes. Increasingly elderly psychiatric patients are included in that percentage. For example, 20% of state hospital patients are elderly (Moak, 1990). As the number of such impaired persons increases, issues relating to their mental health are of greater concern. The staff of the institutions caring for the elderly mentally ill must develop and implement interventions to maintain the psychological functioning of their residents.

The primary therapeutic responsibility for nurses in these settings is to prevent the deterioration that results from withdrawal and disuse that often accompanies institutional life. It has been found that isolation leads to sensory deprivation, loss of mental functions, and personality disintegration in the elderly. Therefore therapeutic approaches should be based on the premise that human beings have need for continuing contacts, social participation, and meaningful work to maintain function (Kermis, 1986). Communicating a sense of unconditional acceptance as a fellow human being may be the most important intervention nurses can provide for a depressed elderly patient (Ronsman, 1987).

Effective milieu management changes the quality of life in the institutional environment by allowing the patients to bring such items as their own furniture, family pictures, and bedspreads to personalize their rooms. The decor of the day-rooms can be changed to deinstitutionalize the atmosphere. For instance, furniture can be placed into conversational groups to provide a homey atmosphere. The staff members may wear street clothes rather than traditional uniforms to encourage social interchange with residents and to break down barriers. The goal of this approach is to prevent the breakdown of personal initiative and autonomy that often occurs in a total-care institution. It also seeks to encourage independent activity and group participation by residents (Burnside, 1988; Kermis, 1986).

**Reality orientation.** Reality orientation is a specific treatment modality used to counter intellectual and sensory losses in confused elderly patients. Reality orientation is generally conducted in a group setting by staff members using natural conversation to discuss important events or items with patients. A bulletin board can be used to include such things as the name of the facility, day, month, year, next meal, and weather. The staff can use memory games that are not difficult but require recall ability.

Reminiscence therapy, as a part of the reality orientation concept, focuses on the patient's self-concept and self-perception through reminiscences of the person's past life, which are shared by the group. In the session, participants are encouraged to share past events, such as vacations, sports, and family experiences. This therapy can establish a warm, friendly relationship in the group. Reminiscence may be a beginning of a more dignified and fulfilling life for those who participate in this therapy (Burnside, 1988; Ebersole and Hess, 1990; Kermis, 1986).

**Pet therapy.** Pet therapy is generally used to help the resident break through apathy and depression. Pet therapy consists of a brief session in which well-behaved small animals, such as dogs, cats, rabbits, and birds, are brought to the institution for residents to play with and hold. The animals provide unconditional love and affection and are blind to the afflictions of the elderly. In some cases the animals may bring about positive changes in the patient's clinical or mental status (Ebersole and Hess, 1990 Kermis, 1986).

## ELECTROCONVULSIVE THERAPY

Electroconvulsive therapy (ECT) (see Chapter 27) is a treatment of choice for severely depressed patients who fail to respond to other treatment or who are poor candidates for drug therapy. ECT may also be effective in treating suicidal patients. With the use of muscle relaxants and anesthesiological assistance, ECT is safe and effective treatment (Coffey and Weiner, 1990). However, it should not be used on elderly persons with dementia of the Alzheimer's type, as it increases confusion associated with this disease (Cohen and Eisdorfer, 1986).

## KEY CONCEPTS

1. Despite the increase in the population of persons 65 years of age and older, this group experiences major barriers to obtaining quality mental health care: ageism, their own attitudes, and costs of care.
2. Depression is the most common mental disorder among the elderly, but it is often overlooked, misdiagnosed, and inadequately treated.

3. Symptoms of other illnesses may mask depression because the elderly may be preoccupied with physical rather than emotional symptoms.
4. Age-related life events, losses, changes, and physical decline are associated with the onset of depression.
5. A skillful comprehensive psychosocial assessment is needed to identify the elderly patient's functioning in a particular social environment.
6. A thorough physical examination is essential for differential diagnosis.
7. The nurse-patient relationship focuses on providing care for the patient and helping his family manage the activities and demands of daily living.
8. Adequate nutrition, socialization, and achievement of small realistic goals in daily living activities help in reducing anxiety and maintaining or restoring psychological functioning.
9. Use of medications with the elderly involves risks associated with polypharmacy, noncompliance, and altered pharmacokinetics.
10. Effective strategies of milieu management can improve the quality of life and prevent deterioration of the elderly in institutional settings.

## REFERENCES

Burnside IM: Reminiscence and other therapeutic modalities. In Burnside IM, editor: Nursing and the aged: a self-care approach (ed 3), New York, 1988, McGraw-Hill Book Co, pp 645-686.

Chaisson-Stewart GM: The diagnostic dilemma. In Chaisson-Stewart GM, editor: Depression in the elderly—an interdisciplinary approach, New York, 1985, Wiley Medical, pp 18-43.

Coffey CE and Weiner RD: Electroconvulsive therapy: an update, Hosp Community Psychiatry 41:515-521, 1990.

Cohen D and Eisdorfer C: Depression. In Calkins E, Davis PJ, and Ford AB, editors: The practice of geriatrics, Philadelphia, 1986, WB Saunders Co., pp 185-193.

Dreyfus JK: Depression assessment and interventions in the medically ill frail elderly, J Gerontol Nurs 14(9):27, 1988.

Ebersole P and Hess P: Mental health and cognition. Toward healthy aging—human needs and nursing responses, ed 3, St. Louis, 1990, Mosby—Year Book, pp 655-708.

Field WE: Physical causes of depression, J Psychosoc Nurs 23:7, 1985.

Green I and Salzman C: Clozapine: benefits and risks, Hosp Community Psychiatry 41:379-380, 1990.

Hawranik P and Kondratuk B: Depression in the elderly, Can Nurse, 82:25, October 1986.

Kaszniak AW, Sadeh M, and Stern LZ: (1985). Differentiating depression from organic brain syndromes in older people. In Chaisson-Stewart GM, editor: Depression in the elderly—an interdisciplinary approach, New York, 1985, Wiley Medical, pp 161-189.

Kermis MD: Mental health in late life: the adaptive process, Boston, 1986, Jones & Bartlett.

Martilla J and Anderson PL: Geriatrics. In Wiener MB et al, editors: Clinical pharmacology and therapeutics in nursing, New York, 1979, McGraw-Hill Book Co, pp 853-860.

McConnell ES and Matteson MA: Psychosocial problems associated with aging. In Matteson MA and McConnell ES, editors: Gerontological nursing: concepts and practice, Philadelphia, 1988, WB Saunders Co, pp 520-527.

Moak GS: Discharge and retention of psychogeriatric long-stay patients in a state mental hospital, Hosp Community Psychiatry 41:445-447, 1990.

Nickens HW, Crook T, and Cohen GD: Psychotropic drugs, Generations, pp 33-37, Spring 1986.

Osgood NJ: Suicide in the elderly: clues and prevention. Letter 153. Belle Mead, NJ, 1988, Carrier Foundation.

Patrick M: Daily living with cognitive deficits and behavioral problems. In Carnevali DL and Patrick M, editors: Nursing management for the elderly (ed 2), Philadelphia, 1986, JB Lippincott Co, pp 270-286.

Ronsman K: Therapy for depression, J Gerontol Nurs 13(12):18, 1987.

Sloan RW: Practical geriatric therapeutics, Oradell, NJ, 1986, Medical Economics Co, Inc.

St. Pierre J, Craven RF, and Bruno P: Late life depression: a guide for assessment. J Gerontol Nurs 12(7):5, 1986.

Tillman-Jones TK: How to work with elderly patients on a general psychiatric unit, J Psychosoc Nurs 28:27 31, 1990.

Tyler RT and Tyler FM: FIM in treating organic dementia. Geriatrics 39:38, 1984.

Wills R: Psychiatric problems of the elderly. In Carnevali DL and Patrick M, editors: Nursing management for the elderly (ed 2), Philadelphia, 1986, JB Lippincott Co, pp 257-269.

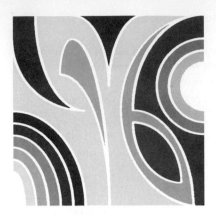

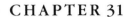

## CHAPTER 31

# Working with Patients with HIV Disease

PEGGY TRACY LEAPLEY AND MARY JO KASSELMAN

LEARNING OBJECTIVES
After reading this chapter you should be able to

- Outline the natural history of the human immunodeficiency virus (HIV).
- Explain the role of the T4 lymphocyte in the progression of HIV infection.
- Understand the consequences of opportunistic infections for the person with AIDS.
- Describe the groups most at risk for HIV transmission in the United States.
- Describe the risk for occupational transmission of HIV.
- List the factors associated with a therapeutic milieu for the patient with HIV dementia.
- Appreciate the ethical responsibility of the nurse in safeguarding the privacy and confidentiality of the person with AIDS.
- Apply the nursing process to care of a patient with AIDS dementia.

**H**uman immunodeficiency virus (HIV) disease is a communicable and progressively fatal condition. The virus attacks the immune system and thus lowers the person's resistance to other diseases. Because transmission in the United States has primarily involved homosexual men and intravenous drug users, stigma and discrimination have aggravated the psychosocial aspects of this disease. In addition, the central nervous system (CNS) can be affected by the virus and thus require highly skilled psychiatric care.

*Human immunodeficiency virus (HIV) disease* is the latest term to describe the entire range of conditions caused by this virus. HIV disease includes infection with the HIV antibody, ARC (AIDS-related complex), and AIDS (acquired immunodeficiency syndrome). A brief review of the immune system, opportunistic diseases, and transmission will provide the foundation for understanding the progression of the disease and the United States Centers for Disease Control (CDC) classification for acquired immunodeficiency syndrome. The overview will provide the background necessary to discuss the psychoemotional aspects of HIV disease, and the related neuropathology includes a case study of AIDS dementia.

## OVERVIEW OF HIV DISEASE
### Causes of HIV disease

In June 1981 the United States Centers for Disease Control published case studies of five men, 29 to 36 years of age, with a diagnosis of *Pneumocystis carinii* pneumonia (PCP) in Los Angeles. PCP is not usually seen in persons with adequate immune response systems. This alerted physicians to unusual opportunistic disease in young males. Additional cases of PCP were reported to the CDC, and Kaposi's sarcoma, a rare form of cancer, was also increasingly diagnosed in young males. The human immunodeficiency virus was initially isolated in 1983 from patients with acquired immune deficiency syndrome (AIDS).

The origin of the virus remains unknown, but the oldest specimen with the HIV antibody was collected in 1959 in Zaire (Clumeck and deWit, 1988). HIV disease in Central Africa was called "wasting disease" because of the extreme weight loss associated with it. The African subcontinent has been implicated as the place of origin for the AIDS virus. A retrovirus similar to HIV has been identified in the African green monkey. One theory suggests that HIV is a mutation of the green monkey retrovirus.

The early history of HIV disease recognized that the disease affected a person's immune system and that it is acquired rather than genetically transmitted. Because it affects the immune system, the disease leaves the person vulnerable to infectious agents the immune system ordinarily can suppress. Diseases that are the result of a compromised immune system are classified as opportunistic infections. Initially, the cause of AIDS was unknown, and thus the diagnosis was based on the presence of certain symptoms within the patient. The symptoms, when seen in combination, were called a syndrome.

HIV disease is caused by exposure to the human immunodeficiency virus, which interacts with other factors in the person. Some of the other factors affecting HIV exposure are dose, entry site, current immune system status, and number of exposures. The human immunodeficiency virus is classified as the lentivirus subfamily of the human retrovirus. It consists of a double-layered envelope full of proteins that surrounds a small amount of ribonucleic acid (RNA). It enters the body from the T4 lymphocyte of an infected person. The infection starts when gp 120, a glycoprotein of the viral envelope, interacts with CD4, a surface antigen present on T lymphocytes, macrophages, glial cells, and neurons. Once the virus enters the cell, it uses reverse transcriptase to maintain its genome in the DNA of the affected cell. The virus may remain dormant for days, weeks, or years, or it may begin replication and thus infect other cells. It is thought that factors related to the immune system affect the dormant or active status. These factors include age, overall health, health-promoting activities such as nutrition and exercise, or health-reducing behaviors such as alcohol. Levy (1990) reports that more virulent HIV strains appear to evolve in the host over time, and some strains show a predilection for certain tissues.

## Opportunistic infections

When the immune system is compromised, certain organisms seize the opportunity to infect the person. Opportunistic infections are those the person would normally resist when the immune system is functional and healthy. Many of the opportunistic diseases are commonly found in the environment and were rarely seen before the HIV disease epidemic. Box 31-1 provides a list of opportunistic diseases and their causative agents.

The most serious opportunistic disease is *Pneumocystis carinii* pneumonia (PCP), which is caused by a protozon. Even with recent prophylactic treatment for PCP, it remains the leading cause of death among persons with AIDS. The second leading cause of AIDS death has been Kaposi's sarcoma (KS). This cancer occurs on the surface of the skin, mouth, or visceral organs, such as the lungs or digestive tract. It causes blue-violet or red-brown nodules or plaques that are distinctive. Another malignancy associated with HIV-infected individuals is a variety of non-Hodgkins lymphoma. Additional common opportunistic infections are *Toxoplasma gondii,* histoplasmosis, coccidioidomycosis, tuberculosis, herpes, *Candida albicans,* and cytomegalovirus.

## HIV disease transmission

HIV disease is transmitted from person to person through sexual contact, intravenously, or in utero from mother to baby. The presence of HIV has been reported in blood, semen, blood plasma, bone marrow, cervical secretions, saliva, breast milk, lymph nodes, brain tissue, tears, and cerebrospinal and amniotic fluid. Although the virus can be isolated in many body fluids, a number of body fluids have not been implicated in any cases of HIV transmission. There have been no documented cases of HIV transmission by insect vectors, handshaking, tears, or saliva. Research overwhelmingly indicates the following as three main means of transmission:

1. Intimate sexual contact with an HIV-infected person
2. Parenteral injection of blood or blood products infected with HIV
3. Transfer of the HIV from mother to baby.

**Box 31-1**
## OPPORTUNISTIC INFECTIONS

### Cancers

1. Kaposi's sarcoma (KS)
2. Primary lymphoma of brain
3. Burkitt's lymphoma
4. Non-Hodgkin's lymphoma
5. Hodgkin's disease

### Protozoan and Helminth (parasitical) infections

1. Cryptosporidiosis, intestinal: causing diarrhea for more than 1 month
2. *Pneumocystis carinii* pneumonia (PCP)
3. Strongyloidosis: pneumonia, central nervous system infection, or disseminated infection
4. *Toxoplasma gondii:* pneumonia or central nervous system infection
5. *Isospora belli:* diarrhea for more than 1 month

### Fungal Infections

1. Aspergillosis: central nervous system or disseminated infection
2. *Candida albicans:* esophagitis
3. Cryptococcosis: pulmonary, central nervous system or disseminated
4. *Hisotoplasma capsulatum*

### Mycobacterial infections

1. Atypical mycobacteriosis *(Mycobacterium avium)*
2. *Mycobacterium tuberculosis* (M.TB)

### Viral infections

1. Cytomegalovirus (CMV)
2. Herpes simplex virus—persisting more than 1 month—or pulmonary, gastrointestinal, or disseminated Epstein-Barr virus (another herpes virus) increased
3. Progressive multifocal leukoencephalopathy
4. Varicella zoster virus (VZV)

### Populations at risk

Various groups have been identified as at risk for HIV infection. One must remember that it is not the group identification that results in HIV infection but rather a behavior common to the at-risk group. Thus determining at-risk status involves not only identification of the risk group but also assessment for specific risk behaviors. This is particularly important since many of the prominent risk groups have changed their behavior or instituted preventive measures.

In the United States the groups most at risk are homosexual and bisexual men, intravenous drug users, infants with HIV-infected mothers, persons with hemophilia, and persons who received blood transfusions before March 1985. Health care providers are not in the high-risk category but do need to be aware of special precautions to avoid exposure.

Initially, in the United States, most transmission of HIV occurred between homosexual men. The risk of infection in this population increased with the number of male sex partners and the frequency with which they were the receptive partner in anal intercourse. More recently, the rate of new infection in homosexual men has declined as a result of such behavioral changes as mutual monogamy of sexual partners and the increased use of safer sex practices.

Intravenous drug users (IVDUs) represent the fastest-growing percentage of AIDS cases. At present, the highest rate of new HIV infection in the United States occurs in non-white IV drug users. The virus is transmitted through the blood present on needles when IV drug users share paraphernalia. In some cities, such as New York City, IV drug users make up the largest percentage of AIDS cases.

Perinatal transmission of HIV to infants born of HIV-infected mothers is well documented. Evidence suggests that transmission can occur in utero, at delivery, or during the immediate postpartum period. The risk that an HIV-infected woman will infect her baby is estimated to be 40% to 60%.

The risk of acquiring HIV through blood transfusion or blood products such as those used by hemophiliacs has been greatly reduced by the testing of donated blood. Currently all blood donations are screened for the HIV antibody. Since March 1985, when all blood banks in the United States initiated HIV antibody screening, the risk of blood product tranmission has been virtually eliminated. Since conversion from antibody-negative to antibody-positive status takes approximately 6 to 8 weeks, there remains a slight risk of transmission by blood transfusion. However, there is no risk in *donating* blood since individual sterile equipment is used for each donor.

Heterosexual transmission for those not in another high-risk group does occur and most apparently occurs during vaginal intercourse. However, study populations have been too small to determine whether the male-to-female or the female-to-male route is the more prevalent. Many couples included in the studies of heterosexual transmission of HIV had unprotected sex over a long period, but in none of the reported cases were more than 50% of the partners infected. This suggests that biologic as well as behavioral factors contribute to HIV transmission in heterosexual populations (Quinn, 1990).

There is a small but definite occupational risk of HIV infections for health care workers. A study reported by the Centers for Disease Control (CDC) demonstrated that 4 persons, or 0.47%, among 860 health care workers with *known exposure to the blood of HIV-infected persons* and not members of any other high-risk group developed the HIV antibody in association with a needle-stick injury (CDC, 1989b). The potential for occupational transmission of HIV can be reduced by implementing and enforcing infection control procedures.

It is equally important to understand that there is no known risk of HIV transmission through casual contact. Despite prolonged contact with an infected person among 400 family members, none have been infected except those members in a high-risk group. Thus the risk of transmission in schools and the workplace is thought to be even more remote than in the home.

## AIDS diagnosis

In 1983, AIDS first became a CDC reportable disease. Before 1987, the diagnosis of AIDS was based on the presence of one or more opportunistic diseases in a person with no other reasonable explanation for having a compromised immune system. After HIV was discovered to be the cause of AIDS and HIV antibody tests became available and specific manifestations of the disease were better defined, it became necessary to revise the CDC definition of AIDS (CDC, 1987a). The major changes apply to persons with laboratory evidence of HIV infection, inclusion of HIV encephalopathy (dementia), HIV wasting syndrome, and a broader range of AIDS-indicative diseases (CDC, 1987a).

Box 31-2 summarizes the most frequent symptoms of HIV infection. Many of the symptoms are generalized and associated with other diseases. This makes the initial diagnosis more difficult. In addition, persons often delay seeking professional advice because the symptoms are initially mild.

## HIV tests

The normal range of T4 cells is 600 to 1200/mm$^3$. With HIV infection the T4 cell range drops to 0 to 500/mm$^3$. The number of T4 cells correlates with symptoms and clinical course. The normal T4 to T8 ratio is 2:1. This ratio is often inverse with HIV disease. The following functional abnormalities of T cells are present in HIV disease (Bullock and Rosendahl, 1988; Porth, 1990):

- Diminished lymphokine production
- Decreased cytotoxic lymphocyte function
- Decreased ability to provide help to B lymphocytes for immunoglobulin (Ig) production
- Decreased proliferative responses
- Decreased responsiveness to specific antigens

The most helpful and relatively specific laboratory evidence of HIV infection is abnormality of T-lymphocyte subsets. Many viral illnesses cause an increase in the absolute number and percentage of suppressor (T8) lymphocytes, but marked depression of helper-inducer (T4) lymphocytes is highly suggestive of HIV effect. Thus a finding of depressed T4 lymphocytes in the appropriate clinical setting strongly supports a diagnosis of HIV infection. The absolute number of cells in this subset rather than the ratio of T4 to T8 cells is most useful.

The test for HIV most commonly used in the United States is the antibody test. ELISA (enzyme-linked immunosorbent assay) detects the HIV antibody that develops in the infected person within 6 to 8 weeks after exposure to HIV. The ELISA is a screening test. If the test is positive, most laboratories use the Western blot or IFA

**Box 31-2**
## HIV-ORIENTED REVIEW OF SYSTEMS

**General:**

Weight loss, anorexia, fever sweats

**Skin:**

New rashes or pigmented lesions, generalized drying, pruritus

**Lymphatics:**

Localized or generalized lymph node enlargement, change in size (increase or decrease) in any previously enlarged lymph nodes

**Head, eyes, ears, nose, and throat:**

Headaches, nasal discharge, sinus congestion, changes in visual acuity, sore throat, whitish or painful lesions of the oral mucosa

**Cardiopulmonary:**

Cough or shortness of breath

**Gastrointestinal:**

Abdominal pain, change in bowel habits, diarrhea

**Musculoskeletal:**

Myalgias, arthralgias

**Neurologic:**

Symptoms of depression, change of personality, cognitive difficulties, bowel or bladder dysfunction, peripheral weakness or paresthesias

From Hollander H: Work-up of the HIV-infected patient. In Sande M and Volberding P, editors: The medical management of AIDS, Philadelphia, 1988, WB Saunders Co.

(immunofluorescent antibody) test to confirm the results. These tests are relatively inexpensive.

New tests are able to detect evidence of the virus (antigen) rather than the antibody. These new tests include the polymerase chain reaction (PCR), p24 antigen, and reverse transcriptase assay. However, these tests are more expensive and thus are not used for screening purposes.

Since babies have immature immune response systems and therefore often delayed development of antibodies, the new tests that detect the virus are valuable for diagnosing babies of HIV-infected mothers. These newer tests will be necessary if early prophylactic treatment against the virus is found to be effective.

With HIV testing, the nurse is responsible for the confidentiality or anonymity of the test and the person's psychological safety. (The psychological safety of HIV testing is discussed under Psychoemotional Implications.)

The ANA Code of Ethics (1985) states that the "nurse safeguards the client's right to privacy by judiciously protecting information of a confidential nature." All tests and diagnoses are confidential and should not be revealed to those not involved in the patient's care without the patient's permission. Most states have enacted laws to promote health provider compliance with maintenance of testing and diagnostic confidentiality. Thus confidentiality becomes an ethical and legal matter for nurses caring for persons with AIDS. In this respect, HIV disease and confidentiality are an ethical responsibility and are the same as for all persons requiring nursing care.

## Progression of HIV disease

The phases of HIV infection can progress rapidly or over years:

- *Acute HIV infection:* Days to weeks
- *Asymptomatic HIV infection but HIV positive:* Years
- *Chronic symptomatic HIV disease:* Months to years
- *Advanced HIV disease—AIDS:* Months to years

The incubation period from initial infection to diagnosis as AIDS can average 8 to 10 years. The initial infection following exposure to HIV results in an acute phase called *acute retroviral syndrome.* From 2 days to several weeks after exposure to HIV, the person may experience symptoms including fever, malaise, sore throat, arthralgia, lymphadenopathy, headache, photophobia, gastrointestinal disturbance, neurologic symptoms, weight loss, and an elevated serum transaminase level (Fang et al., 1989). Often the person does not realize the significance of the symptoms until a later date. The acute phase can last days to weeks.

This is followed by an asymptomatic phase. The person is HIV antibody positive and thus can transmit the disease to others through sexual contact, blood transfusions, or from mother to child during the perinatal period. The asymptomatic phase can last for years.

The chronic symptomatic phase of HIV disease was previously called AIDS related complex (ARC). Although the public still uses the ARC diagnosis, the expanded definition of AIDS has resulted in physicians' limiting this phase to persistent generalized lymphadenopathy symptoms. This phase can last months to years.

The advanced HIV disease phase is present with the AIDS diagnosis. During this phase it is common for the person to develop one or more opportunistic diseases. The progressive symptoms most commonly experienced with HIV disease are listed in Box 31-3.

A number of laboratory tests are used to monitor the immune system for progression of the disease. Commonly ordered tests include a complete blood count (CBC) with differential, platelet count, erythrocyte sedimentation rate (ESR), biochemistry profile, and T-cell counts.

### Box 31-3
### FACTORS ASSOCIATED WITH PROGRESSION OF HIV DISEASE

**Symptoms**

Fevers
Weight loss >10% of ideal body weight
Persistent diarrhea
Cognitive changes
History of dermatomal zoster, candidiasis, hairy leukoplakia

**Signs**

Generalized wasting
Oral findings: candidiasis, hairy leukoplakia
Encephalopathy

**Laboratory abnormalities**

Anemia
Elevated erythrocyte sedimentation rate
Decreased T4 lymphocytes

From Hollander H: Work-up of the HIV-infected patient. In Sande M and Volberding P, editors:
The medical management of AIDS, Philadelphia, 1988, WB Saunders Co.

### Box 31-4
### CLASSIFICATION SYSTEM FOR HIV INFECTION

Group I:    Acute infection
Group II:   Asymptomatic infection
Group III:  Persistent generalized lymphadenopathy
Group IV:   Other diseases
            Subgroup A:   Constitutional disease
            Subgroup B:   Neurological disease
            Subgroup C:   Secondary infection disease
            Subgroup D:   Secondary cancers
            Subgroup E:   Other conditions

From Centers for Disease Control: Classification system for HTLV-III/LAV, MMWR 35:335-340,
May 23, 1986.

The International Classification System for HIV infection as shown in Box 31-4 closely follows the earlier description of the phases of HIV infection. These classifications are useful in both prevention strategies and treatment considerations.

## Incidence and distribution

HIV disease was the primary public health problem of the 1980s. It is projected to continue as a worldwide problem throughout the 1990s. In the United States, as of May 1990, almost 120,000 cases of AIDS have been reported to the federal Centers for Disease Control. The CDC reports 72,000 deaths due to AIDS since 1981. The CDC estimates that more than 1.5 million persons in the United States are infected with HIV. The progression of the disease indicates a major impact on the health care system if the number of persons with HIV infection is not reduced through education, change of risk behaviors, and development of new treatments. The geographical distribution of the disease within the United States is shown in Fig. 31-1.

## Risk-behavior prevention

Nurses need to know the strategies for preventing risk behavior for transmission involving sexual, intravenous drugs, and the health care worker.

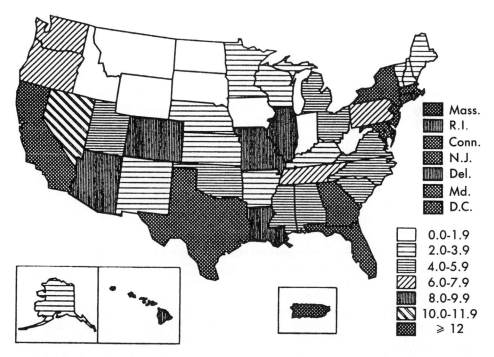

**FIGURE 31-1** AIDS incidence rates per 100,000 population, United States, 1988. *(From Centers for Disease Control: AIDS and HIV infection in the U.S., MMWR 38:S-4:32.)*

**Sexual transmission prevention.** Since early in the AIDS epidemic, "safe sex" has been suggested as an effective prevention strategy. As more information became available on transmission of the virus, the sexual practices that are safe and unsafe have been more clearly described. While the only truly "safe sex" is abstinence, this is not a behavior pattern that will be maintained by many persons over a lifetime. The next option is monogamous relationships between noninfected couples. Persons who do not select these options should take additional precautions, such as use of a latex condom, a spermicide with nonoxynol-9, and water-based lubricant. Studies indicate that use of drugs and alcohol can influence one's judgment of safe sexual behavior.

Identifying an individual, group, or community risk of HIV infection is the first step in risk-reduction education and counseling. Once risk behaviors are identified, the nurse can develop strategies for risk-reduction education and counseling. HIV infection education frequently involves information about the realities and myths of this disease. It is not unusual to encounter personal fear and discrimination or prejudice against persons with AIDS. Following are some risk-reduction strategies:

- Target high-risk groups where high-risk behavior is present.
- Remember that HIV-infected persons may demonstrate no physical or psychological symptoms during a long incubation period.
- Any person participating in high-risk behavior is at risk during each behavior. The risk with each reexposure is not known but is assumed to increase the person's chance of infection.
- Changing to low-risk behaviors requires lifelong change and is enhanced when supported by sexual or drug-using partners.
- Use of condoms is important in realistically reducing certain risk behaviors.

**IVDU transmission prevention.** The most common means of IVDU transmission is through the sharing of drug paraphernalia (intravenous equipment) contaminated with HIV. Second, HIV-infected drug users can infect their sexual partners. Third, HIV-infected women who are either IVDUs or sexual partners of IVDUs can infect their newborn infants. In addition, drugs and alcohol have been implicated as cofactors in HIV transmission through lowered immune system response and reduction in inhibitions so that risky sexual behavior occurs.

IVDUs' risk-reduction strategies include, first, efforts to eliminate and treat the substance-abuse problem and, second, efforts to prevent the spread of HIV or other viruses such as hepatitis B. IVDUs should be encouraged to seek treatment for their problem. For IVDUs who refuse drug treatment programs, emphasis should be placed on education either to not share needles and syringes or to clean their works as described in Fig. 31-2 to reduce their risk. Following are some guidelines for reducing the risk of HIV transmission:

- Never share IV drugs or equipment (works).
- If a needle or syringe must be shared, remember to clean the works (Fig. 31-2).

## BLEACH

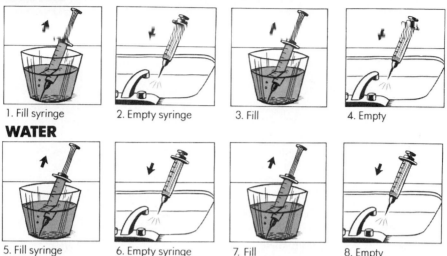

1. Fill syringe      2. Empty syringe      3. Fill      4. Empty

## WATER

5. Fill syringe      6. Empty syringe      7. Fill      8. Empty

**FIGURE 31-2** Cleaning the works. *1,* Flush with bleach. Pour bleach into glass. Fill syringe with bleach. Empty bleach from syringe. Repeat. *2,* Flush with water. Fill glass with clean water. Fill syringe with water. Empty water from syringe. Repeat. (CAUTION: Be sure the client knows not to omit this important step.) *(Courtesy the San Francisco AIDS Foundation.)*

- Do not practice risky sexual behavior.
- If you are a woman who has engaged in risk behaviors, get medical advice before any pregnancy.

**Universal precautions for health care workers.** Fear is a common reaction of health care workers to the initial experience of caring for a person with HIV disease. Without sufficient knowledge and emotional support the nurse's initial reaction is often avoidance and neglect (Zook and Davidhizar, 1989; Rothberg et al., 1990). The first step in resolving the fears of health care workers is to provide information about HIV disease.

Preexisting policies and plans for care of persons with HIV disease assist the nurse in handling her anxiety and fears and also in thinking about her role and responsibilities. Guidelines for care of persons with HIV disease need to be available for all health care workers and auxiliary personnel. Even nurses with persistent fears and prejudice are ethically expected to provide competent care. The ANA Code of Ethics (1985) requires that nursing service be provided "unrestricted by considerations of social or economic status, personal attributes, or the nature of health problems."

The HIV epidemic has probably aggravated the nursing shortage. Chow (1989) reports that "nurses are on the frontline in the war against this epidemic." Nurses

### Box 31-5
## UNIVERSAL INFECTION PRECAUTIONS

Any patient can be infected with HIV (the AIDS virus), even with no symptoms. It takes 6 weeks to 6 months after exposure for a person to develop HIV antibodies. Therefore, nurses must use precautions with blood and body fluids from all patients to protect themselves against other infectious organisms.

1. Wash hands before and after all patient or specimen contact.
2. Handle the blood of all patients as potentially infectious.
3. Wear gloves for potential contact with blood and body fluids.
4. Place used syringe immediately in nearby impermeable container; do *not* recap or manipulate needle in any way.
5. Wear protective eyewear and mask if splatter with blood or body fluids is possible (e.g., bronchoscopy, oral surgery).
6. Wear gown when splash with blood or body fluid is anticipated (e.g., L and D).
7. Handle all linen soiled with blood or body secretions as potentially infectious.
8. Process all laboratory specimens as potentially infectious.
9. Wear mask for TB and other respiratory organisms (HIV is not airborne).
10. Place resuscitation equipment where respiratory arrest is predictable.

From California Nurses Association: AIDS education and training, San Francisco, 1988, The Association.

desiring current knowledge and support may be interested in a recently formed specialty organization, the Association of Nurses in AIDS Care.

Universal precautions mean that all patients are assumed to be potentially infected with HIV or hepatitis B virus (HBV). Both viruses involve blood-borne transmission and common measures for prevention. For the health care worker, hepatitis B virus has been demonstrated to be the much greater risk. The risk of infection with HIV following one needle-stick exposure to blood from an HIV-infected person is approximately 0.5%.

In 1985 the CDC developed the strategy of Universal Blood and Body Fluid Precautions. In 1989 the CDC published Guidelines for Prevention of Transmission of HIV and HBV to health care and public-safety workers. Box 31-5 summarizes the guidelines pertaining to health care workers. Specialty settings, such as psychiatric or mental health facilities, need to develop strategies that ensure that health provider precautions are taken during treatment of the special problems of persons with psychiatric or mental illness (Cournos et al., 1990).

## Treatment and research

A large number of medications are currently in the clinical trial stage for treatment of HIV or one of the associated opportunistic diseases. Zidovudine (often called AZT) has been used extensively to treat persons with AIDS. This drug appears to interfere with the proliferation of the virus and thus extends the life span of the person with AIDS. In addition, zidovudine is being used to reduce the risk of developing AIDS in HIV-infected persons who have no symptoms or mild symptoms (CDC, 1989a). These benefits may be extended by new treatments currently being evaluated (CDC, 1989a).

Other antiviral drugs are now available. Dideoxyinosine (ddI) is a reverse transcriptase inhibitor and is less toxic than zidovudine. It is presently available to persons with AIDS on a compassionate-use basis that does not require the person to meet stringent clinical trial participant requirements. Another option is a combination therapy of zidovudine and dideoxycytidine (ddC), an antiviral drug. Over 90 drugs are now being investigated for the treatment of related opportunistic diseases.

Since the onset of AIDS-related opportunistic diseases, increased effort has been made to treat or prevent these previously uncommon diseases. For example, prophylaxis for *Pneumocystis carinii* pneumonia has involved the use of oral sulfamethoxazole (Bactrim) or inhalation therapy with aerosolized pentamidine.

There is still no known cure for AIDS. Research efforts focus on medication that will prolong the life span, reduce symptoms, treat or prevent AIDS-related diseases, and boost the immune system. Information on AIDS clinical trials can be obtained through the National Institute of Allergy and Infection Diseases (NIAID, telephone 1-800-TRIALS-A).

Extensive research effort has been invested in development of a vaccine. Previous vaccines, such as the polio vaccine, averaged 15 years from initial prototype to human testing. Since the AIDS virus was first isolated in 1983, researchers have worked diligently to understand the biogenetic nature of HIV. Even so, the availability of an HIV vaccine is probably years away.

Initially, nurse researchers were slow to study HIV disease. This has changed in recent years, and the Center for Nursing Research of the National Institute of Health (NIH) has identified HIV disease research as a high priority.

## PSYCHOEMOTIONAL IMPLICATIONS
### HIV testing

Careful and thoughtful pretest and posttest counseling is critical in all HIV testing procedures. The context of the HIV testing situation is an important consideration. Is the testing voluntary or mandatory? Is the testing confidential or anonymous? Does the person being tested demonstrate symptoms? Is he aware of risk behaviors? Does he have family or friends who have AIDS or who are HIV antibody positive? Is he psychologically prepared and able to cope with a positive test result? Persons who request an HIV test but who are free of symptoms can be considered to be "worried well." These worried-well persons may exhibit symptoms of anxiety and depression.

A recent study of HIV-positive diagnoses at an army medical center reports suicidal ideation in more than 90% of the newly diagnosed HIV-positive soldiers (Rothberg et al., 1990). Other symptoms experienced in newly diagnosed HIV-positive persons are anxiety, depression, fear, anger, sleeplessness, obsessions, helplessness, hopelessness, and guilt. Psychiatric referral and management are indicated for these psychoemotional symptoms.

A positive HIV antibody test, or even one of the new HIV tests, is often the first step in diagnosis. Further medical history and examination are often necessary to determine the person's classification status for HIV disease. Some may be totally free of symptoms and unaware of any risk behavior, whereas others may have already experienced advanced symptoms and be very aware of risk behaviors. Thus some persons with a positive test result may be in emotional shock while others are taking the first step toward acceptance of the disease after a long period of denial.

The pretest and posttest counselor needs to be skilled in assessing the emotional status of the patient and in taking appropriate action through immediate treatment and referral when indicated. Suicidal risk should be assessed routinely. Because of the psychological interventions, posttest counseling should be done only by persons with advanced educational preparation in HIV counseling.

Because a person may be infected with HIV for years before symptoms develop, many symptom-free HIV-positive patients are sensitive to any symptoms indicative of the progression of the disease. This continual fear can be emotionally debilitating. In addition, the symptom-free person with HIV infection will need intensive education to eliminate his risk of transmitting the virus. The required changes in behavior may aggravate his psychological status. In rare cases, the person may persist in risky behavior as a defense mechanism of denying the HIV infection or the seriousness of the situation.

### Diagnosis

Diagnosis of AIDS can be initiated as a result of a positive HIV antibody test or one of the newer HIV disease tests or on the basis of symptoms of HIV disease as listed in the CDC definition. Diagnosis will result in classification of the person according to the progression of the disease. A diagnosis of AIDS often results in an initial reaction of denial, disbelief, numbness, inability to concentrate or make decisions, and anger.

The stages of grief and loss are common following a diagnosis of AIDS. The stigma and discrimination of society toward persons with AIDS aggravate the fear and loss experienced. The person with AIDS (PWA) may be concerned about the reactions of family, friends, and coworkers. Many PWAs report problems with health care coverage by their insurance companies which adds to their financial concern and psychoemotional symptoms.

Referral for psychiatric treatment should be made for PWAs who exhibit symptoms of depression, suicidal ideation, denial that is maladaptive by increasing the person's or another's risk, extreme anxiety, or delirium (Zook and Davidhizar, 1989). Extreme depression is treated with the standard protocol of antidepressants and psychotherapy. Safety precautions must be instituted for those with suicidal ideation.

Delirium has been reported in more than 50% of medically hospitalized PWAs. These psychoemotional symptoms can interfere with the treatment plan and nursing care for a PWA and thus require psychiatric nursing skills.

## Living with HIV disease

Society continues to discriminate against PWAs, on the basis of whether the affected person is viewed as a victim (a child or a victim of transfusion transmission) or has practiced unacceptable behavior (homosexual or IVDU transmission). Because of societal attitudes of anger and hostility, the PWA often experiences discrimination and injustice. These experiences can produce strong psychological reactions. A healthy reaction to discrimination and injustice is the political activism of the person with AIDS. Empowerment, decision making, and a support network can help the PWA maintain a reality, goal-directed orientation toward living with HIV disease.

It has become easier for PWAs to remain in their community for care and services. Hospitalizations have become fewer and shorter as treatments for the disease tend to be available through clinics and private health care providers. Nurses frequently provide case-management services to the PWA. The nurse case manager helps coordinate service necessary for the home treatment of the PWA.

Although the medical profession projects that AIDS will become more of a chronic disease, it is still a progressively fatal disease. Therefore decisions are necessary on resuscitation desires, wills, and powers of attorney. These are difficult decisions, but it is best that they be discussed with family, friends, and health care providers throughout the illness.

**Family and friends of persons with HIV disease.** As more family and friends have been affected by the HIV epidemic, empathy and support have increased. For many family and friends of a person with AIDS or HIV disease, there remains uncertainty as to whether others will understand and sympathize. Although societal acceptability of this disease is changing, there is still considerable fear. This fear triggers concern of rejection by others.

Often the family's and friends' initial reactions to the diagnosis of HIV disease in a loved one involves not only feelings about the diagnosis but also feelings about the risk behavior that resulted in HIV infection, particularly homosexuality or IV drug use. This can reduce the support given to the PWA during the period when he is particularly in need of emotional support.

Family and friends of a PWA or an HIV-infected person will need information on the disease process, transmission, and prevention. Lack of education can trigger unreasonable fears that may result in rejection of the HIV-infected person. For the same reason a community or group may reject the PWA or his family and friends.

The PWA needs to discuss concerns about death and dying. Decisions often need to be conveyed to family and friends regarding resuscitation efforts, wills, and powers of attorney. Family and friends often need assistance with skills required for care of the terminally ill. A referral to a hospice nurse, community health nurse, or home health nurse may assist the PWA and his family. Special emotional support is needed to care for a PWA. Caregivers may require respite care services. Support groups may help the caregivers to understand the nature of the disease, the feelings of the PWA, and their own psychological reaction.

## HIV infection among psychiatric patients

Mentally ill patients may be at increased risk for acquiring HIV (Sacks et al., 1990). Poor judgment, hypersexuality, and impulsivity are associated with many psychiatric disorders—behaviors that increase the risk for HIV-infection. Sacks et al. (1990) found that 20% of psychiatric patients were engaging in high-risk behavior. They found that bipolar illness correlated significantly with high-risk behavior and suggested that these patients in particular receive HIV counseling.

## NEUROPATHOLOGY
## AIDS dementia

HIV infection, particularly in its late phase, is complicated by a variety of central nervous system (CNS) and peripheral nervous system (PNS) disorders. These disorders lead to considerable morbidity. They relate not only to opportunistic infec-

## Case Study

Ron Jackson, a 28-year-old married Afro-American man, was admitted to a public hospital after an episode of confusion, hallucination, and memory problems. His admitting diagnosis included AIDS dementia. He was admitted to a medical-surgical unit and placed in a private room. His T4 count was low and his physical condition was aggravated by anorexia and rapid weight loss. His psychological symptoms varied according to his degree of confusion. Confusion was noted to be more severe during the late evenings. The confusion was complicated by poor memory and disorientation to place and time.

Mr. Jackson had a history of IV drug use since the age of 18. He was found to be HIV antibody positive when he was incarcerated for selling drugs. Previous hospitalization included two episodes of PCP. He was

released from jail 1 month before the current hospitalization. His probation officer reports Mr. Jackson was unable to find employment and thus remained on Medicaid and Social Security. Mr. Jackson lives with his 45-year-old mother and his two sisters, age 22 and 17. His family is very concerned and supportive. Currently, Mr. Jackson is not using illegal drugs and has no sexual partners.

Universal precautions were hospital policy, but additional measures were needed when diagnostic tests were done because Mr. Jackson became agitated and resistant to the procedures. The community has a nursing case management program available for PWAs.

One-to-one supervision was found to be the most therapeutic in providing for safety and reality orientation. Visitors were also encouraged.

## Nursing Care Plan

WEEKLY UPDATE: __7/20/90__

NAME: _____Ron Jackson_____          ADMISSION DATE: __7/1/90__

DSM-III-R DIAGNOSIS: _____AIDS Dementia_____

### *ASSESSMENT:*

***Areas of strength:*** Supportive family. Earlier AIDS diagnosis has resulted in Medicaid and Social Security benefits. Currently not abusing drugs.

***Problems:*** Confusion, hallucinations, and memory problems. Physical problems of anorexia and related weight loss. Agitation when diagnostic tests done.

***DIAGNOSES:*** Potential for infection related to presence of HIV. Altered nutrition less than body requirement related to anorexia. Altered thought process related to AIDS dementia.

                                                                                       **Date met**

### *PLANNING:*

***Short-term goals:*** Weight maintenance and improved nutri-          _____
tional status.

Administration of antiviral and antipsychotic medications as or-          _____
dered.

Ongoing assessment of mental status.          _____

***Long-term goals:*** Monitor for opportunistic infections related          _____
to presence of HIV.

Prevention of HIV transmission.          _____

### *IMPLEMENTATION/INTERVENTIONS:*

***Nurse-patient relationship:*** Use simple, short sentences to minimize confusion. Provide high-calorie, high-protein diet. One-to-one care during periods of patient confusion and disorientation. Maintain universal precautions. Obtain assistance, if patient becomes agitated.

***Psychopharmacology:*** Haldol and zidovudine. If giving IM medication, use a retractable needle and follow universal precautions for needle and syringe disposal.

***Milieu management:*** Encourage visitors. Use calendar and clock to provide orientation to time and also reality. Follow daily routine. Use lists and written communication, such as a posted schedule. Remove potentially dangerous objects from environment.

***EVALUATION:*** No opportunistic infection symptoms noted. No health care worker exposed to HIV. Body weight maintained. Interacting with others appropriately. Reduction in disorientation noted.

tions and neoplasms but also to direct HIV infection of the nervous system. AIDS dementia is the most common late CNS dysfunction, and it is characterized by cognitive, motor, and behavioral dysfunction. More often it appears after major opportunistic infections have developed in AIDS patients. However, AIDS dementia may appear before the appearance of major systemic complications, and in recognition of this fact AIDS dementia complex has been added to the diagnostic criteria for AIDS (Burgess, 1990; Johnson, 1989). Between 50% and 85% of PWAs and between 5% and 10% of those with symptomatic HIV disease develop clinical signs of AIDS dementia (Dickson and Ranseen, 1990). Price (1990) reported at the Sixth International AIDS Conference that early HIV infection of the CNS is limited but can be detected. The severity of CNS infection is progressive.

AIDS dementia often is manifested by decreased concentration and forgetfulness, followed by decreased alertness, psychomotor retardation, withdrawal, apathy and reduced interest in work and usual activities, and loss of libido. Later symptoms of AIDS dementia may include hallucinations, confusion, disorientation, possibly seizures, mutism, profound dementia, and finally coma leading to death (Porth, 1990).

Neuroimaging procedures and cerebrospinal fluid evaluations are essential in establishing a diagnosis of AIDS dementia. CT and MRI scans show universal findings of cerebral atrophy, widened cortical sulci, and enlarged ventricles. Accumulated evidence from a multitude of sources supports the contention that the AIDS dementia complex is directly attributable to brain infection by HIV.

The treatment for AIDS often includes a methylphenidate for those with depression, apathy, and withdrawal. Haloperidol may be used in small doses for the management of paranoia and hallucinations (Polk-Walker, 1989). Reality testing and safety precautions should be used on the basis of the nurse's assessment of the psychoemotional status of the PWA.

For patients with AIDS dementia, nurses face a challenge in creating and maintaining a therapeutic milieu. Nurses may need to institute additional measures to ensure that universal precautions are maintained to protect the staff and other patients. For example, retractable needles are necessary for giving emergency medication to severely mentally ill patients who are infected with HIV.

It is uncommon for nurses to wear gloves in caring for psychiatric patients. This universal precaution measure may raise questions by the PWA and other patients. In addition, clear, concise explanations are needed to prevent the triggering of paranoid feelings. The patient with AIDS dementia may require one-to-one nursing care to ensure the safety of the patient, the staff, and other patients.

## KEY CONCEPTS

1. *Acquired immune deficiency syndrome* was the term initially used to describe the effects of a set of rare symptoms occurring in young homosexual men.
2. The human immunodeficiency virus was initially isolated in 1983 from patients with acquired immune deficiency syndrome (AIDS).
3. HIV enters the body from the T4 lymphocyte of an infected person. The normal range of T4 cells is 600 to 1200/mm$^3$. With HIV infection the accepted range is 0 to 500/mm$^3$. The number of T4 cells correlates with symptoms and clinical

course. The normal T4 to T8 ratio is 2:1. This ratio is often inverse with HIV disease. The normal function of the T4 cell is absent or depressed in HIV disease.

4. Opportunistic infections are those the person would normally resist when the immune system is functional and healthy. Many of the opportunistic diseases are commonly found in the environment and were rarely seen before the HIV disease epidemic. The most serious opportunistic disease is *Pneumocystis carinii* pneumonia (PCP), caused by a protozoan. Even with recent prophylactic treatment for PCP it remains the leading cause of death among persons with AIDS.

5. The second leading cause of AIDS deaths has been from Kaposi's sarcoma (KS). This cancer occurs on the surface of the skin, mouth, or visceral organs, such as the lungs or digestive tract. It causes blue-violet or red-brown nodules or plaques that are distinctive.

6. In the United States the groups at highest risk are homosexual and bisexual men, intravenous drug users, perinatal infants, hemophiliacs, and persons who received blood transfusions before March 1985. Health care providers are not in the high-risk category but do need to be aware of special precautions to avoid exposure.

7. The potential for occupational transmission of HIV can be reduced by implementing and vigorously enforcing infection-control procedures.

8. AIDS dementia, the most common late CNS dysfunction, is characterized by cognitive, motor, and behavioral dysfunction.

9. Most states have enacted laws to promote health care provider compliance with maintenance and diagnostic confidentiality. HIV disease and confidentiality are an ethical responsibility and are the same as for all patients requiring nursing care.

10. For the patient with HIV dementia the nurse can maintain a therapeutic milieu by ensuring that measures to safeguard the patient, staff, and other patients are employed. These measures include universal precautions, one-to-one supervision, reality orientation, use of daily routine, posted schedules, clocks, and calendars to minimize confusion.

## REFERENCES

American Nurses' Association: Code for nurses, Kansas City, 1985, The Association.

Bullock B and Rosendahl P: Pathophysiology: adaptations and alterations in function, Boston, 1988, Scott, Foresman & Co.

Burgess AW: Psychiatric nursing in the hospital and community, ed 5, Norwalk, Conn, 1990, Appleton & Lange.

California Nurses' Association: Ethics: principles and issues, San Francisco, 1985, The Association.

California Nurses' Association: Universal infection precautions: AIDS education and training, San Francisco, 1988, The Association.

Centers for Disease Control: Pneumocystic pneumonia—Los Angeles, MMWR 30:250, 1981.

Centers for Disease Control: Classification system for HTLV-III/LAV, MMWR 35:335, May 23, 1986.

Centers for Disease Control: Revision of the CDC surveillance case definition for acquired immunodeficiency syndrome, MMWR 36:1S, Aug. 14, 1987a.

Centers for Disease Control: Recommendations for prevention of HIV transmission in health care settings, MMWR 36:25, Aug. 21, 1987b.

Centers for Disease Control: Update: acquired deficiency virus infection among health care workers, MMWR 37:15, April 22, 1988.

Centers for Disease Control: AIDS and human immunodeficiency virus infection in the United States, 1988 Update, MMWR 38:S4, May 12, 1989a.

Centers for Disease Control: Guidelines for prevention of transmission of human immunodeficiency virus and hepatitis B virus to health care and public safety workers, MMWR 38:46, June 23, 1989b.

Centers for Disease Control: Estimation of HIV prevalence and projected AIDS cases: a summary workshop, MMWR 39:7, October 31-November 1, 1989c.

Chow M: Nursing's response to the challenge of AIDS, Nurs Outlook 37(2):82, 1989.

Clumeck N and de Wit S: AIDS in Africa. In Sande M and Volberding P, editors: The medical management of AIDS, Philadelphia, 1988, WB Saunders Co.

Cournos F et al: HIV infection in state hopsitals: case reports and long-term care strategies, Hosp Community Psychiatry 41:163, 1990.

Dickson LR and Ranseen JD: An update on organic mental syndromes, Hosp Community Psychiatry 41:290, 1990.

Fang C et al: HIV testing and patient counseling, Patient Care 23(17):18, 1989.

Johnson B: Adaptation and growth: psychiatric mental health nursing, ed 2, Philadelphia, 1989, JB Lippincott Co.

Kubler-Ross E: AIDS: the ultimate challenge, New York, 1987, Macmillan Publishing Co.

Levy J: Changing concepts in HIV research: state-of-the-art planning session, paper presented at the Sixth International Conference on AIDS, June 21, 1990, San Francisco, Calif.

McArthur J: AIDS dementia, RN 53:36, 1990.

Polk-Walker G: Treatment of AIDS in a psychiatric setting, Perspect Psychiatr Care 25:9-13, 1989.

Porth CM: Pathophysiology: concepts of altered human health states, ed 3, Philadelphia, 1990, JB Lippincott Co.

Price R: HIV brain infection treatments: state-of-the-art planning session, Sixth International Conference on AIDS, June 22, 1990, San Francisco, Calif.

Quinn TC: Global epidemiology of HIV infections. In Sande M and Volberding P, editors: The medical management of AIDS, Philadelphia, 1990, WB Saunders Co.

Rothberg J et al: Dealing with stress of an HIV positive diagnosis at an Army medical center, Milit Med 155:98, 1990.

Sacks MH et al: HIV-related risk factors in acute psychiatric in patients, Hosp Community Psychiatry 41:449-451, 1990.

Sande MA and Volberding A, editors: The medical management of AIDS, ed 2, Philadelphia, 1990, WB Saunders Co.

Zook R and Davidhizar R: Caring for the psychiatric in-patient with AIDS, Perspect Psychiatr Care 25(2):3, 1989.

# APPENDIXES

# Diagnostic Criteria for Mental Disorders

All official DSM-III-R codes are included in ICD-9-CM. Codes followed by an asterisk (*) are used for more than one DSM-III-R diagnosis or subtype in order to maintain compatibility with ICD-9-CM.

A long dash following a diagnostic term indicates the need for a fifth digit subtype or other qualifying term.

The term *specify* following the name of some diagnostic categories indicates qualifying terms that clinicians may wish to add in parentheses after the name of the disorder.

NOS = Not Otherwise Specified

The current severity of a disorder may be specified after the diagnosis as:

Mild
Moderate
Severe

Currently meets diagnostic criteria

In partial remission (or residual state)
In complete remission

## Disruptive behavior disorders

| | |
|---|---|
| 314.01 | Attention-deficit hyperactivity disorder |
| | Conduct disorder |
| 312.20 | group type |
| 312.00 | solitary agressive type |
| 312.90 | undifferentiated type |
| 313.81 | Oppositional defiant disorder |

## Anxiety disorders of childhood or adolescence

| | |
|---|---|
| 309.21 | Separation anxiety disorder |
| 313.21 | Avoidant disorder of childhood or adolescence |
| 313.00 | Overanxious disorder |

## Eating disorders

| | |
|---|---|
| 307.10 | Anorexia nervosa |
| 307.51 | Bulimia nervosa |
| 307.52 | Pica |
| 307.53 | Rumination disorder of infancy |
| 307.50 | Eating disorder NOS |

## Gender identity disorders

| | |
|---|---|
| 302.60 | Gender identity disorder of childhood |
| 302.50 | Transsexualism *Specify* sexual history: asexual, homosexual, heterosexual, unspecified |

Reprinted with permission from the *Diagnostic and Statistical Manual of Mental Disorders, Third Edition, Revised*, Copyright 1987 American Psychiatric Association.

## DISORDERS USUALLY FIRST EVIDENT IN INFANCY, CHILDHOOD, OR ADOLESCENCE

### DEVELOPMENTAL DISORDERS
NOTE: *These are coded on Axis II*

### Mental retardation
317.00    Mild mental retardation
318.00    Moderate mental retardation
318.10    Severe mental retardation
318.20    Profound mental retardation
319.00    Unspecified mental retardation

### Pervasive developmental disorders
299.00    Autistic disorder
          *Specify* if childhood onset
299.80    Pervasive developmental disorder NOS

### Specific developmental disorders
*Academic skills disorders*
315.10    Developmental arithmetic disorder
315.80    Developmental expressive writing disorder
315.00    Developmental reading disorder

*Language and speech disorders*
315.39    Developmental articulation disorder
315.31*   Developmental expressive language disorder
315.31*   Developmental receptive language disorder

*Motor skills disorder*
315.40    Developmental coordination disorder
315.90*   Specific developmental disorder NOS

### Other developmental disorders
315.90*   Developmental disorder NOS

302.85*   Gender identity disorder of adolescence or adulthood, nontranssexual type
          *Specify* sexual history: asexual, homosexual, heterosexual, unspecified

302.85*   Gender identity disorder NOS

### Tic disorders
307.23    Tourette's disorder
307.22    Chronic motor or vocal tic disorder
307.21    Transient tic disorder
          *Specify*: single episode or recurrent
307.20    Tic disorder NOS

### Elimination disorders
307.70    Functional encopresis
          *Specify*: primary or secondary type
307.60    Functional enuresis
          *Specify*: primary or secondary type
          *Specify*: nocturnal only, diurnal only, nocturnal and diurnal

### Speech disorders not elsewhere classified
307.00*   Cluttering
307.00*   Stuttering

### Other disorders of infancy, childhood, or adolescence
313.23    Elective mutism
313.82    Identity disorder
313.89    Reactive attachment disorder of infancy or early childhood
307.30    Stereotype/habit disorder
314.00    Undifferentiated attention deficit disorder

## ORGANIC MENTAL DISORDERS

### Dementias arising in the senium and presenium
          Primary degenerative dementia of the Alzheimer type, senile onset
290.30    with delirium
290.20    with delusions
290.21    with depression
290.00*   uncomplicated
          (Note: code 331.00 Alzheimer's disease on Axis III)

Code in fifth digit:
1 = with delirium, 2 = with delusions,
3 = with depression, 0* = uncomplicated

| 290.1x | Primary degenerative dementia of the Alzheimer type presenile onset, _____ (Note: code 331.00 Alzheimer's disease on Axis III) |
|---|---|
| 290.4x | Multi-infarct dementia, _____ |
| 290.00* | Senile dementia NOS *Specify* etiology on Axis III if known |
| 290.10* | Presenile dementia NOS *Specify* etiology on Axis III if known (e.g., Pick's disease, Jakob-Creutzfeldt disease) |

**Psychoactive substance-induced organic mental disorders**

Alcohol

| 303.00 | intoxication |
|---|---|
| 291.40 | idiosyncratic intoxication |
| 291.80 | Uncomplicated alcohol withdrawal |
| 291.00 | withdrawal delirium |
| 291.30 | hallucinosis |
| 291.10 | amnestic disorder |
| 291.20 | Dementia associated with alcoholism |

Amphetamine or similarly acting sympathomimetic

| 305.70* | intoxication |
|---|---|
| 292.00* | withdrawal |
| 292.81* | delirium |
| 292.11* | delusional disorder |

Caffeine

| 305.90* | intoxication |
|---|---|

Cannabis

| 305.20* | intoxication |
|---|---|
| 292.11* | delusional disorder |

Cocaine

| 305.60* | intoxication |
|---|---|
| 292.00* | withdrawal |
| 292.81* | delirium |
| 292.11* | delusional disorder |

Hallucinogen

| 305.30* | hallucinosis |
|---|---|
| 292.11* | delusional disorder |
| 292.84* | mood disorder |
| 292.89* | Posthallucinogen perception disorder |

Inhalant

| 305.90* | intoxication |
|---|---|

Nicotine

| 292.00* | withdrawal |
|---|---|

Opioid

| 305.50* | intoxication |
|---|---|
| 292.00* | withdrawal |

Phencyclidine (PCP) or similarly acting arylcyclohexylamine

| 305.90* | intoxication |
|---|---|
| 292.81* | delirium |
| 292.11* | delusional disorder |
| 292.84* | mood disorder |
| 292.90* | organic mental disorder NOS |

Sedative, hypnotic, or anxiolytic

| 305.40* | intoxication |
|---|---|
| 292.00* | Uncomplicated sedative, hypnotic, or anxiolytic withdrawal |
| 292.00* | withdrawal delirium |
| 292.83* | amnestic disorder |

Other or unspecified psychoactive substance

| 305.90* | intoxication |
|---|---|
| 292.00* | withdrawal |
| 292.81* | delirium |
| 292.82* | dementia |
| 292.83* | amnestic disorder |
| 292.11* | delusional disorder |
| 292.12 | hallucinosis |
| 292.84* | mood disorder |
| 292.89* | anxiety disorder |
| 292.89* | personality disorder |
| 292.90* | organic mental disorder NOS |

**Organic mental disorders associated with Axis III physical disorders or conditions, or whose etiology is unknown**

| 293.00 | Delirium |
|---|---|
| 294.10 | Dementia |
| 294.00 | Amnestic disorder |
| 293.81 | Organic delusional disorder |
| 293.82 | Organic hallucinosis |
| 293.83 | Organic mood disorder *Specify*: manic, depressed, mixed |
| 294.80* | Organic anxiety disorder |
| 310.10 | Organic personality disorder *Specify* if explosive type |
| 294.80* | Organic mental disorder NOS |

## PSYCHOACTIVE SUBSTANCE USE DISORDERS

Alcohol
303.90    dependence
305.00    abuse
Amphetamine or similarly acting sympathomimetic
304.40    dependence
305.70*   abuse
Cannabis
304.30    dependence
305.20*   abuse
Cocaine
304.20    dependence
305.60*   abuse
Hallucinogen
304.50*   dependence
305.30*   abuse
Inhalant
304.60    dependence
305.90*   abuse
Nicotine
305.10    dependence
Opioid
304.00    dependence
305.50*   abuse
Phencyclidine (PCP) or similarly acting arylcyclohexylamine
304.50*   dependence
305.90*   abuse
Sedative, hypnotic, or anxiolytic
304.10    dependence
305.40*   abuse
304.90*   Polysubstance dependence
304.90*   Psychoactive substance dependence NOS
305.90*   Psychoactive substance abuse NOS

## SCHIZOPHRENIA

Code in fifth digit:
1 = subchronic, 2 = chronic, 3 = subchronic with acute exacerbation,
4 = chronic with acute exacerbation,
5 = in remission, 0 = unspecified

Schizophrenia
295.2x    catatonic, _____
295.1x    disorganized, _____
295.3x    paranoid, _____
          *Specify* if stable type

295.9x    undifferentiated, _____
295.6x    residual, _____
          *Specify* if late onset

## DELUSIONAL (PARANOID) DISORDER

297.10    Delusional (Paranoid) disorder
          *Specify* erotomanic, grandiose, jealous, persecutory, somatic, unspecified

## PSYCHOTIC DISORDERS NOT ELSEWHERE CLASSIFIED

298.80    Brief reactive psychosis
295.40    Schizophreniform disorder
          *Specify:* without good prognostic features or with good prognostic features
295.70    Schizoaffective disorder
          *Specify:* bipolar type or depressive type
297.30    Induced psychotic disorder
298.90    Psychotic disorder NOS (Atypical psychosis)

## MOOD DISORDERS

Code current state of Major Depression and Bipolar Disorder in fifth digit:
1 = mild, 2 = moderate, 3 = severe, without psychotic features, 4 = with psychotic features (*specify* mood-congruent or mood incongruent), 5 = in partial remission, 6 = in full remission, 0 = unspecified.

For major depressive episodes, *Specify* if chronic and *specify* if melancholic type.

For Bipolar Disorder, Bipolar Disorder NOS, Recurrent Major Depression, and Depressive Disorder NOS, *specify* if seasonal pattern.

### Bipolar disorders

Bipolar disorder
296.6x    mixed, _____
296.4x    manic, _____
296.5x    depressed, _____
301.13    Cyclothymia
296.70    Bipolar disorder NOS

### Depressive disorders

Major depression
296.2x    single episode, _____
296.3x    recurrent, _____

300.40    Dysthymia (or Depressive neurosis)
          *Specify:* primary or secondary type
          *Specify:* early or late onset
311.00    Depressive disorder NOS

## ANXIETY DISORDERS (or Anxiety and Phobic Neuroses)

          Panic disorder
300.21    with agoraphobia
          *Specify* current severity of agoraphobic avoidance
          *Specify* current severity of panic attacks
300.01    without agoraphobia
          *Specify* current severity of panic attacks
300.22    Agoraphobia without history of panic disorder
          *Specify* with or without limited symptom attacks
300.23    Social phobia
          *Specify* if generalized type
300.29    Simple phobia
300.30    Obsessive compulsive disorder (or Obsessive compulsive neurosis)
309.89    Post-traumatic stress disorder
          *Specify* if delayed onset
300.02    Generalized anxiety disorder
300.00    Anxiety disorder NOS

## SOMATOFORM DISORDERS

300.70*   Body dysmorphic disorder
300.11    Conversion disorder (or Hysterical neurosis, coversion type)
          *Specify:* single episode or recurrent
300.70*   Hypochondriasis (or Hypochondriacal neurosis)
300.81    Somatization disorder
307.80    Somatoform pain disorder
300.70*   Undifferentiated somatoform disorder
300.70*   Somatoform disorder NOS

## DISSOCIATIVE DISORDERS (or Hysterical Neuroses, Dissociative Type)

300.14    Multiple personality disorder
300.13    Psychogenic fugue

300.12    Psychogenic amnesia
300.60    Depersonalization disorder (or Depersonalization neurosis)
300.15    Dissociative disorder NOS

## SEXUAL DISORDERS
### Paraphilias

302.40    Exhibitionism
302.81    Fetishism
302.89    Frotteurism
302.20    Pedophilia
          *Specify:* same sex, opposite sex, same and opposite sex
          *Specify* if limited to incest
          *Specify:* exclusive type or nonexclusive type
302.83    Sexual masochism
302.84    Sexual sadism
302.30    Transvestic fetishism
302.82    Voyeurism
302.90*   Paraphilia NOS

### Sexual dysfunctions

*Specify:* psychogenic only, or psychogenic and biogenic
(Note: If biogenic only, code on Axis III)
*Specify:* lifelong or acquired
*Specify:* generalized or situational
          Sexual desire disorders
302.71    Hypoactive sexual desire disorder
302.79    Sexual aversion disorder
          Sexual arousal disorders
302.72*   Female sexual arousal disorder
302.72*   Male erectile disorder
          Orgasm disorder
302.73    Inhibited female orgasm
302.74    Inhibited male orgasm
302.75    Premature ejaculation
          Sexual pain disorders
302.76    Dyspareunia
306.51    Vaginismus
302.70    Sexual dysfunction NOS

### Other sexual disorders

302.90*   Sexual disorder NOS

## SLEEP DISORDERS
### Dyssomnias

          Insomnia disorder
307.42*   related to another mental disorder (nonorganic)

| | |
|---|---|
| 780.50* | related to known organic factor |
| 307.42* | Primary insomnia |
| | Hypersomnia disorder |
| 307.44 | related to another mental disorder (nonorganic) |
| 780.50* | related to a known organic factor |
| 780.54 | Primary hypersomnia |
| 307.45 | Sleep-wake schedule disorder |
| | *Specify:* advanced or delayed phase type, disorganized type, frequently changing type |
| | Other dyssomnias |
| 307.40* | Dyssomnia NOS |

### Parasomnias

| | |
|---|---|
| 307.47 | Dream anxiety disorder (Nightmare disorder) |
| 307.46* | Sleep terror disorder |
| 307.46* | Sleepwalking disorder |
| 307.40* | Parasomnia NOS |

## FACTITIOUS DISORDERS

| | |
|---|---|
| | Factitious disorder |
| 301.51 | with physical symptoms |
| 300.16 | with psychological symptoms |
| 300.19 | Factitious disorder NOS |

## IMPULSE CONTROL DISORDERS NOT ELSEWHERE CLASSIFIED

| | |
|---|---|
| 312.34 | Intermittent explosive disorder |
| 312.32 | Kleptomania |
| 312.31 | Pathological gambling |
| 312.33 | Pyromania |
| 312.39* | Trichotillomania |
| 312.39* | Impulse control disorder NOS |

## ADJUSTMENT DISORDER

| | |
|---|---|
| | Adjustment disorder |
| 309.24 | with anxious mood |
| 309.00 | with depressed mood |
| 309.30 | with disturbance of conduct |
| 309.40 | with mixed disturbance of emotions and conduct |
| 309.28 | with mixed emotional features |
| 309.82 | with physical complaints |
| 309.83 | with withdrawal |
| 309.23 | with work (or academic) inhibition |
| 309.90 | Adjustment disorder NOS |

## PSYCHOLOGICAL FACTORS AFFECTING PHYSICAL CONDITION

| | |
|---|---|
| 316.00 | Psychological factors affecting physical condition |
| | *Specify* physical condition on Axis III |

---

*PERSONALITY DISORDERS*
*NOTE: These are coded on Axis II*

### Cluster A

| | |
|---|---|
| 301.00 | Paranoid |
| 301.20 | Schizoid |
| 301.22 | Schizotypal |

### Cluster B

| | |
|---|---|
| 301.70 | Antisocial |
| 301.83 | Borderline |
| 301.50 | Histrionic |
| 301.81 | Narcissistic |

### Cluster C

| | |
|---|---|
| 301.82 | Avoidant |
| 301.60 | Dependent |
| 301.40 | Obsessive compulsive |
| 301.84 | Passive aggressive |
| 301.90 | Personality disorder NOS |

---

**V CODES FOR CONDITIONS NOT ATTRIBUTABLE TO A MENTAL DISORDER THAT ARE A FOCUS OF ATTENTION OR TREATMENT**

| | |
|---|---|
| V62.30 | Academic problem |
| V71.01 | Adult antisocial behavior |

---

| | |
|---|---|
| V40.00 | Borderline intellectual functioning (Note: This is coded on Axis II) |

---

| | |
|---|---|
| V71.02 | Childhood or adolescent antisocial behavior |
| V65.20 | Malingering |
| V61.10 | Marital problem |
| V15.81 | Noncompliance with medical treatment |
| V62.20 | Occupational problem |
| V61.20 | Parent-child problem |
| V62.81 | Other interpersonal problem |
| V61.80 | Other specified family circumstances |
| V62.89 | Phase of life problem or other life circumstance problem |
| V62.82 | Uncomplicated bereavement |

**ADDITIONAL CODES**

| | |
|---|---|
| 300.90 | Unspecified mental disorder (nonpsychotic) |
| V71.09* | No diagnosis or condition on Axis I |
| 799.90* | Diagnosis or condition deferred on Axis I |

---

| | |
|---|---|
| V71.09* | No diagnosis or condition on Axis II |
| 799.90* | Diagnosis or condition deferred on Axis II |

---

**MULTIAXIAL SYSTEM**

| | |
|---|---|
| Axis I | Clinical Syndromes |
| | V Codes |
| Axis II | Developmental Disorders |
| | Personality Disorders |
| Axis III | Physical Disorders and Conditions |
| Axis IV | Severity of Psychosocial Stressors |
| Axis V | Global Assessment of Functioning |

## SEVERITY OF PSYCHOSOCIAL STRESSORS SCALE: ADULTS

| CODE | TERM | EXAMPLES OF STRESSORS | |
|------|------|-----------------------|---|
| | | **Acute Events** | **Enduring Circumstances** |
| 1 | None | No acute events that may be relevant to the disorder | No enduring circumstances that may be relevant to the disorder |
| 2 | Mild | Broke up with boyfriend or girlfriend; started or graduated from school; child left home | Family arguments; job dissatisfaction; resident in high-crime neighborhood |
| 3 | Moderate | Marriage; marital separation; loss of job; retirement; miscarriage | Marital discord; serious financial problems; trouble with boss; being a single parent |
| 4 | Severe | Divorce; birth of first child | Unemployment; poverty |
| 5 | Extreme | Death of spouse; serious physical illness diagnosed; victim of rape | Serious chronic illness in self or child; ongoing physical or sexual abuse |
| 6 | Catastrophic | Death of child; suicide of spouse; devastating natural disaster | Captivity as hostage; concentration camp experience |
| 0 | Inadequate information, or no change in condition | | |

## SEVERITY OF PSYCHOSOCIAL STRESSORS SCALE: CHILDREN AND ADOLESCENTS

| CODE | TERM | EXAMPLES OF STRESSORS | |
|------|------|-----------------------|---|
| | | **Acute Events** | **Enduring Circumstances** |
| 1 | None | No acute events that may be relevant to the disorder | No enduring circumstances that may be relevant to the disorder |
| 2 | Mild | Broke up with boyfriend or girlfriend; change of school | Overcrowded living quarters; family argument |
| 3 | Moderate | Expelled from school; birth of sibling | Chronic disabling illness in parent; chronic parental discord |
| 4 | Severe | Divorce of parents; unwanted pregnancy; arrest | Harsh or rejecting parents; chronic life-threatening illness in parent; multiple foster home placements |
| 5 | Extreme | Sexual or physical abuse; death of a parent; | Recurrent sexual or physical abuse |
| 6 | Catastrophic | Death of both parents | Chronic life-threatening illness |
| 0 | Inadequate information, or no change in condition | | |

## GLOBAL ASSESSMENT OF FUNCTIONING SCALE (GAF Scale)

Consider psychological, social, and occupational functioning on a hypothetical continuum of mental health-illness. Do not include impairment in functioning due to physical (or environmental) limitations.

**Note:** use intermediate codes when appropriate, e.g., 45, 68, 72.

*Code*

90 | **Absent or minimal symptoms** (e.g., mild anxiety before an exam), **good functioning in all areas, interested and involved in a wide range of activities, socially effective, generally satisfied with life, no more than everyday problems or**
81 | **concerns** (e.g., an occasional argument with family members).

80 | **If symptoms are present, they are transient and expectable reactions to psychosocial stressors** (e.g., difficulty concentrating after family argument); **no more than slight impairment in social, occupational, or school functioning** (e.g.,
71 | temporarily falling behind in school work).

70 | **Some mild symptoms** (e.g., depressed mood and mild insomnia) **OR some difficulty in social, occupational, or school functioning** (e.g., occasional truancy, or theft within the household), **but generally functioning pretty well, has some mean-**
61 | **ingful interpersonal relationships.**

60 | **Moderate symptoms** (e.g., flat affect and circumstantial speech, occasional panic attacks) **OR moderate difficulty in social, occupational, or school functioning**
51 | (e.g., few friends, conflicts with co-workers).

50 | **Serious symptoms** (e.g., suicidal ideation, severe obsessional rituals, frequent shoplifting) **OR any serious impairment in social, occupational, or school function-**
41 | **ing** (e.g., no friends, unable to keep a job).

40 | **Some impairment in reality testing or communication** (e.g., speech is at times illogical, obscure or irrelevant) **OR major impairment in several areas, such as work or school, family relations, judgment, thinking, or mood** (e.g., depressed man avoids friends, neglects family, and is unable to work; child frequently beats up
31 | younger children, is defiant at home, and is failing at school).

30 | **Behavior is considerably influenced by delusions or hallucinations OR serious impairment in communication or judgment** (e.g., sometimes incoherent, acts grossly inappropriately, suicidal preoccupation) **OR inability to function in almost**
21 | **all areas** (e.g., stays in bed all day; no job, home, or friends).

20 | **Some danger of hurting self or others** (e.g., suicide attempts without clear expectation of death, frequently violent, manic excitement) **OR occasionally fails to maintain minimal personal hygiene** (e.g., smears feces) **OR gross impairment in com-**
11 | **munication** (e.g., largely incoherent or mute).

10 | **Persistent danger of severely hurting self or others** (e.g., recurrent violence) **OR persistent inability to maintain minimal personal hygiene OR serious suicidal**
1 | **act with clear expectation of death.**

# Classification of Human Responses of Concern for Psychiatric Mental Health Nursing Practice (PND-I)*

01. Human response patterns in activity processes
    01.01 Altered motor behavior
        01.01.01 Bizarre motor behavior
        01.01.02 Catatonia
        01.01.03 Impaired coordination
        01.01.04 Hyperactivity
        01.01.05 Hypoactivity
        01.01.06 Muscular rigidity
        01.01.07 Psychomotor retardation
    01.02 Altered recreation patterns
        01.02.01 Inadequate diversional activity
    01.03 Altered self-care
        01.03.01 Altered eating
      *01.03.02 Altered grooming
        01.03.03 Altered health maintenance

      *01.03.04 Altered hygiene
        01.03.05 Altered participation in health care
      *01.03.06 Altered toileting
    01.04 Altered sleep/arousal patterns
        01.04.01 Difficult transition to and from sleep
        01.04.02 Hypersomnia
        01.04.03 Insomnia
        01.04.04 Nightmares
        01.04.05 Somnolence
    01.97 Undeveloped activity processes
    01.98 Altered activity processes not otherwise specified
    01.99 Potential for altered activity/ processes
02. Human response patterns in cognition processes
    02.01 Altered decision making

*NANDA diagnosis.
This classification is based on previous work of the Phenomenon Task Force and the Advisory Panel on Classifications for Nursing Practice of the American Nurses' Association.
From ANA Classification of Individual Human Responses by M. Loomis, A. O'Toole, M. Brown, P. Pothier, P. West, H.S. Wilson. Copyright 1986. Published by the American Nurses' Association and reprinted with permission.

05.02.01.02  Aggressive/violent behaviors toward others
05.02.01.03  Aggressive/violent behaviors toward self
05.02.02  Dysfunctional behaviors
05.02.02.01  Age-inappropriate behaviors
05.02.02.02  Bizarre behaviors
05.02.02.03  Compulsive behaviors
05.02.02.04  Disorganized behaviors
05.02.02.05  Unpredictable behaviors
05.03  Altered role performance
05.03.01  Altered family role
05.03.02  Altered leisure role
*05.03.03  Altering parenting role
05.03.04  Altered play role
05.03.05  Altered student role
05.03.06  Altered work role
05.04  Altered sexuality processes
05.05  Altered social interaction
05.05.01  Social intrusiveness
*05.05.02  Social isolation/withdrawal
05.97  Undeveloped interpersonal processes
05.98  Altered interpersonal processes not otherwise specified
05.99  Potential for altered interpersonal processes
*05.99.01  Potential for violence
06.  Human response patterns in perception processes
06.01  Altered attention
06.01.01  Distractibility
06.01.02  Hyperalertness

06.01.03  Inattention
06.01.04  Selective attention
*06.02  Altered comfort patterns
06.02.01  Discomfort
06.02.02  Distress
06.02.03  Pain
06.03  Altered self-concept
*06.03.01  Altered body image
06.03.02  Altered gender identity
*06.03.03  Altered personal identity
*06.03.04  Altered self-esteem
06.03.05  Altered social identity
06.03.06  Undeveloped self-concept
06.04  Altered sensory perception
*06.04.01  Auditory
*06.04.02  Gustatory
06.04.03  Hallucinations
06.04.04  Illusions
*06.04.05  Kinesthetic
*06.04.06  Olfactory
*06.04.07  Tactile
*06.04.08  Visual
06.97  Undeveloped perception processes
06.98  Altered perception processes not otherwise specified
06.99  Potential for altered perception processes
07.  Human response patterns in physiological processes
07.01  Altered circulation processes
07.01.01  Altered vascular circulation
*07.01.01.01  Tissue perfusion
*07.01.01.02  Altered fluid volume
07.01.02  Altered cardiac circulation
07.02  Altered elimination processes

*07.02.01 Altered bowel elimination
  *07.02.01.01 Constipation
  *07.02.01.02 Diarrhea
  *07.02.01.03 Incontinence
  07.02.01.04 Encopresis
*07.02.02 Altered urinary elimination
  *07.02.02.01 Incontinence
  *07.02.02.02 Retention
  07.02.02.03 Enuresis
07.02.03 Altered skin elimination
07.03 Altered endocrine/metabolic processes
  07.03.01 Altered growth
  07.03.02 Altered hormone regulation
    07.03.02.01 Premenstrual stress syndrome
07.04 Altered gastrointestinal processes
  07.04.01 Altered absorption
  07.04.02 Altered digestion
07.05 Altered neurosensory processes
  07.05.01 Altered levels of consciousness
  07.05.02 Altered sensory acuity
  07.05.03 Altered sensory processing
  07.05.04 Altered sensory integration
    07.05.04.01 Learning disabilities
07.06 Altered nutrition processes
  07.06.01 Altered cellular processes
  07.06.02 Altered systemic processes
    *07.06.02.01 More than body requirements
    *07.06.02.02 Less than body requirements

07.06.03 Altered eating processes
  07.06.03.01 Anorexia
  07.06.03.02 Pica
07.07 Altered oxygenation processes
  07.07.01 Altered respiration
    07.07.01.01 Altered gas exchange
    *07.07.01.02 Ineffective airway clearance
    *07.07.01.03 Ineffective breathing pattern
07.08 Altered physical integrity processes
  *07.08.01 Altered skin integrity
  *07.08.02 Altered tissue integrity
07.09 Altered physical regulation processes
  07.09.01 Altered immune responses
    07.09.01.01 Infection
07.10 Altered body temperature
  *07.10.01 Hypothermia
  *07.10.02 Hyperthermia
  *07.10.03 Ineffective thermoregulation
07.97 Undeveloped physiological processes
07.98 Altered physiological processes not otherwise specified
07.99 Potential for altered physiological processes
08. Human response patterns in valuation processes
  *08.01 Altered meaningfulness
    *08.01.01 Hopelessness
    08.01.02 Helplessness
    08.01.03 Loneliness
    *08.01.04 Powerlessness
  08.02 Altered Spirituality
    *08.02.01 Spiritual distress
    08.02.02 Spiritual despair

08.03 Altered values
    08.03.01 Conflict with social order
    08.03.02 Inability to internalize
        values
    08.03.03 Unclarified values

08.97 Undeveloped valuation processes
08.98 Altered valuation processes not otherwise specified
08.99 Potential for altered valuation processes

# The Mini-Mental State Examination

|  | Score | Points |
|---|---|---|

**Orientation**

| 1. What is the | Year? | | 1 |
|---|---|---|---|
| | Season? | | 1 |
| | Date? | | 1 |
| | Day? | | 1 |
| | Month? | | 1 |
| 2. Where are we? | State? | | 1 |
| | County? | | 1 |
| | Town or city? | | 1 |
| | Hospital? | | 1 |
| | Floor? | | 1 |

**Registration**

3. Name three objects, taking one second to say each. Then ask the patient all three after you have said them. Give one point for each correct answer. Repeat the answers until the patient learns all three.  **3**

**Attention and calculation**

4. Serial sevens.* Given one point for each correct answer. Stop after five answers. *Alternative:* Spell WORLD backwards.  **5**

**Recall**

5. Ask for names of three objects learned in Question 3. Give one point for each correct answer.  *Continued.*  **3**

*Serial seven-subtracting 7 from 100, i.e., $100 - 7 = 93$; $93 - 7 = 86$; $86 - 7 = 79$; $79 - 7 = 72$; $72 - 7 = 65$; and so on.

From Folstein MF, Folstein SE, and McHugh PR: Mini-mental state. A practical method of grading the cognitive state of patients for the clinician. J Psychiatr Res 12:189-198, 1975. By permission.

|  | Score | Points |
|---|---|---|

## Language

6. Point to a pencil and a watch. Have the patient name them as you point.                                                                      2

7. Have the patient repeat "No ifs, ands, or buts."                                   1

8. Have the patient follow a three-stage command: "Take the paper in your right hand. Fold the paper in half. Put the paper on the floor."                                                                       3

9. Have the patient read and obey the following: "CLOSE YOUR EYES." (Write it in large letters.)                                          1

10. Have the patient write a sentence of his or her own choice. (The sentence should contain a subject and an object and should make sense. Ignore spelling errors when scoring.)            1

11. Enlarge the design printed below to 1 to 5 cm per side and have the patient copy it. (Give one point if all sides and angles are preserved and if the intersecting sides form a quadrangle.)         1

_____ = Total 30

A score of 23 or less suggests cognitive impairment in a person with eighth grade education or better.

# The Geriatric Depression Scale

Choose the best answer for how you felt over the past week.

| | | |
|---|---|---|
| 1. | Are you basically satisfied with your life? | Yes/No |
| 2. | Have you dropped many of your activities and interests? | Yes/No |
| 3. | Do you feel that your life is empty? | Yes/No |
| 4. | Do you often get bored? | Yes/No |
| 5. | Are you hopeful about the future? | Yes/No |
| 6. | Are you bothered by thoughts you can't get out of your head? | Yes/No |
| 7. | Are you in good spirits most of the time? | Yes/No |
| 8. | Are you afraid that something bad is going to happen to you? | Yes/No |
| 9. | Do you feel happy most of the time? | Yes/No |
| 10. | Do you often feel helpless? | Yes/No |
| 11. | Do you often get restless and fidgety? | Yes/No |
| 12. | Do you prefer to stay at home, rather than going out and doing new things? | Yes/No |
| 13. | Do you frequently worry about the future? | Yes/No |
| 14. | Do you feel you have more problems with memory than most? | Yes/No |
| 15. | Do you think it is wonderful to be alive right now? | Yes/No |
| 16. | Do you often feel downhearted and blue? | Yes/No |
| 17. | Do you feel pretty worthless the way you are now? | Yes/No |
| 18. | Do you worry a lot about the past? | Yes/No |
| 19. | Do you find life very exciting? | Yes/No |
| 20. | Is it hard for you to get started on new projects? | Yes/No |
| 21. | Do you feel full of energy? | Yes/No |
| 22. | Do you feel that your situation is hopeless? | Yes/No |
| 23. | Do you think that more people are better off than you are? | Yes/No |
| 24. | Do you frequently get upset over little things? | Yes/No |

A score of 14 points or more suggests the presence of depression, which needs to be confirmed by clinical evaluation.

From Yesavage JA, Brink TL, Rose TL, Lum O, Huang V, Adey M, and Leirer VO: Development and validation of a geriatric depression screening scale: a preliminary report. J Psychiatr Res 17:37-49, 1983. By permission.

25. Do you frequently feel like crying?                    Yes/No
26. Do you have trouble concentrating?                     Yes/No
27. Do you enjoy getting up in the morning?                Yes/No
28. Do you prefer to avoid social gatherings?              Yes/No
29. Is it easy for you to make decisions?                  Yes/No
30. Is your mind as clear as it used to be?                Yes/No

# Hamilton Psychiatric Rating Scale for Depression

For each item, select the one "answer" that best characterizes the patient and check the corresponding numbered box.

---

### 1. Depressed mood (sadness, hopeless, helpless, worthless)

0 = Absent
1 = These feeling states indicated
only on questioning
2 = These feeling states spontaneously reported verbally

| 0 | 1 | 2 | 3 | 4 |
|---|---|---|---|---|

3 = Communicates feeling states nonverbally—i.e., through facial expression, posture, voice, and tendency to weep
4 = Patient reports VIRTUALLY ONLY these feeling states in his spontaneous verbal
and nonverbal communication

### 2. Feelings of guilt

0 = Absent
1 = Self-reproach, feels he has let
people down

| 0 | 1 | 2 | 3 | 4 |
|---|---|---|---|---|

2 = Ideas of guilt or rumination
over past errors or sinful deeds
3 = Present illness is a punishment. Delusions of guilt
4 = Hears accusatory or denunciatory voices and/or experiences threatening visual
hallucinations

This scale is used for rating the severity of depression. A score of less than 11 suggests that no depression is present.
Reprinted with permission of author from Hamilton, M (1967). Development of a rating scale for primary depressive illness. Br J Soc Clin Psychol, 6:278-296.

### 3. Suicide

0 = Absent
1 = Feels life is not worth living
2 = Wishes he were dead or any
   thoughts of possible death to self
3 = Suicide ideas or gesture
4 = Attempts at suicide (any serious attempt rates 4)

| 0 | 1 | 2 | 3 | 4 |
|---|---|---|---|---|

### 4. Insomnia early

0 = No difficulty falling asleep
1 = Complains of occasional difficulty falling asleep—i.e., more
   than ½ hour
2 = Complains of nightly difficulty falling asleep

| 0 | 1 | 2 |
|---|---|---|

### 5. Insomnia middle

0 = No difficulty
1 = Patient complains of being
   restless and disturbed during
   the night
2 = Waking during the night—any getting out of bed rates 2 (except for purposes of voiding)

| 0 | 1 | 2 |
|---|---|---|

### 6. Insomnia late

0 = No difficulty
1 = Waking in early hours of the
   morning but goes back to
   sleep
2 = Unable to fall asleep again if he gets out of bed

| 0 | 1 | 2 |
|---|---|---|

### 7. Work and activities

0 = No difficulty
1 = Thoughts and feelings of incapacity, fatigue or weakness related to activities, work or
   hobbies

| 0 | 1 | 2 | 3 | 4 |
|---|---|---|---|---|

2 = Loss of interest in activity—hobbies or work—either directly reported by patient, or indirect in listlessness, indecision, and vacillation (feels he has to push
   self to work or activities)
3 = Decrease in actual time spent in activities or decrease in productivity. In hospital, rate 3 if patient does not spend at least three hours a day in activities (hospital job or hobbies) exclusive of ward chores
4 = Stopped working because of present illness. In hospital rate 4 if patient engages
   in no activities except ward chores, or if patient fails to perform ward chores
   unassisted

8. **Retardation (slowness of thought and speech; impaired ability to concentrate; decreased motor activity)**

   0 = Normal speech and thought
   1 = Slight retardation at interview
   2 = Obvious retardation at interview
   3 = Interview difficult
   4 = Complete stupor

| 0 | 1 | 2 | 3 | 4 |
|---|---|---|---|---|

9. **Agitation**

   0 = None
   1 = "Playing with" hands, hair, etc.
   2 = Hand-wringing, nail-biting, hairpulling, biting of lips

| 0 | 1 | 2 |
|---|---|---|

10. **Anxiety psychic**

    Physiological concomitants of anxiety, such as:
    Gastrointestinal—dry mouth, wind, indigestion, diarrhea, cramps, belching
    Cardiovascular—palpitations, headaches
    Respiratory—hyperventilation, sighing
    Urinary frequency
    Sweating
    0 = Absent
    1 = Mild
    2 = Moderate
    3 = Severe
    4 = Incapacitating

| 0 | 1 | 2 | 3 | 4 |
|---|---|---|---|---|

11. **Somatic symptoms—gastrointestinal**

    0 = None
    1 = Loss of appetite, but eating without staff encouragement. Heavy feelings in abdomen
    2 = Difficulty eating without staff urging. Requests or requires laxatives or medication for bowels or medication for GI symptoms

| 0 | 1 | 2 |
|---|---|---|

12. **Somatic symptoms—general**

    0 = None
    1 = Heaviness in limbs, back of head. Backaches, headaches, muscle aches. Loss of energy and fatigability
    2 = Any clear-cut symptom rates 2

| 0 | 1 | 2 |
|---|---|---|

### 13. Genital symptoms

Symptoms such as: loss of libido, menstrual disturbances
0 = Absent
1 = Mild
2 = Severe

| 0 | 1 | 2 |
|---|---|---|

### 14. Hypochondriasis

0 = Not present
1 = Self-absorption (bodily)
2 = Preoccupation with health
3 = Frequent complaints, requests
   for help, etc.
4 = Hypochondriacal delusions

| 0 | 1 | 2 | 3 | 4 |
|---|---|---|---|---|

### 15. Loss of weight—rate either A or B

**A. When rating by history:**
0 = No weight loss
1 = Probable weight loss associated with present illness
2 = Definite (according to patient) weight loss
3 = Not assessed

| 0 | 1 | 2 | 3 |
|---|---|---|---|

**B. On weekly ratings by ward psychiatrist, when actual weight changes are measured:**
0 = Less than 1 lb. weight loss
   in week
1 = Greater than 1 lb. weight
   loss in week
2 = Greater than 2 lb. weight
   loss in week
3 = Not assessed

| 0 | 1 | 2 | 3 |
|---|---|---|---|

### 16. Insight

0 = Acknowledges being depressed
   and ill
1 = Acknowledges illness but attributes cause to bad food, climate, overwork, virus, need for
   rest, etc.
2 = Denies being ill at all

| 0 | 1 | 2 |
|---|---|---|

## 17. Diurnal variation

A. Note whether symptoms are worse in morning or evening. If NO diurnal variation, mark "None."

0 = No variation
1 = Worse in A.M.
2 = Worse in P.M.

| 0 | 1 | 2 |
|---|---|---|

B. When present, mark the severity of the variation. Mark "None" if NO variation.

0 = None
1 = Mild
2 = Severe

| 0 | 1 | 2 |
|---|---|---|

## 18. Depersonalization and derealization

Such as: feelings of unreality, nihilistic ideas

0 = Absent
1 = Mild
2 = Moderate
3 = Severe
4 = Incapacitating

| 0 | 1 | 2 | 3 | 4 |
|---|---|---|---|---|

## 19. Paranoid symptoms

0 = None
1 = Suspicious
2 = Ideas of reference
3 = Delusions of reference and persecution

| 0 | 1 | 2 | 3 |
|---|---|---|---|

## 20. Obsessional and compulsive symptoms

0 = Absent
1 = Mild
2 = Severe

| 0 | 1 | 2 |
|---|---|---|

# Brief Psychiatric Rating Scale

### 1. SOMATIC CONCERN:

Degree of concern over present bodily health. Rate the degree to which physical health is perceived as a problem by the patient, whether complaints have a realistic basis or not.

### 2. ANXIETY-ANXIETY STATEMENTS:

Worry, fear, or overconcern for present or future. Rate solely on the basis of verbal report of patient's own subjective experiences. Do not infer anxiety from neurotic defense mechanisms.

### 3. EMOTIONAL WITHDRAWAL:

Deficiency in relating to others; seclusiveness. Rate only the degree to which the patient gives the impression of failing to be in emotional contact with other people.

### 4. CONCEPTUAL DISORGANIZATION/DISORGANIZATION IN SPEECH:

Degree to which the thought processes are confused, disconnected, or disorganized. Rate on the basis of integration of the verbal products of the patient; do not rate on the basis of the patient's subjective impression of his own level of functioning.

### 5. GUILT FEELING/GUILT STATEMENTS:

Overconcern or remorse for past behavior. Rate on the basis of the patient's subjective experiences of guilt as evidenced by verbal report with appropriate affect; do not infer guilt feelings from depression, anxiety, or neurotic defenses.

### 6. TENSION/TENSION BEHAVIOR:

Physical and motor manifestations of tension, "nervousness," and heightened activation level. Tension should be rated solely on the basis of physical signs and motor behavior and not on the basis of subjective experiences of tension reported by the patient.

| Not present | Mild | Moderate | Severe | Not ratable |
|:---:|:---:|:---:|:---:|:---:|
| | OCCAS. | EXAG. | PREOCC. | |
| 1 | 2 3 | 4 5 | 6 7 | 0 |
| | WORRIED | FEARFUL | PANICKED | |
| 1 | 2 3 | 4 5 | 6 7 | 0 |
| | DOESN'T INITIATE | WITHDRAWS FROM | REPELS CONTACT | |
| 1 | 2 3 | 4 5 | 6 7 | 0 |
| | VAGUE | UNCLEAR | INCOHERENT TALK | |
| 1 | 2 3 | 4 5 | 6 7 | 0 |
| | OVER-CONCERN | PRE-OCCUPIED | DELUSIONS OF GUILT | |
| 1 | 2 3 | 4 5 | 6 7 | 0 |
| | SEEMS TENSE | RESTLESS | AGITATED | |
| 1 | 2 3 | 4 5 | 6 7 | 0 |

*Continued.*

### 7. MANNERISMS AND POSTURING:

Unusual and unnatural motor behavior which causes certain mental patients to stand out in a crowd of normal people. Rate only abnormality of movements; do not rate simple heightened motor activity.

### 8. GRANDIOSITY/GRANDIOSE STATEMENTS:

Exaggerated self-opinion, conviction of unusual ability or powers. Rate only on the basis of patient's statements about himself or self in relation to others, not on the basis of his demeanor.

### 9. DEPRESSIVE MOOD:

Despondency in mood, sadness. Rate only degree of despondency; do not rate on the basis of inferences concerning depression based upon general retardation and somatic complaints.

### 10. HOSTILITY—STATEMENTS AND BEHAVIOR:

Animosity, contempt, threats, belligerence, disdain for other people. Rate solely on the basis of reported feelings and of actions of the patient toward others; do not infer hostility from neurotic defenses, anxiety, or somatic complaints.

### 11. SUSPICIOUSNESS:

Belief (delusional or otherwise) that others have now, or have had in the past, malicious or discriminatory intent toward the patient. On the basis of verbal report and behavior, rate only those suspicions currently held, whether they concern past or present circumstances.

### 12. HALLUCINATORY BEHAVIOR/HALLUCINATION STATEMENTS:

Perceptions without normal external stimulus correspondence. Rate only those experiences which are reported to have occurred during the rating period and which are described as distinctly different from the thought and imagery process of normal people.

### 13. MOTOR RETARDATION/BEHAVIOR:

Reduction in energy level, evidenced in slowed movements and speech, reduced body tone, decreased number of movements. Rate on the basis of observed behavior of the patient only; do not rate on the basis of patient's subjective impression of own energy level.

| Not present | Mild | Moderate | Severe | Not ratable |
|---|---|---|---|---|
| | OCCAS. | FREQUENT | PERVASIVE | |
| 1 | 2 3 | 4 5 | 6 7 | 0 |
| | EXPAN-SIVE | SPECIAL ABILITIES | DELUSIONAL STATE | |
| 1 | 2 3 | 4 5 | 6 7 | 0 |
| | SAD | DESPONDENT | DESPAIRING | |
| 1 | 2 3 | 4 5 | 6 7 | 0 |
| | ANNOYED | HOSTILE | RAGING | |
| 1 | 2 3 | 4 5 | 6 7 | 0 |
| | SEEMS GUARDED | SAYS DOESN'T TRUST | PARANOID DELUSIONS | |
| 1 | 2 3 | 4 5 | 6 7 | 0 |
| | OCCAS. WITH INSIGHT | OFTEN AND NO INSIGHT | PERVASIVE | |
| 1 | 2 3 | 4 5 | 6 7 | 0 |
| | SLOWED | RETARDED | CATATONIC | |
| 1 | 2 3 | 4 5 | 6 7 | 0 |

*Continued.*

### 14. UNCOOPERATIVENESS:

Evidences of resistance, unfriendliness, resentment, and lack of readiness to cooperate with ward procedures and with others.

### 15. UNUSUAL THOUGHT CONTENT:

Unusual, odd, strange, or bizarre thought content. Rate here the degree of unusualness, not the degree of disorganization of thought processes.

### 16. BLUNTED AFFECT:

Reduced emotional tone, apparent lack of normal feeling or involvement.

### 17. EXCITEMENT:

Heightened emotional tone, increased reactivity, agitation, impulsivity.

### 18. DISORIENTATION:

Confusion or lack of proper association for person, place, or time.

### 19. LOSS OF FUNCTIONING*:

Rate general level of functioning

---

*Item 19 is a global scale that is not added in with the other items. Items 1 to 18 are added together to give the total score.

Reprinted with permission of the authors and publisher from Overall JE and Gorham DR: The brief psychiatric rating scale, Psychol Rep 10:799–812, 1962. (Modified, 1966.)

| Not present | Mild | Moderate | Severe | Not ratable |
|---|---|---|---|---|
| | RESENTS | HEARTH | RECOST3 | |
| 1 | 2  3 | 4  5 | 6  7 | 0 |
| | ODD | BIZARRE | IMPOSSIBLE | |
| 1 | 2  3 | 4  5 | 6  7 | 0 |
| | LOWERED FEELING | FLAT | MECHANICAL | |
| 1 | 2  3 | 4  5 | 6  7 | 0 |
| | IN-CREASED EMOTION | INTENSE | OFF THE WALL | |
| 1 | 2  3 | 4  5 | 6  7 | 0 |
| | MUDDLED | CONFUSED | DISORI-ENTED | |
| 1 | 2  3 | 4  5 | 6  7 | 0 |
| | MILD LOSS | MODERATE LOSS | SEVERE LOSS | |
| 1 | 2  3 | 4  5 | 6  7 | 0 |

# A Simple Method to Determine Tardive Dyskinesia Symptoms: AIMS* Examination Procedure

Patient Identification _____  Date _____

Rated by _____

Either before or after completing the examination procedure, observe the patient unobtrusively at rest (eg, in waiting room).

The chair to be used in this examination should be a hard, firm one without arms.

After observing the patient, he may be rated on a scale of 0 (none), 1 (minimal), 2 (mild), 3 (moderate) and 4 (severe) according to the severity of symptoms.

Ask the patient whether there is anything in his/her mouth (ie, gum, candy, etc) and if there is to remove it.

Ask patient about the *current* condition of his/her teeth. Ask patient if he/she wears dentures. Do teeth or dentures bother patient *now?*

Ask patient whether he/she notices any movement in mouth, face, hands or feet. If yes, ask to describe and to what extent they *currently* bother patient or interfere with his/her activities.

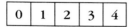

Have patient sit in chair with hands on knees, legs slightly apart and feet flat on floor. (Look at entire body for movements while in this position.)

*Abnormal Involuntary Movement Scale
†Activated movements
From Sandoz Pharmaceuticals, East Hanover, N.J. 07936.

| 0 | 1 | 2 | 3 | 4 |
|---|---|---|---|---|

Ask patient to sit with hands hanging unsupported. If male, between legs, if female and wearing a dress, hanging over knees. (Observe hands and other body areas.)

| 0 | 1 | 2 | 3 | 4 |
|---|---|---|---|---|

Ask patient to open mouth. (Observe tongue at rest within mouth.) Do this twice.

| 0 | 1 | 2 | 3 | 4 |
|---|---|---|---|---|

Ask patient to protrude tongue. (Observe abnormalities of tongue movement.) Do this twice.

| 0 | 1 | 2 | 3 | 4 |
|---|---|---|---|---|

Ask patient to tap thumb, with each finger, as rapidy as possible for 10-15 seconds; separately with right hand, then with left hand. (Observe facial and leg movements.)

| 0 | 1 | 2 | 3 | 4 |
|---|---|---|---|---|

Flex and extend patient's left and right arms. (One at a time.)

| 0 | 1 | 2 | 3 | 4 |
|---|---|---|---|---|

Ask patient to stand up. (Observe in profile. Observe all body areas again, hips included.)

| 0 | 1 | 2 | 3 | 4 |
|---|---|---|---|---|

†Ask patient to extend both arms outstretched in front with palms down. (Observe trunk, legs and mouth.)

| 0 | 1 | 2 | 3 | 4 |
|---|---|---|---|---|

†Have patient walk a few paces, turn and walk back to chair. (Observe hands and gait.) Do this twice.

# A Rating Scale for Extrapyramidal Side Effects

1. **Gait**—The patient is examined as he walks into the examining room, his gait, the swing of his arms, his general posture, all form the basis for an overall score for this item. This is rated as follows:
   0—normal
   1—diminution in swing while the patient is walking
   2—marked diminution in swing with obvious rigidity in the arm
   3—stiff gait with arms held rigidly before the abdomen
   4—stooped shuffling gait with propulsion and retropulsion

2. **Arm Dropping**—The patient and the examiner both raise their arms to shoulder height and let them fall to their sides. In a normal subject a stout slap is heard as the arms hit the sides. In the patient with extreme Parkinson's syndrome the arms fall very slowly:
   0—normal, free fall with loud slap and rebound
   1—fall slowed slightly with less audible contact and little rebound
   2—fall slowed, no rebound
   3—marked slowing, no slap at all
   4—arms fall as though against resistance; as though through glue

3. **Shoulder Shaking**—The subject's arms are bent at a right angle at the elbow and are taken one at a time by the examiner who grasps one hand and also clasps the other around the patient's elbow. The subject's upper arm is pushed to and fro and humerus is externally rotated. The degree of resistance from normal to extreme rigidity is scored as follows:
   0—normal
   1—slight stiffness and resistance
   2—moderate stiffness and resistance
   3—marked rigidity with difficulty in passive movement
   4—extreme stiffness and rigidity with almost a frozen shoulder

4. **Elbow Rigidity**—The elbow joints are separately bent at right angles and passively extended and flexed, with the subject's biceps observed and simultaneously palpated. The resistance to this procedure is rated. (The presence of cogwheel rigidity is noted separately.) Scoring is from 0-4 as in Shoulder Shaking test.

5. **Fixation of position or *Wrist Rigidity***—The wrist is held in one hand and the fingers held by the examiner's other hand, with the wrist moved to extension flexion and both ulner and radial deviation. The resistance to this procedure is ᴜᴀᴛᴇᴜ ᴀꜱ ɪɴ ɪᴛᴇᴍꜱ .ɪ ᴀɴᴜ 4,

6. ***Leg Pendulousness***—The patient sits on a table with his legs hanging down and swinging free. The ankle is grasped by the examiner and raised until the knee is partially extended. It is then allowed to fall. The resistance to falling and the lack of swinging form the basis for the score on this item:
   0—the legs swing freely
   1—slight diminution in the swing of the legs
   2—moderate resistance to swing
   3—marked resistance and damping of swing
   4—complete absence of swing

7. ***Head Dropping***—The patient lies on a well-padded examining table and his head is raised by the examiner's hand. The hand is then withdrawn and the head allowed to drop. In the normal subject the head will fall upon the table. The movement is delayed in extrapyramidal system disorder, and in extreme parkinsonism it is absent. The neck muscles are rigid and the head does not reach the examining table. Scoring is as follows:
   0—the head falls completely with a good thump as it hits the table
   1—slight slowing in fall, mainly noted by lack of slap as head meets the table
   2—moderate slowing in the fall quite noticeable to the eye
   3—head falls stiffly and slowly
   4—head does not reach examining table

8. ***Glabella Tap***—Subject is told to open his eyes wide and not to blink. The glabella region is tapped at a steady, rapid speed. The number of times patient blinks in succession is noted:
   0—0-5 blinks         3—16-20 blinks
   1—6-10 blinks        4—21 and more blinks
   2—11-15 blinks

9. ***Tremor***—Patient is observed walking into examining room and then is reexamined for this item:
   0—normal
   1—mild finger tremor, obvious to sight and touch
   2—tremor of hand or arm occuring spasmodically
   3—persistent tremor of one or more limbs
   4—whole body tremor

10. ***Salivation***—Patient is observed while talking and then asked to open his mouth and elevate his tongue. The following ratings are given:
    0—normal
    1—excess salivation to the extent that pooling takes place if the mouth is open and the tongue is raised
    2—when excess salivation is present and might occasionally result in difficulty in speaking
    3—speaking with difficulty because of excess salivation
    4—frank drooling

# Mental Health Systems Act Recommended Bill of Rights

1. The right to appropriate treatment in a setting and under conditions most supportive of and least restrictive to personal liberty.
2. The right to an individualized, written treatment plan, periodic review of treatment, and revision of plan.
3. The right to ongoing participation in the planning of services and the right to a reasonable explanation of general mental condition, treatment objective, adverse effects of treatment, reasons for treatment, and available alternatives.
4. The right to receive treatment except in an emergency or as permitted by law.
5. The right not to participate in experimentation.
6. The right to freedom from restraint or seclusion.
7. The right to a human treatment environment.
8. The right to confidentiality of records.
9. The right of access to records unless provided by third parties or unless access would be detrimental to health.
10. The right of access to telephone use, mail, and visitors.
11. The right to know these rights.
12. The right to assess grievances when rights are infringed.
13. The right to referral when discharged.

Adapted from Mental Health Systems Act, PL 96-398, Section 9501, U.S. Congress, 96th Congress, 1980.

# Schedules of Controlled Drugs

SCHEDULE I: All nonresearch use forbidden
  *Narcotics*
    Heroin
  *Hallucinogens*
    LSD
    MDA, STP, DMT, mescaline,
      peyote, bufotenine, psilocybin
  *Marijuana*, tetrahydrocannabinols
SCHEDULE II: No telephoned prescriptions; no refills
  *Narcotics*
    Opium
    Opium alkaloids and derived
      phenanthrene alkaloids:
      Morphine, codeine,
      hydromorphone (Dilaudid),
      oxymorphine (Numorphan)
    Designated synthetic drugs:
      Meperidine (Demerol),
      methadone (Dolophine),
      levorphanol (Levo-Dromoran)
  *Stimulants*
    Coca leaves and cocaine
    Amphetamine
    Dextroamphetamine
    Methamphetamine
    Phenmetrazine (Preludin)
    Methylphenidate (Ritalin)

Adapted from Knoben JE and Anderson PO: Handbook of clinical drug data, Hamilton, Ill. 1983, Drug Intelligence Publications, Inc., pp. 238-240.

*Depressants*
Amobarbital
Pentobarbital
Secobarbital
Methaqualone
Phencyclidine (PCP)
SCHEDULE III: Prescription must be rewritten after 6 months or 5 refills
*Narcotics:* The following opiates in
combination with one or more
active nonnarcotic ingredients,
provided the amount does not
exceed that shown:
Codeine: not to exceed 1800 mg/
dl or 90 mg/tablet or other
dose unit.
Opium: 500 mg/dl, or 25 mg/5
ml, or other dosage unit
*Narcotic antagonist*
Nalorphine (Nalline)
*Depressants*
Schedule II barbiturates in
mixtures with noncontrolled
drugs or in suppository dose
form
Butabarbital (Butisol)
Glutethimide (Doriden)
Methyprylon (Noludar)
*Stimulants*
Benzphetamine (Didrex)
Diethylpropion (Tenuate)
Mazindol (Sanorex)
Phendimetrazine (Plegine)
SCHEDULE IV: Prescription must be rewritten after 6 months or five refills.
Differs from Schedule III in penalties for illegal possession.
*Narcotics*
Pentazocine (Talwin)
Propoxyphene (Darvon)
*Stimulants*
Phentermine
Fenfluramine (Pondimin)

*Depressants*
- Benzodiazepines
  - Alprazolam (Xanax)
  - Chlordiazepoxide (Librium)
  - Clonazepam (Clonopin)
  - Clorazepate (Tranxene)
  - Diazepam (Valium)
  - Flurazepam (Dalmane)
  - Lorazepam (Ativan)
  - Oxazepam (Serax)
  - Temazepam (Restoril)
  - Triazolam (Halcion)
- Choral hydrate
- Ethchlorvynol (Placidyl)
- Meprobamate
- Mephobarbital (Mebaral)
- Paraldehyde
- Phenobarbital

SCHEDULE V: As any other nonnarcotic prescription drug: may also be dispensed without prescription unless additional state regulations apply

*Narcotics*
- Diphenoxylate (not more than 2.5 mg and not less than 0.025 mg of atropine per dosage unit, as in Lomotil)
- The following drugs in combination with other active, nonnarcotic ingredients and provided the amount per 100 ml or 100 g does not exceed that shown:
- Codeine: 200 mg
- Dihydrocodeine: 100 mg
- Ethylmorphine: 100 mg

# Glossary

**abstract thinking** the ability to find meaning in proverbs. The ability to conceptualize.

**acquired immune deficiency syndrome (AIDS)** a contagious and fatal viral disease that affects the immune system.

**active listening** verbal and nonverbal skills used by the examiner to demonstrate interest and concern to the patient.

**addiction** psychological and physiological symptoms indicating that an individual cannot control his use of psychoactive substances; termed psychoactive substance dependence in the *DSM-III-R*.

**affect** emotional range attached to ideas; outwardly manifested.

> **appropriate a.** emotional tone in harmony with the accompanying idea, thought, or verbalization.
>
> **blunted a.** a disturbance manifested by a severe reduction in the intensity of affect.
>
> **flat a.** absence or near absence of any signs of affective expression.
>
> **inappropriate a.** incongruence between the emotional feeling tone and the idea, thought, or speech accompanying it.

> **labile a.** rapid changes in emotional feeling tone, unrelated to external stimuli.

**affective disorders** a group of psychiatric diagnoses characterized by mood disturbances on a continuum of depression to mania; termed mood disorders in the *DSM-III-R*.

**aggression** forceful verbal or physical action; that is, the motor counterpart of the affect of anger, rage, or hostility.

**agitation** anxiety associated with severe motor restlessness.

**agnosia** difficulty in recognizing familiar objects; a symptom of organic brain disease.

**agoraphobia** the fear of being in a place or situation in which escape might be difficult or embarrassing or in which help might not be available in case of a panic attack.

**akathisia** motor restlessness generally expressed as the inability to sit still; caused by the dopamine blockade of certain types of neuroleptic medications. An extrapyramidal side effect (EPS).

**alcoholic** an individual whose compulsive use of alcohol causes problems at home, at work, or socially and who

675

continues to use alcohol despite these adverse consequences.

**Alcoholics Anonymous (AA)** a self-help organization that uses a 12-step program to assist alcoholics to achieve and maintain sobriety; Al-Anon is concerned with spouses of alcoholics; Alateen is concerned with the teenage children of alcoholics.

**alertness** an awareness and attentiveness to surroundings.

**Alzheimer's disease** an organic mental disorder resulting in dementia that is related to a progressive deterioration of brain tissue, described as plaques and neurofibrillary tangles.

**ambivalence** opposing impulses or feelings directed toward the same person or object at the same time.

**amnesia** partial or total inability to recall past information.

> **anterograde a.** recent memory loss, as in the early stages of Alzheimer's disease.
>
> **global a.** total memory loss as in advanced stages of Alzheimer's disease.
>
> **retrograde a.** remote memory loss, as in later stages of Alzheimer's disease.
>
> **short-term a.** memory loss observed in alcoholic blackouts.

**anger** an emotion or feeling expressed as a result of anxiety aroused by a real or perceived threat to one's rights, values, possessions, or significant others.

**anhedonia** loss of pleasure in activities or interests previously enjoyed. A symptom noted in depression and schizophrenia.

**anorexia nervosa** a disturbance in body image accompanied by decreased food intake leading to abnormally low weight.

**Antabuse (disulfiram)** a drug given to alcoholics that blocks the breakdown of acetylaldehyde, producing nausea, vomiting, dizziness, flushing, and tachycardia if alcohol is consumed.

**antisocial personality** a personality disorder characterized by blatant disregard for social norms. Behavior is demonstrated on a continuum of mild to pathological. Psychoanalytic theory attributes this disorder to an underdeveloped superego.

**anxiety** nonspecific, unpleasant feeling of discomfort, with physiological and psychological symptoms that generally have no identifiable cause.

**anxiety disorders** patterns of symptoms and behaviors in which anxiety is either the primary disturbance or a secondary problem that is recognized when the primary symptoms are removed.

**apathy** lack of feeling, interest, or emotion. Indifference.

**aphasia** difficulty in searching for words.

> **motor a.** impaired speech due to organic brain disorder in which understanding remains.
>
> **nominal a.** difficulty in finding the correct words in their proper sequence.
>
> **sensory a.** loss of ability to comprehend the meaning of words.

**appropriate** suitable or fitting for a particular person, purpose, occasion, or situation. Examples: appropriate affect, response, or attire.

**apraxia** inability to perform once known, purposeful, skilled activities in the absence of loss of motor function.

**attitude** a pattern of mental views and feelings accumulated through past experiences and affected by present stimuli. A manner, disposition, tendency, or orientation with regard to a person or situation.

**autistic thinking** thoughts, ideas, or desires derived from internal, private stimuli or drives that often are incongruent with reality; most often applied to persons with schizophrenia.

**axon** the part of the neuron that conducts impulses away from the cell body.

**behavior** any observable, recordable, and measurable movement, response, or act of an individual (verbal and nonverbal)

**bipolar disorder** an affective or mood disorder characterized by at least one episode of mania with or without a history of depression.

**bizarre** markedly unusual in appearance, thought, style, character, or behavior. Absurd.

**blocking** unconscious interruption in train of thoughts.

**borderline personality disorder** a personality disorder with the essential feature of a pervasive pattern of unstable self-image, interpersonal relations, and mood.

**bulimia** compulsive binge eating accompanied by purging and overconcern with body shape and weight.

**catalepsy** state of unconsciousness in which immobility is constantly maintained.

**catatonic behavior** motor anomalies in nonorganic disorders such as schizophrenia.

**excitement** excited motor activity.

**rigidity** assumption of an inappropriate posture.

**circumstantiality** digression of inappropriate thoughts into ideas, eventually reaching the desired goal.

**clang associations** words similar in sound but not in meaning that conjure up new thoughts.

**clarification** a communication skill that helps to define a patient's responses through use of direct questions.

**closed-ended questions** questions that generally elicit a yes or no response. Useful in gathering factual data.

**clouding of consciousness** incomplete clearmindedness, with disturbance in perception and attitude. Example: stupor.

**cognition** the act or process of knowing and perceiving.

**cognitive processes** pertaining to perception, judgment, memory, and reasoning.

**Community Mental Health Centers Act 1963** legislation authorizing federal funds for construction of comprehensive mental health centers.

**comprehension** the capacity to perceive and understand.

**compulsion** uncontrollable impulse to perform an act or ritual repeatedly; may be in response to an obsession (unwilled, persistent thought), as in obsessive-compulsive disorder. The act or ritual serves to decrease anxiety. Examples of rituals: handwashing, cleaning, and checking.

**concrete communication** inability to think and communicate abstractly.

**confabulation** unconscious filling of gaps in memory with imagined or untrue experiences that the person believes but has no basis for in reality.

**confidentiality** treating the information about and from patients in a private manner; information about patients is "confidential" and requires their approval before disclosure.

**confused state** bewildered, perplexed, or unclear. The type and degree of confusion need to be specified.

**congruence** accordant states. Example: mood-congruence in which the person's visible emotional state correlates with his mood or feeling state.

**consciousness** state of awareness.

**consultant-liaison nurse** A psychiatric mental health nurse who provides expert consultation for patients and staff in other parts of the hospital agency.

**conversion** process by which a psychic event, idea, feeling, memory, or impulse is represented by a bodily change or symptom such as blindness or paralysis.

**custodial care** the process of caring for hygienic and nutritional needs in an institution but not providing treatment for mental disorder.

cyclothymia a chronic mood disturbance of at least 2 years duration involving numerous hypomanic episodes and numerous periods of depression. Cyclothymia does not meet the criteria for a manic episode or major depression.

delirium a reversible (usually) bewildered state of clouded consciousness, generally accompanied by restlessness, disorientation, and fear. May include periods of hallucinations.

delusion fixed, false belief, not consistent with the person's intelligence and culture, unamenable to reason.

bizarre d. an absurd belief.

control d. false feeling that one is being controlled by others.

grandeur d. exaggerated conception of importance.

nihilistic d. the false belief that the self, part of the self, or another object has ceased to exist.

paranoid d. oversuspiciousness leading to persecutory delusions.

persecution d. false belief that one is being persecuted.

reference d. false belief that the behavior of others in the environment refers to oneself; derived from ideas of reference in which one falsely feels he is being talked about.

somatic d. false belief involving functioning of one's body.

dementia organic loss of mental functioning, generally with a clear sensorium. Most notable in organic mental disorders.

denial avoidance of disagreeable realities or threats by ignoring or refusing to recognize them. An unconscious defense mechanism that may or may not be adaptive.

depersonalization a feeling of unreality or strangeness related to one's self, body parts, bodily functions, or the external environment.

depression a lowered or saddened mood state or major affective disorder, listed as a mood disorder in the *DSM-III-R.*

derailment gradual or sudden deviation in train of thought without blocking.

derealization distortion of spatial relationships so that the environment becomes unfamiliar.

*Diagnostic and Statistical Manual III-R, 1987* a taxonomy of mental disorders by the American Psychiatric Association.

disoriented disturbance in orientation of time, place, or person.

displacement shift of emotion from an object or person who incites the emotion to a less threatening source. An unconscious defense mechanism that may or may not be adaptive.

dissociation the splitting or separation of any group of mental or behavioral processes from the rest of the person's consciousness or identity.

dissociative reaction process by which an individual blocks off a part of his life from conscious recognition because of severe anxiety (multiple personality disorder).

distractibility inability to concentrate attention.

dopamine a brain neurotransmitter that influences muscle movement and emotions. Dopamine theory states that persons with schizophrenia may have too much dopamine, which may account for their sensory-perceptual alterations.

dysarthria difficulty in articulating single sounds or phonemes of speech.

dyskinesia disturbed coordination and motor activity. A side effect of neuroleptic medications related to dopamine blockade. See also *tardive dyskinesia.*

dyslexia difficulty in reading due to a central lesion.

dysphoria an unpleasant mood state.

**dystonia** muscle spasms of head, neck, and tongue. A side effect of neuroleptic medications that block dopamine.

**echolalia** psychopathological repeating of words of one person by another. Noted in types of schizophrenia.

**echopraxia** initiation of the body position of another.

**ego state** structure of the mind that correlates with one's sense of self. A construct of Freud's psychoanalytic theory.

**emotion** a complex feeling state with psychic, somatic, and behavioral components related to affect and mood.

**euphoria** a false sense of elation or well-being; pathological elevation of mood. Most notable in the manic phase of bipolar disorder.

**euthymia** a normal, homeostatic mood state.

**expansive mood** unrestrained expression of feelings.

**extrapyramidal side effects (EPS)** involuntary muscle movements resulting from the effects of neuroleptic drugs on the extrapyramidal nerve tracts (dopamine blockade).

**eye contact** occasional glancing into the patient's eyes to demonstrate interest during an interaction.

**fantasy** an imaginary sequence of events. Common in childhood. Appropriate as long as a person is aware of reality.

**fear** anxiety due to consciously recognized and realistic danger.

**flight of ideas** a speech pattern manifested by a rapid transition from topic to topic, frequently without completing any of the preceding ideas. Prominent in manic states.

**fugue** a period of personality dissociation with memory loss.

**gait** the manner of progression in walking. Example: ataxic gait, in which the foot is raised high and the sole strikes down suddenly.

**general leads** interactive skills that facilitate the communication process by encouraging the patient to continue.

**grimacing** contortion of facial muscles, may be extrapyramidal side effect.

**hallucination** false sensory perceptions not associated with real external stimuli. May involve any of the five senses: auditory, visual, olfactory, gustatory, or tactile. *Auditory hallucinations* are most prevalent in schizophrenia. The sounds may be perceived as thoughts or voices coming from any type of transmitter or the patient's mind. The messages may be condemning or accusatory or complimentary and encouraging. It is critical that the examiner be aware that the messages may be directing the patient toward harming himself or others, so their content cannot be ignored. *Visual hallucinations* are often associated with organic conditions. *Tactile hallucinations* are common in alcohol withdrawal. Hallucinations may also be an effect of certain types of drugs, such as amphetamines, hallucinogens, and *Cannabis*.

**holistic** pertaining to totality or the whole (holistic care).

**hostile** a feeling of intense anger and resentment, manifested by destructive behavior.

**Huntington's chorea** a genetically transmitted disease that includes motor and cognitive changes.

**hyperactivity** (hyperkinesis) restless, aggressive, often destructive activity. Prominent in manic states.

**hypoactivity** (hypokinesis) decreased activity or retardation (psychomotor retardation); slowing of psychologic and physical functions.

**hypomania** a clinical syndrome similar to but less severe than that demonstrated in a full-blown manic episode.

**illogical (thinking)** thinking containing erroneous conclusions or internal contradictions (irrational thoughts).

**illusion** misinterpretation of a sensory input. Observed in alcoholic withdrawal and anesthesia states.

**insight** the recognition of motivational sources behind one's thoughts, actions, or behavior.

**intellectual functioning** the individual's general fund of knowledge, orientation, memory, mastery of simple mathematical equations, and capacity for abstract thinking.

**intellectualization** one of the unconscious defense mechanisms. A process of thinking excessively about the philosophical or theoretical to the extent that the stream of thought is interrupted and anxiety-provoking issues are avoided.

**judgment and comprehension** the ability to understand, recall, mobilize, and constructively integrate previous learning in meeting new situations.

**Korsakoff's psychosis (Korsakov)** an organic mental disorder with memory loss related to alcohol abuse.

**Kraepelin** German psychiatrist who initiated a classification system for psychiatry in 1896. Used the term *dementia praecox.*

**labile (mood, affect, or behavior)** subject to frequent or unpredictable changes.

**lithium** an element or salt used in the treatment and prevention of manic episodes.

**looseness of associations** vague, unfocused, illogical flow or stream of thought. Notable in schizophrenia.

**magical thinking** belief that thoughts, words, or actions can cause or prevent an occurrence by some magical means.

**mania** a disordered mental state of extreme excitement, hyperactivity, euphoria, and hyperverbal behavior.

**memory** function by which information stored in the brain is later recalled to the conscious mind.

**mental disorder** "A clinically significant behavioral or psychological syndrome or pattern . . . typically associated with a painful symptom . . . or impairment, in one or more important areas of functioning" (*DSM-III-R,* 1987).

**mental retardation** a lack of intelligence so great that it interferes with social and occupational performance.

**mental status examination** a record of current findings that includes a description of a patient's appearance, behavior, motor activity, speech, alertness, mood, cognition, intelligence, reactions, views, and attitudes.

**milieu** the environment.

**mood disorder** a diagnostic category in the *DSM-III-R* that includes the affective disorders.

**NANDA** abbreviation for the North American Nursing Diagnosis Association.

**narcissism** extreme self-centeredness and self-absorption (narcissistic personality disorder).

**neologism** a new word created by the patient for psychological reasons. Noted in some types of schizophrenia.

**neuroleptics** antipsychotic medications.

**neurotransmitter** a chemical found in the nervous system (e.g., norepinephrine, serotonin, dopamine) that facilitates the transmission of nerve impulses across synapses between neurons. Implicated in affective and schizophrenic disorders.

**nursing diagnosis** a statement that describes a patient's illness or response to illness treatable by nurses.

**obsession** the pathological persistence of an unwilled thought, feeling, or impulse to the extent that it cannot be eliminated from consciousness by a logical effort.

**obsessive-compulsive disorder** recurrent obsessions (thoughts) alternating with compulsions (behaviors). Both are unwilled and painful.

**open posture** a relaxed, yet attentive position, with arms uncrossed. Enhances patient's trust in the examiner.

**open-ended statement** a statement that elicits further exploration of the patient's problem by encouraging communication. Can also be in the form of a question.

**organic mental disorders** a class of disorders of mental functioning caused by permanent brain damage or temporary brain dysfunction. The cause is known and may be primary (originating in the brain) or secondary to systemic disease. Cognition, emotions, and motivation are affected.

**orientation** conscious awareness of person, place, and time.

**panic** a state of extreme, acute, intense anxiety, accompanied by disorganization of personality and function.

**paranoid thinking** oversuspiciousness. May lead to persecutory delusions or projectile behavior patterns.

**parkinsonism symptoms** masked facies, muscle rigidity, and shuffling gait; common in patients taking neuroleptic drugs; extrapyramidal side effects related to dopamine blockade.

**perception** awareness of objects and relations that follows stimulation of peripheral sense organs.

**perseveration** psychopathological repetition of the same word or idea in response to different questions.

**personality disorder** exaggerated, pathological behavior patterns destructive to the individual and others.

**phobia** exaggerated, pathological dread or fear of some specific type of stimulus or situation.

    **acrophobia** dread of high places.

    **agoraphobia** dread of open places.

    **claustrophobia** dread of closed places.

**phobic disorder** severe phobic behavior patterns that render the individual dysfunctional. Avoidance of the feared object or situation serves to assuage anxiety.

**schizophrenia** a syndrome, illness, or mental health disorder heterogeneous in cause, pathogenesis, presenting picture, response to treatment, and prognosis. Symptoms generally reflect a progressive deterioration and disorganization of the individual's personality structure, affect, and cognition. The *DSM-III-R* lists the following types: paranoid, catatonic, disorganized, undifferentiated, and residual.

**shuffling gait (parkinsonism gait)** a style of walking typically demonstrated by individuals whose dopamine stores have been blocked or depleted as a result of Parkinson's disease or antipsychotic medications.

**somatization** the conversion of mental states or experiences into bodily symptoms; associated with anxiety.

**stereotypy** continuous repetition of speech or physical activities.

**stressor** a stimulus perceived by the individual or the organism as challenging, threatening, or damaging.

**suicidal ideation** verbalization of a person's inclination to do self-injury or self-destruction.

**suicidal plan** a specific method designed to inflict self-injury or self-destruction as verbalized by an individual.

**superego** psychoanalytic structure of the mind equivalent to the conscience (sense of right and wrong). Develops in early childhood.

**tangentiality** inability to have goal-directed associations of thought; never gets to desired goal from desired point.

**tardive dyskinesia** an extrapyramidal syndrome that usually emerges late in the course of long-term antipsychotic drug therapy. Includes grimacing, buccolingual movements, and dystonia (impaired muscle tonus). May be irreversible in some persons.

**therapeutic communication** interactive verbal and nonverbal strategies that focus on the needs of the patient and facilitate a goal-directed, client-oriented communication process.

**thinking** the process of following a goal-directed flow of ideas, symbols, and associations to a logical conclusion in accordance with the person's developmental stage.

**thought disorder** thinking characterized by loose associations, neologisms, and illogical constructs and conclusions.

**undoing** a defense mechanism by which a person symbolically acts out to reverse a previously committed act or thought. A common ritual in obsessive-compulsive disorder.

**validation** the process of confirming an individual's intent by questioning the content of his message.

**withdrawal** the act or process of turning inward to avoid a perceived environmental threat. Also, a physiological response to cessation of an addictive substance.

**word salad** incoherent mixture of words or phrases.

# Study Questions

## Chapter 1

1. The forces behind deinstitutionalization started gaining momentum during what period?
   a. 1940s and 1950s
   b. 1960s
   c. 1970s
   d. Early 1980s

2. Which of the following are part of the convergence of forces that created the groundswell for deinstitutionalization?
   a. Opponents of state hospitals
   b. Confidence in psychopharmacology
   c. New emphasis on civil rights
   d. Economic forces, e.g., ATD, SSI
   e. All of the above

3. There is general agreement that four benchmarks in the history of psychiatric care are significant. Which item below includes a legitimate representive from each benchmark era?
   a. Tuke, Pinel, Freud, ECT
   b. Pinel or Tuke, Freud, chlorpromazine (Thorazine), community mental health centers

4. The decline of interest in inpatient psychiatric nursing may be attributed to which of the following?
   a. Community mental health centers and consequent outpatient care
   b. The advent of newer roles for psychiatric nurses
   c. Both of the above

## Chapter 2

Match the examples with the most appropriate defense mechanism.

1. _____ I told you that I do not want to talk about         a. Denial
   my boss now, maybe tomorrow.                                   b. Suppression
2. _____ I do not have my list of goals because my pen       b. Reaction formation
   ran out of ink.                                                d. Repression

3. _____    Despite knowing about her husband's affair,    e. Rationalization
the patient tells the nurse, "I love my hus-
band, he's such a good man."

4. Mr. Lawrence, a 29-year-old patient, tells the nurse that he has had three factory
jobs in the last 8 months. His bosses have told him that he is too slow for the
assembly line, and none of his coworkers would help him. Mr. Lawrence feels
alone and is having difficulty with his ceramics project. With which developmental stage is he struggling?
a. Autonomy vs. shame and doubt
b. Initiative vs. guilt
c. Industry vs. inferiority

5. According to Selye's General Adaptation Syndrome (GAS), which behaviors can
occur in the stage of exhaustion?
a. Personality disorganization, immobilization, or suicide
b. Increased alertness, mild anxiety, and mobilization of resources
c. Problem solving with assistance and moderate anxiety

Mark the following statements true or false.

6. _____    The nurse teaches the patient that he is responsible for himself and
can make appropriate choices or decisions.

7. _____    Irrational beliefs based on feelings of self-blame and guilt do not produce feelings of anxiety and hostility toward self.

8. Describe how concepts from various theoretical models can assist the nurse with
understanding patient behaviors and problems.

## Chapter 3

1. Psychotherapeutic management includes
a. A therapeutic nurse-patient relationship
b. Appropriate use of psychopharmacology
c. A well-managed milieu
d. All of the above

2. Upon what foundation are the components of psychotherapeutic management
based?
a. Knowledge of drugs
b. Knowledge of psychopathology
c. Knowledge of the client-centered approach
d. Knowledge of mental mechanisms

3. According to the premise on which psychotherapeutic management is based,
which of the following components is most important?
a. A therapeutic nurse-patient relationship
b. Appropriate use of psychopharmacology
c. A well-managed milieu
d. All are equally important functions of the psychiatric nurse

4. When the nurse uses structured times for working with the patient, contracts with the patient for length and number of sessions, and implements a specific therapeutic model, the nurse is
   a. Being therapeutic
   b. Providing therapy
   c. Engaging in psychotherapeutic management
   d. None of the above

## Chapter 4

1. Our fundamental rights flow from which of the following?
   a. Amendments to the Constitution of the United States
   b. Constitutions of individual states
   c. Neither of the above
   d. Both a and b

2. The specific rights accorded mental patients are derived from which of the following basic rights?
   (1) Freedom from unreasonable search and seizure
   (2) Right of privacy
   (3) Freedom of choice and self-determination
   (4) Freedom of speech
   (5) Freedom to bear arms
       a. (1), (2), (3)
       b. (1), (2), (3), (4)
       c. (2), (3), (4)
       d. All of the above

3. *Griswold v. Connecticut* was a court case that considered the issue of
   a. Exemption from guilt by reason of insantiy
   b. Right to treatment
   c. Right of personal privacy
   d. Right to refuse treatment

4. *Wyatt v. Stickney* was a court case that considered the issue of
   a. Exemption from guilt by reason of insanity
   b. Right to treatment
   c. Right of personal privacy
   d. Right to refuse treatment

5. *Tarasoff v. The Regents of the University of California* was a court case that considered the issue of
   a. Right to refuse treatment
   b. Duty to warn of threatened suicide
   c. Duty to warn of threatened harm to self or others
   d. Right to refuse treatment

6. Individuals can be treated involuntarily if they are
   (1) Dangerous to self
   (2) Dangerous to others
   (3) Gravely disabled
   (4) Unable to provide food and shelter for self (i.e., homeless)
      a. All of the above
      b. Only (1) and (2) in about half the states
      c. (1), (2), (3) in a majority of the states
      d. (1) and (4)

7. An important nursing concern when one is caring for the patient involuntarily detained for evaluation and emergency care is
   (1) Basic nursing assessment documentation
   (2) Adherence to legal time constraints
   (3) Developing a nursing care plan
      a. All of the above
      b. (1) and (3)
      c. (2) only
      d. (3) only

8. The probable cause statement is required by the
   a. Fourth Amendment of the Constitution of the United States
   b. *Wyatt v. Stickney*
   c. Mental Health Code
   d. *Griswold v. Connecticut*

9. Which of the following patient rights can be suspended with good cause?
   a. Right to treatment in least restrictive alternative
   b. Right to freedom from restraint and seclusion
   c. Right to confidentiality of records
   d. Right to daily exercise

## Chapter 5

1. Therapeutic communication
   a. Involves intimacy and equal opportunities for spontaneity between a patient and nurse
   b. Resembles the "give and take" of social communication
   c. Is structured with a plan and purpose
   d. Is dominated by the therapist

2. One general goal of therapeutic communication is to
   a. Assist the patient to learn problem-solving skills
   b. Express anger and hostility whenever he or she feels these emotions
   c. Become friends
   d. Use a wide variety of techniques

3. Reflection is a technique that facilitates therapeutic communication by
   a. Giving approval for behavior that the nurse wants to reward
   b. Demonstrating the skills of the nurse

   c. Restating or repeating the patient's statement to encourage clarification or
      continuation of the same thoughts
   d. Serving as a "mirror" where the nurse takes on the patient's feelings

4. Listening is an aspect of therapeutic communication
   a. That can be done by anyone
   b. Aims to understand, integrate, and guide the conversation with a few carefully
      selected words
   c. Allows the patient to direct the conversation and "subject-hop" as desired
   d. That results in few benefits for the patient

5. Limit setting helps the patient by
   a. Modifying behavior
   b. Enlisting the patient's opinion about acceptable behavior
   c. Adopting socially acceptable responses
   d. Establishing rules and boundaries that incorporate honesty and safety

6. One of the common barriers to therapeutic communication is
   a. Feedback
   b. Objectivity
   c. Rhythms or patterns
   d. Evasion

## Chapter 6

1. The nurse-patient relationship is
   a. Based on a single theoretical model that explains dynamics of the patient's
      needs
   b. Conducted by a nurse psychotherapist who offers specialized techniques for
      specialized problems
   c. Based on a foundation of companionship, mutual support, and interest
   d. A series of goal-directed interactions conveying respect and a willingness to
      help the patient with his needs and problems

Match the stage of the nurse-patient relationship with the appropriate description.

2. _____   Exploring problems, identifying solutions, testing          a. Preparaton
              new behaviors                                                b. Orientation
3. _____   Facilitating trust, collecting information, defining         c. Working
              tentative goals                                             d. Termination
4. _____   Discussing feelings about the relationship and iden-
              tifying resources in the community and long-term
              goals

5. Mrs. Jackson was admitted to the unit a week ago with complaints of fatigue,
   inability to get out of bed to get to work, and low self-esteem. During a phone
   call to her husband she begins screaming, "Don't leave me, I need you." She then
   runs to her room and while throwing all of her clothes into her suitcase, she
   says repeatedly, "Home ... Dan ... he can't ...." Your assessment and immediate
   intervention is

    a. The patient is experiencing a crisis situation. You allow her to cry and en-
courage her to talk about what just happened but let her know you will not
let her leave the unit at this time.

    b. The patient is angry at her husband. You encourage her to discuss her feelings
and what she can do on her weekend pass when she sees him.

    c. The patient does not want her husband to leave her. You encourage her to
identify ways of reconciling with her husband and call her doctor for an order
for a pass.

    d. The patient is out of control because of stresses. You let her cry for a few
minutes and then ask her to put her clothes and suitcase away.

6. When nursing interventions are being planned, the nursing diagnoses are
    a. Based on what the patient identifies as issues for him to work on
    b. Specific patient problems that point to a desired patient outcome
    c. Specific behavioral goals the patient needs to work on during this admission
    d. Specific nursing activities needed to assist the patient in achieving goals

7. Issues and patient behaviors interfering with progress in the nurse-patient relationship are which of the following?
    a. Generally ignored until the patient is more stable
    b. Usually not significant enough to address directly
    c. Most often assessed and then a specific intervention designed
    d. Generally not charted because of a need for confidentiality

8. Briefly discuss strategies used by the nurse in the roles of facilitator and educator.

## Chapter 7

1. Which of the following statements about anger is true?
    a. Open displays of anger should be discouraged.
    b. Verbalization of anger is detrimental to relationships.
    c. Anger is a normal response to frustration of desires and needs.
    d. Suppression of anger helps decrease the potential for violence.

2. Which of the following is the major guide in dealing with the overt expression
of aggression?
    a. The ANA Standards for Psychiatric Nursing
    b. The social norms defining assault and battery
    c. The hospital protocols for seclusion and restraints
    d. The principle of least restrictive alternative

3. Which of the following statements is accurate?
    a. Verbal aggression is a safe alternative to physical aggression.
    b. Assertiveness allows expression of feelings while protecting the rights of self
and others.
    c. Passive-aggressive individuals are usually turning their anger inward.
    d. Passive individuals rarely cause trouble with others.

Mark the following statements true or false.

4. _____    Expression of anger tends to change as a child gets older.

5. _____ Alcohol and drugs have little effect on expressions of anger.

Match the phase of the assault cycle with the most appropriate nursing intervention.

6. _____ Escalation phase
7. _____ Recovery phase

a. Encouraging ventilation of feelings and a description of the situation
b. Offering p.r.n. medications and time out in a quiet room
c. Staff control by use of seclusion and restraints
d. Debriefing among staff and with the patient

8. Identify the nursing care required for a patient in restraints.

## Chapter 8

1. The leadership functions of the psychiatric nurse are
   a. Observed only in formal, planned, and structured group meetings
   b. Seldom demonstrated on an inpatient unit
   c. Inherent in the role of a psychotherapeutic manager

2. Which of the following statements best describes how patients benefit from groups?
   a. Patients gain support from the group leader.
   b. Testing out new behaviors can occur when the patient is discharged.
   c. Feelings of powerlessness are not addressed.
   d. Patients learn how their behaviors affect others.

Match each of the following groups with its appropriate description.

3. _____ Support group
4. _____ Remotivation group
5. _____ Education or problem-solving group

a. Helps patients to cope and negotiate problems in living
b. Reinforces patient strengths and behaviors
c. Facilitates communication and interaction with each other

6. Discuss the positive factors of coleadership.

7. Give an example of a nursing intervention for a hostile patient.

## Chapter 9

Mark the following statements true or false.

1. A psychiatric nurse consultant may be useful to an organization when a major change is needed or when an area is not functioning well.

2. Orginally, the role of the liaison nurse focused on the mental health needs of patients and their families in health care facilities.

3. Key factors in the success of the role of the consultant are
   a. Being in a supervisory position facilitates change.
   b. The consultee is ultimately responsible for the patient.
   c. The roles are the same regardless of setting.
   d. The focus is personal not professional concerns.

4. List the three main types of consultation.

5. Which of the following statements is accurate concerning the phases of a consultation relationship?
   a. Assessment includes identifying the perception of the problem by the people involved as well as that of the consultant.
   b. Goal setting identifies a contact person, a time frame for activities, and the means for reporting progress.
   c. Formulation of agreement involves development of an action plan that is realistic and practical.
   d. Disengagement is the process of evaluating whether the desired outcomes were achieved.

6. Describe ways in which the consultant functions as an educator, facilitator, and researcher.

## Chapter 10

1. Psychotropic medications were partially responsible for the development of which of the following concepts?
   a. Least restrictive alternative
   b. Psychotherapeutic management
   c. Psychoeducation
   d. Noncompliance

2. A substance that changes the resting potential of a postsynaptic membrane is a
   a. Psychoactive drug
   b. Cerebrospinal agent
   c. Poison
   d. Neurotransmitter

3. Neurotransmitters
   a. Are synthesized from natural precursors
   b. Are stored in storage vesicles in the presynaptic terminals
   c. Combine with specific receptors
   d. All of the above

4. Psychotropic drugs affect neurotransmitters in several ways. They can
   (1) Release stored neurotransmitters
   (2) Block neurotransmitters
   (3) Affect the response of a neurotransmitter
   (4) Terminate the inactivation of a neurotransmitter
   (5) Increase the number of neurons releasing neurotransmitters
       a. (1), (2), (3), (5)
       b. (1), (2), (3), (4)
       c. (2), (4), (5)
       d. (1), (2), (4)
       e. All of the above

5. The brain is protected from fluctuations in the body by the
   a. Spinal cord
   b. CNS
   c. Blood-brain barrier
   d. All of the above

6. The most important chemical property influencing a drug's ability to pass easily through the blood-brain barrier is
   a. Water solubility
   b. Lipid solubility
   c. Transport systems

7. Which of the following drugs can most easily pass the blood-brain barrier?
   a. Penicillin
   b. Ethanol
   c. Dopamine
   d. Potassium

## Chapter 11

1. Parkinsonism can be caused by
   a. An imbalance between dopamine and acetylcholine
   b. Age-related degeneration of the extrapyramidal system
   c. Dopamine-depleting drugs such as antipsychotic drugs
   d. All of the above

2. A decreased availability of dopamine in the brain is responsible for
   a. Parkinsonism
   b. Schizophrenia
   c. Tardive dyskinesia

3. Which of the following drugs (assuming dosage is the same) when taken by mouth has the greatest potential for aggravating schizophrenia (hint: has the greatest potential to increase dopamine levels)?
   a. Dopamine
   b. L-dopa
   c. Levodopa-carbidopa (Sinemet)
   d. Chlorpromazine

4. The pharmacological goal in treating parkinsonism is to
   (1) Increase acetylcholine to balance dopamine
   (2) Increase dopamine to balance acetylcholine
   (3) Decrease acetylcholine to balance dopamine
   (4) Decrease dopamine to balance acetylcholine
        a. (1), (2)
        b. (1), (3)
        c. (2), (3)
        d. (2), (4)
        e. All of the above

5. Extrapyramidal side effects are related to parkinsonism because
   a. Both are related to decreased availability of dopamine.
   b. Both are related to increased availability of dopamine.
   c. They are not related.

6. The antiparkinsonism drug that blocks the conversion of L-dopa to dopamine in the peripheral nervous system is
   a. Amantadine (Symmetrel)
   b. Carbidopa-levodopa (Sinemet)
   c. Bromocriptine
   d. Trihexyphenidyl (Artane)

7. The antiparkinsonism drug that decreases the availability of acetylcholine is
   a. Amantadine (Symmetrel)
   b. Carbidopa-levodopa (Sinemet)
   c. Bromocriptine
   d. Trihexyphenidyl (Artane)

## Chapter 12

1. A man being treated for schizophrenia enters the nurses' station with his eyes fixed upward. You know he has been involved in group therapy, is on haloperidol (Haldol), 10 mg t.i.d., and has been attending occupational therapy. He screams, "I can't move my eyes. I'm going crazy." What is going on? What should you do?
   a. Call the doctor. This could be a life-threatening seizure.
   b. He is having a dystonic reaction. Check the chart for a p.r.n. anticholinergic to give him.
   c. Ignore him and do not reinforce attention-seeking behaviors.
   d. He is having a bizarre manifestation of his psychosis. Talk to him in a calm voice and check the chart for a p.r.n. antipsychotic to give him.

2. The first psychotropic drug introduced in the U.S. was
   a. Chlorpromazine in about 1954.
   b. Imipramine (Tofranil) in about 1959.
   c. Lithium in 1949.
   d. Haloperidol in 1963

3. High-potency antipsychotic drugs are more likely to have more severe _____ side effects than low-potency antipsychotics.
   a. Sedative
   b. Orthostatic hypotension
   c. Extrapyramidal
   d. Anticholinergic

4. If in preparing the nursing care plan for a 65-year-old man you learn that he has symptoms of prostatic hypertrophy, which of the following side effects of low-potency antipsychotic drugs would concern you most?

a. Sedative
b. Orthostatic hypotension
c. Extrapyramidal
ii    iiiiiiiiiiiiiiiiiiiijiii

5. Inability to sit coupled with complaints of "something is going on inside my legs" would indicate which EPS?
   a. Parkinsonism
   b. Dystonia
   c. Akathisia
   d. Tardive dyskinesia

6. Mr. Jones reports hearing voices and beginning to feel "crazy." He admits that he has not been taking his antipsychotic medication. Which of the following medications would be most effective for Mr. Jones if he cannot see the nurse daily?
   a. Chlorpromazine
   b. Fluphenazine (Prolixin decanoate)
   c. Haloperidol
   d. Fluphenazine (Prolixin)

7. If only drugs are provided and the nurse does not establish a therapeutic nurse-patient relationship nor a well-managed milieu, the patient will
   a. Decompensate
   b. Become violent
   c. Receive only custodial care

8. Mr. Smith is prescribed haloperidol, 10 mg t.i.d. After 5 days he complains of tremor, rigidity, and difficulty in initiating movement. These symptoms are
   a. Antiadrenergic effects
   b. Extrapyramidal side effects
   c. Anticholinergic side effects
   d. All of the above

9. Mr. Smith has a tough time of it. The medication makes him feel terrible, but these side effects are effectively alleviated by reducing the dosage and adding an anticholinergic. He says to you, "My medication almost killed me. What am I going to do if I get real sick and have to take a large dose again?" Your best response would be
   a. "I understand your concern. I would like for you to know however that other people have resumed their medications along with Cogentin (an anticholinergic) without suffering these symptoms again."
   b. "I would be concerned too. Your best bet is to take life as it comes and not worry about the future."
   c. "I know you are scared, but the chances of your getting sick like this again are remote."
   d. "There is no free lunch. If you want to play, you gotta pay."

10. Mr. Smith calls you 10 days after discharge. He was given a prescription for haloperidol (Haldol), 5 mg t.i.d., and benztropine (Cogentin), 2 mg q.d. He says, "My legs are on fire. I cannot sit still." Based on these few comments you
    a. Cannot make an assessment—there is simply not enough information.
    b. Believe he is experiencing akathisia and tell him to hold the Haldol and come into the outpatient department.
    c. Assess that he is experiencing an intense but not serious side effect and ask the patient to call back in 2 days.
    d. Ask the patient to hold the Cogentin and call his doctor.

## Chapter 13

1. During the first day of treatment with a TCA you could expect
   a. An improvement in appetite
   b. An improvement in mood
   c. Anticholinergic side effects (dry mouth)
   d. Signs of toxicity

2. An elderly male patient receiving TCAs should be especially observed for
   a. Mania
   b. Constipation
   c. Dry mouth
   d. Urinary retention

3. All of the following are true statements about TCAs except
   a. They can be given once daily.
   b. They have a narrow therapeutic index.
   c. Beneficial, therapeutic effects occur immediately after administration.
   d. Many side effects disappear after a few weeks.

4. During therapy with amitriptyline
   a. A patient's sleep disturbance will often improve immediately.
   b. One should watch for symptoms of physical addiction.
   c. Anticholinergic side effects are rare.
   d. The patient should be cautioned about eating tyramine-containing foods.

5. Depression treated with TCAs should be relieved within
   a. 24 hours
   b. 1 week
   c. 2 to 4 weeks
   d. 6 to 8 weeks

6. Amitriptyline is a TCA drug that
   a. Has no anticholinergic properties
   b. Causes tardive dyskinesia as a long-term side effect
   c. Has more sedating and antianxiety properties than other TCAs
   d. Has to be given 3 times per day

7. Tom is placed on phenelzine sulfate (Nardil), 60 mg q.d. Which of the following is contraindicated (theoretically)?

(1) Old cheese, figs, certain wines
(2) Indirect-acting stimulants
(3) Mixed-acting stimulants
(4) Direct acting stimulants
    a. (1), (2), (3)
    b. (1), (4)
    c. (2), (3), (4)
    d. All of the above

8. According to the chapter discussion, TCAs exert their effect by
    a. Primarily blocking the reuptake of serotonin and norepinephrine at the pre-synaptic neuron.
    b. Primarily blocking postsynaptic dopamine receptors.
    c. Inhibiting the enzyme monoamine oxidase.
    d. Increasing brain levels of endorphins.

9. Which of the following statements about lithium are true?
    (1) Lithium is a naturally occurring element.
    (2) Lithium has always been used for treating elevated moods.
    (3) Lithium levels should be taken once per month initially.
    (4) A fine hand tremor is an early side effect.
        a. (1), (2)
        b. (1), (4)
        c. (1), (2), (3)
        d. All of the above

10. The serum parameters for a therapeutic response to lithium are
    a. 0.2 to 0.6 mmol/L
    b. 0.6 to 1.2 mmol/L
    c. 1.0 to 1.6 mmol/L
    d. 2.0 to 3.0 mmol/L

11. Monoamine oxidase inhibitors are effective because they
    a. Block the metabolism of norepinephrine and serotonin
    b. Block the reuptake of norepinephrine and serotonin
    c. Increase the availability of dopamine

## Chapter 14

1. Benzodiazepines are abused because
    a. They increase inhibitions.
    b. They blur reality.
    c. They can be safely mixed with other drugs like alcohol.

2. Benzodiazepines work by
    a. Exciting the CNS
    b. Depressing the reticular activating system
    c. Increasing inhibitory feelings

3. Benzodiazepines given alone can usually cause all but one of the following:
   a. Dependence
   b. Withdrawal
   c. Death from overdose
   d. Abuse problems

4. Valium interacts with alcohol to cause
   a. CNS depression
   b. CNS excitement
   c. An increase in tolerance to alcohol
   d. A depletion of neuronal stores

5. Which benzodiazepine is most prescribed for elderly patients?
   a. Diazepam (Valium)
   b. Lorazepam (Ativan)
   c. Chlordiazepoxide (Librium)

6. Which of the following antianxiety drugs is not a benzodiazepine and shows no cross tolerance with sedatives and alcohol and no withdrawal symptoms?
   a. Diazepam (Valium)
   b. Buspirone (Buspar)
   c. Oxazepam (Serax)
   d. Alprazolam (Xanax)

## Chapter 15

1. Milieu management is the purposeful use of all interpersonal and environmental forces to enhance mental health.
   a. True
   b. False

2. Which discipline provides 24-hour-a-day care for psychiatric patients?
   a. Nursing
   b. Medicine
   c. Social work
   d. Psychology

3. When only psychotropic drugs are offered, the patient receives
   a. Routine nursing care
   b. Only custodial care
   c. Psychotherapeutic management

4. The first professional to conceptualize the need for all aspects of the patient's environment to be therapeutic was
   a. Sigmund Freud
   b. Emil Kraepelin
   c. Maxwell Jones
   d. Hildegard Peplau

## Chapter 16

1. The framework around which the therapeutic environment revolves and takes direction is referred to as
   a. Unit structure
   b. Unit norms
   c. Limit setting
   d. Unit modification

2. The expectation of nonviolence is an example of
   a. Unit structure
   b. Unit norms
   c. Limit setting
   d. Unit modification

3. When the psychiatric nurse clearly identifies acceptable and unacceptable behavior, she is instituting
   a. Unit structure
   b. Unit norms
   c. Limit setting
   d. Unit modification

4. An example of balance is
   a. Choosing orange juice for a patient
   b. Articulating the competing forces in deciding whether to go into the bathroom with a suicidal patient
   c. Developing personal interests along with one's professional interests
   d. All of the above

5. Providing a large orientation board for patients is an example of
   a. Unit structure
   b. Unit norms
   c. Limit setting
   d. Unit modification

## Chapter 17

1. The place where patients are discussed individually and decisions regarding treatment are developed is called
   a. A community meeting
   b. A team meeting
   c. A group meeting
   d. All of the above

2. Which of the following groups do psychiatric nurses typically supervise?
   a. New nurses
   b. Student nurses
   c. Psychiatric technicians

   d. Psychiatric aides

   e. All of the above

3. Which professional group typically leads team meetings?

   a. Nursing

   b. Psychiatry

   c. Psychology

   d. Social work

## Chapter 18

1. The most common mental disorders are

   a. Anxiety disorders

   b. Substance abuse

   c. Schizophrenia

   d. Mood disorders

2. Approximately what percentage of the population suffers from schizophrenia?

   a. 10%

   b. 5%

   c. 1%

   d. 0.5%

3. There are several diagnostic systems available for nurses. The system most commonly used in the United States is the

   a. Feighner Criteria

   b. Research Diagnostic Criteria (RDC)

   c. *Diagnostic and Statistical Manual of Mental Disorders (DSM-III-R)*

   d. *ICD-9*

4. Signs and symptoms of mental disorders are criteria used by clinicians to establish a diagnosis. When a patient reports hearing voices, the nurse understands this to be a(n)

   a. Objective sign

   b. Subjective symptom

   c. Diagnostic proof of schizophrenia

   d. All of the above

5. When clinicians debate whether schizophrenia is caused by life experiences or by a dopamine imbalance, they are engaging in which of the following arguments?

   a. Nature vs nurture

   b. Organic vs functional

   c. Biological vs environmental

   d. All of the above

## Chapter 19

1. Bleuler conceptualized four symptoms he thought were always present in the patient with schizophrenia. Bleuler's 4 As are

    a. Flat affect, anhedonia, loose associations, anergia
    b. Affective problems, loose associations, ambivalence, autism
    c. Anergia, anhedonia, alogia, ambivalence
    d. Ambivalence, autism, loose associations, agoraphobia

2. An excessive level of dopamine may be responsible for
    a. Parkinson's disease
    b. Extrapyramidal symptoms
    c. Tardive dyskinesia
    d. Schizophrenia

3. A person is brought into the county emergency room laughing inappropriately, talking silly, and not making sense. The patient is dirty, and his clothes are torn. Which of the following *DSM-III-R* subtypes of schizophrenia would most likely be used for the diagnosis?
    a. Disorganized
    b. Catatonia
    c. Paranoid
    d. Undifferentiated

4. Type II schizophrenia is best described as
    a. Cortical, dopamine-related, responsive to drugs
    b. Cortical, structurally related, not as responsive to drugs

5. A patient states that he hears a voice telling him that he is Jesus. He believes the voice. The belief is best described as a(n)
    a. Hallucination
    b. Paranoid delusion
    c. Delusion of grandeur
    d. Illusion

6. The patient being reviewed during morning report is described as having bizarre delusions and hallucinations. Based on this limited information, you are
    a. Optimistic because antipsychotic drugs should help this type I schizophrenia
    b. Optimistic because type II schizophrenia will respond to milieu management
    c. Pessimistic because type I schizophrenia is slow to respond to antipsychotic drugs
    d. Pessimistic because the bizarre nature of the symptoms indicates a very sick person

7. Mr. Smith, a 36-year-old, single salesman, is admitted to the unit for the first time. He reportedly beat up a female acquaintance and was brought to the hospital by the city police. On arriving on the unit in leather restraints he screams, "Get them away from me. Can't you hear those ...." This symptom is best described as

    a. Regression
    b. A flight of ideas
    c. A hallucination
    d. A delusion

8. You find out from the emergency room admitting nurse that Mr. Smith has grown to distrust his neighbors in the apartment building where he resides. He is convinced that they were talking about him. He states that the staff are going to kill him, "going to crucify me again." Mr. Smith's symptom picture would probably carry the diagnosis of
    a. Anxiety reaction
    b. Schizophrenia, paranoid type
    c. Schizophrenia, catatonic type
    d. Manic depression

9. The *DSM-III-R* lists all the following subtypes for schizophrenia except
    a. Simple
    b. Disorganzied
    c. Catatonic
    d. Paranoid
    e. Undifferentiated

10. A hallucination is an alteration of
    a. Affect
    b. Memory
    c. Orientation
    d. Perception

11. Which of the early psychiatric investigators had the most pessimistic view of the prognosis for schizophrenia?
    a. Bleuler
    b. Freud
    c. Kraepelin
    d. Sullivan

## Chapter 20

1. Which of the following classifications of mood disorders reflects the most current thinking in psychiatric nursing?
    a. Reactive depression vs endogenous depression
    b. Primary vs secondary depression
    c. Unipolar vs bipolar depression
    d. Psychotic vs neurotic depression
    e. Major depression vs dysthymic disorder

2. Which of the following classifications of mood disorders best explains the effectiveness and appropriate use of antidepressants?
    a. Reactive depression vs endogenous depression
    b. Primary vs secondary depression

    c. Unipolar vs bipolar depression
    d. Psychotic vs neurotic depression
    e. Major depression vs dysthymic disorder

3. Subjective symptoms of major depression include
    a. Alterations in activity
    b. Altered social interactions
    c. Alterations in affect

4. Pessimism, self-blame, and self-deprecating thoughts are examples of
    a. Alterations in affect
    b. Altered cognition
    c. Alterations in activity
    d. Altered perceptions

5. Endogenous depression is thought to be related to low levels of
    a. Norepinephrine
    b. Epinephrine
    c. Taraxein
    d. Enkephalins

6. Psychodynamic theories of depression include all but
    a. Debilitating early life experiences
    b. Nonsuppressor status on the DST
    c. Intrapsychic conflict
    d. Reaction to life events

7. Ms. Long is taking lithium and has a lithium serum level of 1.5 mmol/L. You would expect which of the following?
    a. Some manic behavior since this blood level is below the therapeutic range of lithium
    b. That she would be doing well since her serum level is within the normal range
    c. That she would have mild symptoms of toxicity since her blood level is slightly higher than recommended

8. The important parameters for a suicidal patient are
    a. Whether he means to hurt himself or not
    b. Whether he has a plan, has chosen a lethal method, and has attempted to block rescue efforts
    c. Whether his suicidal attempt is a cry for help or merely represents a manipulation

9. John, who is 70 years old, is admitted to the unit for depression. He has been a successful businessman for many years. He complains of weight loss, early morning awakening, fatigue, slowed gait, pain, and feeling blue and sad for several months. He cannot think of anything that has happened to make him sad. John should be told

    a. Depression often occurs "out of the blue," without a precipitating life event.

    b. Depression is a symptom of old age.

    c. Many patients feel sad all their lives.

    d. Depression is a form of punishment.

10. Flight of ideas, insomnia, grandiosity, and intense irritability are symptoms that best describe

    a. Bipolar illness, manic type

    b. Bipolar illness, depressed type

    c. Major depression

    d. Dysthymia

## Chapter 21

1. In assessing methods used to cope with anxiety, the nurse evaluates

    a. How effective a method of coping is in relation to reducing anxiety

    b. Whether the coping behavior solves the problem

    c. Effectiveness and outcome of each coping behavior

2. Secondary gain refers to

    a. The benefits received from others while one is sick

    b. Decreasing and relieving anxiety

    c. Increased ability to cope with anxiety in the future

3. Before a patient with an anxiety-related disorder can problem solve and develop adaptive coping responses, the nurse must first

    a. Confront the patient with his maladaptive behaviors

    b. Assist the patient with managing and reducing anxiety

    c. Administer p.r.n. lorazepam (Ativan) to eliminate subjective symptoms of discomfort

Match each of the following disorders with its appropriate description

4. _____  Panic disorder

5. _____  Phobic disorder

6. _____  Obsessive-compulsive disorder

    a. Characterized by a persistent fear of specific places or things. Anxiety is displaced or externalized.

    b. Neutralizes anxiety by performing repetitive behaviors or experiencing recurrent persistent thoughts that cannot be controlled or stopped.

    c. Spontaneous attacks of intense fear and discomfort.

7. The most characteristic symptom of posttraumatic stress disorder and the one that distinguishes it from other disorders is

    a. Depression

    b. Suspiciousness of others

    c. Lack of interest in family and activities

    d. Reexperiencing the trauma in nightmares or flashbacks

8. Which intervention would *not* be appropriate in planning care for a patient with a somatoform disorder?
   a. Push insight or awareness to connect conflict with need for physical symp-
   |ιιιιι
   b. Set limits by withdrawing attention from patient when he persists in complaining about physical symptoms.
   c. Encourage patient to verbalize negative as well as positive feelings.
   d. Decrease patient's focus about physical complaints by involving him in milieu activities.

## Chapter 22

1. The major symptoms of delirium include
   a. Primarily cognitive disturbances developing gradually with age
   b. A wide-spread cerebral dysfunction affecting thinking, attention, perception, memory, consciousness, and activity level
   c. Transient, pathological neurological symptoms such as ataxia and diplopia
   d. Changes in motor functioning, rigidity, and tremor

2. The major symptoms of dementia include
   a. Depression, aphasia, restlessness, and wandering
   b. Vision and hearing disturbances and ataxia
   c. Impaired intellectual function and judgment and changes in personality and perceptions
   d. Disturbances in reflexes, memory, and impulse control

Match each of the following organic mental disorders with its primary characteristics:

3. _____    Alzheimer's disease
4. _____    Parkinson's disease
5. _____    Huntington's disease

a. Neurological disorder causing tremor, rigidity, and weakness in voluntary movement
b. Deterioration of neurological, motor, and intellectual functions
c. Progressive nonreversible CNS disorder affecting cognitive function

Mark the following statements true or false.

6. _____    Antipsychotic medications are not particularly effective in treating symptoms of delirium and dementia.

7. _____    The primary goal of nursing care for a patient with dementia is an individualized approach that maintains an optimal level of functioning.

8. Describe the major characteristic of a milieu that is safe for a patient with an organic mental disorder.

## Chapter 23

Mark the following statements true or false.

1. _____    Traits are temporary approaches used to deal with others.

2. _____ Individuals with personality disorders experience discomfort and distress because of others' reactions toward them.

3. _____ Individuals with personality disorders use rigid, inflexible, and maladaptive coping responses.

4. Which nursing approach is most appropriate for a patient with a paranoid personality disorder?
   a. Involve the patient in groups as much as possible.
   b. Use a light-hearted manner in interacting with the patient.
   c. Confront the patient's use of projection and need to control.
   d. Use clear, simple explanations when making requests.

5. A patient with a borderline personality disorder uses self-destructive behavior
   a. As a means to get attention
   b. To express intense feelings of anger or frustration
   c. To express feelings of being "bad"
   d. As a means to manipulate staff

6. Mrs. Cannon withdraws from everyone on the unit. She refuses to go to activities because no one will talk to her, and she feels she is unable to initiate conversation with others. The nurse would
   a. Escort Mrs. Cannon to her activity and leave her there
   b. Tell the patient that she should rest in her room until she feels more comfortable with others
   c. Include Mrs. Cannon in a conversation with the nurse and the patient's roommate
   d. Suggest to the patient that she discuss these difficulties with her doctor

7. Mr. Brand constantly bends rules to meet his needs and then gets angry when other patients and staff confront him on his behavior. He threatens patients and manipulates staff to get what he wants. Which is the best nursing approach to use with Mr. Brand?
   a. Administer p.r.n. medication everytime Mr. Brand does not follow the rules.
   b. Ignore his behavior and privately tell the other patients to let Mr. Brand switch the television channels as much as he wants.
   c. Encourage the other staff to take turns watching Mr. Brand.
   d. Set firm limits for Mr. Brand and be consistent in confronting behaviors and enforcing unit rules.

## Chapter 24

1. Physiological dependence, development of tolerance, and withdrawal symptoms are best referred to as
   a. Addiction
   b. Substance abuse
   c. Substance dependency
   d. Habitual use

2. The oldest and most widely abused drug is
   a. Alcohol
   b. Opium
   c. Cocaine
   d. Marijuana

3. Alcohol abuse accounts for approximately how many deaths per year in the United States?
   a. 50,000
   b. 100,000
   c. 200,000
   d. 1,000,000

4. About what percentage of fatal automobile accidents can be traced to alcohol abuse?
   a. 80%
   b. 25%
   c. 50%
   d. 70%

5. Alcohol is metabolized at about what rate per hour?
   a. 10 ml every 90 minutes
   b. 10 g per 10 kg body weight per hour
   c. 5 g per 10 kg of body weight per hour
   d. None of the above

6. Alcohol is classified as a(n)
   a. CNS stimulant
   b. CNS depressant
   c. Opioid
   d. Hallucinogen

7. The legal definition of intoxication in most states is a blood alcohol level of
   a. 0.10%
   b. 0.08%
   c. 0.8%
   d. 0.01%

8. Which of the following is a common example of denial?
   a. The patient states that he does not drink.
   b. The patient claims to drink only on the weekend.
   c. The patient states that concerning alcohol he can take it or leave it.
   d. None of the above.

9. A common effect of CNS stimulants is
   a. Hypotension
   b. Anorexia
   c. Sedation
   d. All of the above

10. In which of the following ways does "crack" cocaine differ from "regular" cocaine?
    a. More rapid high
    b. Stronger effect
    c. Is less expensive per purchase
    d. All of the above

11. Which of the following are opioids?
    a. Opium
    b. Morphine
    c. Heroin
    d. All of the above

12. Opioids are best classified as
    a. CNS depressants
    b. CNS stimulants
    c. agonists
    d. antagonists

13. Overdose of heroin is more lethal than withdrawal from heroin.
    a. True
    b. False

14. Death from opioids usually occurs from
    a. Hypertension
    b. CNS stimulation
    c. Respiratory depression
    d. Cardiac arrhythmia

15. Withdrawal from barbiturates is
    a. About as severe as withdrawal from stimulants
    b. About as severe as withdrawal from opioids
    c. More severe than withdrawal from heroin

16. If opioid overdose is suspected, the patient can be given
    a. Antabuse
    b. Narcan
    c. Elavil
    d. Librium

17. When developing a nursing care plan for the substance abuser, which of the following best evaluates goal accomplishment?
    a. Routine urinalysis
    b. Patient teaching
    c. Psychotherapy
    d. All of the above

18. Which of the following short-term effects have often been found in users of hallucinogens?

   a. Dystonic reactions
   b. Time distortion
   c. Sexual disinterest
   d. None of the above.

19. Deaths related to PCP are usually due to
   a. Overdose
   b. Perceptual distortions
   c. The pain producing quality of the drug

## Chapter 25

1. Characteristics of anorexia include
   a. Loss of appetite, amenorrhea, and weight loss
   b. Episodes of binging and purging, use of laxatives, and concern about body shape
   c. Self-inflicted weight loss, a distorted body image, and amenorrhea
   d. Intense fear of becoming fat, a feeling of lack of control over eating, and self-induced vomiting

2. The intense need of an anorectic to control her weight usually stems from which of the following factors?
   a. Failure in academic work
   b. A sense of helplessness and feelings of abandonment or inadequacy
   c. Lack of parental attention
   d. A desire to be sexually attractive

3. The characteristics most typical of bulimia are
   a. Unsuccessful efforts to control weight with normal methods
   b. Persistent overconcern with body shape and weight combined with periods of strict dieting
   c. Self-induced vomiting alternating with periods of normal eating
   d. Episodes of binge eating and self-induced vomiting or other severe weight control methods

4. Emotions commonly experienced by bulimics are
   a. Being torn between two conflicting feelings: the fear of being fat and the love of food
   b. A compelling desire for intimacy
   c. A fear of asking for help
   d. Feeling intense anger just before a binge episode

5. In addition to family and group therapy, nursing interventions for the patient with anorexia nervosa include
   a. Regulating what, where, and when the patient eats and monitoring urine output
   b. Ignoring the patient's effort to manipulate the staff

    c. Facilitating a positive self-esteem, rewarding weight gain, and setting limits on inappropriate behaviors

    d. Inserting a feeding tube each time the patient does not eat a complete meal

6. Important nursing interventions for patients with bulimia are to
    a. Negatively reinforce binging or purging with withdrawal of attention
    b. Encourage vigorous exercise as an alternative to vomiting
    c. Help the patient identify feelings, her positive qualities, and relationship issues
    d. Correcting body image disturbances and set limits on inappropriate eating behaviors

7. List some possible physiological outcomes of anorexia nervosa and bulimia.

## Chapter 26

1. Which of the following statements most accurately describes the classical conditioning?
    a. When a neutral stimulus is paired repeatedly with an eliciting stimulus, the neutral stimulus alone will elicit the respondent behavior.
    b. Reinforcers control whether a behavior will be repeated.
    c. Deprivation decreases the chance of a behavior's occurring.

2. Operant conditioning emphasizes which of the following?
    a. Human reflexes
    b. Stimulus generalization
    c. Primary and secondary reinforcers
    d. Internal factors influencing behaviors

Match the technique with the desired behavioral outcome.

3. _____  Increasing a behavior      a. Reinforcing successive approximations and negative reinforcement

4. _____  Decreasing a behavior      b. Reinforcing opposite behaviors and removing secondary reinforcers

5. List two major techniques used in skills training.

Mark the following statement true or false.

6. _____  In token economy, tangible reinforcers for positive behaviors may be exchanged for other reinforcers that patients desire.

7. When a patient has an unpleasant response to a stimulus, respondent conditioning is useful. Which techniques are useful in this case?
    (1) Relaxation techniques
    (2) Gradual exposure to progressively fearful stimuli
    (3) Imagining the fearful situation and placing oneself in that situation
    (4) Developing a self-control program
        a. (1), (3), and (4)
        b. (1) and (2)

c. (3) and (4)

d. (1), (2), and (3)

e. All of the above

8. Describe the six steps in the protocol for behavioral nursing interventions.

## Chapter 27

1. Anectine given immediately preceding electroconvulsive therapy (ECT) produces
   a. Muscle relaxation (paralysis)
   b. Anesthesia
   c. Decreased amounts of secretions (decreases possibility of aspiration)
   d. Convulsive activity

2. During effective ECT the nurse might expect the patient to
   a. Have a full grand mal seizure
   b. Have only a "brain" seizure
   c. Become apprehensive immediately before the electrical stimulus
   d. Have a brief seizure (10 seconds or less)

3. ECT is appropriate for which of the following?
   a. Major depression
   b. Catatonia
   c. Manic-depressive illness
   d. All of the above

4. Approximately how many people are given ECT in the United States each year?
   a. 10,000 to 20,000
   b. 20,000 to 30,000
   c. 30,000 to 50,000
   d. 100,000

5. The most controversial somatic therapy is
   a. Electroconvulsive therapy
   b. Psychosurgery
   c. Hydrotherapy
   d. Psychopharmacology

## Chapter 28

1. Victims of crime experience emotional violation even when not physically injured. This initial violation involves
   a. A loss of trust and sense of autonony
   b. Destruction of property
   c. "Blaming the victim"
   d. Depression

For most crime victims the type of resource needed depends on the stage of recovery with which they are struggling. Match the stage of recovery with the most appropriate resource.

2. _____     Impact                          a. Long-term counseling
3. _____     Recoil                          b. Support groups
                                                 c. Crisis intervention

4. Which of the following needs and rights of the rape victim must be addressed immediately during emergency room procedures?
   a. A medical release to return to work
   b. The presence of a representative of the prosecutor's office
   c. A referral for long-term counseling
   d. Privacy, confidentiality, and information about crisis counseling, support groups, and legal rights

5. Which of the following statements about incest is the most accurate?
   a. Incest involves physical assault and rape by an older relative.
   b. Most incest victims are able to report the abuse when they reach adolescence.
   c. Coercion is the means used to get the victim to conceal the abuse.
   d. The best intervention for the adult supervisor of incest is to help her confront the perpetrator.

Match the behaviors of the cycle of violence with the appropriate nursing interventions

6. _____     Escalation of tension,          a. Discretely giving her a card with emergency
                 efforts to comply                  phone numbers and a few facts about her
                 with demands, frantic              rights
                 attempt to withdraw            b. Assisting her with getting transporation to
7. _____     Lying about causes of             a shelter if she wants to leave
                 injuries, shame, hu-
                 miliation, denial of
                 need for help

8. Make a list of the agencies and resources in your city for victims of rape, incest, and wife abuse.

## Chapter 29

1. Which of the following are risk factors for childhood emotional disorders?
   a. Genetic predisposition
   b. Biological factors
   c. Adverse environmental factors
   d. Social and cultural factors
   e. All of the above

2. The child who is fidgeting and restless, inattentive, impulsive, and hyperactive may suffer from:
   a. ADA
   b. AHDH
   c. ADHD
   d. AAD

3. Approximately what percentage of school-age children most likely experience attention-deficit hyperactivity disorder?
   a. 20%
   b. 10%
   c. 1% to 3%
   d. 0.5% to 1%

4. Boys are more likely to be treated for ADHD than girls are.
   a. True
   b. False

5. The most commonly prescribed drug for ADHD?
   a. Methylphenidate (Ritalin)
   b. Amphetamine
   c. Pemoline (Cylert)

6. Schizophrenia is more common in
   a. Early childhood      (0-6 y)
   b. Young children       (6-12 y)
   c. Adolescence          (12-17 y)

7. The milieu management of the psychotic or autistic child might include
   a. Providing a predictable environment
   b. Providing physical and emotional safety
   c. Orientation
   d. Providing helmets and arm pads
   e. All of the above

8. As the nurse develops the nurse-patient relationship with the depressed child, the nurse's primary task is to:
   a. Help the patient examine self perceptions related to low self-esteem
   b. Assess for suicidal ideation
   c. Accept the patient
   d. Help the patient evolve from a dependent lifestyle to a more independent lifestyle

9. According to Martin and Agran (1988) a heart rate over _____ in a child taking TCAs is cause for alarm
   a. 70
   b. 90
   c. 110
   d. 130

## Chapter 30

1. Which of the following are the major barriers to mental health care for the elderly?
   a. Age discrimination, costs, attitudes of the elderly
   b. Transportation, finances, lack of research

c. Misdiagnosis, disorientation, disabilities

d. Ageism, attitudes of health professionals, lack of available services

2. Although major depression is the most common illness among the elderly, it is often overlooked or misdiagnosed because

a. Depression is just a normal response to other diseases.

b. The elderly deny they have any problems.

c. The elderly are often preoccupied with bodily functions and physical complaints more than emotional symptoms.

d. Memory loss interferes with remembering depressing situations.

3. It is useful to modify the psychosocial assessment to fit the special needs of the elderly in which of the following ways?

a. Making a list of skills and behaviors that would be expected of a person that age

b. Scheduling the interview in the late afternoon or evening

c. Discouraging reminiscing that gets off the main point

d. Compensating for vision or hearing impairments and allowing extra time for answers

4. In the elderly the onset of depression is most often associated with

a. Onset of dementia and disorientation

b. Loss of friends and declines in income and health

c. A serious accident or injury

d. The sixtieth birthday

5. A major focus of a nursing care plan for an elderly person would be

a. Helping the family select a long-term care facility

b. Allowing the patient to sleep as often as possible

c. Encouraging reminiscence about the patient's past life

d. Helping the patient and his family manage the activities and demands of daily living

Mark the following statements true or false.

6. _____ Levels of intervention with the elderly include prevention of impairment, restoration of mental functioning, or slowing the rate of deterioration.

7. _____ Most elderly in institutions benefit from staying in their rooms rather than participating in activities such as reality orientation, remotivation therapy, and pet therapy.

8. Describe the major problems in use of medications in the elderly.

## Chapter 31

1. Nursing care measures found to be helpful for the person with AIDS (PWA) dementia may include

a. Relaxation of universal precaution measures to avoid triggering feelings of paranoia

   b. Isolating the PWA from family and friends to provide quiet and rest

   c. Clear, concise explanations with one-to-one patient supervision

   d. Recommendation of a low-calorie, weight-reduction diet to reduce joint strain

2. High-risk behaviors include all of the following *except*
   a. Sharing needles or drug paraphernalia
   b. Anal intercourse without a condom
   c. Social kissing (dry)
   d. Vaginal intercourse without a condom

3. There have been reported cases of HIV transmission by which of the following means
   a. Insect bites
   b. Toilet seats
   c. Handling objects touched by the PWA
   d. Shaking hands or touching the PWA
   e. None of the above

4. The most serious opportunistic infection for the PWA is
   a. Kaposi's sarcoma
   b. *Pneumocystis carinii* pneumonia
   c. Coccidioidomycosis
   d. Tuberculosis

5. Family members of a PWA dementia may need information counseling or referral for
   a. Information about hospice care
   b. Their concerns about HIV transmission to other family members
   c. Information about wills and powers of attorney and insurance coverage
   d. Their feelings about the risk behavior leading to the HIV infection
   e. All of the above

**ANSWER KEY**

**Chapter 1**

1. a
2. e
3. b
4. c

**Chapter 2**

1. b
2. e
3. c
4. c
5. a
6. True
7. False

**Chapter 3**

1. d
2. b
3. d
4. b

**Chapter 4**

1. d
2. a
3. c
4. b
5. c
6. b
7. a
8. a
9. b

**Chapter 5**

1. c
2. a
3. c
4. b
5. d
6. d

**Chapter 6**

1. d
2. c
3. b
4. d
5. a
6. b
7. c

**Chapter 7**

1. c
2. d
3. b
4. True
5. False
6. b
7. d

**Chapter 8**

1. c
2. d
3. b
4. c
5. a

**Chapter 9**

1. True
2. True
3. b
4. Patient-focused, consultee-focused, organization-focused
5. a

**Chapter 10**

1. a
2. d
3. d
4. b
5. c
6. b
7. b

**Chapter 11**

1. d
2. a
3. c
4. c
5. a
6. b
7. d

**Chapter 12**

1. b
2. a
3. c
4. d
5. c

6. b
7. c
8. b
9. a
10. b

## Chapter 13

1. c
2. d
3. c
4. a
5. c
6. c
7. a
8. a
9. b
10. b
11. a

## Chapter 14

1. b
2. b
3. c
4. a
5. b
6. b

## Chapter 15

1. a
2. a
3. b
4. c

## Chapter 16

1. a
2. b
3. c
4. b
5. d

## Chapter 17

1. b
2. e
3. a

## Chapter 18

1. a
2. c
3. c

4. b
5. d

## Chapter 19

1. b
2. d
3. a
4. b
5. c
6. a
7. c
8. b
9. a
10. d
11. c

## Chapter 20

1. e
2. a
3. c
4. b
5. a
6. b
7. c
8. b
9. a
10. a

## Chapter 21

1. c
2. a
3. b
4. c
5. a
6. b
7. d
8. a

## Chapter 22

1. b
2. c
3. c
4. a
5. b
6. False
7. True

## Chapter 23

1. False

2. True
3. True
4. d
5. b
6. c
7. d

**Chapter 24**

1. c
2. a
3. b
4. c
5. a
6. b
7. a
8. c
9. b
10. d
11. d
12. a
13. a
14. c
15. c
16. b
17. a
18. b
19. b

**Chapter 25**

1. c
2. b
3. d
4. a
5. c
6. c
7. *Anorexia nervosa:* amenorrhea, lanugo hair, hypotension, bradycardia, hypothermia, constipation, polyuria, electrolyte imbalances. *Bulimia:* dental caries, ECG changes, parotid gland enlargement, esophagitis, gastric dilatation, menstrual irregularity, electrolyte imbalances

**Chapter 26**

1. a
2. c
3. a
4. b
5. Reinforcement, shaping, modeling, or imitation

6. True
7. d
8. Baseline observations, analysis of behaviors, problem specification, formulation of treatment, intervention, and evaluation

**Chapter 27**

1. a
2. b
3. d
4. c
5. b

**Chapter 28**

1. a
2. c
3. b
4. d
5. c
6. b
7. a

**Chapter 29**

1. e
2. c
3. c
4. a
5. a
6. c
7. e
8. b
9. d

**Chapter 30**

1. a
2. c
3. d
4. b
5. d
6. True
7. False
8. Polypharmacy, patient compliance, altered pharmacokinetics

**Chapter 31**

1. c
2. c
3. e
4. b
5. e

# Index

**A**

AA; *see* Alcoholics Anonymous
Abandonment
   suicide rate and, 336
   withdrawn parent and, 422
A-B-C theory of personality, rational-emotive
     therapy and 32
Abdominal pain, bulimia nervosa and, 505
Abnormal involuntary movement scale, 198
Abnormal protein model, Alzheimer's disease
     and, 400
Absorption
   alcohol and, 448, 450
   antipsychotic drugs and, 194-196
Abuse
   aggressive patient and, 113
   antisocial personality disorder and, 418
   drug; *see* Drug abuse
   history of psychiatry and, 12
   mandatory reporting of child, 559
   therapeutic skills and, 78
Abusive male; *see* Victim of violence, wife abuse
     and
Acceptance, empathy and, 261
Accident; *see* Posttraumatic stress disorder
Acetaldehyde, metabolism of alcohol and, 448,
     452, 454
Acetazolamide, lithium and, 224
Acetylcholine
   Alzheimer's disease and, 398, 400
   anticholinergic agents and, 176, 182-183
   parkinsonism and, 174, 175
Acid, buffered, Alzheimer's disease and, 398
Acidifying agent, urinary, 467
ACoAs; *see* Adult Children of Alcoholics
Acquired immunodeficiency syndrome, 614-630;
     *see also* Human immunodeficiency virus
     disease
   dementia and, 630-632
   diagnosis of, 619-621
Activities of daily living
   dementia and, 394

Activities of daily living—cont'd
   depression and, 323-325
   Parkinson's disease and, 400
Activity
   altered
     antipsychotic drugs and, 193
     manic episodes and, 343
     schizophrenia and, 291, 305
   limited, manic patient and, 348
Activity group
   group therapy and, 139-140
   unit structure and, 257
Acute-care setting, 85
Acutely ill patient, deinstitutionalization and,
     10-11
Adapin; *see* Doxepin
Adaptive coping; *see* Coping
Addiction, dependency and, 444
ADHD; *see* Attention-deficit hyperactivity dis-
     order
Adjustment disorder, posttraumatic stress disor-
     der versus, 376
ADL; *see* Activities of daily living
Admission process
   aggressive patient and, 124, 125
   assault cycle and, 130
   voluntary, 49
Adolescent; *see also* Child and adolescent psychi-
     atric nursing
   adult survivors of childhood incest and, 553
   anorexia nervosa and, 493, 494
   bulimia nervosa and, 502, 503; *see also* Buli-
     mia nervosa
Adrenocortical function, dexamethasone suppres-
     sion test and, 506
Adult Children of Alcoholics, 593
Adult home, elderly mentally ill and, 610-611
Adult manifestation, Erikson's developmental
     model and, 26-29
Adulthood, fear of, anorexia nervosa and, 495
Advice
   prohibitions against, 69, 70